T0343427

BIOACTIVE FOOD AS DIETARY INTERVENTIONS FOR CARDIOVASCULAR DISEASE

ACKNOWLEDGMENTS FOR BIOACTIVE FOODS IN CHRONIC DISEASE STATES

The work of editorial assistant, Bethany L. Stevens and the Oxford-based Elsevier staff in communicating with authors, working with the manuscripts and the publisher was critical to the successful completion of the book and is much appreciated. Their daily responses to queries, and collection of manuscripts and documents were extremely helpful. Partial support for Ms Stevens' work, graciously provided by the National Health Research Institute as part of its mission to communicate to scientists about bioactive foods and dietary supplements, was vital (http://www.naturalhealthresearch.org). This was part of their efforts to educate scientists and the lay public on the health and economic benefits of nutrients in the diet as well as supplements. Mari Stoddard and Annabelle Nunez of the Arizona Health Sciences library were instrumental in finding the authors and their addresses in the early stages of the book's preparation.

BIOACTIVE FOOD AS DIETARY INTERVENTIONS FOR CARDIOVASCULAR DISEASE

Edited by

**RONALD ROSS WATSON AND
VICTOR R. PREEDY**

ELSEVIER

BOSTON   HEIDELBERG   LONDON   NEW YORK   OXFORD
PARIS   SAN DIEGO   SAN FRANCISCO   SINGAPORE   SYDNEY   TOKYO

Academic Press
Academic Press is an imprint of Elsevier
525 B Street, Suite 1900, San Diego, CA 92101-4495, USA
32 Jamestown Road, London NW1 7BY, UK
225 Wyman Street, Waltham, MA 02451, USA

First edition 2013

Copyright © 2013 Elsevier Inc. All rights reserved.

No part of this publication may be reproduced, stored in a retrieval system, or transmitted in any form
or by any means electronic, mechanical, photocopying, recording or otherwise without the prior
written permission of the publisher.

Permissions may be sought directly from Elsevier's Science & Technology Rights,
Department in Oxford, UK: phone (+44) (0) 1865 843830; fax (+44) (0) 1865 853333;
email: permissions@elsevier.com. Alternatively, visit the Science and Technology Books
website at www.elsevierdirect.com/rights for further information.

Notice
No responsibility is assumed by the publisher for any injury and/or damage to persons, or property as a
matter of products liability, negligence or otherwise, or from any use or, operation of any methods,
products, instructions or ideas contained in the material herein. Because of rapid advances in the medical
sciences, in particular, independent verification of diagnoses and drug dosages should be made.

British Library Cataloguing-in-Publication Data
A catalogue record for this book is available from the British Library

Library of Congress Cataloging-in-Publication Data
A catalog record for this book is available from the Library of Congress

ISBN: 978-0-12-396485-4

For information on all Academic Press publications
visit our website at elsevierdirect.com

Typeset by SPi Global
www.spi-global.com

Printed and bound in the United Kingdom and United States of America

13 14 15 16 17   10 9 8 7 6 5 4 3 2 1

Working together to grow
libraries in developing countries

www.elsevier.com | www.bookaid.org | www.sabre.org

ELSEVIER   BOOK AID International   Sabre Foundation

CONTENTS

The historical records defining the beneficial and preventative effects of consumption of vegetables, fruits, and herbs in cardiovascular disease are extensive. Some benefits may be due to a class of compounds like antioxidants and others to specific molecules such as a particular polyphenol. Major emphasis is placed on potential or likely mechanisms of action, spurring further research. These summaries provide well documented materials and foods for health promotion in business, research and for the individual. Contributors are primarily experts in supplements and heart disease with international standing as leaders in the field. Plant extracts as dietary supplements are an 18–22 billion dollar business in the United States affecting many individuals' health. However, the overall goal is to provide the most current, scientific appraisal of the efficacy of key foods, nutrients, herbs, and dietary supplements in preventing the primary cause of death in older adults, cardiovascular disease.

One major example of the synergism of bioactive foods and their extracts is antioxidant remediation of heart disease. Cardiovascular disease affects more than 5 million Americans with heart failure, with 550 000 new cases a year. Despite the recommendations of various evidence-based guidelines and current established medications, mortality, and morbidity rates due to this syndrome remain high. The American Heart Association estimates the economic burden of managing heart failure in the United States at $29.6 billion. There is compelling evidence that oxidative stress is implicated in the path physiology of this and other cardiovascular diseases. Increased free radical formation and reduced antioxidant defenses in heart failure may contribute to increased oxidative stress. Importantly diets rich in antioxidants in human dietary studies reduce the incidence of congestive heart failure, suggestive of potential cardio protective roles of antioxidant nutrients. This book investigates the role of foods, herbs, and novel extracts in moderating the pathology leading to heart failure.

This book has 41 chapters written by more than 100 experts on various dietary foods, herbs, and extracts as modulators of heart function or lacking such actions. A variety of small molecules are described in 14 chapters as modulators of cardiovascular disease. These range from nutrients like vitamins D and K, as well as a general review of bioactive nutrients in heart protection, with one chapter emphasizing their benefits in preventing infarction in diabetics. Other supplements containing nutrients such as fish and palm oils, and their isolated omega fatty acids are reviewed in chapters relating to heart disease. Non-nutritive small molecules also show benefits in heart function modification. Thus chapters review taurine, L-carnitine, quercetin, and production of homocysteine in humans in their heart health promotion.

A variety of larger, non-nutritive molecules such as polyphenols, flavonoids, plant statins, phytoestrogens, polysterols, and phytochemicals are reviewed in 12 chapters for their cardio protective actions. These reviews include an overview of complementary and alternative therapeutics, as well as focused chapters on myocyte regeneration and sterols in artery disease. India has a history of plants, herbs and food uses in health. Therefore a chapter reviews individual constituents in Indian diets and heart health. Non-Indian food bioactive compounds are broadly reviewed in heart disease. Flavonoids in protection from ischemia-reperfusion injury are discussed. Some benefits from such molecules are still developing. Thus the roles of phytoestrogens in heart health are discussed to answer the question as to whether they should be consumed. Chapters also focus on a range of bioactive compounds.

Some specific foods are receiving special and developing research attention. Two chapters review dairy products including probiotics in heart health. Clearly, foods and herbs with often unknown active ingredients are historically and traditionally thought to be important in cardiovascular disease prevention and treatment and are covered in 11 chapters. A range of plants are reviewed in individual chapters including ginger, garlic, fish proteins, blueberry, and cacao for specific, defined effects. Ethnomedical validation was applied in understanding their actions. Reviews of herbal supplements and herbs in coronary heart disease cover a broad range of materials. Traditional Chinese medicine has a long history in possibly modifying heart disease and is clarified. Finally, the benefits of fruit and vegetable consumption in non communicable diseases like heart disease are defined as the overall basis for this book.

CONTRIBUTORS

M. Akhlaghi
Shiraz University of Medical Sciences, Shiraz, Iran

C. Angeloni
University of Bologna, Bologna, Italy

R. Arora
Staff Officer to Chief Controller Research and Development (Life Sciences and International Cooperation), New Delhi, India; Institute of Nuclear Medicine and Allied Sciences, Delhi, India

F. Azizi
Nutrition and Endocrine Research Center, Research Institute for Endocrine Sciences, Shahid Beheshti University of Medical Sciences, Tehran, Iran

M.S. Baliga
Father Muller Medical College, Kankanady, Mangalore, Karnataka, India

B. Bandy
University of Saskatchewan, Saskatoon, SK, Canada

S.N. Batchu
University of Alberta, Edmonton, AB, Canada

A.J.S. Benadé
Cape Peninsula University of Technology, Cape Town, South Africa

J.W.J. Beulens
University Medical Center Utrecht, Utrecht, The Netherlands

A. Bhatia
PGIMER, Chandigarh, India

S.F. Bolling
University of Michigan Health System, Ann Arbor, MI, USA

W. Cai
Shanghai Rundo Biotech Japan Co., Ltd., Kobe, Hyogo, Japan

N.O.S. Câmara
Universidade de São Paulo, São Paulo, Brazil

M. Celik
Gulhane Military Medical Academy, Etlik, Ankara, Turkey

T. Celik
Gulhane Military Medical Academy, Etlik, Ankara, Turkey

K.R. Chaudhary
University of Alberta, Edmonton, AB, Canada

P. Chedraui
Universidad Católica de Santiago de Guayaquil, Guayaquil, Ecuador

H. Chen
University of Arizona, Tucson, AZ, USA

J. Chen
Shanghai Rundo Biotech Japan Co., Ltd., Kobe, Hyogo, Japan

N.J. Correa-Matos
Brooks College of Health, University of North Florida, Jacksonville, FL, USA

G.W. Dalmeijer
University Medical Center Utrecht, Utrecht, The Netherlands

J.J. Dsouza
Father Muller Medical College, Kankanady, Mangalore, Karnataka, India

A.M. Fernández-Alonso
Hospital Torrecárdenas, Almeria, Spain

D. Fuchs
Innsbruck Medical University, Innsbruck, Austria

J.J. Gormley
Gormley NPI Consulting, Riverdale, NY, USA

J.M. Gostner
Innsbruck Medical University, Innsbruck, Austria

B. Goswami
Institute of Nuclear Medicine and Allied Sciences, Delhi, India

J.A. Goudevenos
University of Ioannina, Ioannina, Greece

H. Gylling
University of Helsinki, Helsinki, Finland

R. Haniadka
Father Muller Medical College, Mangalore, Karnataka, India

F. Hosseini-Esfahani
Nutrition and Endocrine Research Center, Research Institute for Endocrine Sciences, Shahid Beheshti University of Medical Sciences, Tehran, Iran

S. Hrelia
University of Bologna, Bologna, Italy

T.-C. Hsieh
New York Medical College, Valhalla, NY, USA

S.L. Hummel
University of Michigan Health System, Ann Arbor, MI, USA

H. Hwang
University of Arizona, Tucson, AZ, USA

K.G. Jackson
University of Reading, Reading, UK

R. Jaffe
Fellow, Health Studies Collegium, Ashburn, VA, USA

T. Jaxa-Chamiec
Postgraduate Medical School, Grochowski Hospital, Warsaw, Poland

M. Jenny
Innsbruck Medical University, Innsbruck, Austria

P.J.H. Jones
University of Manitoba, Winnipeg, Manitoba, Canada

V. Juturu
United Bio-Med Inc., Dobbs Ferry, NY, USA; Avon Products, Inc., Suffern, NY

C.-M. Kastorini
University of Ioannina, Ioannina, Greece; Harokopio University, Athens, Greece

J. Katz
Dr. Katz's Cardiology Center, New York, NY, USA; Columbia University, New York, NY, USA

P.B. Kaufmanz
University of Michigan Health System, Ann Arbor, MI, USA

A. Kirakosyan
University of Michigan Health System, Ann Arbor, MI, USA

M.G. Kondoleon
University of Michigan Health System, Ann Arbor, MI, USA

J.P. Konhilas
University of Arizona, Tucson, AZ, USA

S. Kumar
University of Pittsburgh, Pittsburgh, PA, USA

Y. Kumar
Chhuttani Medical Centre, Chandigarh, India

D.S. MacKay
University of Manitoba, Winnipeg, Manitoba, Canada

S. Maggini
Bayer Consumer Care AG, Basel, Switzerland

B. Mathai
St. John's Pharmacy College, Bangalore, Karnataka, India

N. Mathew
Father Muller Medical College, Mangalore, Karnataka, India

S.K. Maulik
All India Institute of Medical Sciences, New Delhi, Delhi, India

L.M. McCune
BotanyDoc Education and Consulting Services, Tucson, AZ, USA

T.A. Miettinen
University of Helsinki, Helsinki, Finland

H.J. Milionis
University of Ioannina, Ioannina, Greece

A.M. Minihane
University of East Anglia, Norwich, UK

P. Mirmiran
Nutrition and Endocrine Research Center, Research Institute for Endocrine Sciences, Shahid Beheshti University of Medical Sciences, Tehran, Iran

R.J. Moffatt
Florida State University, Tallahassee, FL, USA

M.R. Movahed
University of Arizona Sarver Heart Center, Tucson, AZ, USA

P.L. Palatty
Father Muller Medical College, Kankanady, Mangalore, Karnataka, India

D.B. Panagiotakos
Harokopio University, Athens, Greece

D.M. Periera
Father Muller Medical College, Kankanady, Mangalore, India

A.N. Prabhu
Father Muller Medical College, Mangalore, Karnataka, India

D. Prabhu
Manipal University, Manipal, Karnataka, India

F.R. Pérez-López
Universidad de Zaragoza, Zaragoza, Spain

F.J.O. Rios
Universidade de São Paulo, São Paulo, Brazil

S. Roysommuti
Khon Kaen University, Khon Kaen, Thailand

S. Schroecksnadel
Innsbruck Medical University, Innsbruck, Austria

J.M. Seubert
University of Alberta, Edmonton, AB, Canada

E.M. Seymour
University of Michigan Health System, Ann Arbor, MI, USA

R. Sharma
Amity University Uttar Pradesh, Noida, India; Dr Katz's Cardiology Center, New York, NY, USA; Columbia University, New York, NY, USA; Florida State University, Tallahassee, FL, USA

A.R. Shivashankara
Father Muller Medical College, Kankanady, Mangalore, Karnataka, India

T. Simoncini
University of Pisa, Pisa, Italy

R.B. Singh
Halberg Research Center, Moradabad, India

J.E. Slemmer
Department of Biology, University of Prince Edward Island, Charlottetown, PE, Canada; Department of Applied Human Sciences, University of Prince Edward Island, Charlottetown, PE, Canada

V. Spitzer
Bayer Consumer Care AG, Basel, Switzerland

M.I. Sweeney
Department of Biology, University of Prince Edward Island, Charlottetown, PE, Canada

G.R. Tummuri
New York Medical College, Valhalla, NY, USA

F. Ueberall
Innsbruck Medical University, Innsbruck, Austria

S.B. Vaghefi
University of North Florida, St. Johns, FL, USA

Y.T. van der Schouw
University Medical Center Utrecht, Utrecht, The Netherlands

J. van Rooyen
Cape Peninsula University of Technology, Cape Town, South Africa

G.J. Wiebe
University of Alberta, Edmonton, AB, Canada

J.M. Wu
New York Medical College, Valhalla, NY, USA

J.M. Wyss
University of Alabama at Birmingham, Birmingham, AL, USA

Omega-3 Fatty Acids in Prevention of Cardiovascular Disease in Humans: Intervention Trials, Healthy Heart Concept, Future Developments

R. Sharma*,†,‡, R.J. Moffatt§, R.B. Singh¶, J. Katz†,‡

*Amity University Uttar Pradesh, Noida, India
†Dr Katz's Cardiology Center, New York, NY, USA
‡Columbia University, New York, NY, USA
§Florida State University, Tallahassee, FL, USA
¶Halberg Research Center, Moradabad, India

1. INTRODUCTION

In the twentieth century, dietary intake and lifestyles have changed significantly to cause increased intake of saturated fatty acids (SFAs), linoleic acid, and a decrease in omega-3 fatty acids, from grain-fed cattle, farm houses, and inbreeding in animals. Such changes marked a reduction in the consumption of omega-3 fatty acids, vitamins, minerals, and proteins, and a significant increase in the intake of refined carbohydrates and fat (saturated, *trans* fat, and linoleic acid). As a result, less availability of omega-3 fatty acids in the diet or improper fatty acid omega-6/omega-3 ratio modulates or enhances blood pressure, obesity, diabetes, dyslipidemia, and coronary risk in patients with high risk of cardiovascular disease (CVD). It is believed that the proper omega-6/omega-3 ratio in the diet and a lifestyle with plenty of physical exercise may be protective because of the antioxidant, anti-inflammatory, and anti-arrhythmic action of omega fatty acids. This chapter describes the role of omega fatty acids in CVD and as functional foods, omega fatty acid supplementation, its safety, global guidelines of fatty acid intake, its lipid lowering mechanisms, ancient or tribal practices, and future developments, in the following sections.

2. ROLE OF OMEGA-3 FATTY ACIDS IN CVD

Evidence shows that reducing the incidence of coronary heart disease (CHD) with omega-3 fatty acid therapy is possible (Calder, 2004). National Cholesterol Education Program Adult Treatment Panel III (ATP III) suggested dietary changes (saturated fat

© 2013 Elsevier Inc.
All rights reserved.

1

$<7\%$; polyunsaturated fat $<10\%$; monounsaturated fat $<20\%$; total fat 25%; carbohydrates 50%; fiber 30 g day^{-1}; protein 15% of total calories; cholesterol <200 mg day^{-1}) to reduce the risk factors of coronary atherosclerosis with physical activity for 30–60 min (NCEP ATP III, 2001).

2.1 Role of Omega Fatty Acids in Dietary Fat and Vascular Health

Intake of dietary SFAs, *trans* fatty acids (TFAs), and cholesterol has been shown to increase serum total cholesterol and low-density lipoprotein-cholesterol (LDL-C) levels in a dose-dependent manner. Recommendations specify reduced dietary saturated fat, *trans* fats, and cholesterol, and fat limited to 13% of energy (Van Horn et al., 2008). National Cholesterol Education Program Adult Treatment Panel III (ATP III) suggested dietary changes (saturated fat $<7\%$; polyunsaturated fat $<10\%$; monounsaturated fat $<20\%$; total fat 25%; carbohydrates 50%; fiber 30 g day^{-1}; protein 15% of total calories; cholesterol <200 mg day^{-1}) to reduce the risk factors of coronary atherosclerosis with physical activity for 30–60 min. TFAs have the strongest effect on raising the ratio of serum total cholesterol to high-density lipoprotein (HDL) (Mensink et al., 2003)-cholesterol (HDL-C) of CHD risk. *Trans* fats account for 2.6% or 5.3 g day^{-1} of total energy intake in US populations. The American Heart Association's (AHA's) diet and lifestyle recommendations include limiting *trans* fats to ≤ 1 g day^{-1}, a decrease from past consumption levels (Lichtenstein et al., 2006).

2.2 Role of Omega-3 Fatty Acids in CVD Prevention

Giugliano et al. (2006) recommended omega-3 dietary strategies to prevent CHD by increasing consumption of omega-3 fatty acids from fish or plant sources. In another study, increased omega-3 fats reduced generation of a proinflammatory milieu or anti-inflammatory activity (Connor, 2000).

Two major studies on omega-3 fatty acids in CVD prevention are GISSI and Japan EPA Lipid Intervention Study (JELIS) as described in section 1. Other small studies also support the role of omega fatty acids in CVD prevention (Daviglus et al., 1997; Galan et al., 2003; Heidarsdottir et al., 2010; Kowey et al., 2010; Marchioli et al., 2009). There is limited research evaluating the relationship between ALA and risk of CHD, but lower doses may enhance the risk of cardiac fibrillation (Aarsetøy et al., 2008). Investigations are needed to determine optimal dietary intake of omega-3 fatty acids (EPA, DHA, and ALA) and the ratio of omega-6 to omega-3 fatty acids. Current omega-3 fatty acid therapy is ambiguous or fishy protection for the heart (Albert et al., 2010).

2.3 Therapeutic Lifestyle Changes Diet: A Multifaceted Lifestyle Approach to Reduce Risk of CHD

Epidemiological, experimental, and clinical trials have pointed to a positive correlation between lifestyle and dietary factors, especially omega-3/omega-6 fatty acids, as they relate to blood lipid levels, blood pressure, and CHD. Western dietary patterns, which are high in red and processed meat, sweets and desserts, potatoes and French fries, and refined grains, have been found to warm up inflammation, whereas prudent dietary practices, which are high in fruits, vegetables, legumes, whole grains, poultry, and fish, have been found to cool it down. Dietary patterns high in refined starches, sugar, and SFAs and TFAs and poor in natural antioxidants and fiber from fruits, vegetables, and whole grains have been found to predispose susceptible people to increased incidence of CHD (Giugliano et al., 2006). The following section highlights the role of key nutrients and lifestyle factors in preventing CVD and identifies practical applications for clinicians.

2.4 Omega-Fatty-Acid-Rich Functional Foods and CVD Risk

Over the past decade, a 'heart-healthy food strategy' has been the cornerstone of the AHA's dietary recommendations for combating CVD and related diseases. It is challenging to include heart-healthy foods into the diet without increasing energy intake beyond that required for a healthy body weight (Kris-Etherton et al., 2002). In relation to food, the AHA's four goals for people are to achieve a healthy overall diet, achieve a healthy body weight, promote desirable blood lipid levels, and achieve desirable blood pressure levels. To meet these goals, omega-fatty-acid-rich nuts have been added to the list of heart-healthy foods. Monounsaturated fats, such as olive oil or canola oil, and polyunsaturated fats are found in nuts and seeds.

Consumption of 0.75–1 oz of unsalted nuts daily (almonds or walnuts) is thought to confer cardiovascular benefits. In more than 86 000 women in the Nurses Health Study, the consumption of 5 oz of nuts per week resulted in significantly lower CHD risk than those who rarely ate nuts in favor of primary cardioprotective action (Kris-Etherton et al., 2002). In a randomized, crossover trial of 28 men and women, the mean (SD) levels of total cholesterol and LDL-C were 6.0 (1.1) $mmol\,l^{-1}$ and 4.1 (1.0) $mmol\,l^{-1}$, respectively, with a mean body mass index (BMI) of 26.9 (3.2) $kg\,m^{-2}$. Participants were fed a low-saturated-fat 'nut diet' of 30 g day^{-1} of nuts or a cereal diet containing canola oil for two periods of 6 weeks, separated by a 4-week gap (Chisholm et al., 2005). Investigators showed that a 30 g day^{-1} serving of nuts had the same effect that canola-based cereal has because the same omega-3 fatty acid profile in both diets may produce decreases in lipoprotein-mediated cardiovascular risk. A serving of almonds or walnuts gives 140 kcal and discretionary calories can add up quickly and cause weight gain, obesity, a risk factor for CVD. The authors recommend the intake of fruits and vegetables (9–11 servings per day) and dietary fiber (25 g day^{-1}) with omega-3 fatty acids from cold-water fish at least two times per week, and plant sterol/stanols (2 g day^{-1}) and nuts (1 oz day^{-1}) while maintaining the energy balance, weight status, BMI, and waist circumference will keep cardiovascular health and wellness.

2.5 Cardioprotective Effects of Omega-3 Fatty Acids

Polyunsaturated fatty acids (P-OM3) are approved for use in postmyocardial infarction (MI) patients to prevent CHD events. The AHA advises ~ 1 g day^{-1} of EPA plus DHA for cardiovascular protection in patients with documented CHD, and in those without documented CHD, consumption of a variety of fatty fish at least twice per week. The AHA recommends that treatment of elevated TGs with omega-3 fatty acids at higher doses (2–4 g day^{-1}) can be taken under a physician's supervision (Kris-Etherton et al., 2002). Recent clinical data strongly support the cardioprotective effect of omega-3 fatty acids (Aarsetøy et al., 2008; Bays et al., 2008; Calo et al., 2005; Cleland et al., 2004; de Roos et al., 2009; Geelen et al., 2005; Geppert et al., 2005; Grundt et al., 2003, 2004; Hamaad et al., 2006; Harrison and Abhyankar, 2005; Lindman et al., 2004; London et al., 2007; Madsen et al., 2007; Metcalf et al., 2008; O'Keefe et al., 2006; Raitt et al., 2005; Rajaram et al., 2009; Sanders et al., 2006; von Schacky et al., 2001; Walser and Stebbins, 2008). Main findings are summarized in favor of fatty acids in cardioprevention as following.

- Meta-analyses of primary and secondary CHD prevention trials have shown that omega-3 fatty acids can significantly decrease the risk of all-cause mortality, CHD death, and sudden death (Ramsden et al., 2010).
- GISSI study showed efficacy of omega-3 fatty acid for secondary prevention of CHD in Prevenzione Study (GISSI, 1999). Patients who had survived a heart attack ($n = 11\,324$) were randomized to 300 mg of vitamin E, 850 mg of omega-3 fatty acid ethyl esters, both, or usual care alone. After 3.5 years, the group given the omega-3 fatty acid alone experienced a 20% reduction in all-cause mortality ($p = 0.01$) and a 45% reduction in sudden death ($p < 0.05$) compared to the usual care group. Vitamin E provided no additional benefit. This trial, although very large and carried out in a relatively 'real-life' setting, did not include a placebo arm and drop-out rates were high (>25%) in both the omega-3 and vitamin E groups. Thus, there remains a need for further research to determine the efficacy, the optimal dose, and the mechanism of action of omega-3 fatty acids in the prevention of CHD death.
- A secondary prevention, JELIS, was conducted on a high-fish-consuming population in Japan included 18 645 patients (14 981 patients with no history of coronary artery disease and 3664 patients with a history), all on statin treatment, who were randomized to 1.8 g day^{-1} EPA (no DHA) or to usual care and followed for 4.6 years for major coronary events (Yokoyama et al., 2007). Compared with the statin-only group, the EPA-plus-statin group demonstrated a 19% reduction in major coronary events ($p = 0.011$). The effect was virtually the same in both the primary and secondary subgroups, but reached statistical significance only in the secondary group ($p = 0.048$). The beneficial effect of EPA on CHD events was not associated with changes in the levels of total cholesterol, TG, HDL-C, or LDL-C, indicating that nonlipid factors played a major role in the cardioprotective effect of EPA (Calder,

2004). Cardioprotective effects of omega-3 fatty acids were antiarrhythmic effects, decreased platelet aggregation, stabilization of atherosclerotic plaques, and lowering of blood pressure (Kris-Etherton et al., 2002).

- The Chicago Western Electric Study cohort of 1822 free-living men aged 40–55 years reported that men consuming >35 g fish per day had a significantly decreased relative risk of death from CHD. In studies examining how blood levels of DHA and EPA affect cardiovascular health, the Cardiovascular Health Study, which examined free-living adults >65 years old, found that a higher concentration of combined plasma DHA and EPA was associated with a lower risk of fatal ischemic heart disease (Daviglus et al., 1997).

- ALA and risk of CHD is less known and needs information about the efficacy of marine and plant-derived omega-3 fatty acids in women and in high-risk populations with a detailed optimal dietary intake of omega-3 fatty acids (EPA, DHA, and ALA) and the ratio of omega-6 to omega-3 fatty acids (Van Horn et al., 2008).

- An FDA-approved health claim needs recommendation of 3 g day^{-1} of maximum omega-3 fatty acids to reduce the risk of CHD because no conclusive research shows that consumption of EPA and DHA omega-3 fatty acids may reduce the risk of CHD (Albert et al., 2010). The AHA recommends ≥ 2 servings (~4 oz per serving) of oily fish per week and inclusion of foods and oils rich in ALA, such as walnuts and soy or other vegetable oils (US FDA, 2004).

- The 'Tsim Tsoum concept' proposes the need for exercise, lifestyle change, behavioral counseling, and dietary intervention when medication fails and the concept integrates with modern nutrition and lifestyle in mind–body diseases. The focus is on dietary fatty acid balance in which 'mother nature' recommends the ingestion of fatty acids in a balanced ratio (polyunsaturated (P):saturated (S) = ω-6:ω-3 = 1:1) as part of a dietary lipid pattern where monounsaturated fatty acids (MUFA) are the major fatty acids (P:M:S = 1:6:1) in the background of other dietary factors: antioxidants, vitamins, minerals, and fibers, cereal grains (refined), and vegetable oils that are rich in omega-6 fatty acids, as well as physical activity and low mental stress. Excess of alphalinolenic acid, TFAs, saturated and total fat, as well as refined starches and sugar is proinflammatory. Low dietary MUFA and n-3 fatty acids and other long-chain polyunsaturated fatty acids are important in the pathogenesis of metabolic syndrome. Approximately 30–50% of the omega-3 fatty acids in the brain are low-carbon chain-PUFA in membrane phospholipids, and it is possible that their supplementation may be protective for stroke. The 'Tsim Tsoum concept' explains blood lipid composition as a marker of holistic health, important in the pathogenesis of CVDs. Blood lipid composition does reflect one's health status: (1) circulating serum lipoproteins and their ratio provide information on their atherogenicity to blood vessels and (2) circulating plasma fatty acids, such as the omega-6/omega-3 fatty acid ratio, give an indication about the proinflammatory status of blood vessels, cardiomyocytes, liver cells, and neurons (Singh et al., 2010). Cholesterol and saturated fats constitute primary risk factors, whereas omega-6 fatty acids are the secondary risk factors.

2.6 Who Needs Initial Treatment with Omega-3 Fatty Acid Supplementation?

- Initially if TC, LDL-C, non-HDL-C, or TG are elevated or HDL-C is low followed by repeat lipid profile 3 weeks later to confirm the first lipid profile as shown in Table 1.1.
- If one or more of the lipid or lipoprotein values remain above the elevated cutoff point or HDL-C is low, secondary causes of dyslipidemia – need of omega-3/omega-6 in diet in all ages.
- If repeated lipoprotein profile in 6–8 weeks shows dyslipidemia, it needs <3 g day^{-1} maximum in all ages (US FDA, 2004).

2.7 Safety and Efficacy of Omega Fatty Acid Therapy in Infants, Children, and Adolescents

Human milk remains the gold standard for infant feeding. A low-fat, omega-3 fatty acid-supplemented diet with micronutrients, such as calcium, zinc, vitamin E, and phosphorus, is safe from the age of 7 months to 11 years as advocated by the Special Turku Coronary Risk Factor Intervention Project (Simell et al., 2009) and from the ages of 8–10 years throughout adolescence by the Dietary Intervention Study in Children

Table 1.1 Acceptable, Borderline, and High Plasma Lipid, Lipoprotein, and Apolipoprotein Concentrations for Children and Adolescents

Category	Acceptable	Borderline	High[a]	Low[a]
TC	<170	170–199	≥200	
LDL-C	<110	110–129	≥130	
Non-HDL-C	<123	123–143	≥144	
ApoB	<90	90–109	≥110	
TG				
0–9 years	<75	75–99	≥100	
10–19 years	<90	90–129	≥130	
HDL-C	>45	35–45		<35
ApoA-I	>120	110–120		<110

Sources: National Cholesterol Education Program (NCEP) Expert Panel on Cholesterol. Values for plasma apoB and apoA-I are from the National Health and Nutrition Examination Survey III (NHANES III); US Food and Drug Administration, 2004. FDA Announces Qualified Health Claims for Omega-3 Fatty Acids 2004. http://www.fda.gov/bbs/topics/news/2004/new01115.html.
[a] The cutoff points for a high or low value represent approximately the 95th and 5th percentiles, respectively.

(Schwartz et al., 2009). However, the efficacy and safety of a low-fat diet is based on epidemiological reports and insulin resistance; endothelial functions in adolescents are factors to interfere with lipid lowering.

3. MODERN VIEW OF OMEGA FATTY ACID THERAPY IN CVD

In the modern world, fatty fish, fish oil, walnuts, oatmeal, and oat bran, and foods fortified with plant sterols or stanols are advocated to help control cholesterol. Several studies have shown that omega-3-fatty-acid-rich fish (salmon, tuna, and sardine) bring down triglycerides and total cholesterol (Brouwer et al., 2003, 2006; Christensen et al., 1999; Harris and Isley, 2001; Harris and Von Schacky, 2004; Harris et al., 2004; Jones and Lau, 2002; Kris-Etherton et al., 2002, 2003; Leaf et al., 2003a,b; Marchioli et al., 2001, 2002, 2005, 2007, 2009, 2010; McLennan and Abeywardena, 2005; Mozaffarian, 2008; Rauch et al., 2006; Verboom et al., 2006; Zhao et al., 2009).

The authors believe that claims of lipid-lowering effects are based on the mixed reports of verbal testimonies or epidemiological surveys and as such are insufficient to validate lipid lowering by omega fatty acids. However, scientific evidence supporting these effects do exist (Kris-Etherton et al., 2002, 2004). Supplementation of a low-fat diet with an omega-3 fatty acid (docosahexaenoic acid 1.2 g day^{-1}) increased the large-sized LDL by 91% and reduced the small-sized LDL by 48%. However, the standard prescription of omega-3 fatty acids is not yet approved by the FDA. Fish oils (1–2 g day^{-1}) lower TG by decreasing TG biosynthesis.

3.1 National Guidelines

Guidelines indicate that patients with elevated LDL cholesterol should consume <7% calories from saturated fat and <200 mg cholesterol means limited TFAs and supplementation of monounsaturated omega-3 fatty acids and stanol-rich margarine, soy products, and cereals with vegetables as shown in Tables 1.2 and 1.3 (Fonarow, 2008; Kris-Etherton et al., 2004). The major goal is lowering LDL-C, raising HDL-C, and limiting serum triglycerides (representative of very low-density lipoprotein (VLDL)) to control dyslipidemia and avoid atherogenesis and diabetes with the aim of cutting down dietary fat, as shown in Table 1.4.

3.2 Mechanisms

At the molecular level, omega-3 fatty acids can prevent free cholesterol from being absorbed into the bloodstream. Instead of clogging up arteries, the 'bad' cholesterol just goes out with the other wastes. The metabolic mechanistic basis of clearance can be described at various end points including LDL receptor activity (Goldstein et al., 2011), inability of ApoB-100 to bind with LDL-R (Rader et al., 2003), autosomal recessive

Table 1.2 Food Supplements in Dyslipidemia Management and Control

Bioactive foods	Nutrition contents	Readymade recipes
Plant sterols and stanols (2 g a day)	Grains, vegetables, fruits, legumes, nuts, and seeds	Margarine spreads, orange juice, cereals, granola bars, some cooking oils, salad dressings, milk, yogurt, snack bars, and juices
Nuts (a handful daily intake)	Walnuts, almonds rich in protein, fiber, healthy monounsaturated fats, vitamins, nutrients, and antioxidants	Salty, fatty, and high calorie snack bowls of dingy, smoky bars
Salmon, tuna, sardines, herring, mackerel, and trout (50–80 g or 3 oz a day)	Omega-3 fatty acids – 750–900 cal (total 2000 cal)	Fish fry, fish chips, and fish oils (50–80 g or 15 tsp)
Oatmeal fiber or bran (25 g of fiber a day)	Soluble fibers	Boiled pudding cup
Soya bean (50 g day^{-1})	Soy meal, a side dish, a snack, or drink	Tofu, soy nuts, soy burger, soy cheese, edamame, tempeh, miso, and soy flour

Sources: Third Adult Treatment Panel of National Cholesterol Education Program. 2001; Kris-Etherton, P.M., Harris, W.S., Appel, L.J., et al., 2002. Fish consumption, fish oil, omega-3 fatty acids, and cardiovascular disease. Circulation 106, 2747–2757; Kris-Etherton, P.M., Lichtenstein, A.H., Howard, B.V., Steinberg, D., Witztum, J.L., Nutrition Committee of the American Heart Association Council on Nutrition, Physical Activity, and Metabolism, 2004. Antioxidant vitamin supplements and cardiovascular disease. Circulation 110 (5), 637–641.

Table 1.3 Web Sites Helpful for Patient Education and Information

Web address	Materials available
http://www.bellinstitute.com/ nutrition/hn/nem.htm	Behavior change focused based on the ATP III with a focus on soluble fiber from oat cereal
	Brochure – destination: healthy heart brochure
http://www.ndep.nih.gov	National Diabetes Education Program
	Brochure – be smart about your heart: control the ABCs of diabetes
http://www.nhlbi.nih.gov/chd/ lifestyles.htm	Therapeutic lifestyle changes information for consumers
http://www.deliciousdecisions. org	Interactive AHA materials including advice on cooking and shopping
http://www.nhlbi.nih.gov/ about/oei/index.htm	Obesity education initiative; weight control information for consumers and health professionals
http://www.soyfoods.com	Information on soy products and amounts of soy protein and recipes

AHA, American Heart Association; ATP III, Third Adult Treatment Panel of the National Cholesterol Education Program.

hypercholesterolemia (Arca et al., 2002), and mutations in proprotein convertase subtil-isin-like kexin type 9 (Horton et al., 2007). Briefly, abnormal omega fatty acid (PUFA) metabolism in FCHL and other small, dense LDL syndromes may reflect the primary defect in these patients or impaired insulin-mediated suppression of hormone-sensitive lipase in adipocytes leads to an elevation in fatty acids (Kwiterovich, 2002). Elevated PUFA may drive hepatic overproduction of TG and ApoB, leading to a two- to threefold increased production of VLDL and the dyslipidemic triad. Insulin resistance also inter-feres with normal upregulation of lipoprotein lipase (LPL) by insulin, leading to de-creased lipolysis of TG in VLDL, as well as in intestinally derived TG-rich lipoproteins. This paradigm may also result from a defect in the normal effect of acylation stimulatory protein, which is to stimulate the normal incorporation of FFA into TG in the adipocyte (Maslowska et al., 2005).

3.3 Clinical Trials to Modify Residual Cardiovascular Risk by LDL Cholesterol Lowering

A diet limited in the LDL-raising nutrients, such as SFAs, cholesterol, and *trans*-unsaturated fatty acids, was suggested by NCEP's ATP III and the ADA's nutrition prin-ciples for the benefit of low dietary saturated fat to maintain a serum LDL-C below 100 mg dl^{-1} (NCEP ATP III, 2001). The following advice is described for each diet sup-plement in the following sections based on NCEP and ADA recommendations.

3.3.1 Saturated fatty acids

Dietary SFAs decrease synthesis and activity of LDL receptors, providing elevated serum LDL-C conducive to atherogenesis (Grundy et al., 2004b). Every 1% increase in calories from saturated fat (butter, cream) increases serum LDL-C by ~2%. ATP III guidelines limit this saturated fat to <7% of calories. A meta-analysis concluded that the previous NCEP Step 1 diet (30% calories from total fat, <10% calories from saturated fat, and 300 mg of cholesterol) lowered LDL by 12%, but the further limitations of the Step 2 diet (7% calories from saturated fat, 200 mg of cholesterol) lowered LDL to an average of 16% (Yu-Poth et al., 2005). *Diet advice*: keep low saturated fat to <7% of calories; select animal products low in fat, such as skim or 1% fat milk and other low-fat dairy products; keep to a daily meat intake of lean beef, poultry, or fish <6 oz; take less of saturated veg-etable fats (palm and coconut oils; see Table 1.4).

3.3.2 Trans *fatty acids*

In the American diet, 2.6% of the calories comes from TFAs and 11% comes from saturated fat (NCEP ATP III, 2001). *Trans*-unsaturated fatty acids are formed from poly-unsaturated fats, such as corn and soybean oil, upon hydrogenation to produce stick mar-garine and fats with greater shelf life. These elevate LDL-C and HDL-C. However, an omega–3 fatty acid (docosahexaenoic acid 1.2 g day^{-1})-supplemented low-fat diet did

Table 1.4 Approximate LDL-C Reduction Achievable by Dietary Modification

Dietary component	Dietary change	Approximate LDL reduction (%)
Saturated fat	<7% of calories	8–10
Mono-/polyunsaturated fatty acids	<3%	8–10
Dietary cholesterol	<200 mg day^{-1}	3–5
Weight reduction	Lose 10 lb	5–8
Soluble fiber	5–10 g day^{-1}	3–5
Plant sterol or stanol esters	2 g day^{-1}	6–15
Cumulative estimate	–	20–30

Source: National Cholesterol Education Program, Third Adult Treatment Panel; http://www.nhlbi.nih.gov/guidelines/cholesterol/atp3_rpt.htm.
LDL, low-density lipoprotein.

not lower LDL-C but significantly increased the largest LDL subclass by 91% and decreased the smallest LDL subclass by 48% (Engler et al., 2005). Metabolic diets containing various fat sources (e.g., butter, soybean oil, semiliquid margarine, shortening, or stick margarine) elevate LDL-C levels and reduce LDL by 5% on stick margarine, 9% on tub margarine, 12% on soybean oil, and 11% on margarine (Denke et al., 2000). *Diet advice:* less saturated fat and TFAs–polyunsaturated and monounsaturated fat intake (7% in tub margarine, and <1% in semiliquid margarine); cookies, crackers, and doughnuts, French fries or chicken (FDA HHS, 2002).

3.3.3 Dietary cholesterol

Cholesterol in the diet increases total serum cholesterol (10 mg dl^{-1} for every 100 mg per dietary cholesterol per 1000 calories; Grundy et al., 2004a,b). The best example is limited egg yolk intake (AHA recommends one yolk per day and NECP ATP III recommends two per week) to keep dietary cholesterol to <200 mg day^{-1}.

3.3.4 Monounsaturated fatty acids

Monounsaturated *cis* fatty acids in olive oil, canola oil, avocado oil, pecan oil, and peanut oil lower LDL and triglyceride. *Diet advice*: olive or canola oil and salad dressing with avocado on sandwiches, snack on pecans, or pack a peanut butter sandwich for lunch.

3.3.5 Wild foods

Wild foods are mainly wild plants, wild vegetables, wild fruits, and wild mushrooms. Mushrooms, flowers, fruits, and wine berries were reported to be beneficial in cardioprotection (He et al., 2007; Heidemann et al., 2008), INTERHEART study (Iqbal et al., 2008). Other epidemiological studies reported other factors such as BMI, waist circumference, alcohol consumption, low physical activity, hypertension, diabetes, C-reactive protein, fetuin-A, and insulin resistance as risks not protected by wild foods.

For a full description of the value of Mediterranean soup (mixture of tomato, grapes, raisins, carrot, spinach, walnuts, almonds, lin/chia seeds, olive oil) in acute coronary syndrome patients with pro-inflammatory effects and challenges, readers are referred to the web document written by the first author (http://www.scribd.com/doc/22527813/Wild-Foods-in-Cardioprotection) highlighting the 'Columbus concept' originally advocated by De Meester (2009).

3.3.6 Supplementation of omega-3 fatty acids in combinatorial therapy

NECP ATP III (Grundy et al., 2004b) estimated that the combination of major dietary principles could lower LDL-C by 20–30%. The scientific basis is that omega-3 fatty acids may reduce the synthesis of TG and VLDL and increase APO-B degradation (transcription of ATP binding protein transporter) to increase HDL-C. So, omega-3 fatty acids facilitate HDL-C mediated cholesterol efflux away from peripheral hepatic cells. A more global approach of combined fatty acid treatment strategies suggested that a low-fat diet, exercise, and vitamin supplementation with statin medication and quarterly visits by a team of physicians, nurses, and dietitians will result in better lipid profiles, better glycemic control, and good cardiovascular protection. As discussed before, it is crucial to modify all the atherogenic risk factors for better outcomes in patients during dyslipidemia or later with atherosclerotic vascular disease. To accomplish it, the options of omega fatty acid alone or in combinatorial therapy are described in the following section. The 2007 National Lipid Association's safety task force concluded that omega therapy is a safe therapeutic option for lowering TG (Bays, 2007). Observational studies have shown several cardiovascular benefits of omega fatty acids such as decrease in cardiac dysrhythmias, sudden cardiac death, and decrease in blood pressure (see in section 1). The mechanism of omega-3 fatty acid action in the reduction of TG is unclear (Bays et al., 2008). Omega-3 fatty acids increase TG clearance from circulating VLDL particles by increasing LPL activity. In the JELIS study, a combination of omega-3 fatty acids and statin was compared with statin monotherapy. There was a 19% reduction in major coronary events by the combination therapy as compared with statin alone. Study showed an increase of HDL-C with high doses of omega-3 fatty acids (Yokoyama et al., 2007). Another trial, COMBOS (COMBination of prescription Omega-3 plus Simvastatin), also showed that a combination of omega-3 fatty acids and simvastatin reduced non-HDL-C, TG, and raised HDL as compared to statin monotherapy (Davidson et al., 2007). The AFFORD trial (atorvastatin factorial with omega-3 fatty acids risk reduction in diabetes) did not show any benefit of residual cardiovascular risk reduction (Holman et al., 2009). However, dietary supplementation with omega-3 fatty acids is not subject to FDA regulation, and thus, higher doses of fish oil supplement may be required to be equivalent to the prescription form of omega-3 fatty acids (Fonarow, 2008). Statin and lipid lowering medications became more controversial in the last 2 years than ever before for their safety as found by the Air Force/Texas Coronary Atherosclerosis Prevention (TCAP) study

(Kendrick et al., 2010); SEAS: first clinical endpoint trial (Hamilton–Craig et al., 2009); PROactive trial (Dormandy et al., 2009); and OCTOPUS trial (Iseki et al., 2009). Omega-3 therapy has issues of side effects and safety (Shah and Mudaliar, 2010). Polypharmacy is still a challenge (Volpe et al., 2010).

4. HEALTHY HEART CONCEPT: LESS-KNOWN FACTS ON OMEGA FATTY ACIDS

Omega fatty acids in the diet have drawn attention based on dietary surveys in tribal areas in India, Australia, and Greenland, as described in the following sections. Eaton et al. (1998) reported a paleolithic diet. Konner and Eaton (2010) estimated that paleolithic diet eaters had lower levels of carbohydrates and sodium, higher levels of proteins and fibers, unsaturated fat with higher physical activity, and high energy throughput quite comparable with the modern-day hunter-gatherer's dietary intake (see Tables 1.5 and 1.6). Our 'healthy heart concept' aims to keep lipids and the risk of CHD/CVD low by the combined approach of 'exercise, low fat calorie intake, higher omega-3 fatty acids >5%

Table 1.5 Estimated Fatty Acid Consumption in the Late Paleolithic Period

Sources	Fatty acids (g day^{-1}) en 35.65 day^{-1}
Plants	
Linoleic acid	4.28
Alpha-linoleic acid	11.40
Animal	
Linoleic acids	4.56
Alpha-linolenic acid	1.21
Total	
Linoleic acid	8.84
Alpha-linolenic acid	12.60
Animal	
Arachidonic acid (ω-6; AA)	1.81
Long chain ω-3 fatty acids	
Eicosapentaenoic acid (ω-3; EPA)	0.39
Docosatetraenoic acid (ω-6; DTA)	0.12
Docosapentaenoic acid (ω-3; DPA)	0.42
Docosahexaenoic acid (ω-3; DHA)	0.27
Total long chain ω-3 fatty acids	1.20
Ratios of ω-6/ω-3	0.70
Linoleic acid/alpha linolenic acid + AA + DTA/ EPA + DPA + DHA	1.79
Total ω-6/ω-3	0.77

Source: Eaton, S.B., Eaton, S.B., III, Sinclair, A.J., Cordain, L., Mann, N.J., 1998. Dietary intake of long-chain polyunsaturated fatty acids during the Paleolithic. World Review of Nutrition and Dietetics 83, 12–23.

Table 1.6 Ethnic Differences in Fatty Acid Levels in Thrombocytes, Phospholipids, and Percentage of All Deaths from Cardiovascular Disease

Fatty acids	Europe and USA (%)	Japan (%)	Greenland Eskimos (%)	Kurichias tribals (%)
Arachidonic acid (20:4ω-6)	26	21	8.3	8.5
Eicosapentaenoic acid (20:5ω-3)	0.5	1.6	8.0	2.4
Ratio of ω-6/ω-3	50	12	1	1.5
Mortality from cardiovascular disease	45	12	7	9

Source: Singh, R.B., et al., in press. Ancient nutrition practices in India: a nutrition survey of Kuchirias. The Open Nutraceutical Journal.

energy, or omega-6/omega-3 ratio <1, nonsmoking, nonalcoholic habits, a healthy, positive attitude, and a spiritual lifestyle' under the supervision of a nutritionist and regular lipid profile checks. In support, the following less known facts about some communities at very low risk of CHD/CVD are described (Table 1.5).

4.1 Ancient Tribals: Indian Kurichiyas

The recent description of Indian Kurichiyas was published in the first time report on Kurichiyas (Singh et al., in press). He emphasized lifestyle, dietary habits (fatty acid intake), and physical activity as the main factors that keep Kurichiya tribals healthy, as shown in Table 1.6. Kurichias walk for 10–20 miles every day, which is characteristic of hunter-gatherers. Obesity and overweight, cancer, heart attack, hypertension, obesity, and diabetes mellitus are uncommon among Kurichiya hunter-gatherers.

Recently, the dietary practices in the paleolithic age were highlighted in the form of the Mediterranean diet, the Indo-Mediterranean diet, the Japanese diet, and the DASH diet documented in several studies (Aratti et al., 2004; Fung et al., 2008; Singh et al., 2002; Trichopoulou et al., 2009).

4.2 Australian Tribals

Kimberley aboriginals were reported for their diet and eating patterns of 1200 kcal per person per day, two-third quantity of meat; total fat intake (13% energy from balanced saturated, unsaturated, and P-OM3); 54% energy from proteins; and 33% energy from carbohydrates (O'Dea, 1988). The 'hunter-gatherer lifestyle' was associated with in-creased physical activity and a low-fat, high-fiber diet of low energy density and high nutrient density derived from very lean wild meat, and uncultivated vegetable foods. It was shown that low carbohydrates and high proteins in the diet with extensive physical activity kept fat in the body under the control of the 'thrifty gene,' driving hepatic gluconeogenesis to convert dietary protein into glucose and available fat energy precursors without therisk of diabetes (O'Dea, 1991).

4.3 Greenlandic Eskimos

Eskimos live in Greenland and have extremely low incidence of heart disease. Their dietary fat intake (18% fat energy) and intake of omega-3 PUFAs from seal and fish was about sixfold higher than that found in western diets without coronary thrombosis (Côté et al., 2004; Kristensen et al., 2001). Recently, enzyme modulatory mechanisms of omega-3-fatty-acid-induced cardiac prevention were described (Siddiqui et al., 2008).

- In addition to the high fat, the seal meat also provided high amounts of omega-3 fatty acids and low amount of omega-6 fatty acids.
- All lipoproteins, except HDL, were significantly lower in the Greenland Eskimos who ate lots of fat and had lower LDL-C and higher good cholesterol (HDL).
- Ekismos' blood had higher EPA and DHA, two of the three types of omega-3 fatty acids.
- Electrical activity in the heart muscle is stabilized by omega-3 PUFAs as PUFAs are 'antiarrhythmic.' Heart rhythm remains stable and the chances of 'sudden death' are greatly diminished.
- Omega-3 PUFAs also prevent blood from clotting or occluding a hardened coronary artery with a blood clot is greatly reduced by omega-3 PUFAs.
- Inuit Eskimo diet has six times more omega-3s than the typical western diet. Omega-3 PUFAs maintain low total cholesterol and 'bad' LDL-C levels.
- L-type calcium channels, role of the Na^+–Ca^{2+} exchanger to mobilize calcium out, activation of phospholipases, synthesis of eicosanoids, and regulation of receptor-associated enzymes and protein kinases play roles in mediating n-3 PUFA effects on cardiovascular health.

4.4 Dietary Fat Intake and Fatty Acid Ratio

Recently, the 'fatty acid ratio' was highlighted based on unsaturated and saturated fats in the diet and overall distribution to explain good health or risk of atherogenesis after oxidative stress in various continents as the Indian paradox, French paradox, and Israeli paradox (de Lorgeril et al., 2002; Dubnov and Berry, 2003; Pella et al., 2003). The fatty acid ratio is described in this section and oxidative stress in the next section.

4.4.1 Columbus concept

De Meester et al. (2009) developed and marketed the Columbus concept (www.columbus-concept.com) at BNL food, a concept that stands for the return of the evolutionary lipid pattern (omega-6:omega-3 = 1:1) in the human diet. The fatty acid ratio in the 'Columbus concept' of diet means that humans evolved on a diet that was low in saturated fat and the amount of omega-3 and omega-6 fatty acids was quite equal. In the lines of the 'Columbus concept' "Nature recommends the ingestion of fatty acids in a balanced ratio (polyunsaturated:saturated $= \omega$-6:ω-3 $= 1$:1) as part of a dietary lipid pattern in which monounsaturated fatty acid (M) is the major fat (P:M: S $= 1$:6:1). These ratios represent the overall distribution of fats in a natural untamed environment." (www.columbus-concept.com) (Dubnov and Berry, 2003)

According to the 'Columbus concept,' ancient foods included egg, milk, meat, oil, and whole grain foods, all rich in omega-3 fatty acids, similar to wild foods consumed about 150 years ago from now. Furthermore, blood lipid composition reflects one's health status predicted by: (1) circulating serum lipoproteins, and their (LDL + VLDL)/ total cholesterol ratio provides information on their atherogenicity to blood vessels; and (2) circulating plasma fatty acids, such as the omega-6/omega-3 fatty acid ratio, indicates the proinflammatory status of blood vessels. Both factors (1) and (2) are phenotype related and depend on several genetic, environmental, and developmental factors. Hence, they appear as universal markers reflecting physical, mental, social, and spiritual health. The author has described in detail other contributory factors that influence mind–body interactions and lifestyle against environmental factors (http://www.scribd.com/doc/ 19575964/Traditional-Therapies-Lessons).

4.4.2 Oxidative stress and fatty acid ratio

Long-term intervention with high doses of omega-3 fatty acids (PUFA) following an acute MI was reported to increase lipid peroxidation (Grundt et al., 2003). Another group's study showed reduced oxidative stress by omega fatty acid intake (Mori et al., 2000). The author with Pella et al. (2003) reported the 'Indian Paradox,' the shift from an affluent fat-rich diet (vegetable ghee, butter, cream, refined oils, and refined bread) to a less fat-rich diet (mustard oil, whole grains, walnuts, and vegetables rich in ALA) in both urban and rural populations. It enhanced the ALA content in diet and reduced omega-6/ omega-3 ratio, now believed to be protective against CVD (Dubnov and Berry, 2003; Pella et al., 2003). Moreover, supplementation of omega-3 fatty acids was also reported to influence the 'arachidonic acid and eicosapentanoic acid ratio' resulting in more safety and less oxidative stress in stable CHD patients (Burns et al., 2007).

5. GUIDELINES ON OMEGA FATTY ACID IN CVD TO PHYSICIANS, NURSES: HEALTHY HEART CONCEPT

Available omega-3 PUFA food supplements contain EPA and DHA derived from marine oils in varying proportions, and contain 180 mg EPA and 120 mg DHA per capsule. Typical cod liver oil supplements contain 173 mg EPA and 120 mg DHA. For vegetarians, there is an alternative in the form of DHA oils derived from algae, 100 mg DHA per capsule (Kris-Etherton et al., 2000). This section is a guide to medical and health-care workers who are actively involved in cardiovascular care and cardioprevention. The awareness of both dietary fat intake along with side effects of statins and their safe use is important while practicing them to perform lipid lowering in prospective patient population. The lipid dysfunction includes mainly hypercholesterolemia, hypertriglyceridemia, low HDL-cholesterol, and apolipoprotein changes. The target lipid levels (LDL-C <2.5 mmol l^{-1}, <3.5 mmol l^{-1}, <4.5 mmol l^{-1}, and total cholesterol/HDL-C ratio <6.0, <5.0, <4.0) indicate the high risk, moderate risk, and low risk of dyslipidemia, respectively. The triglycerides >1.7 mmol l^{-1} with HDL-C <1.0–1.3 mmol l^{-1} indicate metabolic syndrome. Dietary PUFA fat intake (2.5–12%) to improve serum lipid profile includes mainly the intake of unsaturated omega-3 (0.5–2 energy % or 8 g day^{-1}) and omega-6 fatty acids (2–10 energy % or 6 g day^{-1}) with antioxidants, L-arginine, and folic acid. Table 1.7 shows that omega-6/omega-3 PUFA ratio varies between 2:1 and 10:1, depending on whether adequate or upper level values are selected. There is no consensus about the optimal omega-6/omega-3 PUFA ratio in the diet (Table 1.7).

The best fish sources of omega-3 PUFAs are mackerel, herring, halibut, and salmon. Plant sources of omega-3 PUFAs are some of the legumes (especially pinto beans and soy beans) and nuts or seeds (especially walnuts and flaxseed). Leeks and leafy purslane are also excellent sources. Canola, flaxseed, and soybean oils in salad dressings are also good sources. Cod liver oil is a good supplemental source, but it is also very high in vitamin D and vitamin A. For those who do not like fish or vegetable sources of omega-3 PUFAs, omega-3 PUFAs may be taken in capsular form (750–1000 mg total EPA) as dietary supplements. The authors recommend vegetable sources in capsular form (750–1000 mg

Table 1.7 Fatty Acids Ratio in the Daily Diet Intake

Subjects	ω-6/ω-3 (2001)	ω-6/ω-3 (prior to 1960)
Paleolithic	0.79	Estimated
Greece	7.10	1.00–2.00
Japan	4.00	1–2
India, rural	5–6.1	3–4
India urban	38–50	5–10
UK	15.00	10.00
Northern Europe	15.00	10.00
USA (FNB)	8.0 (5–10/06–1.2)	7–8
Eastern Europe	20–25	Estimated
Indian hunter-gatherers	1.00–2.00	Estimated
D-A-CH	5.0 (2.5/05)	Estimated
France (ANC)	4 (4/1)	Estimated
Netherlands (DRI)	2 (2/1)	Estimated
Nordic countries (NNR)	>4 (>4/>1)	Estimated
SCF	4 (2/0.5)	Estimated

Source: Singh, R.B., et al., in press. Ancient nutrition practices in India: a nutrition survey of Kuchirias. The Open Nutraceutical Journal.

total EPA) as dietary supplements or Res-Q 1250 rich in omega-3 marine oil. Olive oil in the 'Mediterranean diet' is rich in P-OM3 (omega-3 fatty acids and omega-6 fatty acids). MUFA derived from olive oil keeps the heart healthy. Of specific mention, whole foods, such as garlic, spirulina, fenugreek, ginkgo, soy, and genistein, have been on nonprescription counters as cardioprotective food supplements popular for reducing low and moderate risks.

The high-risk category (LDL-C <2.5 mmol l^{-1} and TC/HDL-C ratio <4.0) needs immediate attention for lipid lowering medication, preferably statins. Other choices may be BSA, fibrates (benzo-, phenol-), gemfibrozil (400–1200 mg day^{-1}), and niacin (1–3 g). Moreover, health workers need to be aware of the prescribed limits for beneficial effects of these omega PUFA supplements and persistent risk of antioxidants and cancer promoters (Kearney, 1987; Pearce and Dayton, 1971). MUFA are more effective than PUFA (Wolk et al., 1998). It is important to keep low the risks of ventricular tachycardia and ventricular fibrillation in patients with implanted defibrillators if they are being treated with fish oil supplementation (Raitt et al., 2005). On the other hand, statins have gained popularity in acute hyperlipidemia and acute CVDs to combat them within time, but our advice is 'keep statins low as much as possible with 'spiritual acceptance'[1] of active fat-smoking-alcohol-free lifestyle and a positive attitude (healthy heart concept).' Statin therapy is not free from side effects and it needs the right prescription[2] and safe use under supervision. The Canadian Cardiovascular Society 2009 recommendations advocated new hs-CRP, ApoB/ApoI, TC/HDL-C, carotid intima-media thickness biomarkers of risk with heavy emphasis on a restricted diet (low sodium and simple sugars, with substitution of unsaturated fatty acids for saturated and *trans* fats, as well as increased consumption of fruits and vegetables), smoke/alcohol cessation, calorie restriction, and least psychological stress. For full description, readers are referred to read guidelines (Genest et al., 2009; Goldstein et al., 2011).

5.1 Omega Fatty Acids in CHD: Treating Beyond LDL-C

The most common adverse affects include gastrointestinal discomfort and nausea in patients receiving high EPA doses. The gastrointestinal events are most likely in response to the ingestion of such a large volume of an oily substance or actual omega-3 PUFA. Very high doses (>20 g day^{-1}) of omega-3 PUFA might be associated with increased bleeding times. However, moderate consumption (ranging up to 7.5 g day^{-1}) does not appear to cause delayed bleeding time (Hathcock et al., 2006). However, PUFA amounts in commonly used supplements are safe (Dall and Bays, 2009). More progress in support of the 'healthy heart concept' is highlighted for an understanding of the influence of the diet-induced blood/tissue omega-6 status on premetabolic disorders (VVDs and

---

[1] http://www.appbrain.com/app/hindu-vrat-calendar/com.pm.HinduVratCalendar.
[2] www.cmaj.ca/cgi/content/full/169/9/921/DC1/.

SPDs) in different age groups in representative sample populations in different continents; to determine the lifespan of omega fatty acid intake influence, psychological, and chronological factors in maintaining good homeostasis & biorhythms; to understand the interactive relationship between the cardiac clock and diet and lifestyle, human behavior, development with lifespan, new insights into human/environment mutual interactions, biological rhythms; and to determine the complex relationships of human biological, psychosocial functions versus age/time structures (Okuyama et al., 2000).

6. IMPLICATIONS AND FUTURISTIC PROSPECTIVE

In brief, CVD is a major health hazard and ancient concepts of nutrition appear based on eating natural foods; fruits, vegetables, roots, and tubers, sprouted whole grains, nuts, cow milk, and curd and honey to combat adverse effects of dietary fats and fat-rich foods seem to be sound. However, less is known about the secret of high cardiac protection among tribals and Eskimos. The biochemical mechanisms of fatty acid transport regulation, LDL-transport, and their relation with cardiac arrhythmia and electrical activity are less understood. There is no clear advice in modern concepts for fresh animal foods; eggs, fresh fish, and meat from running animals commonly consumed by tribals and hunter-gatherers.

Nowadays, clinical trials suggest the success of a low-fat dietary lifestyle. Supervised dietary intervention to reduce low risk of both coronary and carotid artery disease and cardiac prevention are anticipated more rigorously. Large trials such as JELIS, GISSI, and AFFORD have suggested the importance of omega-3 fatty acids, fish oil efficacy, and the need for more investigations on reducing cardiac injury in prevention of CVD. Ongoing trials are needed to demonstrate the incremental CVD benefits and the safety of combination dietary regimens. In future, more omega-3 fatty acid variants and combinatorial products will be available in CVD therapy for more extensive prophylactic prescription in normolipidemic patients with new definitions advocated by government or research agencies if patients have other conventional risk factors such as hypertension, diabetes mellitus, or other new factors identified under medical supervision. To identify new risk factors related with hyperlipidemia or cardiovascular risks, is a kind of a race to pick up the thread early and advise interventions such as omega-3 fatty acids capsules, exercise, or lifestyle changes. It remains to be established whether prolonged lipid-lowering omega-3 fatty acid treatment is risk free from any lipid lowering omega-3-fatty-acid-induced immunosuppression, or cancer in the body after long duration especially in infants, children, adolescents, and elderly of different ethnicities. It will be clear if a monounsaturated or polyunsaturated fatty-acid-rich-diet in childhood can prevent CVD in adulthood or obesity due to insulin resistance and whether it can enhance endothelial function in teenaged boys and girls, with clear information as to how much TC or LDL-C or HDL-C is the culprit.

This chapter suggested the following broader implications: (1) low fat, low sodium with a high PUFA-rich diet or capsules may cause significant cholesterol and triglyceride lowering in serum but small change; (2) omega-3 and omega-6 fatty acid intervention or fish oil supplementation in combination therapy causes lipid lowering and improves serum lipid profile more than dietary intervention alone; (3) dietary low-fat energy intake or omega-6/omega-3 fatty acid supplementation may cause significant change in HDL cholesterol; and (4) combination of low fat, low salt with omega fatty acids may show limited benefit but combination with statin therapy may contribute more to the effect of therapeutic intervention on other factors such as mortality from CVD and ischemic heart disease. However, two issues remain unclear: (1) whether prolonged low fat and higher omega fatty acids given to low socio-economic populations may further the risk of malnutrition or immunity loss or immunosuppression because of less available energy or resistance to clearance of nutrients as added risk; (2) whether omega fatty acid-rich fish oils recommended for prolonged periods may contribute to any less known adverse effect. No perfect means of lipid lowering or clear lipid regulatory mechanism exists today to explain complete cure without adverse effects. No clear information is available on consumption of omega fatty acids in correct ratio due to wide variation of omega-6 and omega-3 fatty acid ratio in daily intake among different populations in different continents (see Table 1.7). The authors propose a novel approach – 'keep the daily dietary fat intake to the minimum, low salt, combined omega-3 fatty acids with optimal cardiovascular drugs,' which may keep dyslipidemia and CVD in control within normal limits of blood pressure, BMI, and serum lipids (Sharma et al., 2010a). Our idea is to highlight the implication of 'low fat optimal omega-drug combination therapy' approach to manage dyslipidemia and reduce the mortality from hypertension, coronary, or ischemic heart disease and cardiovascular disorders as shown in Figure 1.1.

This chapter is focused on two main purposes: first, to introduce the mechanism of omega-fatty-acid-induced changes in plasma lipids and cardioprotection; clinical evidence of combinatorial drug + omega-3 fatty acid therapy to observe the subtle benefits or limited cardiac protection in different social populations at risk; the 'Columbus concept' and 'Tsi-Tom concept' as new concepts of balanced fatty acids in the diet. This chapter advocates the importance of omega fatty acids in reducing CVD and preventing heart disease with wider implications including rapid beta oxidation and active fatty acid transport, scavenging LDL-C transport, stabilizing electrical activity in cardiac nodes and smoothening muscle activity, reducing platelet aggregation and triglycerides, and increasing HDL-C. Still, less is known for mechanisms and long-term regulation of fatty acid and lipid transport across cardiovascular systems. Role of fatty acids and effects of low dietary fat energy intake are less known in the light of modern views and clinical trials in favor of lifestyle change and importance of social behavior. Moreover, definition of

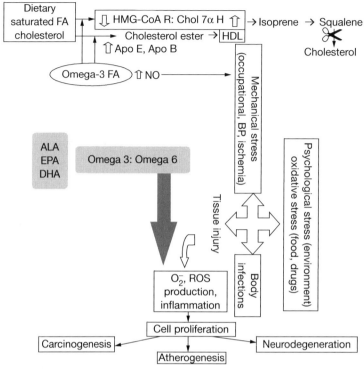

Figure 1.1 The figure represents the role of omega-3 fatty acids and the importance of the omega-3/omega-6 ratio (1:1) prescribed in limit for heart disease. Notice the effect of omega fatty acids in neuroprotection and inflammation and cancer.

cardiovascular risks and lipid profile interpretation has own limitations in different age groups and ethnicities. Western multiracial population or mixed racial population further warrants establishing relationship between diet modification and omega fatty acid therapy in dyslipidemic population with CVD risk in terms of serum lipid changes in different ethnicities. Our recent preliminary survey showed clear differences in plasma lipid and lipoprotein levels (Sharma et al., 2010b). Another important issue is the rapidly changing lifestyle among intracountry or international migratory white collar employees. Supervised dietary or omega fatty acid intervention as primary management is anticipated in such populations or individuals to reduce the risk of high omega-3 intake in both coronary or carotid artery disease and cardiac prevention.

To accomplish these goals, attention needs to be paid to the following issues in future. First, more accurate body lipid diagnostic methods or in vivo biomarkers for early detection of cardiovascular risk or dyslipidemia must be established and standardized to assess the need of omega fatty acid alone or in combinatorial nutrition + statin option. Similarly, in advanced dyslipidemic population at high cardiovascular risk, accurate body lipid imaging and sensitive cardiac tissue diagnostic methods are must to establish sequential 'cardiovascular incapability' before any omega fatty acid intervention to assess the effectiveness of different dosage of omega fatty acids or need of combinatorial therapies or immediate surgical intervention in time. It is believed that the degree of association between 'dyslipidemia switch to hypertension or CVD or atherosclerosis or diabetes' and 'abnormal serum lipids and size of LDL lipoproteins' will serve as a criteria and surrogate endpoint(s) to evaluate the pleiotropic effects of omega fatty acids and/or statins in different stages to improve both dyslipidemia and cardiovascular incapability in time. Next, it is believed that one must reevaluate normal and vulnerable limits of serum lipid profiles and cardiac physiological functions carefully in populations under study with details of lifestyle, social factors, and nutrition factors at a specific place and environment (independent from specific study report or specific Government guidelines) before intervention of omega fatty acids or drugs and/or dietary fat restriction in different ethnicities, cultures, and age groups along with careful consideration of dyslipidemia resistance in populations, if any, in order to reduce the side effects of existing or new drugs. In future, possibly rigorous lipid lowering drug therapy and optimized cardioprotective dietary or omega fatty acid supplementation will be extensively applied even in normolipidemic patients to keep good health with suggestions of dietary low fat intake if they have any conventional risk factors such as hypertension, diabetes mellitus, or others under medical supervision. Furthermore, other alternate cardioprotective medication will be rationalized such as more effective omega fatty acid derivatives, antidiabetic regimens, antihypertensive therapy to intervene in early stage dyslipidemia risks such as postprandial hyperlipidemia or hyperglycemia, insulin resistant state, masked hypertension, or metabolic syndrome to further reduce mortality or morbidity of both coronary artery disease and cardiac heart disease. More facts of dyslipidemia at risk of CVD and CHD in infants, children, and adulthood will be revealed with clear recognition and definitions of blood lipids with cut-off values in different ethnicities. New foods and omega-fatty-acid-rich dietary regimens have more scope in controlling dyslipidemia to keep away hypertension and CVD, as indicated in a recent study on the prospects of the NORDIET trial (Adamsson et al., 2011).

7. CONCLUSIONS

This chapter presents the current view of the role of omega fatty acid in reducing CVD or heart disease in the light of new experiences and clinical trials in different parts of the world and ethnicities in different age groups. Present state of the art on dyslipidemia control and cardiovascular prevention by omega fatty acids still remains controversial because of lack of comparisons of omega fatty acid usage in different populations and no common agreement on dyslipidemia management risk reduction of CVD. As a result, primary management of dyslipidemia and consequences remain inconclusive bottlenecks in prevention of CVD with lot of new side effects of newly introduced omega fatty acids or new pharmaceutical drugs. Omega-6/omega-3 ratio seems a key in cardiac prevention. The growing and advanced techniques of lipid science have opened up new vistas in the characterization of different lipid molecule sizes, visualization, fatty acid and lipoprotein metabolism, metabolic regulation, and molecular basis of lipoprotein disease during sequential progress of CVD, either atherosclerosis, heart disease, or diabetes with renal complications, but medical treatment approaches remain frustrating on reversing disease or complete cure of CVD. A new 'healthy heart concept' is proposed with guidelines on low fat or omega fatty acid dietary therapies to show some promise because of less or no side effects due to them if used as exclusive nutrition therapy or combinatorial regimens with change in lifestyle, positive behavior. For a better understanding of omega fatty acids and the healthy heart concept, this chapter surveys the views and needs of ancient life-styles that provided better life expectancy and good health. Evidence of Australian, Asian Indian, and Greenland Eskimo tribal practices of traditional diets and their life expectancy without any significant cardiac diseases is examined. Awareness of new practices among tribals is an exciting and explorable frontline area in both nutrition and social research. New dietary fatty acid intake information and typical lifestyles of tribals pose a challenge to both nutritionists and doctors if personal and spiritual acceptance can give some benefits.

ACKNOWLEDGMENTS

The authors acknowledge the support of Indian Council of Medical Research for the postgraduate studies program in Applied Nutrition, and for the training and the opportunity for patient data collection given to the first author at the National Institute of Nutrition, Hyderabad. The authors acknowledge the manuscript preparation at Department of Exercise, Food, and Nutrition, Florida State University, Tallahassee, and the discussions included in this chapter.

REFERENCES

Aarsetøy, H., Pönitz, V., Nilsen, O.B., Grundt, H., Harris, W.S., Nilsen, D.W., 2008. Low levels of cellular omega-3 increase the risk of ventricular fibrillation during the acute ischaemic phase of a myocardial infarction. Resuscitation 78 (3), 258–264.

Adamsson, V., Reumark, A., Fredriksson, I.B., et al., 2011. Effects of a healthy Nordic diet on cardiovascular risk factors in hypercholesterolaemic subjects: a randomized controlled trial (NORDIET). Journal of Internal Medicine 269 (2), 150–159.

Albert, C., Anderson, M., Nattel, S., 2010. Omega-3 oil: a fishy protection for the heart. Community corner. Nature Medicine 16 (11), 1192–1193.

Aratti, P., Peluso, G., Nicolai, R., Calvani, M., 2004. Polyunsaturated fatty acids: biochemical, nutritional, and epigenetic properties. Journal of the American College of Nutrition 23, 281–302.

Arca, M., Zuliani, G., Wilund, K., et al., 2002. Autosomal recessive hypercholesterolemia in Sardinia, Italy, and mutations in ARH: a clinical and molecular genetic analysis. Lancet 359 (2002), 841–847.

Bays, H.E., 2007. Safety considerations with omega-3 fatty acid therapy. The American Journal of Cardiology 99 (6A), 35C–43C.

Bays, H.E., et al., 2008. Prescription omega-3 fatty acids and their lipid effects: physiologic mechanisms of action and clinical implications. Expert Review of Cardiovascular Therapy 6 (3), 391–409.

Brouwer, I.A., Zock, P.L., Camm, A.J., et al., 2006. Effect of fish oil on ventricular tachyarrhythmia and death in patients with implantable cardioverter defibrillators: the study on omega-3 fatty acids and ventricular arrhythmia (SOFA) randomized trial. Journal of the American Medical Association 295 (22), 2613–2619.

Brouwer, I.A., Zock, P.L., Wever, E.F., et al., 2003. Rationale and design of a randomised controlled clinical trial on supplemental intake of *n*-3 fatty acids and incidence of cardiac arrhythmia: SOFA. European Journal of Clinical Nutrition 57 (10), 1323–1330.

Burns, T., Maciejewski, S.R., Hamilton, W.R., Zheng, M., Mooss, A.N., Hilleman, D.E., 2007. Effect of omega-3 fatty acid supplementation on the arachidonic acid: eicosapentaenoic acid ratio. Pharmacotherapy 27 (5), 633–638.

Calder, P.C., 2004. *n*-3 Fatty acids and cardiovascular disease: evidence explained and mechanisms explored. Clinical Science 107, 1–11.

Calo, L., Bianconi, L., Colivicchi, F., et al., 2005. *n*-3 Fatty acids for the prevention of atrial fibrillation after coronary artery bypass surgery: a randomized controlled trial. Journal of the American College of Cardiology 45, 1723–1728.

Chisholm, A., Mc Auley, K., Mann, J., Williams, S., Skeaff, M., 2005. Cholesterol lowering effects of nuts compared with a Canola oil enriched cereal of similar fat composition. Nutrition, Metabolism, and Cardiovascular Diseases 15 (4), 284–292.

Christensen, J.H., Dyerberg, J., Schmidt, E.B., 1999. *n*-3 Fatty acids and the risk of sudden cardiac death assessed by 24-hour heart rate variability. Lipids 34 (Suppl.), S197.

Cleland, J.G., Freemantle, N., Kaye, G., et al., 2004. Clinical trials update from the American Heart Association meeting: omega-3 fatty acids and arrhythmia risk in patients with an implantable defibrillator, ACTIV in CHF, VALIANT, the Hanover autologous bone marrow transplantation study, SPORTIF V, ORBIT, and PAD and DEFINITE. European Journal of Heart Failure 6 (1), 109–115.

Connor, W.E., 2000. Importance of *n*-3 fatty acids in health and disease. American Journal of Clinical Nutrition 71 (1 Suppl.), 171S–175S.

Côté, S., Dodin, S., Blanchet, C., et al., 2004. Very high concentrations of *n*-3 fatty acids in peri- and postmenopausal Inuit women from Greenland. International Journal of Circumpolar Health 63 (Suppl. 2), 298–301.

Dall, T.L., Bays, H., 2009. Addressing lipid treatment targets beyond cholesterol: a role for prescription omega-3 fatty acid therapy. Southern Medical Journal 102 (40), 390–396.

Davidson, M.H., et al., 2007. Efficacy and tolerability of adding prescription omega-3 fatty acids 4 g/d to simvastatin 40 mg/d in hypertriglyceridemic patients: an 8-week, randomized, double-blind, placebo-controlled study. Clinical Therapeutics 29 (7), 1354–1367.

Daviglus, M.L., Stamler, J., Orencia, A.J., et al., 1997. Fish consumption and the 30-year risk of fatal myocardial infarction. The New England Journal of Medicine 336, 1046–1053.

de Lorgeril, M., Salen, P., Paillard, F., Laporte, F., Boucher, F., de Leiris, J., 2002. Mediterranean diet and the French paradox: two distinct biogeographic concepts for one consolidated scientific theory on the role of nutrition in coronary heart disease. Cardiovascular Research 54 (3), 503–515.

De Meester, F., 2009. Progress in lipid nutrition: the Columbus concept addressing chronic diseases. World Review of Nutrition and Dietetics 100, 110–121.

de Roos, B., Mavrommatis, Y., Brouwer, I.A., 2009. Long-chain *n*-3 polyunsaturated fatty acids: new insights into mechanisms relating to inflammation and coronary heart disease. British Journal of Pharmacology 158 (2), 413–428.

Denke, M.A., Adams-Huet, B., Nguyen, A.T., 2000. Individual cholesterol variation in response to a margarine- or butter-based diet: a study in families. Journal of the American Medical Association 284, 2740–2747.

Dormandy, J., Bhattacharya, M., van Troostenburg de Bruyn, A.R., 2009. PROactive investigators: Safety and tolerability of pioglitazone in high-risk patients with type 2 diabetes: an overview of data from PROactive. Drug Safety 32 (3), 187–202.

Dubnov, G., Berry, E.M., 2003. Omega-6/omega-3 fatty acid ratio: the Israeli paradox. World Review of Nutrition and Dietetics 92, 81–91.

Eaton, S.B., Eaton III, S.B., Sinclair, A.J., Cordain, L., Mann, N.J., 1998. Dietary intake of long-chain polyunsaturated fatty acids during the paleolithic. World Review of Nutrition and Dietetics 83, 12–23.

Engler, M.M., Engler, M.B., Malloy, M.J., Paul, S.M., Kulkarni, K.R., Mietus-Snyder, M.L., 2005. Effect of docosahexaenoic acid on lipoprotein subclasses in hyperlipidemic children (the EARLY study). The American Journal of Cardiology 95, 869–871.

Fonarow, G.C., 2008. Statins and n-3 fatty acid supplementation in heart failure. Lancet 372 (9645), 1195–1196.

Food and Drug Administration, HHS, 2002. Food labeling: *trans* fatty acids in nutrition labeling, nutrient content claims, and health claims; reopening of the comment period. Federal Registration 67, 69171–69172.

Fung, T.T., Chiuve, S.E., McCullough, M.L., Rexrode, K.M., Logroscino, G., Hu, F.B., 2008. Adherence to DASH-style diet and risk of coronary heart disease and stroke in women. Archives of Internal Medicine 168, 713–720.

Galan, P., De Bree, A., Mennen, L., et al., 2003. Background and rationale of the SU.FOL.OM3 study: double-blind randomized placebo-controlled secondary prevention trial to test the impact of supplementation with folate, vitamin B6 and B12 and/or omega-3 fatty acids on the prevention of recurrent ischemic events in subjects with atherosclerosis in the coronary or cerebral arteries. The Journal of Nutrition, Health & Aging 7 (6), 428–435.

Geelen, A., Brouwer, I.A., Schouten, E.G., Maan, A.C., Katan, M.B., Zock, P.L., 2005. Effects of n-3 fatty acids from fish on premature ventricular complexes and heart rate in humans. American Journal of Clinical Nutrition 81 (2), 416–420.

Genest, J., McPherson, R., Frohlich, J., Anderson, T., Campbell, N., 2009. 2009 Canadian Cardiovascular Society/Canadian guidelines for the diagnosis and treatment of dyslipidemia and prevention of cardiovascular disease in the adult – 2009 recommendations. Canadian Journal of Cardiology 25 (10), 567–579.

Geppert, J., Kraft, V., Demmelmair, H., Koletzko, B., 2005. Docosahexaenoic acid supplementation in vegetarians effectively increases omega-3 index: a randomized trial. Lipids 40 (8), 807–814.

GISSI-Prevenzione Investigators, 1999. Dietary supplementation with n-3 polyunsaturated fatty acids and vitamin E after myocardial infarction: results of the GISSI-Prevenzione trial. Lancet 354, 447–455.

Giugliano, D., Ceriello, A., Esposito, K., 2006. The effects of diet on inflammation: emphasis on the metabolic syndrome. Journal of the American College of Cardiology 48, 677–685.

Goldstein, L.B., Bushnell, C.D., Adams, R.J., et al., 2011. Guidelines for the primary prevention of stroke: a guideline for healthcare professionals from the American Heart Association/American Stroke Association. Stroke 42 (2), 517–584.

Grundt, H., Nilsen, D.W., Hetland, Ø., Mansoor, M.A., 2004. Clinical outcome and atherothrombogenic risk profile after prolonged wash-out following long-term treatment with high doses of n-3 PUFAs in patients with an acute myocardial infarction. Clinical Nutrition 23 (4), 491–500.

Grundt, H., Nilsen, D.W., Mansoor, M.A., Nordøy, A., 2003. Increased lipid peroxidation during long-term intervention with high doses of n-3 fatty acids (PUFAs) following an acute myocardial infarction. European Journal of Clinical Nutrition 57 (6), 793–800.

Grundy, S.M., et al., 2004a. Clinical management of metabolic syndrome: report of the American Heart Association/National Heart, Lung, and Blood Institute/American Diabetes Association conference on scientific issues related to management. Circulation 109 (4), 551–556.

Grundy, S.M., et al., 2004b. Implications of recent clinical trials for the National Cholesterol Education Program Adult Treatment Panel III guidelines. Circulation 110 (2), 227–239.

Hamaad, A., Kaeng Lee, W., Lip, G.Y., MacFadyen, R.J., 2006. Oral omega n3-PUFA therapy (Omacor) has no impact on indices of heart rate variability in stable post myocardial infarction patients. Cardiovascular Drugs and Therapy 20 (5), 359–364.

Hamilton-Craig, I., Kostner, K., Colquhoun, D., Woodhouse, S., 2009. At sea with SEAS: the first clinical endpoint trial for ezetimibe, treatment of patients with mild to moderate aortic stenosis, ends with mixed results and more controversy. Heart, Lung & Circulation 18 (5), 343–346.

Harris, W.S., Isley, W.L., 2001. Clinical trial evidence for the cardioprotective effects of omega-3 fatty acids. Current Atherosclerosis Reports 3 (2), 174–179.

Harris, W.S., Sands, S.A., Windsor, S.L., et al., 2004. Omega-3 fatty acids in cardiac biopsies from heart transplantation patients. Circulation 110, 1645–1649.

Harris, W.S., Von Schacky, C., 2004. The Omega-3 Index: a new risk factor for death from coronary heart disease? Preventive Medicine 39 (1), 212–220.

Harrison, N., Abhyankar, B., 2005. The mechanism of action of omega-3 fatty acids in secondary prevention post-myocardial infarction. Current Medical Research and Opinion 21 (1), 95–100.

Hathcock, J., Richardson, D., Shao, A., Jennings, S., 2006. The Risk Assessment and Safety of Bioactive Substances in Food Supplements, pp. 52–57. IADSA.

He, F.J., Nowson, C.A., Lucas, M., MacGregor, G.A., 2007. Increased consumption of fruit and vegetables is related to a reduced risk of coronary heart disease: meta-analysis of cohort studies. Journal of Human Hypertension 21, 717–728.

Heidarsdottir, R., Arnar, D.O., Skuladottir, G.V., et al., 2010. Does treatment with n-3 polyunsaturated fatty acids prevent atrial fibrillation after open heart surgery? Europace 12 (3), 356–363.

Heidemann, C., Schulze, M.B., Franco, O.H., et al., 2008. Dietary patterns and risk of mortality from cardiovascular disease, cancer, and all causes in a prospective cohort of women. Circulation 118, 230–237.

Holman, R.R., et al., 2009. Atorvastatin in factorial with omega-3 EE90 risk reduction in diabetes (AFORRD): a randomised controlled trial. Diabetologia 52 (1), 50–59.

Horton, J.D., Cohen, J.C., Hobbs, H.H., 2007. Molecular biology of PCSK9: its role in LDL metabolism. Trends in Biochemical Sciences 32, 71–77.

Iqbal, R., Anand, S., Ounpuu, S., et al., 2008. Dietary patterns and the risk of acute myocardial infarction in 52 countries. Circulation 118, 1929–1937.

Iseki, K., Tokuyama, K., Shiohira, Y., et al., 2009. Olmesartan clinical trial in Okinawan patients under OKIDS (OCTOPUS) study: design and methods. Clinical and Experimental Nephrology 13 (2), 145–151.

Jones, P.J., Lau, V.W., 2002. Effect of n-3 polyunsaturated fatty acids on risk reduction of sudden death. Nutrition Reviews 60 (12), 407–409.

Kearney, R., 1987. Promotion and prevention of tumour growth – effects of endotoxin, inflammation, and dietary lipids. International Clinical Nutrition Review 7, 157.

Kendrick, J., Shlipak, M.G., Targher, G., Cook, T., Lindenfeld, J., Chonchol, M., 2010. Effect of lovastatin on primary prevention of cardiovascular events in mild CKD and kidney function loss: a post hoc analysis of the Air Force/Texas Coronary Atherosclerosis Prevention Study. American Journal of Kidney Diseases 55 (1), 42–49.

Konner, M., Eaton, S.B., 2010. Paleolithic nutrition: twenty-five years later. Nutrition in Clinical Practice 25 (6), 594–602.

Kowey, P.R., Reiffel, J.A., Ellenbogen, K.A., Naccarelli, G.V., Pratt, C.M., 2010. Efficacy and safety of prescription omega-3 fatty acids for the prevention of recurrent symptomatic atrial fibrillation: a randomized controlled trial. Journal of the American Medical Association 304 (21), 2363–2372.

Kris-Etherton, P.M., Harris, W.S., Appel, L.J., Nutrition Committee, 2003. Fish consumption, fish oil, omega-3 fatty acids, and cardiovascular disease. Arteriosclerosis, Thrombosis, and Vascular Biology 23 (2), e20–e30.

Kris-Etherton, P.M., Harris, W.S., Appel, L.J., et al., 2002. Fish consumption, fish oil, omega-3 fatty acids, and cardiovascular disease. Circulation 106, 2747–2757.

Kris-Etherton, P.M., Lichtenstein, A.H., Howard, B.V., Steinberg, D., Witztum, J.L., 2004. Nutrition Committee of the American Heart Association Council on Nutrition, Physical Activity, and Metabolism: Antioxidant vitamin supplements and cardiovascular disease. Circulation 110 (5), 637–641.

Kris-Etherton, P.M., Taylor, D.S., Yu- Poth, S., et al., 2000. Polyunsaturated fatty acids in the food chain in the United States. American Journal of Clinical Nutrition 71 (1 Suppl.), 179S–188S.

Kristensen, S.D., Iversen, A.M., Schmidt, E.B., 2001. n-3 Polyunsaturated fatty acids and coronary thrombosis. Lipids 36 (Suppl.), S79–S82.

Kwiterovich Jr., P.O., 2002. Clinical relevance of the biochemical metabolic, and genetic factors that influence low-density lipoprotein heterogeneity. The American Journal of Cardiology 90 (8A), 30i–47i.

Leaf, A., Kang, J., Xiao, Y., Billman, G., 2003. Clinical preservation of sudden cardiac death by *n*-3 poly-unsaturated fatty acids and mechanism of prevention of arrhythmias by *n*-3 fish oils. Circulation 107, 2646–2652.

Leaf, A., Xiao, Y.F., Kang, J.X., Billman, G.E., 2003. Prevention of sudden cardiac death by *n*-3 polyun-saturated fatty acids. Pharmacology and Therapeutics 98 (3), 355–377.

Lichtenstein, A.H., Appel, L.J., Brands, M., et al., 2006. Diet and lifestyle recommendations revision 2006: a scientific statement from the American Heart Association Nutrition Committee. Circulation 114, 82–96.

Lindman, A.S., Pedersen, J.I., Hjerkinn, E.M., et al., 2004. The effects of long-term diet and omega-3 fatty acid supplementation on coagulation factor VII and serum phospholipids with special emphasis on the R353Q polymorphism of the FVII gene. Thrombosis and Haemostasis 91 (6), 1097–1104.

London, B., Albert, C., Anderson, M.E., et al., 2007. Omega-3 fatty acids and cardiac arrhythmias: prior studies and recommendations for future research: a report from the National Heart, Lung, and Blood Institute and Office Of Dietary Supplements Omega-3 Fatty Acids and their Role in Cardiac Arrhyth-mogenesis Workshop. Circulation 116 (10), e320–e335.

Madsen, T., Christensen, J.H., Schmidt, E.B., 2007. C-reactive protein and *n*-3 fatty acids in patients with a previous myocardial infarction: a placebo-controlled randomized study. European Journal of Nutrition 46 (7), 428–430.

Marchioli, R., Barzi, F., Bomba, E., et al., 2002. Early protection against sudden death by *n*-3 polyunsat-urated fatty acids after myocardial infarction: time-course analysis of the results of the Gruppo Italiano per lo Studio della Sopravvivenza nell'Infarto Miocardico (GISSI)-Prevenzione. Circulation 105 (16), 1897–1903.

Marchioli, R., Levantesi, G., Macchia, A., et al., 2005. Antiarrhythmic mechanisms of *n*-3 PUFA and the results of the GISSI-Prevenzione trial. Journal of Membrane Biology 206 (2), 117–128.

Marchioli, R., Levantesi, G., Silletta, M.G., et al., 2009. Effect of *n*-3 polyunsaturated fatty acids and rosu-vastatin in patients with heart failure: results of the GISSI-HF trial. Expert Review of Cardiovascular Therapy 7 (7), 735–748.

Marchioli, R., Marfisi, R.M., Borrelli, G., et al., 2007. Efficacy of *n*-3 polyunsaturated fatty acids according to clinical characteristics of patients with recent myocardial infarction: insights from the GISSI-Prevenzione trial. Journal of Cardiovascular Medicine (Hagerstown) 8 (Suppl. 1), S34–S37.

Marchioli, R., Schweiger, C., Tavazzi, L., Valagussa, F., 2001. Efficacy of *n*-3 polyunsaturated fatty acids after myocardial infarction: results of GISSI-Prevenzione trial. Gruppo Italiano per lo Studio della Sopravvivenza nell'Infarto Miocardico. Lipids 36 (Suppl.), S119–S126.

Marchioli, R., Silletta, M.G., Levantesi, G., Pioggiarella, R., Tognoni, G., 2010. *n*-3 Polyunsaturated fatty acids in heart failure: mechanisms and recent clinical evidence. Cellular and Molecular Biology (Noisy-le-Grand, France) 56 (1), 110–130.

Maslowska, M., Wang, H.W., Cianflone, K., 2005. Novel roles for acylation stimulating protein/C3a desArg: a review of recent in vitro and in vivo evidence. Vitamins and Hormones 70, 309–332.

McLennan, P.L., Abeywardena, M.Y., 2005. Membrane basis for fish oil effects on the heart: linking natural hibernators to prevention of human sudden cardiac death. Journal of Membrane Biology 206 (2), 85–102.

Mensink, R.P., Zock, P.L., Kester, A.D., Katan, M.B., 2003. Effects of dietary fatty acids and carbohydrates on the ratio of serum total to HDL cholesterol and on serum lipids and apolipoproteins: a meta-analysis of 60 controlled trials. American Journal of Clinical Nutrition 77, 1146–1155.

Metcalf, R.G., Sanders, P., James, M.J., Cleland, L.G., Young, G.D., 2008. Effect of dietary *n*-3 polyun-saturated fatty acids on the inducibility of ventricular tachycardia in patients with ischemic cardiomy-opathy. The American Journal of Cardiology 101 (6), 758–761.

Mori, T.A., Puddey, I.B., Burke, V., et al., 2000. Effect of omega 3 fatty acids on oxidative stress in humans: GC–MS measurement of urinary F2-isoprostane excretion. Redox Report 5 (1), 45–46.

Mozaffarian, D., 2008. Fish and *n*-3 fatty acids for the prevention of fatal coronary heart disease and sudden cardiac death. American Journal of Clinical Nutrition 87 (6), 1991S–1996S.

NCEP ATP III, 2001. NCEP REPORT: Executive summary of the third report of the National Cholesterol Education Program (NCEP) Expert Panel on Detection, Evaluation, and Treatment of High Blood

Cholesterol in Adults (Adult Treatment Panel III). Journal of the American Medical Association 285, 2486–2497.

O'Dea, K., 1988. The hunter gatherer lifestyle of Australian aborigines: implications for health. In: McLean, A.J., Wahlqvist, M.L. (Eds.), Current Problems in Nutrition, Pharmacology, and Toxicology. John Libbey Nutrition, London, pp. 27–36.

O'Dea, K., 1991. Cardiovascular disease risk factors in Australian aborigines. Clinical and Experimental Pharmacology and Physiology 18 (2), 85–88.

O'Keefe Jr., J.H., Abuissa, H., Sastre, A., Steinhaus, D.M., Harris, W.S., 2006. Effects of omega-3 fatty acids on resting heart rate, heart rate recovery after exercise, and heart rate variability in men with healed myocardial infarctions and depressed ejection fractions. The American Journal of Cardiology 97 (8), 1127–1130.

Okuyama, H., Fujii, Y., Ikemoto, A., 2000. N-6/N-3 ratio of dietary fatty acids rather than hypercholesterolemia as the major risk factor for atherosclerosis and coronary heart disease. Journal of Health Sciences 46 (3), 157.

Pearce, M.L., Dayton, S., 1971. Incidence of cancer in men on a diet high in polyunsaturated fat. Lancet 7697, 464–467.

Pella, D., Dubnov, G., Singh, R.B., Sharma, R., Berry, E.M., Manor, O., 2003. Effects of an Indo-Mediterranean diet on the omega-6/omega-3 ratio in patients at high risk of coronary artery disease: the Indian paradox. Omega-6/Omega-3 Essential Fatty Acids ratio: The Scientific Evidence. World Review of Nutrition and Dietetics 92, Karger, Basel, pp. 74–80.

Rader, D.J., Cohen, J., Hobbs, H.H., 2003. Monogenic hypercholesterolemia: new insights in pathogenesis and treatment. Journal of Clinical Investigation 111 (12), 1795–1803.

Raitt, M.H., Connor, W.E., Morris, C., et al., 2005. Fish oil supplementation and risk of ventricular tachycardia and ventricular fibrillation in patients with implantable defibrillators: a randomized controlled trial. Journal of the American Medical Association 293 (23), 2884–2891.

Rajaram, S., Haddad, E.H., Mejia, A., Sabaté, J., 2009. Walnuts and fatty fish influence different serum lipid fractions in normal to mildly hyperlipidemic individuals: a randomized controlled study. American Journal of Clinical Nutrition 89 (5), 1657S–1663S.

Ramsden, C.E., Hibbeln, J.R., Majchrzak, S.F., Davis, J.M., 2010. n-6 Fatty acid-specific and mixed polyunsaturate dietary interventions have different effects on CHD risk: a meta-analysis of randomised controlled trials. British Journal of Nutrition 104 (11), 1586–1600.

Rauch, B., Schiele, R., Schneider, S., et al., 2006. Highly purified omega-3 fatty acids for secondary prevention of sudden cardiac death after myocardial infarction-aims and methods of the OMEGA-study. Cardiovascular Drugs and Therapy 20 (5), 365–375.

Sanders, T.A., Lewis, F., Slaughter, S., et al., 2006. Effect of varying the ratio of n-6 to n-3 fatty acids by increasing the dietary intake of alpha-linolenic acid, eicosapentaenoic, and docosahexaenoic acid, or both on fibrinogen and clotting factors VII and XII in persons aged 45–70 y: the OPTILIP study. American Journal of Clinical Nutrition 84 (3), 513–522.

Schwartz, J., Dube, K., Sichert-Hellert, W., et al., 2009. Modification of dietary polyunsaturated fatty acids via complementary food enhances n-3 long-chain polyunsaturated fatty acid synthesis in healthy infants: a double blinded randomised controlled trial. Archives of Disease in Childhood 94 (11), 876–882.

Shah, P., Mudaliar, S., 2010. Pioglitazone: side effect and safety profile. Expert Opinion on Drug Safety 9 (2), 347–354.

Sharma, R., Raghuram, T.C., Rao, U.B., Moffatt, R.J., Krishnaswamy, K., 2010. The effect of fat intake and antihypertensive drug therapy on serum lipid profile: a cross-sectional survey of serum lipids in male and female hypertensives. Molecular and Cellular Biochemistry 343 (1–2), 37–47.

Sharma, R., Singh, R.B., Moffatt, R.J., Katz, J., 2010. Dietary fat intake: promotion of disease in carotid artery disease: lipid lowering versus side effects of statins. In: Meester, F.D., Zibadi, S., Watson, R.R. (Eds.), Modern Dietary Fat Intakes in Disease Promotion (Nutrition and Health), pp. 151–185. Springer Science + Business Media, New York.

Siddiqui, R.A., Harvey, K.A., Zaloga, G.P., 2008. Modulation of enzyme activities by n-polyunsaturated fatty acids to support cardiovascular health. The Journal of Nutritional Biochemistry 19 (7), 417–437.

Simell, O., Niinikoski, H., Rönnemaa, T., et al., 2009. Cohort profile: the STRIP study (special Turku Coronary Risk Factor Intervention Project), an infancy-onset dietary and life-style intervention trial. International Journal of Epidemiology 38 (3), 650–655.

Singh, R.B., De Meester, F., Wilczynska, A., 2010. The tsim tsoum approaches for prevention of cardiovascular disease. Cardiology Research and Practice. 10.4061/2010/824938.

Singh, R.B., Dubnov, G., Niaz, M.A., et al., 2002. Effect of an Indo-Mediterranean diet on progression of coronary disease in high risk patients: a randomized single blind trial. Lancet 360, 1455–1461.

Singh, R.B., et al., in press. Ancient nutrition practices in India: a nutrition survey of Kurichiyas. The Open Nutraceutical Journal.

Trichopoulou, A., Bamia, C., Trichopoulos, D., 2009. Anatomy of health effects of Mediterranean diets. Greek epic prospective heart study. British Medical Journal 338, b2337.

US Food and Drug Administration, 2004. FDA Announces Qualified Health Claims for Omega-3 Fatty Acids 2004. http://www.fda.gov/bbs/topics/news/2004/new01115.html.

Van Horn, L., McCoin, M., Kris-Etherton, P.M., et al., 2008. The evidence for dietary prevention and treatment of cardiovascular disease. Journal of the American Dietetic Association 108, 287–331.

Verboom, C.N., Critical Analysis of GISSI-Prevenzione Trial, 2006. Highly purified omega-3 polyunsaturated fatty acids are effective as adjunct therapy for secondary prevention of myocardial infarction. Herz 31 (Suppl. 3), 49–59.

Volpe, M., Chin, D., Paneni, F., 2010. The challenge of polypharmacy in cardiovascular medicine. Fundamental and Clinical Pharmacology 24 (1), 9–17.

von Schacky, C., Baumann, K., Angerer, P., 2001. The effect of n-3 fatty acids on coronary atherosclerosis: results from SCIMO, an angiographic study, background, and implications. Lipids 36 (Suppl.), S99–S102.

Walser, B., Stebbins, C.L., 2008. Omega-3 fatty acid supplementation enhances stroke volume and cardiac output during dynamic exercise. European Journal of Applied Physiology 104 (3), 455–461.

Wolk, A., et al., 1998. A prospective study of association of monounsaturated fat and other types of fat with risk of breast cancer. Archives of Internal Medicine 158, 41–45.

Yokoyama, M., Origasa, H., Matsuzaki, M., et al., 2007. Effects of eicosapentaenoic acid on major coronary events in hypercholesterolaemic patients (JELIS): a randomised open-label, blinded endpoint analysis. Lancet 369, 1090–1098.

Yu-Poth, S., Yin, D., Kris-Etherton, P.M., Zhao, G., Etherton, T.D., 2005. Long-chain polyunsaturated fatty acids upregulate LDL receptor protein expression in fibroblasts and HepG2 cells. Journal of Nutrition 135, 2541–2545.

Zhao, Y.T., Chen, Q., Sun, Y.X., et al., 2009. Prevention of sudden cardiac death with omega-3 fatty acids in patients with coronary heart disease: a meta-analysis of randomized controlled trials. Annali Medici 41 (4), 301–310.

CHAPTER 2

Herbal Supplements or Herbs in Heart Disease: History, Herbal Foods, Coronary Heart Disease

R. Sharma
Florida State University, Tallahassee, FL, USA
Amity University, Uttar Pradesh, Noida, Uttar Pradesh, India

1. INTRODUCTION

Herbs are natural form of dry whole plants or their parts such as dry flower, root, oil, and stem rich in bioactive chemical compounds so-called Herbiceuticals. The main difference between pharmaceutic drug and herbal principles is their isolation method and purification level. The pharmaceutical drugs are available with high purity as artificial chemical(s) while herbs are rich in natural complex chemicals in mixture. Herbal 'mixtures' are prepared by simple extraction, filtration, and powder making to test it by high performance chromatography and other techniques. Bioactive herbal principles (whole herbs, extracts, or concentrates) may be used as 'bioactive herbal formulations' as combinations of different active isolated chemicals of plants or their parts combined with known enzyme inhibitors, vitamins, and alkalizing minerals that have value in health promoting, disease preventing, or semimedicinal properties. Herbal 'extracts' may be fortified with vitamin, proteins, amino acids, minerals, and carbohydrates.

Since World War II, it became necessary to reduce death causalities due to high lipids in body as major cardiovascular risk. With all available technological advances, still today high lipids in blood and severe cardiac arrests remain as major threat to the human. With this fact, our motivation was to search other alternate herbal therapy possibilities and catching attention of federal and regulatory agencies to watch the concerns of side effects after long-term cardiovascular lipid lowering pharmaceutical drugs and need of consistent new awareness on less-known herbal supplements. In 1994, the United States implemented Dietary Supplement Health and Education Act (DSHEA) that sparked an upsurge in 'herbal' use as alternative medicine and continues today (Brazier and Levine, 2003). Different food companies have advocated their natural herbal products from herbs available from (a) the food industry, (b) the herbal and dietary supplement, (c) pharmaceutical industry, and (d) the newly emerged bioengineered microorganisms, agroproducts, or active biomolecules. It may range from isolated nutrients, herbal products, dietary supplements, and diets to genetically engineered 'custom' foods and processed products

Bioactive Food as Dietary Interventions for Cardiovascular Disease
http://dx.doi.org/10.1016/B978-0-12-396485-4.00001-3

© 2013 Elsevier Inc.
All rights reserved.

29

such as cereals, soups, and beverages. Chemically the active components in bioactive herbs may be classified as isoprenoid derivatives (terpenoids, carotenoids, saponins, tocotrienols, tocopherols, terpenes), phenolic compounds (couramines, tannins, lignins, anthrocynins, isoflavones, flavonones, flavanoids), carbohydrate derivatives (ascorbic acid, oligosaccharides, nonstarch polysaccharides), fatty acids and structural lipids (n-3 polyunsaturated fatty acids PUFA, CLA, MUFA, sphingolipids, lecithins), amino acid derivatives (amino acids, allyl-S compounds, capsaicnoids, isothiocyanates, indols, folate, choline), microbes (probiotics, prebiotics), and minerals (Ca, Zn, Cu, K, Se; Butterweck and Winterhoff, 2001).

1.1 Symptoms of Coronary Heart Disease

The most common symptom of coronary artery disease (CAD) is angina or chest pain. Angina can be described as a discomfort, heaviness, pressure, aching, burning, fullness, squeezing, or painful feeling in your chest. It can be mistaken for indigestion or heartburn. Angina is usually felt in the chest, but may also be felt in the shoulders, arms, neck, throat, jaw, or back (4). Symptoms are summarized in Table 2.1.

Other symptoms of CAD include
- Shortness of breath
- Palpitations (irregular heart beats, skipped beats, or a 'flip-flop' feeling in your chest)
- A faster heartbeat
- Weakness or dizziness
- Nausea
- Sweating.

1.2 Biochemical Basis of CHD

In general, increase in blood cholesterol and lipoproteins cause lipid deposition in cardiovascular tissues with reduced HDL–cholesterol. With advanced imbalance in blood lipids, it leads to uncontrolled dyslipidemia and heart disease (Apple and Jaffe, 2008).

Heart disease is known as Acute Ischemic Heart Disease due to myocardial injury and leakage of troponin, CK-MB enzymes and continuous release of nitric oxide (NO), cyclooxygenase-2 (COX-2), cardial output (CO), superoxide dismutase (SOD), malondialdehyde (MDA), atrial natriuretic peptide-sensitive superoxide dismutase (ANPSOD), and atrial natriuretic peptide (ANP) proteins. After advanced heart disease development, congestive heart failure (CHF) occurs with abrupt release of beta-natriuretic peptide (BNP), N-terminal proBNP as shown in Figure 2.1. Following metabolites are secreted from the damaged cardiac muscle (Apple and Jaffe, 2008):
- Cardiac troponins cTn-I and cTn-T: cTn-T is 11 amino acid residue on N-terminal of molecule. It is specific in cardiac muscles.
- BNP: It is the hormone released from cardiac ventricles from cardiac myocytes as a counter regulatory hormone in response to a variety of cardiac stress. Circulating

Table 2.1 Symptoms of Coronary Heart Disease at Various Stages

Symptoms of arrhythmias

Arrhythmias, abnormal heart rhythm

- Palpitations (a feeling of skipped heart beats, fluttering or 'flip-flops,' or feeling that your heart is 'running away')
- Pounding in your chest
- Dizziness or feeling light-headed
- Fainting
- Shortness of breath
- Chest discomfort
- Weakness or fatigue (feeling very tired)

Symptoms of atrial fibrillation

Atrial fibrillation (AF): Aymptomatic or symptomatic

- Heart palpitations (a sudden pounding, fluttering, or racing feeling in the heart)
- Lack of energy; tired
- Dizziness (feeling faint or light-headed)
- Chest discomfort (pain, pressure, or discomfort in the chest)
- Shortness of breath (difficulty breathing during activities of daily living)

Symptoms of heart valve disease

- Shortness of breath and/or difficulty catching your breath
- Weakness or dizziness
- Discomfort in your chest, feel a pressure or weight in chest with activity or when going out in cold air
- Palpitations (this may feel like a rapid heart rhythm, irregular heartbeat, skipped beats, or a flip-flop feeling in your chest)

If valve disease causes heart failure:

- Swelling of ankles or feet, abdomen, which may cause feel bloated
- Quick weight gain

Symptoms of heart failure

- Shortness of breath noted during activity (most commonly) or at rest, especially when you lie down flat in bed
- Cough that is productive of a white mucus
- Quick weight gain (a weight gain of two or three pounds in 1 day is possible)
- Swelling in ankles, legs, and abdomen
- Dizziness
- Fatigue and weakness
- Rapid or irregular heartbeats
- Other symptoms include nausea, palpitations, and chest pain

Symptoms of a heart attack (myocardial infarction or MI)

- Discomfort, pressure, heaviness, or pain in the chest, arm, or below the breastbone
- Discomfort radiating to the back, jaw, throat, or arm
- Fullness, indigestion, or choking feeling (may feel like heartburn)
- Sweating, nausea, vomiting, or dizziness
- Extreme weakness, anxiety, or shortness of breath
- Rapid or irregular heartbeats

Continued

Table 2.1 Symptoms of Coronary Heart Disease at Various Stages—cont'd

Symptoms of congenital heart defects
- Shortness of breath
- Limited ability to exercise
- Symptoms of heart failure (see above) or valve disease (see above)

Congenital heart defects in infants and children
- Cyanosis (a bluish tint to the skin, fingernails, and lips)
- Fast breathing and poor feeding
- Poor weight gain
- Recurrent lung infections
- Inability to exercise

Symptoms of heart muscle disease (cardiomyopathy)
- Chest pain or pressure
- Heart failure symptoms (see above)
- Swelling of the lower extremities
- Fatigue
- Fainting
- Palpitations (fluttering in the chest due to abnormal heart rhythms)

Symptoms of pericarditis
- Chest pain. Sharp and located in the center of the chest
- Low-grade fever
- Increased heart rate

concentration of BNP hormone is high in ventricles in patients with moderate to severe CHF.

- Creatine kinase isozymes: CK-MB or CK-3 is prominent in heart muscles as four isoenzymes especially in left ventricular hypertrophy (LVH) with CAD as a result of aortic stenosis.
- Myoglobin in serum is increased after acute myocardial infarction (AMI) muscle injury.
- C-reactive protein (CRP) is an indicator of inflammation and atherosclerosis.
- Choline is released after stimulation by phospholipase D during ischemia as test of acute coronary syndrome (ACS).
- Elevated sCD40 ligand, a transmembrane protein related with myocardial necrosis factor-alpha to indicate ACS.
- Ischemia modified albumin (IMA) is the FDA-approved test as negative value for ischemia.
- Myeloperoxidase is released in active inflammatory response in chronic CAD and ACS.
- Oxidized low-density lipoprotein molecule and lipoprotein A concentrations are high in atherosclerosis.
- Lipoprotein-associated phospholipase A2 is associated with inflammation and increases before AMI develops and phospholipase A2 measures acute phase reactants differently from CRP.

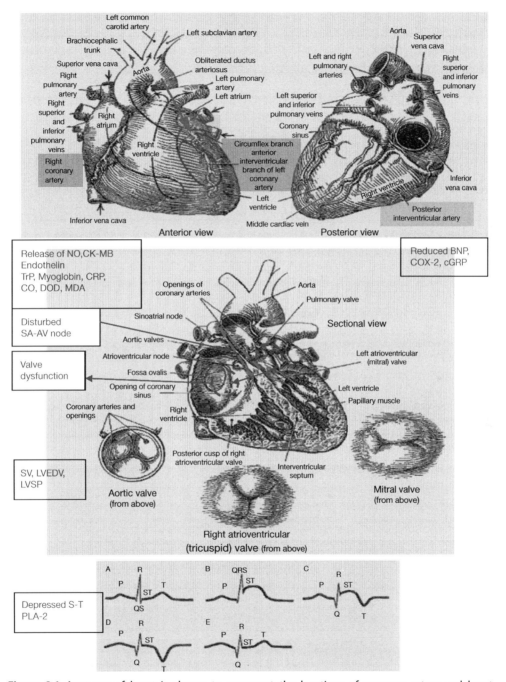

Figure 2.1 Anatomy of heart is shown to represent the locations of coronary artery and heart territories during CHD. Notice the plaque formation in coronary arteries shown in color either removed or treated by bypass, EKG patterns and ventricular functions are main indicators of heart disease. *Reproduced from Apple, F.S., Jaffe, A.S., 2008. Cardiovascular diseases. Part V: pathophysiology. In: Burtis, C.A., Ashwood, E.R., Bruns, D.E., Sawyer, B.G. (Eds.), Tietz Fundamentals of Clinical Chemistry, sixth ed. Saunders Elsevier Companay, St Louis, MO, pp. 614–630 (Chapter 33).*

- Pregnancy-associated plasma protein A (PAPP-A) metalloproteinase enzyme is released from high-risk plaques to rupture in ACS.

In the following section, the events of cardiac metabolism and release of molecules are described (Apple and Jaffe, 2008).

1.2.1 Acute ischemic heart disease

1. Acetylcholine activates endothelial cells, which produce NO from labile substance derived by L-arginine degradation through endothelial NO synthase (eNOS). Nitric oxide is relaxing vasodilator agent and it inhibits platelet aggregation, monocyte adhesion, and smooth muscle cell proliferation. In heart disease or endothelial dysfunction, agonist-induced stimulation of endothelium leads to activation of COX pathway and production of thromboxane A2 or prostaglandin H2 or oxygen free radicals. Two cyclooxygenases 1 and 2 (COX 1 and 2) or prostaglandin endoperoxide synthase 1 and 2 convert arachidonic acid to prostaglandins, thromboxanes, and eicosanoids. COX 1 is responsible in homeostatic function, whereas COX 2 is responsible in proinflammatory conditions with high NO. Cardioprotection strategy is inhibition of COX and NO-mediated vasodilation to restore blood pressure and low inflammation.
2. Myocardium is the thickest layer and myocardial infarction, ischemia, myocarditis, septic shock in heart failure are associated with overexpression of iNOS or large amount of NO (produced by iNOS) inhibit COX 2 metabolites formation and ultimately causes CHF and myocardial dysfunction with hypertrophy.
3. Nitric oxide production.
4. cGRP reduction.
5. Release of troponin T and CK–MB.
6. Release of CO, SOD, and MDA.
   - Heartbeat volume (SV), CO, cardial index (CI), cardial emission fraction (EF), and left ventricle end diastole volume (LVEDV).
   - Higher contents of MDA, ANPSOD, SOD, reduced glutathione peroxidase, and ANP after herbal treatment.
   - Improved systolic capacity of cardial muscle by measuring left ventricle systole pressure value (LVSP), left ventricle maximum systole speed rate $(+dp/dt)$, and left ventricle minimum systole speed rate $(-dp/dt)$.

1.2.2 Congestive heart failure

- CHF weakens heart function with edema, narrowing coronary arteries leading to myocardial infarction and myocardial scar formation to interfere with normal electrocardiac function and high blood pressure.
- CRP is a marker of systemic or vascular inflammation in acute phase, which predicts cardiovascular events and stroke. It promotes expression of adhesion molecules and

pathogenesis of vascular inflammation or coronary artery atherosclerosis or heart disease CHD. Atrial fibrillation (AF) is rapid randomized contractions of atrial myocardium causing irregular, often rapid ventricular rate. AF persists because of structural changes in atria promoted by inflammation.

- BNP hormone release from myocardium.

1.3 Diagnosis of CHD

1.3.1 Acute coronary syndrome

- Elevated ST segment on electrocardiogram (ECG) AMI.
- Increase in troponin T with elevated Q wave non-STEMI.
- Plaque visible in magnetic resonance angiography, MRI, and ultrasound ACS.
- Rise and gradual fall of cardiac troponin T and CK-MB AMI.
- Ischemia with elevated or depressed S-T segment AMI.
- High phospholipase A2 with CRP Pro-AMI.

1.3.2 Congestive heart failure

- Events of heart dysfunction CHF.

Impaired SV, CO, CI, cardial EF, LVEDV, left LVSP, left ventricle maximum systole speed rate $(+\mathrm{d}p/\mathrm{d}t)$, and left ventricle minimum systole speed rate $(-\mathrm{d}p/\mathrm{d}t)$.

1.4 Scientific Basis of Herbal Therapy of Heart Disease

1.4.1 Herbal supplements that open blood vessels

Our research indicates that when it comes to heart disease and dietary supplements used for opening blood vessels, the following are some of the best preventive strategies against heart disease.

Ginkgo biloba is well renowned for improving blood flow throughout the body, including the heart muscle. Ginkgo is also a powerhouse antioxidant and it appears to reduce blood stickiness, which lowers the risk of blood clots.

Policosanol — some studies have shown that policosanol can lower one's bad cholesterol (LDL) by up to 20% and raise beneficial cholesterol (HDL) by 10%.

Guggulipid is prized for its ability to lower bad cholesterol (LDL) levels as well as high blood triglyceride levels. It has also shown to boost the levels of good cholesterol (HDL).

Vitamin B complex, particularly vitamins B6, B12, and folic acid reduce levels of homocysteine.

Chromium is a mineral that plays a role in helping to manage cholesterol levels. In addition, it can help improve blood sugar control for diabetes sufferers.

Garlic is noted to reduce cholesterol and triglyceride levels as well as slightly lower blood pressure. In addition, studies indicate that garlic can help reduce the likelihood of blood clots.

Other nutrients that help open blood vessels include niacin and soy protein.

1.4.2 Supplements that strengthen the heart muscle

Magnesium – this mineral plays a vital role in controlling muscle contraction and relaxation. It is also involved in regulating blood pressure (by relaxing blood vessels) and can help reduce the tendency of blood clotting.

Coenzyme Q10 is prized for its ability to strengthen the heart muscle and help prevents heart attacks and heart disease.

Hawthorn is a powerful heart tonic. It also strengthens the heart's pumping ability (muscle), helping the heart to beat more forcefully and efficiently.

Other possible heart muscle strengtheners include L-carnitine and potassium.

1.4.3 Heart disease and dietary supplements: antioxidants

Antioxidants are believed to help prevent heart disease by fighting free radicals, substances that harm the body when left unchecked. These nutrients are on a constant search and destroy mission, fighting the continuous onslaught of free radicals. The following dietary supplements help fight free radicals and, as such, should be a part of your preventive strategies against heart disease.

Grape seed extract is a rich source of flavonoid compounds (oligomeric proanthocyanidins – OPCs) that perform as potent antioxidants and powerful blood vessel strengtheners.

Green tea contains a particular group of potent antioxidants called polyphenols. Green tea also protects LDL cholesterol and blood vessel linings from oxidative damage.

Fish oil is a rich source of omega-3 fatty acids (docosahexanoic acid and ecosapentanoic acid) that benefits heart health. Fish oil helps prevent platelets in the blood from clumping together, reducing the risk that blood clots will form. It has also been shown to reduce blood pressure, lower triglycerides (blood fats) levels, and improve blood flow. Indeed, fish oil omega 3s are praised by many experts as being one of the best heart disease and dietary supplements, meaning it should be a part of your preventive strategies against heart disease.

Some other antioxidants noted to help with cardiovascular heart health include vitamins C and E, and resveratrol.

1.4.4 Chinese herbs in reduction of HDL catabolism

Radix Panacis Quinquefolii (American ginseng), San-Huang-Hsie-Hsin-Tang for purging fire and clearing three torsos, Scutellaria (Radix Scutellariae), rhizome of coptis (Rhizoma Coptidis), root, rhizome of rhubarb (Radix et Rhizoma Rhei), *Zingiber officinale*, Zizyphi fructus, Radix ginseng, *Rhizoma gingiberis* (ginger). Still search is going for herbs if they can influence cholesterol ester transport protein (CETP). If herb blocks CETP, it may reduce the catalysis of HDL.

The mechanism of possible cardioprotection role of herb in the treatment of atherosclerosis is described. In this process, plasma CETP binds neutral lipids (CE or TG) and PL on HDL3, but CETP selectively promotes an exchange of CE and TG among lipoproteins. As a result, deficiency of CETP in human results in increased HDL levels due to decreased catabolism of HDL apoA-I and decreased LDL levels due to increased catabolism of LDL apoB. Two factors play role in maintaining blood HDL concentration: (1) HDL–TG can be hydrolyzed by hepatic lipase, so plasma CETP reduces HDL particle size via CE/TG exchange between chylomicron (CM)/VLDL and HDL or accelerates catabolic rate of HDL apolipoproteins and (2) genetic polymorphisms of the CETP gene promoter slightly decrease plasma CETP activity (-20%) and increases HDL-C concentration. Such clinical results show decreasing coronary risk in meta-analyses. Although lipoprotein phenotype found in CETP-deficient heterozygotes showed CETP activity by -40–50%, lipoprotein profiles were antiatherogenic in most studies as shown in Figure 2.2. ApoE-rich large HDL and decreased cholesterol esterification rate are characteristics of HDL found in CETP deficiency. CETP inhibitor or antisense therapy may be useful for prevention of atherosclerotic diseases through increasing lipoprotein size of LDL and HDL in addition to lowering LDL and elevating HDL. However, it is unknown if subjects have association of very high HDL (>100 mg dl^{-1}) with homozygous CETP deficiency (Borggreve et al., 2007). Atherogenicity of plasma CETP possibly depends on regulatory factors (liver LDL receptor mRNA, apo A-I mRNA, and apo B mRNA) with coronary artery atherosclerosis and LDL cholesterol levels. CETP mRNA levels ultimately may influence plasma lipoprotein levels and atherogenesis. LDL and HDL cholesterol behave different because

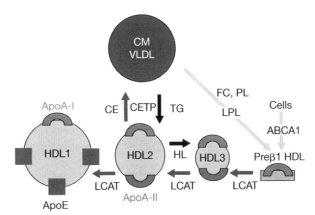

Figure 2.2 Scheme for HDL metabolism. Plasma cholesteryl ester transfer protein (CETP) facilitates the exchange of the neutral lipids CE and TG between chylomicron (CM)/VLDL and HDL2. HDL-TG is provided by CETP, and it is hydrolyzed by hepatic lipase (HL). The synthetic rate of preβ1HDL is positively correlated with lipoprotein lipase (LPL)-mediated lipolysis and increased cholesterol efflux by the ABCA1 transporter. On the other hand, the catabolic rate of preβ1HDL is correlated with the cholesterol esterification rate by lecithin:cholesterol acyltransferase (LCAT). *Reproduced from Mabuchi, H., Inazu, A., 2010. Human cholesteryl ester transfer protein in human HDL metabolism. In: Schaefer, E.J. (Ed.), High Density Lipoproteins, Dyslipidemia, and Coronary Heart Disease. Springer Science+Business Media, New York, pp. 95–110.*

CETP catalyzes the transfer of cholesteryl esters from HDL to LDL to influence the steady-state concentration of cholesterol (mostly cholesteryl ester). Rate of cholesteryl ester transfer from HDL to other lipoproteins or Apo B proteins is a determinant of plasma HDL concentration, determined by the LDL particle size and level of plasma triglycerides under CETP genetic control (Borggreve et al., 2007).

2. RELATION TO TG METABOLISM

HDL-cholesterol is directly transported to the liver by selective uptake of HDL-CE or FC via hepatic lipase and/or SR-BI pathway. CETP pathway appears to be antiatherogenic when LDL levels are low and TRL clearance is rapid as observed with low-fat diets. Subjects with high CETP activity may manifest lower coronary risk when plasma TG levels are low (Borggreve et al., 2007).

However, western type high saturated-fat diets suppress LDL receptor expression, and therefore, the flow of HDL-derived cholesterol back to the liver via the LDL pathway is reduced.

CETP gene mutations and polymorphisms indicate coronary heart disease (CHD) risk. Meta-analysis on CETP gene SNPs of TaqIB2, -629 C>A and Ile 405 Val (I405V) showed that the genotypes with low CETP may have antiatherogenic effects (Thompson et al., 2008). Antiatherogenicity of lower CETP levels in heterozygous CETP deficiency and increased plasma CETP levels associated with coronary artery calcium and intima-media thickness (Okamura et al., 2009). In contrast, no definite CAD has been found in cohort of homozygous CETP deficiency ($n=53$), thus CHD risk needs to be clarified in a larger cohort of homozygous CETP deficiency by a national survey.

However, it is unknown if subjects have association of very high HDL (>100 mg dl^{-1}) with homozygous CETP deficiency.

3. HERBAL FOODS: APPROVED HERBS IN CARDIOVASCULAR DISEASE

3.1 Garlic: The Most-Studied Herbal Food for the Cardiovascular System

Garlic may be the world's most respected medicinal plant – not only does it have thousands of years of historical medicinal usage, but it has also been the subject of numerous research studies published in 1100 scientific articles, of which there have also been about 258 research studies on the cardiovascular effects of garlic, which represents a major amount of research (Calder, 2004). These studies showed the following:

- When fats are eaten, the blood responds by getting thicker – this can lead to increased risk of heart attack and stroke. Adding garlic to the fats (as in stir-frys) cuts fatty obstruction of the arteries by one-half.

- Elevated blood cholesterol and triglyceride levels are thought to be indicators of increased risk of heart attack and stroke. Garlic can increase the elimination of fats and cholesterol through the bile, and overall cholesterol levels can be reduced. In one human study conducted in India, three groups were studied to see how eating garlic and onions would affect blood cholesterol levels. The first group ate one 3/4 ounces of garlic a week, the second group 1/3 ounces, and the third did not eat garlic and had never eaten it. The average blood cholesterol levels for the three groups – (first) 159 mg per 100 ml (of blood), (second) 172 mg, (third) 207 mg – a significant difference. A number of other human studies done in the United States, Germany, and other countries support garlic's efficacy in lowering blood cholesterol by an average of 10–20% with up to a 17% reduction in blood fats when the equivalent of only one clove per day is eaten. Since estimates indicate that from 40 to 75% of the adult population has cholesterol levels that could lead to increased risk of heart disease but are not yet in need of stronger drugs, adding garlic to the diet in meals, or in the form of a supplement, could be of great benefit.
- Studies show that garlic can reduce the tendency of the blood to form life-threatening clots (possibly leading to heart attack or stroke) by adding as little as 2/3 of a clove per day to meals. The ability of the blood to destroy clots that may be forming is increased by 50–80% when using even one clove a day (Zahid et al., 2005).
- Garlic has only moderate blood pressure-lowering effects, and it must be taken regularly for any significant benefits, but even the modest 7–10% that double-blind studies have shown can be helpful for people taking garlic for its other stronger effects.

While garlic's contribution to the health of the heart and cardiovascular system is significant, many people do not like to eat garlic because of the smell it imparts to their breath. Garlic odors can even exude from the pores of some people when eaten regularly. It seems many people would rather die of heart disease than loneliness. For this reason, and also because of convenience, many people wish to get their daily clove or two from garlic capsules or tablets. Because of the controversy about what form of product is best (fresh-dried, allicin-rich, or aged), it is good to know that just about any quality garlic product, whether dried or oil-based, has some beneficial activity on the cardiovascular system. While allicin-rich products are more antibacterial and possibly antiviral, breakdown products such as ajoene, methyl ally trisulphide, and dimethyl trisulphide created during drying and cooking of garlic, can also have beneficial effects on the heart and circulation.

The best advice about taking garlic seems to be – eat it raw, cook with it, or take it as a supplement – but *do* use it every day.

3.2 Hawthorn, Gentle Heart Herb

The best-known herb for the heart in western herbalism is Hawthorn, which is a small tree or shrub that grows throughout the northern hemisphere. The fruits, flowers, and leaves are processed into tinctures and other kinds of extracts available in capsules or tablets in the United States and other parts of the world.

In Europe, both homeopathic and allopathic doctors used the herb for various heart and cardiovascular ailments from the late nineteenth through the early twentieth centuries – and with great clinical success since hawthorn had entered American clinical practice by 1896 (Cleland et al., 2007; Dalli et al., 2011; Holubarsch et al., 2008; Koch and Malek, 2011; Zick et al., 2009).

Today, hawthorn is an official drug in the Pharmacopeias of Brazil, China, Czechoslovakia, France, Germany, Hungary, Russia, and Switzerland. As a measure of its incredible popularity, it is an ingredient of 213 commercial European herbal formulas, mostly for the cardiovascular system such as *Crataegus laevigata* and *Crataegus oxyacantha* (Cleland et al., 2007; Dalli et al., 2011; Holubarsch et al., 2008; Koch and Malek, 2011; Zick et al., 2009).

The extract of hawthorn can increase blood flow to the heart muscle itself, helping to counteract causes of death in industrial countries – heart attack due to lack of blood flow to the heart. In pharmacological tests on both animals and humans, hawthorn has been shown to improve the contractility of the heart muscle (which can lead to a stronger pumping action of the heart), increase cardiac performance and output, lower the peripheral vascular resistance (reducing the workload of the heart), steady the heartbeat (antiarrhythmic effect), as well as increasing the heart's tolerance to oxygen deficiency, such as might happen during stress or excitement, or in diseases where the arteries are partially blocked (Koch and Malek, 2011).

It is considered so safe that it is sometimes prescribed concurrently with heart medications such as digitalis. Hawthorn is also considered a mildly calming herb to the nervous system – an appropriate bonus considering that stress and nervousness often accompany cardiovascular problems (Cleland et al., 2007; Dalli et al., 2011; Holubarsch et al., 2008; Zick et al., 2009).

The extract can be taken long-term, is very safe, and will not interfere with any medications, according to the official European Community monograph (ESCOP) on hawthorn. The daily dose is 1–2 tablets of the standardized extract, morning and evening (Steinhoff and Krenn, 2011).

3.3 Lemon and Soy, Isoflavanoids

Limocitrin derivatives are group of citrus flavanoids occurring naturally in plant. Major flavanoids are limocitrin derivatives, quercitin derivatives, polymethoxyflavones, and tocotrienols (Shukla et al., 2010).

3.4 Scutellaria, Panacea

It is mainly Chinese herb and tested for ameliorating cardiovascular disease (CVD). It is used in preparations of herbal mixture to treat and prevent heart diseases including

Table 2.2 Different Plant Sources are Shown in Scutellaria Herbal Mixture

Radix Scutellariae (Scutellaria) Family: Labiatae (American scutellaria or scute)
Rhizoma Coptidis (*Coptis chinensis*), Franch. C, deltoidea C.Y. Family: Ranunculaceae:
American coptis rhizome
Cheng C, omeiensis (Chen) C. Y. Cheng or C, teetoides C. Y.
Radix et Rhizoma (Rheum), Family: polygonaceae (rhubarb root)
Rhizome, Zingiber family: Zingiberaceae (American ginger) Zingiberis
Radix Panacis (Panax), Family: Araliaceae (American Quinquefolii)
quinquefolium L. (American ginseng)
Radix Ginseng (Panax ginseng) Family: Araliaceae (American ginseng)

arrhythmia, myocardial infarction, atherosclerosis, lipid lowering, and inflammation. It has active ingredients of baicalin, oroxylin, A–glucuronide, wogonin-7-O-glucuronide, baicalin, wogonin, and oroxylin A. Rhizome of coptis is rich in berberastine, columbamine, jatrorrhizine, epiberberine, coptisine, palmitine, and berberine. Rhizome of rhubarb contains sennoside B,A, aloe emodin, rhein, emodin, and chrysophanol. Radix Panacis Quinquefolii (American ginseng) has ginseno-Guangdong, shogaol, zingerone, and gingerol as shown in Table 2.2. It is available as herbal preparation (He et al., 2010). For details, readers are referred to other section on following herbal formula made from scutellaria.

3.5 Radix Salviae Miltiorrhizae, Danshen Herbal Extract

Danshensu acts as dilating smooth muscle cells, reducing creatine phosphokinase (CPK), lactate dehydrogenase (LDH), and malonic diethyl aldehyde (MDA) and promoting SOD enzyme activities of myocardial reperfusion or cardioprotective effect to remoce free radical and lipid peroxidation. Danshensu enhances diastolic pressure with low ventricular arrhythmia events after isopropylnoradrenaline injection but increases the blood flow (Wang et al., 2003).

Components in Danshen extract are described as following:

- Tanshinone acts as improving bile excretion and hepatic biotransformation.
- Matrine and oxymatrine increases right atrial systolic power and reduces left atrial maximum driving force (MDF), increases blood flow capacity of coronary artery with lower heart rate (consistency of atrial autorhythmicity) and extended P–R and Q–T intermission without any calcium antagonism effect.
- Radix Sophorae Flaescentis (RSG), Tanshinone IIA, Matrine, Oxymatrine.
- Puerarin from plant *Pueraria lobota* (Wild) Ohwi reduced LVSD, release of CPK, phosphocreatinase isozyme from myocardium at the time of ischemia, and reperfusion due to myocardial consumption and myocardial water content. All it indicates reduced myocardial infarction event and mitigated angina pectoris. Puerarin slows

down oxygen consumption, decreases main aortic pressure (MAP), tension time in-dex (TTI), ascending rate of left ventricular pressure, coronary lateral branch resis-tance but enhances systolic power, better ischemic ECG and more coronary artery flow volume (Wang et al., 2003; Yuan et al., 1997).

4. REPERTORY OF HERBS AND THEIR PROPERTIES

4.1 Wild yam (*Dioscorea villosa*) or black root

The herb is class I herb, rich in phytosterol such as diosgenin and serves as therapeutic effect on female hormone regulation and relief to menopause (Fugh–Berman, 2000; Russell et al., 2002). The diosgenin is antiproliferative and arrests G2/M cycle with simultaneous downregulating NF-kappa B, Akt, cyclin D, c-myc to result with PARP enzyme cleavage and DNA fragmentation (Leger et al., 2006; Shishodia and Aggarwal, 2006).

4.2 Blood root (*Sanguinaria Canadensis*)

It is known as AHPA-BSH class 2 herb but it is recommended less than $1 \, \text{mg kg}^{-1}$ human body weight. It is caustic agent and is part of 'black salve or can-X' made of zinc chloride with herbal ingredients. However, it showed to have berberine, ouabain side effects of tissue corrosion, basal cell carcinoma. Some examples of blood root pharma products are sanguinarine and viadent.

4.3 Taesal root (*Dipsacus asper*)

It is AHPA-BSH class I herb anticancer formulation. Other uses are in lime disease, fibromyalgia, Alzheimer disease and available as product dose of $6–21 \, \text{g day}^{-1}$ for human use.

4.4 Balm of Gilead bud (*Populus balsamifera*)

It is AHPA-BSH class 1 herb. Its main use is in urinary infections, wounds, pain, and arthritis. However, side effects are liver inflammation, Reye's syndrome, and brain damage.

4.5 Frankincense (*Boswellia carteri*)

It is AHPA-BSH class 1 herb showing topoisomerase I and II inhibitor due to boswellic acid pentacyclic triterpene induced antiproliferation. Other actions are caspase 3/8/9 activation and PARP cleavage (Syrovets et al., 2000); leukotriene/5-lipoxygenase blocker. It is available as Boswellia serrata extract in capsule form of 400 mg ($\times 3$) daily dose as anticancer remedy.

4.6 Bakuchi seeds (*Cyamposis psoraliodes*)
It is an anticancer natural product safe for oral consumption available as bakuchi seed powder for leprosy, infections, tumors, and baldness. FDA has warned for its use.

4.7 Buckthrone bark (*Rhamnus cathatica*)
It is APHA-BSH class 2 herb with anticancer properties. It also shows effective relief for intestinal cramps as laxative, constipation. However, it shows side effects of liver changes, mutagenesis, and electrolyte imbalance (Lichtensteiger and Johnston, 1997). FDA has warned for its use.

4.8 Chaparral (*Larrea tridentate*)
It is APHA-BSH class 2 herb having tumoricidal properties and shows side effects of liver damage and renal disease (Stickel et al., 2001). However, its potentials as anticancer are not confirmed. FDA has warned for its use.

4.9 Dichroa root (*Dichroa febrifuga*)
It is potent antimalaria agent available in dose of 5–10 g day^{-1}. It is also reported as anticancer agent with anti-inflammatory properties (Murata et al., 1998).

4.10 Alkanet root (*Batschia canescens*)
It is APHA-BSH class 2 herb containing toxic pyrrolizidine alkaloids, with promise as anticancer. Owing to presence of alkaloids, the use is limited in human but used as coloring agents for oils, cosmetics, textiles, and hair coloring (German Monographs, 1998). More investigations are needed for its use in human.

4.11 Kochia seed (*Kochia scoparia*)
It is aggressive tumbleweed, noxious seed with no known literature in human use. However, plant Kochia Hay is available for hepatotoxicity caused by saponins, oxalates, and nitrates (German Monographs, 1998; Rankins et al., 1991). Its use is limited because of safety and efficacy in prior use.

4.12 Kanta kari (*Solanum xanthocarpum*)
It is common in India for asthma and respiratory infections without any known side effects. The herb is rich in salasodine with possible antifertility effects (Gupta and Dixit, 2002).

4.13 Sweet myrrh (*Commiphora molmol*)
It is APHA-BSH class 2 herb. It is used for infections, pain, swelling, leprosy with anti-inflammatory, antiparasitic, and antioxidant properties (Haridy et al., 2003). Its use in schistosomiasis, *Dicrocoelium dentriticum* infections is administration of Myrrh for 3 days

at 10 mg kg^{-1} was effective with no side effects on liver or kidney (Sheir et al., 2001). It is approved by German Commission E for tropical treatment such as inflammation. Other uses are of Myrrh are in apoptosis, antiproliferation in lung, pancreas, breast, and prostate cancers under 500 µg ml^{-1} dose.

4.14 Blue cohosh root (*Caulophyllum thalictroides*)
It is APHA–BSH class 2b herb with tumoricidal properties and used for uterine contractions during labor. However, it can give side effects of myocardial infarction, tachycardia, and stroke (Finkel and Zarlengo, 2004; Rao and Hoffman, 2002). The adverse side effects make its use limited.

4.15 Male fern rhizome (*Dryopteris crassirhizoma*)
It is known as rich in kaempferol glycosides that can impair DNA polymerase and act as anticancer agents (Sharma et al., 2007). In *in vitro* cell lines, the plant extracts showed the fatty acid synthase enzyme inhibitor and arrested cancer growth through downregulation of PI3K/AKt and JNK pathways, S-phase arrest, and resulting apoptosis (Sebastiani et al., 2006; Zhao et al., 2006). Little is known about its potentials in human use. It is common in treating tapeworms and influenza infections.

4.16 Garcinia fruit (*Garcinia cambogia*)
It is rich in prenylated xanthones from mangosteen fruit with inhibitory properties against antineoplastic lesions in colon (Jung et al., 2006). It showed cytotoxic effects to leukemia, breast, gastric, lung, and liver cancer cell lines. However, xanthones mediate anticancer effects through downregulation of c-MYC mRNA expression/telomerase reverse transcriptase gene and initiate apoptosis, arresting immortalization, and proliferation of human cancer cells (Zhang et al., 2004). Other component is garcinol, a polyisoprenylated benzophenone with capability of impairing unbridled cell proliferation by inhibiting nuclear histone acetyltransferase p300 and PCAF, capable of initiating apoptotic signaling in HeLa cells (Balasubramanyam et al., 2004). It arrested tumor cell proliferation, migration, cell adhesion, inhibition of MAPK/ERK, PI3K/Akt, membrane adhesion kinase phosphorylation, augmented expression of BAX, caspase 2/3 activation, released cytochrome C, and PARP-1 cleavage in human cancer cell lines (Liao et al., 2005). Recommended dose of garcinia is 3–6 tablets per day of 500–1000 mg per tablet and considered potent and well tolerated.

4.17 Vitex powder (*Vitex agnus-castus*)
It is APHA–BSH class 2b herb and typically known as chasteberry or emmenagogue herb. It is widely known to cause homeopathic regulation of female endocrine system to ameliorate symptoms of PMS, amenorrhea, infertility, and menopause due to estrogenic effects of phytoesterogens present in vitex (Jarry et al., 2003), blocking production of

prolactin from pituitary, shortening luteal phase, and antagonizing hormonal imbalance (low progesterone synthesis in luteal phase; Liu et al., 2001). Its inducing cell death (tumoricidal) action is established in ovarian, cervical, breast, gastric, colon, and lung cancer cells *via* oxidative stress-related induction of proapoptotic caspase 3,8,9 hydroxy oxidase (a reduction in BCL-2, BCL-XL and Bid protein, increased Bad gene expression and induced DNA fragmentation (Ohyama et al., 2003, 2005)). However, it showed side effects of nausea, headache, and rashes. The herb is approved by German Commission E with warnings of chaste tree fruit with irregularities of menstrual cycle, mastodynia under the doses of 30–40 mg day^{-1} in aqueous–alcoholic extracts.

4.18 Dragons blood (*Calamus draco*)

It is commonly known with fruits of dragons blood used along with illicit marijuana use. It is restricted in human use. Its wider use is in coloring industries, varnishes, lacquers, and plasters, incense. It needs investigations if useful in human use.

4.19 Psoralea fruit (*Psoralea corylifolia*)

It is psoralea fruit with side effects of internal burning, allergic responses, and phototoxicity. These adverse effects made its use restricted by UK Committee on Safety of Medicines (CSM) because of predisposition of adverse allergic reactions (Wang et al., 2009).

4.20 Cubeb berry (*Piper cubeba*)

It is traditional black pepper, used as spice known with antimicrobial, antioxidant, and insecticidal properties as food preservative. Traditionally cubeb berry is used in treatment of gonorrhea, bronchitis, hepatitis, inflammation, pain, and oxidative stress-induced biological injury. Still its use is limited as kitchen spice and research is needed for its anticancer properties if any.

4.21 Mace (*Myristica fragans*)

It is the cooking herb from the plant nutmeg and mainly used in bakery. Its use in low dose of less than 300 mg kg^{-1} day is recommended with no serious side effects. However, overdose of 5 g day^{-1} showed nutmeg side effects including psychological hallucinations, delusions, dizziness, psychosis and sedation, and coma. Its action is not much known but predicted as proliferation inhibition in leukemia, lung, and colon cancer induced by myristicin or dihydroguaiaretic acid ingredients (Park et al., 1998). Other actions of anti-inflammatory, antimicrobial, liver detoxification, and cholesterol-lowering effects are known as potential benefits of nutmeg.

4.22 Senna leaf (*Senna alexandria*)

It is APHA-BSH class 2 herb commonly used in intestinal obstruction, hemorrhoids, to promote bowel movement, relief constipation. Its main ingredients are sennosides as nontoxic but other constituents are known as intestinal irritants. So, its use is warranted with caution among individuals with intestinal disorders, liver damage. It was reported to interfere with absorption of therapeutic drugs and allergic response in susceptible individuals (Spiller et al., 2003). German Commission E brought its chronic use in daylight with electrolyte imbalance, potassium deficiency, albuminuria, hematuria, cardiovascular, and muscle weakness. For these reasons, further research is required to elucidate plant constituents responsible for anticancer effects of Senna.

4.23 White sage (*Salvia apiana*)

It is AHPA-BSH class 2b herb widely known as food preservative, flavoring medicinal agent to treat headache, pain, indigestion, heart disease, and influenza. It has ingredients of polyphenolics, rosamarinic acid, camphor, and carnasol with medicinal properties as anti-inflammatory, antioxidant, antimalarial, antibacterial, and antifungal effects (Feres et al., 2005). The administration of essential oil of white sage showed beneficial effects on memory, cognitive function, mood and alertness (Tildesley et al., 2005), and Alzheimer disease (Perry et al., 2003). However, it showed toxicity primarily associated with induced hypoglycemia, tachycardia, convulsions, muscle cramps, and respiratory disorders (Gali-Muhtasib et al., 2000). German Commission E approved its internal use for dyspeptic symptoms and excessive perspiration and external use in oral inflammations with recommended dry leaf intake: 1–3 g three times daily or fluid extract 1:1 (g ml^{-1}) 1–3 ml, three times daily. Owing to reported adverse side effects, its use is limited not more than 4–6 g daily despite of long-known benefits of senna leaves (Kennedy et al., 2006).

4.24 Rosemary leaf (*Rosmarinus oficinalis*)

It is APHA-BSH class 2b/emmenagogue herbs known for cooking applications and treating muscle pain, arteriosclerosis, alopacea, and infections. It has phenolic compound camosol reported as lehal against acute lymphoblastic leukemia, colon cancer (Dörrie et al., 2001), and breast cancer (Plouzek et al., 1999). German Commission E approved its limited internal use for dyspeptic complaints in dose of 4–6 g cut leaves and external use as powder or dry extract for rheumatic diseases and circulatory diseases.

4.25 Eucalyptus leaf (*Eucalyptus globulus*)

It is APHA-BSH class 2 herb and it is contraindicated with liver, gastrointestinal tract, and bile duct disease reported by German commission E. It is known for its internal use to induce convulsions, nausea, vomiting, and blood pressure drop. However, it is reported as potent therapy of cold, headache, infections, inflammation, arthritis, pain, and bacterial infections (Warnke et al., 2006; Zhao et al., 2006). Less data is available and more investigations are needed to establish its value in cancer prevention.

4.26 Feverfew (*Tanacetum pathenium*)

It is a well-known herb with anticancer properties and prophylaxis in migraine. It contains parthenolide as active ingredient. Its action is reported as inducing prostaglandin synthesis to act as antimigraine, antithrombotic, and anti-inflammatory agents (Heptinstall et al., 1985). However, it showed allergic reaction that restricts its use in susceptible individuals for human use.

4.27 Red sandalwood (*Pterocarpus santalinus*)

It is APHA-BSH class 1 herb for potent use in diabetes, wound healing, and dermatitis. The action of sandalwood is less known but well reported in skin papilloma prevention (Dwivedi and Aggarwal, 2009).

4.28 Yellow Dock Root (*Rumex Crispus*)

It is the APHA-BSH class 2 herb rich in oxalate contents and used in chronic skin conditions, psoriasis, jaundice, constipation, and anemia. It shows allergic reactions and side effects of hypocalcaemia, metabolic acidosis, tremors, ataxia, and so on (Panciera et al., 1990). These adverse effects restrict its use in kidney complications such as renal stones.

4.29 White cherry bark (*Prunus serotina*)

It is less-known plant product with proven anticancer properties such as antiproliferative action *via* downregulation of cyclin D1 expression/apoptotic effects in colorectal cancer (Yamaguchi et al., 2006). However, it contains trace levels of cyanide ions less than 0.5% that makes it restricted in pregnancy and persons with liver or kidney disease. It needs more research for its safety in internal use.

4.30 Bushy Knotweed rhizome (*Polygonum cuspidatum*)

It is a known plant with noxious, invasive weed with potentials of anti-ischemic reperfusion injury, cholesterol lowering, antibacterial, antiviral, esterogenic, and blastoma cell cytotoxic anticancer properties (Chang et al., 2005). Unconfirmed report showed the presence of 3,4' dimethoxy-5-hydroxystilbene in this plant which has action of methylation/acid hydrolysis of resveratrol-3-O-glucoside to induce apoptosis in leukemia (Lee et al., 2005). Resveratrol is known to induce proapoptotic/antiproliferative action by inhibiting nuclear factor NF-kappa B, COX-2 in arresting mammary carcinogenesis (Banerjee et al., 2002).

4.31 Birch leaf (*Betula alba*)

It is a kind of tea known to flush kidneys used in 5–10 g in boiled water in routine. Not much known for the possible anticancer properties. Its allergic response also restricts its use in human individuals with known allergies.

4.32 Elecampane root (*Inula helenium*)

It is a known herb for the use in cold, flu, pain, skin infections, parasite infections. It is rich in inulin and helenin components with potentials of anticancer effects. However, it contains chemical alantolactone with allergic response that restricts its use even in skin dermatitis (Paulsen, 2002).

4.33 Ginger (*Zinggiber officinale*)

It is a regular kitchen spice routinely used in cooking. Its properties of antiplatelet aggregation, anti-inflammatory, analgesic, antimicrobial, antiworm, antioxidant, hyperlipidemic, antiarthritic, and hypoglycemic effects are well documented (Smith et al., 1994). In Indian traditional Ayurvedic system, it is known for having antinausea, vomiting effects in pregnancy, arthritis. However, its use in cancer is very less known including its inhibitory effect on angiogenesis, inducing effect on apoptosis in experimental animals (Chun et al., 2002; Wei et al., 2004, 2005). In human use, it is approved by German Commission E in the amount of 5–10 g daily (Boone et al. 2005), APHA-BSH in the amount of 4–6 g day^{-1}.

4.34 Turkey Rhubarb (*Rhenum palmatum*)

It is a APHA-BSH class 2 herb with high oxalate content with contraindications in people with renal stones or intestinal obstruction. It has active anticancer ingredient known as hydroxyanthraquinones and anthraquinone glycosides with antiproliferative/antimutagenic activity (Zhou et al., 2006). However, high oxalate content restricts its long time use because of oxalate's binding property with metals. Very less is known for its anticancer safe use in humans.

4.35 Cinnamon (*Cinnamomum cassia*)

It is a APHA-BSH class 2 herb with known anticancer, antimicrobial, antifungal, and antidiabetic properties (Schoene et al., 2005). However, it also showed inducing hypertension, skin allergy, and cathartic in diabetes that makes its use restricted in sensitive individuals. Both German commission E and APHA-BSH have recommended limited use 2–4 g day^{-1} as bark for appetite loss, dyspepsia, and flatulence.

4.36 Kava Kava (*Piper methysticum*)

It is the herb with active gradient of kavalactones kavain, dihydrokavain, methysticin, dihydromethysticin, yangonin, desmethoxyyangonin, with known to cause psychoactivity and liver toxicity effects. The pharmacological effects are muscle relaxation, anesthetic, anticonvulsive, anxiolysis, with possible therapy of ovarian cancer and leukemia. However, skin rashes and liver toxicity due to piperidine alkaloid restrict its use in humans by CDC.

4.37 Arjun (*Terminalia arjuna*)

It is herb routinely used for angina, hypertension, ecchymosis, gonorrhea, CHD, and hypercholesterolemia.

4.38 Babul chalk bark (*Acacia arabica*)

Acacia Bark also known as *Wattle Bark*, is collected from wild or cultivated trees, seven years old or more. Acacia Bark contains from 24 to 42% of the tannin gallic acid.

Medicinally, Acacia Bark is employed as a substitute for Oak Bark. Acacia Bark has special use in diarrhea, mainly in the form of a decoction, the British Pharmacopia preparation being six parts in 100 administered in doses of 1/2–2 fluid ounces. The decoction also is used as an astringent gargle, lotion, or injection in doses of 1/2–1 fluid ounces. The use of both gum and bark for industrial purposes is much larger than their use in medicine.

4.39 Bhumi Amalaki (*Phyllanthus niruri*)

It is traditional herb in use for viral hepatitis, chronic liver disorders, jaundice, constipation, dyspepsia, anorexia, with known effect of liver detoxification. Its anticancer properties not reported at all.

4.40 Goldenseal (*Hydrastis canadensis*)

Typically known as Goldenseal herb with known effects similar to rifampin and clarithromycin. The action was reported as phytochemical-mediated modulation of p-glycoprotein (Gurley et al., 2007).

These said herbs display antilithogenic and heart protective effects along with other therapeutic actions because of whole herbs without concentrated active ingredient(s) used. The therapeutic action is measured and reported as LC50 dose in normal experimental homogenous cancer cell lines in culture to determine the effective maximum dose tolerance after exposure to herbal extracts or whole concentrates. Although the knowledge of herbal antithrombotic effect is very poorly known, sufficient data is available to design herbal anticancer formula. For simplicity, a gross and tentative list of herbs is presented showing relative strengths of herbs as anticancer supplements. The molecular mode of herbal biochemical action is far from the present discussion on how these herbs could be used and for how long. The following discussion is a window or glimpse to explore the possibility of other antiarrhythmic and herbal therapy.

Green tea is popular in Asia for centuries, green tea helps to keep blood pressure under control. It also may help keep cholesterol from clogging arteries. The tea contains Epigallocatechin Gallate (EGCG) and other substances that protect the body against the dangers of oxidation, while helping to keep the harmful LDL cholesterol down and the helpful HDL cholesterol up. They also assist in keeping blood pressure under control (Zeng et al., 2011).

Garlic (*Allium sativum*) prevents the oxidation of LDL cholesterol, may prevent the liver from producing excess fat and cholesterol. In one study, adding as little as two ounces of garlic juice to a fatty, cholesterol-laden meal was found to actually lower the cholesterol by up to 7%. Another study found that 600 mg of garlic powder a day could push the total cholesterol down by some 10%. Other research has corroborated these findings reporting that garlic can lower both total and LDL cholesterol while raising the HDL ('good') cholesterol.

A 10-month study found that eating three cloves of garlic a day keeps the cholesterol down for extended periods. And because it contains ajoene and other substances, garlic also helps to keep the blood 'thin' and free of potentially deadly blood clots (Zeng et al., 2011).

Hawthorn (*Crataegus* species) contains a combination of flavonoids that can protect the heart against oxygen deprivation and the development of abnormal rhythms. It dilates coronary blood vessels, improving the flow of blood to the heart. It strengthens the heart muscle and works to help the body rid itself of excess salt and water. It reduces blood levels of cholesterol and triglycerides, and brings down high blood pressure. Choose a standardized extract containing 1.8% vitexin-2 rhamnosides (Cleland et al., 2007; Dalli et al., 2011; Holubarsch et al., 2008; Koch and Malek, 2011; Zick et al., 2009).

Arjuna (*Terminalia arjuna*) an important ayurvedic herb, is a coronary vasodilator. It protects the heart, strengthens circulation, and helps to maintain the tone and health of the heart muscle. It is also useful in stopping bleeding and to promote healing after a heart attack (Dwivedi and Aggarwal, 2009). Take 1/2 teaspoon (500 mg to 1 g) three times a day with honey and warm water.

Ginger (*Zingiber officinales*) is an important herb for a healthy heart. Ayurvedic physicians suggest that eating a little bit of ginger every day will help to prevent heart attack. It reduces cholesterol. It also reduces blood pressure and prevents blood clots. Ginger's heart-helping attributes are similar to that of garlic. Ginger interferes with the long sequence of events necessary for blood clots to form. This helps to prevent clots that can lodge in narrowed coronary arteries and set off heart attack (Park et al., 2009a).

Turmeric lowers blood cholesterol levels by stimulating the production of bile. It also prevents the formation of dangerous blood clots that can lead to heart attack (Ghosh et al., 2010).

Onions contain adenosine and other 'blood thinners' that help to prevent the formation of blood clots. In addition to thinning the blood, onions can help keep the coronary arteries open and clear by increasing the HDL. Eating half a raw onion every day can increase HDL by 20–30% (Park et al., 2009b).

Ginkgo biloba improves the flow of blood throughout the body. It is also an antioxidant. It can benefit the cardiovascular system by preventing the formation of free radicals. Take a ginkgo extract containing 24% ginkgo flavone glycosides (Kuller et al., 2010).

Fo-ti (ho shou wu, Polygonum multiflorum), combats the symptoms of heart disease, helping to reduce blood pressure and blood cholesterol levels (Yim et al., 2000).

Alfalfa leaves and sprouts help reduce the blood cholesterol levels and plaque deposits on artery walls (Hwang et al., 2001).

Citrin is an extract from the plant *Garcinia cambogia*, inhibits the synthesis of fatty acids in the liver. It helps to prevent the accumulation of potentially dangerous fats in the body (Shara et al., 2004).

Guggul (*Comniphora mukul*), an ayurvedic herb, is derived from a type of myrrh tree. It has been shown to lower blood-fat levels while raising levels of HDL, the so-called good cholesterol (Mahmood et al., 2010; Singh et al., 1994).

Grape seed extract with OPCs may lower high blood pressure, which can cause heart disease (Willett, 2007).

Soy had been long popular in Asia. It has been proven to be heart antioxidant protector. When people with high cholesterol are put on a low-fat, low-cholesterol diet, their cholesterol levels usually drop. But if you replace the animal protein in their diet with soy protein, their cholesterol levels are found to drop significantly lower. One study has showed that soy protein could cancel out the effect of 500 mg of cholesterol deliberately added to the daily diet (Santo et al., 2010). Although soy can lower cholesterol levels in those with normal levels, it works best in people with elevated cholesterol.

Brewer's yeast can lower the total cholesterol and LDL while raising the helpful HDL. (Brewer's yeast is not the same as the yeast we use in the kitchen.) In one study with normal- and high-cholesterol patients, 11 healthy volunteers were given brewer's yeast. Eight weeks later, 10 of the 11 people with normal cholesterol levels had even lower total cholesterol levels and increased HDL levels. Among the 15 volunteers with high cholesterol, eight enjoyed the same beneficial results (Rayner et al., 2007).

Cordyceps is a Chinese herb. It can slow the heart rate, increase blood supply to the arteries and heart, and lower blood pressure (Zhou et al., 2009).

Artichoke leaf extract reduces blood cholesterol and protects the liver. This herb has antioxidant activity and may inhibit the oxidation of cholesterol, a factor in atherosclerosis (Bonnemeier et al., 2007).

Cat's claw contains a variety of valuable phytochemicals that inhibit the processes involved in the formation of blood clots. It increases circulation and inhibits inappropriate clotting. Thus, it may help to prevent stroke and reduce the risk of heart attack (Sheng and Bryngelsson, 2000).

Oat straw and Kava Kava are tonics for the nervous system (Clough et al., 2004).

White willow bark contains salicin, an aspirin-like compound. It has been used for centuries much as aspirin is today. Aspirin is often recommended for cardiovascular condition. This herb may provide the same protection without stomach upsets associated with aspirin.

Rudraksha are the dried seeds of the rudraksha tree. They are good for the heart both physically and spiritually. They are often used in meditation (like the rosary by Catholics). It is believed to 'open the heart chakra.' Rudraksha can be used in a number of forms such as soaked rudraksha beads or overnight water to drink in the morning. Drinking rudraksha water is believed to reduce blood pressure and strengthen the heart (Dasgupta et al., 1984).

Other ayurvedic herbs used to manage cardiovascular system are ashwagandha, guggul, sandalwood, saffron, hawthorn berries, myrrh, ginger, cinnamon, barberry, black cohosh, butcher's broom, cayenne (capsicum), dandelion, ginseng, and valerian root, alfalfa, astragalus, garlic, ginger, ginkgo, ginseng, hawthorn berry, kelp, kola, mother-wort, myrrh, psyllium (metamucil), passion flower, red pepper, saffron, Siberian ginseng, skullcap, tarragon, turmeric, and valerian, However, *barberry* or black cohosh is not recommended during pregnancy. Ginseng not recommended in high blood pressure. Ephedra (ma huang) and licorice, as they cause a rise in blood pressure.

5. HERBS IN HUMAN USE

Herbs have demonstrated their effect in isolated cultured cells or in patient use mainly by Chinese or Ayurvedic Indian traditional methods.

Garcinia cambogia (garcina fruit) decreased the oxidative stress biomarkers and increased NO level. There were significant positive correlations among BMI, kidney functions (creatinine and urea), TG, and oxidative markers (renal MDA and catalase). Other biomarkers are inhibited MAP kinase, ER kinase, P13K/Akt, membrane adhesion kinase with activated cytochrome C release and PARP-1 cleavage (Amin et al., 2011).

- Oxidative stress induced proapoptosis: Reduced BCL-2, Bcl-XL and Bid protein by Caspase 3,8 9-OH oxidase, enhanced Bad gene expression and induced DNA fragmentation. Example: Vitex (Ohyama et al., 2005).
- Downregulation of Cyclin D1 expression/apoptotic effects: Owing to reduced proliferation, a proapoptosis process initiates to cause cyclin D1 expression. Example: wild cherry bark (Hietala et al., 2008).
- Modulation of p-glycoprotein: Owing to phytochemical-mediated modulation of p-glycoprotein process initiates anticancer behavior of herbs. Example: Goldenseal and Kava Kava (Gurley et al., 2008).
- Expression of gene: Downregulated gene expression of silbinin synthase enzyme causes the activation of nerves and brain activity with enhanced immunity. Example: MTHFR, PAI-1, ACE, PON1, and eNOS gene (Agirbasli et al., 2011).

6. CARDIOPROTECTIVE HERB ACTIVE COMPONENTS IN HUMAN USE APPROVED BY CDC AND REGULATED BY FDA

The herbs are rich in different metabolites plying role in active intermediary metabolism and these are needed in body in a minimum amount daily so-called recommended daily allowances (RDAs) through diets or herbal supplements. Saponoin glycosides, antioxidents, flavanoids, and OPC fractions are major players with other ingredients. Readers are referred to read other separate section on 'biochemical basis of herbiceuticals in cardiac prevention' for details. A number of herbal active ingredients are listed below in Table 2.3 and some of the ingredients are identified abundant in different parts of herbal plants as shown in Table 2.4.

Table 2.3 These Cited Herbs Have Potential as Antiarrhythmic and Tested in Human Use but Not Approved or with Safety Warning

- *Strong herbs*: Alkanet root (0.138); Kochia seed (0.147); Blood root (0.04); Bakuchi seed (0.102); Chaparral (0.124); Cubeb berry (0.263); Dragon blood (0.242); Sweet myrrh (0.158); male fern rhizome (0.232); Dragon blood (0.242); Psoralea fruit (0.243); Senna leaf (0.275); Rosemary (0.299); Black pepper (0.495); Blue cohosh root (0.218); Babul bark (0.492); Buckthrone bark (0.107); Bhumy amalaki (0.497); Butternut bark (0.506); Eucalyptus leaf (0.305); Feverfew (0.307); Osho root (0.509); Sage (0.519); Red sandalwood (0.326); Yellow dock root (0348); Wild cherry bark (0.360); Birch leaf (0.365); Kava Kava (0.491); Elecampane root (0.447); Turkey rhubarb (0.466); Cinnamon (0.479); Green tea (0.507)
- Less known herbs or one time evidence of their anticancer properties are listed below as tentative list (57). It is a handout list to readers interested in to become aware of possible less known herbs either tested one time in preclinical Chinese or ayurvedic use or likely to be the prospective anticancer herbal candidate
- *Potential herbs*: Yam Root, abalone shell, tertraphylla root, ailanthus bark, mimosa bark, alfafa leaf and seeds, alum, angelica, snise seed, Ash bark, Ashwanda root, Astralgus root, Bamboo leaf, Barley grass, Bee pollen, Bilberry fruit, Black Haw, Blue Green Algae, Blue Verian, Borage, Buddleia Flower Bud, Bugleweed, Burdock root, Cardamom, Carob Powder, Carpesium fruit, Cassia seed, Catnip, Chamomile, Chervil, Chicory root, Chickweed, Chinese Holly leaf, Chlorella, Cilantro, Cleavers, Clematis root, Club moss, Codonopsis root, Coix seed, Coltsfoot, Comfry leaf, Corn silk, Cortyceps, Couch grass, Cranberry powder, Dandelion root, Dill seed, Dittany root bark, Dog grass root, Don Quai root, Dulse, Echinechea, Eleuthro root, Erend herb, Eucomnia, Eyebright, False unicorn root, Fennel seed, Fenugreek, Flax seed, Fo ti, Forsythia Fruit, Foxnut barley, Fringe bark tree, Fumitory herb, Gential root, Ginseng, Glaborous greenbrier rhizome, Glehnia, Gloryvine stem, Goats Rue, Goldenseal, Green Clay, Guduchi root powder, Gypsum, Hawthorne berry, Helichrysum flowers, Hibiscus, Homalomena rhizome, Honeysuckle vine, Horsetail, Houttuynia cordata, Hydrangea root, Hylocereus flower, Hyssop, Isatis leaf, Jasmine flower, Kadsura stem, Kelp, Knotweed grass, Kola nut, Kombu, Kudzu root, Kukicha twig, Laminaria (Kelp), Lemon, Lobelia, Lotis leaf or root, Lungwort, Lycii berries, Lycium bark, Lycopodium japonicum vine, Marshmallow root, Melilot herb, Mica-Schist, Milk Thistle seed, Mother-Of-Pearl, Motherwort, MSM, Mugwort, Muirapuama, Mettle root, Noni juice, Onion powder, Orange, Pagoda tree fruit, Paprika, Parsley leaf or root, Passion flower, Peppermint, Perilla leaf or root, Periwinkle, Pigeon pea root, Pivet fruit, Plantain leaf, Pleurisy root, Poke root, Poppy seed, Psylliam seed, Puff-ball/Lasiophaera, Purnarnava herb, Pyrrosia leaf, Red clover, Reed rhizome, Rehmannia root, Rooibos tea, Rosehips, Safflower threads, Saffron, Scrophularia root, Scutellaria barbata herb, Self heal, Shank pushpin herb, Shephards purse, Skull cap, Slippery Elm, Soloman seal, Spearmint, Speranskia herb, Spilanthes, Spirulina, Stone lotus seed, Swalloeort root, Tonka bean, Tribulus, Uncaria vina with hooks, Vanilla root, Vasak leaves powder, Vasma Rochna leaves, Watercress, Wheat grass, White Oak bark, White Peony root, White pine powder, Woolly grass rhizome, Yellow mustard seed, Yohimbe bark, Yucca root, Zedoary rhizome

The list is a comparative account of safe use in human as antiarrhythmic. Effective potency is shown in brackets.
Sharma, R., Singh, R.B., 2010. Bioactive foods and nutraceutical supplementation criteria in cardiovascular protection. The Open Nutraceuticals Journal 3, 141–153.

Table 2.4 Handbook of Herbs is Proposed Showing Potency of Action in Decreasing Order

Anti arrhythmic herbs: Wild Yam (0.19); Teasel root (0.42); Balm of Gilead bud (0.78); Frankincense (0.081); Dichroa root (0.137); Kanta kari (0.157); Garcinia fruit (0.235); Mace (0.271), Myrrh gum (0.283); White sage (0.299); Vitex powder (0.302); Bushy Knotweed rhizome (0.361), Ginger root (0.447), Nutmeg (0.447)

Medicinal plants or their parts are shown below as known with possible anticancer properties

Bark: Buckthrone, Chaparral, Sandalwood, Wild cherry, Babul, Butternut bark, Cramp, White billow, Catuaba, Cascara sagrada, Paul D' Arko, Wood betany, Pygeum

Seeds: Bakuchi, Kochia, Cinnamon, Black pepper, White peppercorn, Black walnut hull, Annatto, Habanero, Celery, Coriander, Guarana, Cumin, Caraway, Lychee pit, California poppy

Roots: Yellow turmeric, Blood root, Alkanet, Yellowdock, Elecampane, Kava Kava, Osho, Redroot, Buplerum, Terragon, Green mosaia, Licorice root, Lovage root, Barberry root, Witch hazel root, Lindera, Blue cohosh, Cranebill, Red henna, Bay berry, Gravel root, Butches broom, Pulsatilla, Blackberry, Galangal, Birch bark root, Rhodiola, costus, Aster, Orris, Sophora, Yarrow root, Calamus, Beet

Leaf: Senna, Rosemary, Eucalyptus, Feverfew, Damiana leaf, Birch, Bhumi amalaki, Green tea, Gymnema, Sage, Pipsissewa, Vidanga, Boldo, Bay leaf, Bilberry leaf, Nageshkar leaf, Damiana, Ashoka, Neem leaf, Papaya leaf, Raspberry, Stevia, Biota, Linden, Patchouili, Strawberry, olive, Buchu, Lemon grass, Blue violet, Lemon verbena, Yerba mate, Black walnut, Artemisia

Whole herb: Dragon blood, Turkey rhubarb, Cynomorium songaricum, Arjun, Horse chestnut, Black henna, Uva ursi, Rabdosia rubescens, Usnea, Brahmi, Sasparilla, Spikenard, Wintergreen, Epidedium, Soap wort, Blessed thistle, Lady's mantle, Pennyroyal, Bladderwrack, Oatstraw, Centipeda, Thyme, Cat claw, Boneset, Iceland moss, Meadow sweet, Savory winter, Wormwood, Mistletoe, Golden rod, Horehound, Luffa sponge, Elsholtzia, Siegesbeckia, Celandine, Basil, Gotu kola

Rhizome: Dryopteris fern, Sweet myrrh, Usnea, Brahmi herb, Maiden hair, Coral calcium, Drynaria, Curculigo

Fruit: Psoralea, Pipli, Karela, Copal resin, Oregon grape, Conchord grape juice, Terminalia

Berry: Cubeb, Schisandra, Cider, Saw palmetto, Sumar

Powder: Superior gun powder, Pomegranate husk, Sambhar, Haritaki fruit powder, Pashanbheda herb powder, Garlic powder, Kutaj bark powder, Satavari, Kachnar, Bringraj, Allspice berry powder, Musta root powder, Bilwa fruit powder, Cayeen, Lavan bhaskar, Maca powder, Psyllium husk, Lemon balm

Flower: Lavender, Calendula, Rose petals, Pyrite, Clove, Agmoni, Oregano, Malva flower, Heather

The therapeutic potency of selected herbs (LC50 values in mg ml^{-1}) indicates the antiarrhythmic potential of herbs in human use. The above list highlights the possible use of different parts of herb plants in developing herbiceuticals and herbal mixture formula.

6.1 Biochemical Basis of Herbiceuticals in Cardiac Prevention

Natural vegetables, herbs, plants, and wild foods are complex in structural composition. The biochemical basis of individual source of these foods is not explored because of their complex nature. Some of the evidences are in favor of the active food principles as herbiceuticals to show cardioprotective or preventive supplements. Some of the herbiceuticals are in the phase of clinical trial or already available as food supplement.

Complementary and alternative medicine is emerging in prevention of chronic coronary and heart diseases as safe practice because of the high risk of mortality and long-term morbidity associated with surgical procedures of CAD and high side effects of chemotherapy. Herbal medicines have shown reduced myocyte cell necrosis in cultured cells. The vitamins, minerals, and dietary fat play a role in relation to cardioprevention and control. The mechanisms of herbiceutical action can be discussed broadly in following categories based on active metabolites present in herbiceuticals.

1. Niacin-bound chromium is reported to enhance myocardial protection from ischemia–reperfusion injury (Thirunavukkarasu et al., 2006).

2. Mechanism of the antithrombotic effect was invented by dietary diacylglycerol in atherogenic mice (Roche and Gibney, 2000).

3. Protective effect of potassium against the hypertensive cardiac dysfunction was associated with reactive oxygen species reduction (Matsui et al., 2006).

4. The atherogenic process is reduced by regulation of coenzyme Q10 biosynthesis and breakdown.

5. The n-3 fatty acids reduce the risk of CVD. The evidence was explained and mechanisms were explored (Dallner et al., 2003; Matsui et al., 2006).

6. Mediterranean diet and optimal diets play a role in the prevention of CHD.

7. Alpha-tocopherol therapy was evidenced to reduce oxidative stress and atherosclerosis (Harris et al., 2002).

8. Genetic deficiency of inducible NO synthase reduces atherosclerosis and lowers plasma lipid peroxides in apolipoprotein E-knockout mice.

9. Glutathione is the liver's most abundant protective constituent of antioxidant glutathione reductase enzyme. Glutathione functions as a substrate for the two key detoxification processes in the liver: (a) transforming toxins into water soluble forms and (b) neutralizing and 'conjugating' with toxins for elimination through the gut or the kidneys. If either of these processes is impaired for any reason, toxins will accumulate in the body and lead to disease. The best nutrition with liver CVD focuses on improving the body's glutathione reserves (Calder, 2004).

10. The Soy isoflavone Haelan951 (genistein and genistin) and garlic allicin were reported to have some role as a cardioprotective in humans (Santo et al., 2010). Beta-glycoside conjugate, genistin is abundant in fermented soybeans, soybean products such as soymilk and tofu. Beta-glycosyl bond of genistin is cleaved to produce genistein by microbes during fermentation to yield miso and natto. Soy sauce has high isoflavone but low miso and natto contents.

    How much soy isoflavones needed? 1.5–4.1 mg per person miso isoflavone and 6.3–8.3 mg per person natto, respectively (Santo et al., 2010).

11. Green tea has always been considered by the Chinese and Japanese peoples as a potent medicine for the maintenance of health, endowed with the power to prolong life (Basu and Lucas, 2007).

12. The CVD has been reported associated with vascular endothelial growth factor (Gurley et al., 2008).

13. Some herbal plants act as cardioprotective medicine. The herbal extracts are known to reduce the circulating markers of inflammation, including CRP, interleukine-6 (IL-6), tumor necrosis factor-α (TNF-α), serum amyloid A (SAA).

14. Combination of garlic, ginko biloba, herbs with reverastrol inhibited a full 92% of age-related gene changes in the heart (Gurley et al., 2008).

7. CONCLUSION

In present paper, herbs are surveyed and introduced to demonstrate their benefits in human health and possible use as antihypertensive, antiarrhythmic, cardioprotective supplements. The pharmacological action and biochemical mechanisms of herbs are highlighted with examples for their possible antihypertensive, antiarrhythmic, cardioprotective effects on heart tissue, and cardioprotective action. A possible antihypertensive, antiarrhythmic, and cardioprotective composition is proposed to make effective cardioprotective herbal formula. The focus of this chapter is to review herbs, survey of herbal hand book type repertory of herbal sources, comparison of anti antihypertensive, antiarrhythmic, and cardioprotective strengths of different herbs in the light of present knowledge. The toxic effects of herbal over intake are highlighted to show their side effects. Finally, the aim is to catch the attention of regulatory government bodies on growing unnoticed use of herbs among large population having no knowledge of herbal side effects they are using so that government or health authorities can remain vigilant in informing public and insurers in time before it is too late.

ACKNOWLEDGMENTS

The author acknowledges the permission to do advanced level internship at Heart and Vascular Surgery Center, Tallahassee Memorial Hospital, Mikusukee Road, Tallahassee, Florida for Cardiovascular Technology Research program under Drs. Julian Hurt, Murrah, Al Saint and Khairullah. He also acknowledges the opportunity of engineering and biotechnology internship under supervision of Dr. Ching J. Chen at FAMU-FSU College of Engineering, Tallahassee, FL.

REFERENCES

Agirbasli, M., Guney, A., Ozturhan, H., et al., 2011. Multifactor dimensionality reduction analysis of MTHFR, PAI-1, ACE, PON1, and eNOS gene polymorphisms in patients with early onset coronary artery disease. European Journal of Cardiovascular Prevention and Rehabilitation 18 (6), 803–809.

Amin, K.A., Kamel, H.H., Abd Eltawab, M.A., 2011. Protective effect of Garcinia against renal oxidative stress and biomarkers induced by high fat and sucrose diet. Lipids in Health and Disease 10, 6.

Apple, F.S., Jaffe, A.S., 2008. Cardiovascular diseases. Part V: pathophysiology. In: Burtis, C.A., Ashwood, E.R., Bruns, D.E., Sawyer, B.G. (Eds.), Tietz Fundamentals of Clinical Chemistry. sixth ed. Saunders Elsevier Company, St Louis, MO, pp. 614–630 (Chapter 33).

Balasubramanyam, K., Altaf, M., Varier, R.A., et al., 2004. Polyisoprenylated benzophenone, garcinol, a natural histone acetyltransferase inhibitor, represses chromatin transcription and alters global gene expression. Journal of Biological Chemistry 279 (32), 33716–33726.

Banerjee, S., Bueso-Ramos, C., Aggarwal, B.B., 2002. Suppression of 7, 12 dimethylbenz(a) anthracene-induced mammary carcinogenesis in rats by resveratrol: role of nuclear factor-kappaB, cyclooxygenase 2, and matrix metalloprotease 9. Cancer Research 62 (17), 4945–4954.

Basu, A., Lucas, E.A., 2007. Mechanisms and effects of green tea on cardiovascular health. Nutrition Reviews 65 (8), 361–375.

Bonnemeier, H., Ortak, J., Burgdorf, C., et al., 2007. 'The artichoke heart': the inverse counterpart of left ventricular apical ballooning. Resuscitation 72 (3), 342–343.

Borggreve, S.E., Hillege, H.L., Dallinga-Thie, G.M., et al., 2007. High plasma cholesteryl ester transfer protein levels may favour reduced incidence of cardiovascular events in men with low triglycerides. European Heart Journal 28 (8), 1012–1018.

Brazier, N.C., Levine, M.A., 2003. Brazier drug–herb interaction among commonly used conventional medicines: a compendium for health care professionals. American Journal of Therapeutics 10 (3), 163–169.

Butterweck, V., Winterhoff, H., 2001. Herkenham M. St John's wort, hypericin, and imipramine: a comparative analysis of mRNA levels in brain areas involved in HPA axis control following short-term and long-term administration in normal and stressed rats. Molecular Psychiatry 6 (5), 547–564.

Calder, P.C., 2004. n-3 Fatty acids and cardiovascular disease: evidence explained and mechanisms explored. Clinical Science 107 (1), 1–11.

Chang, J.S., Liu, H.W., Wang, K.C., et al., 2005. Ethanol extract of Polygonum cuspidatum inhibits hepatitis B virus in a stable HBV-producing cell line. Antiviral Research 66 (1), 29–34.

Chun, K.S., Park, K.K., Lee, J., Kang, M., Surh, Y.J., 2002. Inhibition of mouse skin tumor promotion by anti-inflammatory diarylheptanoids derived from *Alpinia oxyphylla* Miquel (Zingiberaceae). Oncology Research 13 (1), 37–45.

Cleland, J.G., Coletta, A.P., Clark, A.L., 2007. Clinical trials update from the American College of Cardiology 2007: ALPHA, EVEREST, FUSION II, VALIDD, PARR-2, REMODEL, SPICE, COURAGE, COACH, REMADHE, pro-BNP for the evaluation of dyspnoea and THIS-diet. European Journal of Heart Failure 9 (6–7), 740–745.

Clough, A.R., Rowley, K., O'Dea, K., 2004. Kava use, dyslipidaemia and biomarkers of dietary quality in Aboriginal people in Arnhem Land in the Northern Territory (NT), Australia. European Journal of Clinical Nutrition 58 (7), 1090–1093.

Dalli, E., Colomer, E., Tormos, M.C., et al., 2011. *Crataegus laevigata* decreases neutrophil elastase and has hypolipidemic effect: a randomized, double-blind, placebo-controlled trial. Phytomedicine 18, 769–775.

Dallner, G., Brismar, K., Chojnacki, T., Swiezewska, E., 2003. Regulation of coenzyme Q biosynthesis and breakdown. Biofactors 18 (1–4), 11–22.

Dasgupta, A., Agarwal, S.S., Basu, D.K., 1984. Anticonvulsant activity of the mixed fatty acids of *Elaeocarpus ganitrus roxb* (Rudraksh). Indian Journal of Physiology and Pharmacology 28 (3), 245–246.

Dörrie, J., Sapala, K., Zunino, S.J., 2001. Carnosol-induced apoptosis and downregulation of Bcl-2 in B-lineage leukemia cells. Cancer Letters 170 (1), 33–39.

Dwivedi, S., Aggarwal, A., 2009. Indigenous drugs in ischemic heart disease in patients with diabetes. Journal of Alternative and Complementary Medicine 15 (11), 1215–1221.

Feres, M., Figueiredo, L.C., Barreto, I.M., et al., 2005. In vitro antimicrobial activity of plant extracts and propolis in saliva samples of healthy and periodontally-involved subjects. Journal of the International Academy of Periodontology 7 (3), 90–96.

Finkel, R.S., Zarlengo, K.M., 2004. Blue cohosh and perinatal stroke. The New England Journal of Medicine 351 (3), 302–303.

Fugh-Berman, A., 2000. Herb–drug interactions. Lancet 355 (9198), 134–138.

Gali-Muhtasib, H., Himan, C., Khater, C., 2000. Traditional uses of *Salvia libanotica* (East Mediterranean sage) and the effects of its essential oils. Journal of Ethnopharmacology 71 (3), 513–520.

German Monographs, 1998. Bundesinstitut fur Arzneimittel und Medizinproduckte. Complete German Commission E Monographs: the Therapeutic Guide to Herbal Medicines. Lippincott Williams & Wilkins, New York.

Ghosh, S.S., Salloum, F.N., Abbate, A., et al., 2010. Curcumin prevents cardiac remodeling secondary to chronic renal failure through deactivation of hypertrophic signaling in rats. American Journal of Physiology. Heart and Circulatory Physiology 299 (4), H975–H984.

Gupta, R.S., Dixit, V.P., 2002. Effects of short term treatment of solasodine on cauda epididymis in dogs. Indian Journal of Experimental Biology 40 (2), 169–173.

Gurley, B.J., Swain, A., Barone, G.W., et al., 2007. Effect of Goldenseal (*Hydrastis canadensis*) and Kava Kava (*Piper methysticum*) supplementation on digoxin pharmacokinetics in humans. Drug Metabolism and Disposition 35 (2), 240–245.

Gurley, B.J., Swain, A., Hubbard, M.A., et al., 2008. Clinical assessment of CYP2D6-mediated herb-drug interactions in humans: effects of milk thistle, black cohosh, Goldenseal, Kava Kava, St. John's wort, and Echinacea. Molecular Nutrition and Food Research 52 (7), 755–763.

Haridy, F.M., El-Garhy, M.F., Morsy, T.A., 2003. Efficacy of Mirazid (*Commiphora molmol*) against fasioliasis Egyptian sleep. Journal of the Egyptian Society of Parasitology 33 (3), 917–924.

Harris, A., Devaraj, S., Jialal, I., 2002. Oxidative stress, alpha-tocopherol therapy, and atherosclerosis. Current Atherosclerosis Reports 4 (5), 373–380.

Harris, W.S., Reid, K.J., Sands, S.A., Spertus, J.A., 2007. Blood omega-3 and trans fatty acids in middle aged acute coronary syndrome patients. The American Journal of Cardiology 99, 154–158.

He, X., Zhou, N., Lin, Q., et al., 2010. Study on effect of total flavonoids from Scutellaria amoena on experimental arrhythmia. Zhongguo Zhong Yao Za Zhi 35 (4), 508–510.

Heptinstall, S., White, A., Williamson, L., Mitchell, J.R., 1985. Extracts of feverfew inhibit granule secretion in blood platelets and polymorphonuclear leucocytes. Lancet 1 (8437), 1071–1074.

Hietala, A.M., Solheim, H., Fossdal, C.G., 2008. Real-time PCR-based monitoring of DNA pools in the tri-trophic interaction between Norway spruce, the rust *Thekopsora areolata*, and an opportunistic ascomycetous *Phomopsis* sp. Phytopathology 98 (1), 51–58.

Holubarsch, C.J., Colucci, W.S., Meinertz, T., Gaus, W., Tendera, M., 2008. Survival and prognosis: investigation of *Crataegus* extract WS 1442 in CHF (SPICE) trial study group. The efficacy and safety of *Crataegus* extract WS 1442 in patients with heart failure: the SPICE trial. European Journal of Heart Failure 10 (12), 1255–1263.

Hwang, J., Hodis, H.N., Sevanian, A., 2001. Soy and alfalfa phytoestrogen extracts become potent low-density lipoprotein antioxidants in the presence of acerola cherry extract. Journal of Agricultural and Food Chemistry 49 (1), 308–314.

Jarry, H., Spengler, B., Porzel, A., et al., 2003. Evidence for estrogen receptor beta-selective activity of *Vitex agnus-castus* and isolated flavones. Planta Medica 69 (10), 945–947.

Jung, H.A., Su, B.N., Keller, W.J., Mehta, R.G., Kinghorn, A.D., 2006. Antioxidant xanthones from the pericarp of *Garcinia mangostana* (Mangosteen). Journal of Agricultural and Food Chemistry 54 (6), 2077–2082.

Kennedy, D.O., Pace, S., Haskell, C., et al., 2006. Effects of cholinesterase inhibiting sage (*Salvia officinalis*) on mood, anxiety and performance on a psychological stressor battery. Neuropsychopharmacology 31 (4), 845–852.

Koch, E., Malek, F.A., 2011. Standardized extracts from hawthorn leaves and flowers in the treatment of cardiovascular disorders – preclinical and clinical studies. Planta Medica 77 (11), 1123–1128.

Kuller, L.H., Ives, D.G., Fitzpatrick, A.L., et al., 2010. Does Ginkgo biloba reduce the risk of cardiovascular events? Circulation. Cardiovascular Quality and Outcomes 3 (1), 41–47.

Lee, E.B., Kim, O.J., Kang, S.S., Jeong, C., Araloside, A., 2005. An antiulcer constituent from the root bark of *Aralia elata*. Biological and Pharmaceutical Bulletin 28 (3), 523–526.

Leger, D.Y., Liagre, B., Beneytout, J.L., 2006. Role of MAPKs and NFkappaB in diosgenin-induced megakaryocytic differentiation and subsequent apoptosis in HEL cells. International Journal of Oncology 28 (1), 201–207.

Liao, C.H., Sang, S., Ho, C.T., Lin, J.K., 2005. Garcinol modulates tyrosine phosphorylation of FAK and subsequently induces apoptosis through down-regulation of Src, ERK, and Akt survival signaling in human colon cancer cells. Journal of Cellular Biochemistry 96 (1), 155–169.

Lichtensteiger, C.A., Johnston, N.A., 1997. Beasley VR *Rhamnus cathartica* (buckthorn) hepatocellular toxicity in mice. Toxicologic Pathology 25 (5), 449–452.

Liu, J., Burdette, J.E., Xu, H., et al., 2001. Evaluation of estrogenic activity of plant extracts for the potential treatment of menopausal symptoms. Journal of Agricultural and Food Chemistry 49 (5), 2472–2479.

Mabuchi, H., Inazu, A., 2010. Human cholesteryl ester transfer protein in human HDL metabolism. In: Schaefer, E.J. (Ed.), High Density Lipoproteins, Dyslipidemia, and Coronary Heart Disease. Springer Science+Business Media, New York, pp. 95–110.

Mahmood, Z.A., Sualeh, M., Mahmood, S.B., Karim, M.A., 2010. Herbal treatment for cardiovascular disease the evidence based therapy. Pakistan Journal of Pharmaceutical Sciences 23 (1), 119–124.

Matsui, H., Shimosawa, T., Uetake, Y., et al., 2006. Protective effect of potassium against the hypertensive cardiac dysfunction: association with reactive oxygen species reduction. Hypertension 48 (2), 225–231.

McGuffin, M., 2000. American Herbal Products Association's Botanical Safety Hand. CRC Press, Boca Raton, FL HerbalGram Copyright American Botanical Council 48, 42.

Murata, K., Takano, F., Fushiya, S., Oshima, Y., 1998. Chemical constituents from the roots of *Hydrangea chinensis*. Natural Products 61 (6), 729–733.

Ohyama, K., Akaike, T., Hirobe, C., Yamakawa, T., 2003. Cytotoxicity and apoptotic inducibility of *Vitex agnus-castus* fruit extract in cultured human normal and cancer cells and effect on growth. Biological and Pharmaceutical Bulletin 26 (1), 10–18.

Ohyama, K., Akaike, T., Imai, M., et al., 2005. Human gastric signet ring carcinoma (KATO-III) cell apoptosis induced by *Vitex agnus-castus* fruit extract through intracellular oxidative stress. International Journal of Biochemistry and Cell Biology 37 (7), 1496–1510.

Okamura, T., Sekikawa, A., Kadowaki, T., et al., 2009. Cholesteryl ester transfer protein, coronary calcium and intima-media thickness of the carotid artery in middle-aged Japanese men. American Journal of Cardiology 104 (6), 818–822.

Panciera, R.J., Martin, T., Burrows, G.E., Taylor, D.S., Rice, L.E., 1990. Acute oxalate poisoning attributable to ingestion of curly dock (*Rumex crispus*) in sheep. Journal of the American Veterinary Medical Association 196 (12), 1981–1984.

Park, S.J., Choi, K.S., Shin, D.H., et al., 2009a. Effects of mixed herbal extracts from parched *Puerariae radix*, gingered Magnoliae cortex, *Glycyrrhizae radix* and *Euphorbiae radix* (KIOM-79) on cardiac ion channels and action potentials. Journal of Korean Medical Science 24 (3), 403–412.

Park, S., Kim, M.Y., Lee, D.H., et al., 2009b. Methanolic extract of onion (*Allium cepa*) attenuates ischemia/hypoxia-induced apoptosis in cardiomyocytes via antioxidant effect. European Journal of Nutrition 48 (4), 235–242.

Park, S., Lee, D.K., Yang, C.H., 1998. Inhibition of fos-jun-DNA complex formation by dihydroguaiaretic acid and in vitro cytotoxic effects on cancer cells. Cancer Letters 127 (1–2), 23–28.

Paulsen, E., 2002. Contact sensitization from compositae-containing herbal remedies and cosmetics. Contact Dermatitis 47 (4), 189–198.

Perry, N.S., Bollen, C., Perry, E.K., Ballard, C., 2003. Salvia for dementia therapy: review of pharmacological activity and pilot tolerability clinical trial. Pharmacology Biochemistry and Behavior 75 (3), 651–659.

Plouzek, C.A., Ciolino, H.P., Clarke, R., Yeh, G.C., 1999. Inhibition of P-glycoprotein activity and reversal of multidrug resistance in vitro by rosemary extract. European Journal of Cancer 35 (10), 1541–1545.

Rankins Jr., D.L., Smith, G.S., Hallford, D.M., 1991. Altered metabolic hormones, impaired nitrogen retention, and hepatotoxicosis in lambs fed Kochia scoparia hay. Animal Science 67 (7), 2932–2940.

Rao, R.B., Hoffman, R.S., 2002. Nicotinic toxicity from tincture of blue cohosh (*Caulophyllum thalictroides*) used as an abortifacient. Veterinary and Human Toxicology 44 (4), 221–222.

Rayner, K., Chen, Y.X., Hibbert, B., et al., 2007. NM23-H2, an estrogen receptor beta-associated protein, shows diminished expression with progression of atherosclerosis. American Journal of Physiology. Regulatory, Integrative and Comparative Physiology 292 (2), R743–R750.

Roche, H.M., Gibney, M.J., 2000. Effect of long-chain n-3 polyunsaturated fatty acids on fasting and post-prandial triacylglycerol metabolism. American Journal of Clinical Nutrition 71 (1), 232S–237S.

Russell, L., Hicks, G.S., Low, A.K., Shepherd, J.M., Brown, C.A., 2002. Phytoestrogens: a viable option? American Journal of the Medical Sciences 324 (4), 185–188.

Santo, A.S., Santo, A.M., Browne, R.W., et al., 2010. Postprandial lipemia detects the effect of soy protein on cardiovascular disease risk compared with the fasting lipid profile. Lipids 45 (12), 1127–1138.

Schoene, N.W., Kelly, M.A., Polansky, M.M., Anderson, R.A., 2005. Watersoluble polymeric polyphenols from cinnamon inhibit proliferation and alter cell cycle distribution patterns of hematologic tumor cell lines. Cancer Letters 230 (1), 134–140.

Sebastiani, V., Botti, C., Di Tondo, U., et al., 2006. Tissue microarray analysis of FAS, Bcl-2, Bcl-x, ER, PgR, Hsp60, p53 and Her2-neu in breast carcinoma. Anticancer Research 26 (4B), 2983–2987.

Shara, M., Ohia, S.E., Schmidt, R.E., et al., 2004. Physico-chemical properties of a novel (−)-hydroxycitric acid extract and its effect on body weight, selected organ weights, hepatic lipid peroxidation and DNA fragmentation, hematology and clinical chemistry, and histopathological changes over a period of 90 days. Molecular and Cellular Biochemistry 260 (1–2), 171–186.

Sharma, V., Josheph, C., Ghosh, S., et al., 2007. Kaempferol induces apoptosis in glioblastoma cells through oxidative stress. Molecular Cancer Therapeutics 6 (9), 2544–2553.

Sharma, R., Singh, R.B., 2010. Bioactive foods and nutraceutical supplementation criteria in cardiovascular protection. The Open Nutraceuticals Journal 3, 141–153.

Sheir, Z., Nasr, A.A., Massoud, A., et al., 2001. A safe, effective, herbal antischistosomal therapy derived from myrrh. American Journal of Tropical Medicine and Hygiene 65 (6), 700–704.

Sheng, Y., Bryngelsson, C., 2000. Pero RW Enhanced DNA repair, immune function and reduced toxicity of C-MED-100, a novel aqueous extract from *Uncaria tomentosa*. Journal of Ethnopharmacology 69 (2), 115–126.

Shishodia, S., Aggarwal, B.B., 2006. Diosgenin inhibits osteoclastogenesis, invasion, and proliferation through the downregulation of Akt, I kappa B kinase activation and NF-kappa B-regulated gene expression. Oncogene 25 (10), 1463–1473.

Shukla, S.K., Gupta, S., Ojha, S.K., Sharma, S.B., 2010. Cardiovascular friendly natural products: a promising approach in the management of CVD. Natural Product Research 24 (9), 873–898.

Singh, R.B., Niaz, M.A., Ghosh, S., 1994. Hypolipidemic and antioxidant effects of *Commiphora mukul* as an adjunct to dietary therapy in patients with hypercholesterolemia. Cardiovascular Drugs and Therapy 8 (4), 659–664.

Smith, M.C., Holcombe, J.K., Stullenbarger, E., 1994. A meta-analysis of intervention effectiveness for symptom management in oncology nursing research. Oncology Nursing Forum 21 (7), 1201–1210.

Spiller, H.A., Winter, M.L., Weber, J.A., et al., 2003. Skin breakdown and blisters from senna-containing laxatives in young children. Annals of Pharmcotherapy 37 (5), 636–639.

Steinhoff, B., Krenn, L., 2011. Phytotherapy in Europe – 18 years of ESCOP presidency laudation on the occasion of the retirement of Professor Fritz H. Kemper from ESCOP. Phytomedicine 18 (5), 431.

Stickel, F., Seitz, H.K., Hahn, E.G., Schuppan, D., 2001. Liver toxicity of drugs of plant origin. Zeitschrift für Gastroenterologie 39 (3), 225–232 234–237.

Syrovets, T., Büchele, B., Gedig, E., Slupsky, J.R., Simmet, T., 2000. Acetyl-boswellic acids are novel catalytic inhibitors of human topoisomerases I and II alpha. Molecular Pharmacology 58 (1), 71–81.

Thirunavukkarasu, M., Penumathsa, S.V., Juhasz, B., et al., 2006. Niacin-bound chromium enhances myocardial protection from ischemia-reperfusion injury. American Journal of Physiology. Heart and Circulatory Physiology 291 (2), H820–H826.

Tildesley, N.T., Kennedy, D.O., Perry, E.K., et al., 2005. Positive modulation of mood and cognitive performance following administration of acute doses of *Salvia lavandulaefolia* essential oil to healthy young volunteers. Physiology and Behavior 83 (5), 699–709.

Wang, Q., Simonyi, A., Li, W., et al., 2005. Dietary grape supplement ameliorates cerebral ischemia-induced neuronal death in gerbils. Molecular Nutrition and Food Research 49 (5), 443–451.

Wang, J., Wang, Z., Tang, G., 2003. TCM treatment of extrasystole with huanglian shengmai yin – a report of 357 cases. Journal of Traditional Chinese Medicine 23 (1), 35–37.

Wang, H., Ye, X., Gao, Q., et al., 2009. Pharmacovigilance in traditional Chinese medicine safety surveillance. Pharmacoepidemiology and Drug Safety 18 (5), 357–361.

Warnke, P.H., Sherry, E., Russo, P.A.J., et al., 2006. Antibacterial essential oils in malodorous cancer patients: clinical observations in 30 patients. Phytomedicne 13 (7), 463–467.

Wei, F., Li, D., Luo, C., Yue, H., Chen, Q., Huang, Z., 2004. Pharmaceutical composition for the treatment of cardiovascular and cerebrovascular diseases. US Patent 7438935.

Wei, Q.Y., Ma, J.P., Cai, Y.J., Yang, L., Liu, Z.L., 2005. Cytotoxic and apoptotic activities of diarylheptanoids and gingerol-related compounds from the rhizome of Chinese ginger. Journal of Ethnopharmacology 102 (2), 177–184.

Willett, W.C., 2007. Ask the doctor. For the health of my heart and arteries, how does regular consumption of red wine compare with grape juice or the equivalent in grapes? Harvard Heart Letter 17 (7), 7.

Yamaguchi, K., Liggett, J.L., Kim, N.C., Baek, S.J., 2006. Anti-proliferative effect of horehound leaf and wild cherry bark extracts on human colorectal cancer cells. Oncology Reports 15 (1), 275–281.

Yim, T.K., Wu, W.K., Pak, W.F., et al., 2000. Myocardial protection against ischaemia–reperfusion injury by a Polygonum multiflorum extract supplemented 'Dang-Gui decoction for enriching blood', a compound formulation, ex vivo. Phytotherapy Research 14 (3), 195–199.

Yuan, J., Guo, W., Yang, B., et al., 1997. 116 cases of coronary angina pectoris treated with powder composed of radix ginseng, radix notoginseng and succinum. Journal of Traditional Chinese Medicine 17 (1), 14–17.

Zahid, A.M., Hussain, M.E., Fahim, M., 2005. Antiatherosclerotic effects of dietary supplementations of garlic and turmeric: restoration of endothelial function in rats. Life Sciences 77 (8), 837–857.

Zeng, X., Li, Q., Zhang, M., Wang, W., Tan, X., 2011. Green tea may be benefit to the therapy of atrial fibrillation. Journal of Cellular Biochemistry 112 (7), 1709–1712.

Zhang, H.Z., Kasibhatla, S., Wang, Y., et al., 2004. Discovery, characterization and SAR of gambogic acid as a potent apoptosis inducer by a HTS assay. Bioorganic & Medicinal Chemistry 12 (2), 309–317.

Zhao, W., Kridel, S., Thorburn, A., et al., 2006. Fatty acid synthase: a novel target for antiglioma therapy. British Journal of Cancer 95 (7), 869–878.

Zhou, H.L., Deng, Y.M., Xie, Q.M., 2006. The modulatory effects of the volatile oil of ginger on the cellular immune response in vitro and in vivo in mice. Journal of Ethnopharmacology 105 (1–2), 301–305.

Zhou, X., Gong, Z., Su, Y., Lin, J., Tang, K., 2009. Cordyceps fungi: natural products, pharmacological functions and developmental products. Journal of Pharmacy and Pharmacology 61 (3), 279–291.

Zhou, J., Møller, J., Ritskes-Hoitinga, M., et al., 2003. Effects of vitamin supplementation and hyperhomocysteinemia on atherosclerosis in apoE-deficient mice. Atherosclerosis 168 (2), 255–262.

Zick, S.M., Vautaw, B.M., Gillespie, B., Aaronson, K.D., 2009. Hawthorn extract randomized blinded chronic heart failure (HERB CHF) trial. European Journal of Heart Failure 11 (10), 990–999.

CHAPTER 3

Plant Statins and Heart Failure

T. Celik, M. Celik

Gulhane Military Medical Academy, Etlik, Ankara, Turkey

1. HEART FAILURE

Heart failure (HF) is a major public health problem. Approximately 5 million patients have HF, and over 550 000 patients are diagnosed with HF for the first time each year in the United States (US) (Rosamond et al., 2008). Furthermore, there are at least 15 million patients with HF in the 51 countries of the European Society of Cardiology (The Task Force for the Diagnosis et al., 2008).

The most common cause of congestive failure is coronary artery disease (CAD). HF is also associated with untreated hypertension, various abnormalities of the heart valves (particularly aortic and mitral), alcohol abuse, viral infection or inflammation of the heart (myocarditis), primary heart muscle disease (cardiomyopathy), hyperthyroidism, and in rare instances, extreme vitamin deficiencies, and drug abuse (primarily cocaine and amphetamines). The prognosis of HF depends upon the cause of the HF and the overall degree of cardiac dysfunction.

The treatment of HF depends on several factors such as its cause, its severity, and the patient's health condition. Nonpharmacological treatment of HF includes restriction of dietary sodium, a prudent diet, regular exercise, and weight control. Several large number of trials have been published about the pharmacological therapy of HF with all stages of this disease from asymptomatic HF to severe HF. The main classes of drugs used in the management of HF are angiotensin converting enzyme inhibitors, beta-blockers, angiotensin receptor blockers, aldosterone antagonists, diuretics, and digoxin. Such treatments improve ventricular function and patient well-being, reduce hospital admission for worsening HF, and increase survival.

Despite advances in our understanding of pathophysiology and treatment of HF, 20% of patients newly diagnosed with HF will die within 1 year and long-term morbidity and mortality remain high with a mortality rate of 60–70% within 5 years (Rosamond et al., 2008). Thus, different or alternative pharmacological agents are required in the treatment of HF. Statin is one of them.

2. STATINS IN THE TREATMENT OF HF

CAD is the most common etiology of HF in industrialized nations. Hypercholesterolemia is a major risk factor for CAD. Thus, most of patients with HF appear to be

Bioactive Food as Dietary Interventions for Cardiovascular Disease
http://dx.doi.org/10.1016/B978-0-12-396485-4.00002-5

© 2013 Elsevier Inc.
All rights reserved.

candidates for statin therapy. Retrospective analyses of clinical trials of statins have suggested that statin use was associated with improvement of left ventricular ejection fraction (LVEF), reduction in developing new-onset HF, and hospitalization for HF in patients taking statins (Krum et al., 2007a). However, it should not be forgotten that patients with HF have been largely excluded from major randomized clinical trials of statins and there is no direct evidence that statins might be useful for patients with HF. The survival benefit with statins results from the prevention of progression of CAD, and there is no benefit to initiate statin treatment once symptomatic HF is present.

Statins (3-hydroxy-3-methyl-glutaryl-coenzyme A reductase inhibitors) may reduce the risk for cardiovascular events through lipid lowering by reducing the endogenous synthesis of cholesterol. In addition, statins have other biological effects (so-called pleiotropic effects), apart from cholesterol lowering that are of potential benefit for patients with HF.

Overactivity of the immune system has been an ongoing issue of concern in patients with HF. C-reactive protein, tumor necrosis factor-α, IL (interleukin)-1, and IL-6 have been demonstrated to be markers of an adverse prognosis in patients with HF (Anker and von Haehling, 2004). Treatment with statins has been shown to reduce levels of inflammatory biomarkers and cytokines in patients with HF (Tousoulis et al., 2005). Also, statin therapy improves endothelial function and microvascular circulation by stimulating angiogenesis and modulating the synthesis and activity of endothelial nitric oxide synthase and endothelin-1 (Hernandez-Perera et al., 1998). So, the possible beneficial effect of statins in HF appears independent of cholesterol levels.

Three large randomized clinical trials examine the safety and efficacy of statin therapy in patients with HF: the GISSI-HF (Gruppo Italiano per lo Studio della Sopravvivenza nell'Infarto miocardico-Heart Failure), CORONA (Controlled Rosuvastatin Multinational Trial in Heart Failure), and UNIVERSE trials. In the CORONA study, 5011 patients at least 60 years of age with ischemic cardiomyopathy, New York Heart Association (NYHA) class III/IV HF and LVEF of 40% or less, or NYHA II HF and LVEF of 35% or less, were randomized to rosuvastatin 10 mg daily versus placebo (Serebruany, 2008). Although, treatment with rosuvastatin did not result in benefit with respect to the primary endpoint (death from CVD causes, nonfatal myocardial infarction, or nonfatal stroke), it resulted in a significant decrease in HF hospitalizations. In the GISSI-HF study, 4574 patients aged 18 years or older with NYHA II–IV symptomatic HF were randomized to rosuvastatin 10 mg daily versus placebo (Tavazzi et al., 2008). As with the CORONA study, rosuvastatin failed to improve clinical outcomes despite significantly lowering the concentrations of low-density lipoprotein (LDL) cholestrol. However, there was no difference in the primary endpoints of time to death and time to death or hospitalization for cardiovascular reasons between the two study arms. In the UNIVERSE (rosuvastatin impact on ventricular remodeling, cytokines, and neurohormones) trial, 86 patients with chronic systolic HF were randomized to placebo or rosuvastatin at an increasing dose (target: 40 mg once a day) in a double-blind fashion

(Krum et al., 2007b). Despite being safe and effective at decreasing plasma cholesterol, rosuvastatin treatment did not result in a significant improvement in the parameters of LV remodeling compared with placebo. Furthermore, the value of statins in HF patients with a non ischemic etiology is unknown.

Despite statin therapy appears to have several potentially beneficial effects in patients with HF, lipid lowering with statins may have some adverse effects. Advanced HF is a highly catabolic state and is associated with cardiac cachexia, elevated inflammatory markers, and lower cholesterol levels. Further reductions in cholesterol and lipoproteins induced by statins might have adverse outcomes in HF. It occurred mainly by two mechanisms. First, lipoproteins may remove bacterial endotoxins that enter the circulation. Statins might make HF patients more susceptible to infection by lowering lipoprotein levels. Secondly, ubiquinone is an important cofactor in the mitochondrial electron transport chain, and plasma levels of ubiquinone (coenzyme Q10) are reduced during treatment with statins (Molyneux et al., 2008). The reduction of plasma ubiquinone level might adversely affect cardiac muscle. Furthermore, higher cholesterol levels were found in association with better survival in the EuroHeart Failure survey of 10701 hospitalized patients with HF or suspected HF (Velavan et al., 2007).

Although statins have been shown to prevent of progression of the CAD, they can produce some side effects, and several drug interactions have been noted between statins and other HF drugs. Lipid alterations can also be effected by a number of dietary approaches or specific dietary supplements. So, an alternative lipid lowering therapy without statin is considered.

3. COMPLEMENTARY MEDICINE IN HEART FAILURE

The prevention and treatment of cardiovascular diseases is progressive and complementary and alternative medicine other than traditional medical treatment might be required. Complementary medicine (CAM) is a term to describe the use of alternative medicine as an adjunct to, not primarily a replacement for, traditional medical and interventional treatment. Many of the CAMs have been used as herbal supplements for thousands of years in the East.

There has been an increased public interest and use of CAMs for cardiovascular disease over the years. Several forms of CAMs such as vitamins, herbal remedies, and other dietary supplements have been studied in patients suffering from cardiovascular diseases (Frishman et al., 2009). However, these studies have been limited to selected populations. In addition, the results of these clinical studies remain controversial, and risk-versus-benefit ratios are not well defined.

CAMs are used mainly by the white, educated, women, and middle-class population. The most commonly used CAM modalities are herbal products. Echinacea, garlic, ginseng, ginkgo biloba, and glucosamine with or without chondroitin are the most commonly used herbal products for lowering the risk of CVD. Plant sterols, soluble fiber, omega-3 fatty acids, nuts, and soy supplements are also used.

4. PLANT STEROLS/STANOLS (PHYTOSTEROLS)

Whereas cholesterol is an essential constituent of cell membranes in mammalian cells, sterol is present in cell membranes of plants. Plant sterols (also called as phytosterols) are structurally similar to cholesterol, but they differ in their chemical structure only due to the presence of an additional methyl (campesterol) or ethyl (sitosterol) group at the C-24 position of the side chain (Igel et al., 2003). Sitosterol, campesterol, stigmasterol, brassicasterol, and avenosterol are the most known sterols in the literature. On the other hand, plant stanols are the saturated form of plant sterols. Stanols differ from the corresponding sterols due to saturation of the $\Delta 5$ double bond to the 5α position (Frishman et al., 2009).

Plant sterols competitively inhibit the intestinal absorption of cholesterol. Plant stanols and sterols displace cholesterol from micelles, reducing dietary cholesterol uptake at the brush border membrane in the small intestine and increasing fecal loss of cholesterol. The exact molecular mechanisms are not completely understood. Both cholesterol and phytosterols require the Niemann-Pick C1-Like 1 protein to obtain entry in enterocytes. In enterocytes, cholesterol is esterified via the enzyme acetyl-coenzyme A acetyltransferase 2, packed into chylomicrons, and drained into the lymph system via the basolateral membrane. Nonesterified cholesterol and phytosterols are pumped back into the intestinal lumen via the adenosine triphosphate (ATP) proteins, ATP-binding cassette (ABC), and half-transporters ABCG5 and ABCG8 (Katan et al., 2003).

The efficacy of intestinal absorption of plant sterols differs markedly from that of cholesterol. Plasma sterols are transported in serum with lipoproteins and excreted into bile. In contrast with cholesterol, plant sterols are not metabolized to bile acids in the liver. The intestinal absorption ranges from 0.4% to 5% for plant sterols and from 0.02% to 0.3% for their saturated counterparts (Lutjohann et al., 1995). Consequently, plant stanol concentrations in serum are much lower than their respective sterols. The absorption of campesterol is approximately three times lower than that of cholesterol, and sitosterol is three times lower than that of campesterol (Heinemann et al., 1993). They are excreted much faster from the liver into bile compared with cholesterol. Furthermore, the biliary excretion rate of plant sterols is opposite to their absorption rate: sitosterol is excreted faster than campesterol, and campesterol is excreted faster than cholesterol (Sudhop et al., 2002a).

Plant sterols are currently available in a wide variety of foods and drinks. Since they are not synthesized in the human body, they are therefore exclusively derived from the diet in different amounts. Foods that are high in plant sterols are cereals (such as rice bran, wheat germ, oat bran, bran, whole wheat, brown rice), legumes (such as dried peas, dried beans, lentils), nuts, and seeds (such as peanuts, almonds, walnuts, pecans, sunflower seeds, pumpkin seeds, sesame seeds), fruits, and vegetables (such as broccoli, cauliflower, brussels sprouts, dill, apples, avocados, tomato, vegetable oils, wheat germ oil, blueberries).

Plant sterols and stanols occur naturally in small amounts in food, and it can be difficult to get the recommended amount of sterols from the foods. Thus, many manufacturers have started to fortify common foods (such as orange juice, margarine, cookies, energy bars, yogurt drinks) with plant sterols. Cholesterol-lowering margarines enriched with plant sterols are the most studied products. Because of the poor water solubility of plant sterols, esterifying with fatty acid enhances the availability of plant sterol in food fats such as margarines. Sitosterol and campesterol are major saturated plant sterols and are found in one of these products. Although these commercially available margarines lower serum concentrations of cholesterol, they are expensive. The cost of fortified margarines is approximately two to five times that of ordinary margarine.

Furthermore, emulsification with lecithin for increasing absorption of plant sterols is created. Lecithin can be formulated as a spray dried powder, and it has been mixed with egg whites, lemonade drinks, yogurt flavored drinks, and orange juice (Spilburg et al., 2003). Although, these products markedly reduce serum cholesterol concentrations to a similar degree to that seen with cholesterol-lowering margarines, none of these products has been adequately studied for clinical endpoints (Spilburg et al., 2003). Salo and Wester (2005) showed that the cholesterol-lowering efficacy of plant sterols was independent of the food type.

Phytosterols seem to be well tolerated according to most case reports and studies. But, it is possible over the long-term that they can cause reduction in the absorption of fat-soluble vitamins such as β-carotene, vitamin D, and vitamin E. It has been shown that consuming one additional daily serving of a high carotenoid vegetable or fruit counteracted any effects of the margarine in lowering plasma carotenoids (Noakes et al., 2002). Furthermore, there is no report on any adverse interactions between plant sterols/stanols and traditional prescription medications that the patients are taking for their cardiovascular conditions.

Plant sterols or phytosterols have been known to have a cholesterol-lowering effect since the 1950s and have been added to patients' diets for the treatment of hypercholesterolemia. The effects of stanol/sterol esters have been demonstrated in various population groups, including young adults, elderly men, premenopausal and postmenopausal women, children with and without familial hypercholesterolemia, and patients with type II diabetes and CHD. Plant sterols might also protect against certain types of cancer such as colon, breast, and prostate (Awad et al., 2000). Sitosterol has been observed to have greater effects than other phytosterols. Although there have been no studies demonstrating that the consumption of stanol/sterol esters influences cardiovascular risk, there is convincing clinical evidence from over 20 studies showing that plant sterols reduce LDL-cholesterol levels, without affecting HDL-cholesterol or triglycerides (Cater, 2000).

Recent studies have examined the efficacy of plant sterol-enriched margarines for lowering serum cholesterol. In their longer-term (1-year follow-up) double-blind study, Miettinen et al compared the efficacy and tolerability of margarine fortified with sitostanol to unfortified margarine in 153 randomly selected subjects with mild hypercholesterolemia (total cholesterol $\geq$216 mg dl^{-1} and triglycerides <265 mg dl^{-1}) (Miettinen et al., 1995). The average 1-year reduction in serum cholesterol and LDL-cholesterol concentration were significantly lower in the sitostanol ester group compared with the control group. No effect was observed on triglyceride and HDL-cholesterol concentrations. Absorption of fat soluble vitamins did not appear to be affected, although serum β-carotene levels were significantly lowered. Thereby, the investigators concluded that those consuming the fortified margarine as part of the daily fat intake in subjects with mild hypercholesterolemia was effective in lowering serum total cholesterol and LDL cholesterol, and was well tolerated even when administered long term up to 1 year. Another a randomized double-blind placebo-controlled study compared effects of margarines enriched with different vegetable oil sterols or sitostanol ester on plasma total-, LDL-, and HDL-cholesterol concentrations in 100 patients with normal cholesterol or mild hypercholesterolemia (Weststrate and Meijer, 1998). A margarine with sterol esters from soybean oil, mainly esters from sitosterol, campesterol, and stigmasterol, was found as effective as a margarine with sitostanol ester in lowering blood total- and LDL-cholesterol levels without affecting HDL-cholesterol concentrations.

Although phytosterol esters were commercially used in margarines effectively to reduce blood cholesterol, their effectiveness in nonfat moieties is not yet established. A more recent study looked at the effects of sterol-fortified orange juice in 72 mildly hypercholesterolemic healthy subjects (Devaraj et al., 2004). Of 72 subjects, half received regular orange juice and half the fortified orange juice. After just 2 weeks, sterol-fortified orange juice significantly decreased total (7.2%), LDL-cholesterol (12.4%), and HDL-cholesterol (7.8%) compared with baseline and compared with placebo orange juice ($P<0.01$). Nonetheless, plant sterols combined with dark chocolate reduced serum concentrations of cholesterol (Allen et al., 2008). Also, tablets and soft gel capsules containing 1.3–1.9 g of plant sterol are available.

Plant sterol-ester margarines can also have an additive or interactive effect on LDL-cholesterol reduction when ingested in combination with a stable dose of a statin drug. One randomized, 8-week placebo-controlled trial of 167 subjects with an LDL-cholesterol $\geq$130 mg dl^{-1}, despite at least 3 months of statin therapy, found that using plant stanol esters reduced total cholesterol by 12% (vs. 5% for placebo) and LDL-cholesterol by 17% (vs. 7% for placebo) (Blair et al., 2000). A multicenter, randomized, double-blind study with four parallel treatment arms in a balanced 2×2 factorial design (placebo plus regular margarine, placebo plus sterol-ester margarine, cerivastatin plus regular margarine, and cerivastatin plus sterol–ester margarine) was conducted in patients with primary hypercholesterolemia with baseline LDL-cholesterol ≥ 97 mg dl^{-1}. In subjects with primary hypercholesterolemia, the addition of sterol–ester margarine to statin therapy offers LDL cholesterol reduction equivalent to doubling the dose of statin (Simons, 2002). Also, it has been shown that consumption of sitostanol fortified margarine in combination with statins for 12 weeks in postmenopausal women with previous myocardial infarction reduced the needed drug dose of simvastatin necessary to reach the target level of cholesterol (Gylling et al., 1997).

Although there is no clinical evidence of plant stanol/sterol esters consumption as a therapeutic option in the management of HF, it is obvious that plant-derived stanol/sterol esters reduce LDL-cholesterol levels without affecting HDL-cholesterol or triglycerides. Thus, plant stanol/sterol esters may reduce the risk for cardiovascular events through lipid lowering by reducing the intestinal absorption of exogenous cholesterol. Otherwise, the decrease in serum cholesterol is less than that expected by the degree of reduced absorption, probably and likely because of a compensatory increase in hepatic cholesterol synthesis (Miettinen et al., 1995). Therefore, plant sterol may prevent adverse effects of further reductions in cholesterol and lipoproteins induced by statins in patients with HF. More experience and further large-scale randomized studies of the use of plant sterol in patients with HF are needed.

Despite the beneficial effects of plant sterols in lowering blood cholesterol, a few studies hypothesized that plasma plant sterol levels may be an independent risk factor for cardiovascular disease (Sudhop et al., 2002b). The effects of plant sterol esters on endothelial function, stroke, or atherogenesis are not known. A study of dietary supplementation with plant sterols was conducted in mice, and found harmful vascular effects including impaired endothelial function and increased atherogenesis (Weingartner et al., 2008).

Phytosterolemia (or sitosterolemia) is a rare inherited disease. The genetic defect in phytosterolemia has been located to chromosome 2p21 (Patel et al., 1998). This disease shows increased dietary sterol absorption and failure to excrete sterols into bile. All plant sterol species are highly elevated in this condition, and the patients with phytosterolemia are associated with premature atherosclerosis and coronary heart disease. Thus, plant stanol and sterol esters should be avoided in patients with phytosterolemia.

Since they have impressive LDL-cholesterol lowering effects, the US Food and Drug Administration (FDA) gave these products the status of a "health claim" in 2000. The Nutrition Committee of the American Heart Association (AHA) recommends the use of these fortified foods with caution for people with hypercholesterolemia or an atherosclerotic event who require lowering of total and LDL-cholesterol levels. The Third Adult Treatment Panel (ATP III) of the National Cholesterol Education Program (NCEP) guidelines concur with those of the AHA (Executive Summary of the Third Report of the National Cholesterol Education Program (NCEP) Expert Panel on Detection, 2001). Although the FDA has issued a 4.5 g day^{-1} use of plant sterols as a health claim, ATP III and AHA have advised individuals with hypercholesterolemia to consume 2 g day^{-1} of plant-derived stanol/sterol esters as a therapeutic option for LDL-cholesterol lowering (Executive Summary of the Third Report of the National Cholesterol Education Program (NCEP) Expert Panel on Detection, 2001).

The AHA recommends that further studies and large-scale monitoring are needed to determine the long-term safety of phytosterol-containing foods in both normocholesterolemic adults and children. Therefore, people with normal cholesterol levels should not use these products until long-term studies looking at clinical endpoints are available.

5. CONCLUSION

Lipid alterations can also be effected by a number of dietary approaches or specific dietary supplements. Based on current data, plant stanols/sterols lower LDL cholesterol levels in individuals with hypercholesterolemia. Maximum effects are observed at plant stanol/sterol intakes of 2 g day^{-1}. To sustain serum total and LDL cholesterol reductions, patients need to consume these products daily, as they would use lipid-lowering medications. Although there is no evidence for the efficacy of plant stanols/sterols in the treatment of HF, plant stanols/sterols seem to be beneficial by lowering total cholesterol and LDL cholesterol levels. Thence, plant stanols/sterols incorporated into traditional food products can be considered as a complementary adjunctive therapeutic option, in addition to lipid-lowering medicine for individuals with HF and elevated LDL cholesterol levels.

REFERENCES

Allen, R.R., Carson, L., Kwik-Uribe, C., Evans, E.M., Erdman Jr., J.W., 2008. Daily consumption of a dark chocolate containing flavanols and added sterol esters affects cardiovascular risk factors in a normotensive population with elevated cholesterol. Journal of Nutrition 138, 725–731.

Anker, S.D., von Haehling, S., 2004. Inflammatory mediators in chronic heart failure: an overview. Heart 90, 464–470.

Awad, A.B., Downie, A., Fink, C.S., Kim, U., 2000. Dietary phytosterol inhibits the growth and metastasis of MDA-MB-231 human breast cancer cells grown in SCID mice. Anticancer Research 20, 821–824.

Blair, S.N., Capuzzi, D.M., Gottlieb, S.O., Nguyen, T., Morgan, J.M., Cater, N.B., 2000. Incremental reduction of serum total cholesterol and low-density lipoprotein cholesterol with the addition of plant stanol ester-containing spread to statin therapy. The American Journal of Cardiology 86, 46–52.

Cater, N.B., 2000. Plant stanol ester: review of cholesterol-lowering efficacy and implications for coronary heart disease risk reduction. Preventive Cardiology 3, 121–130.

Devaraj, S., Jialal, I., Vega-Lopez, S., 2004. Plant sterol-fortified orange juice effectively lowers cholesterol levels in mildly hypercholesterolemic healthy individuals. Arteriosclerosis, Thrombosis, and Vascular Biology 24, e25–28.

European Society of Cardiology, 2008. The task force for the diagnosis and treatment of acute and chronic heart failure 2008 of the European Society of Cardiology. European Heart Journal 29, 2388–2442.

Frishman, W.H., Beravol, P., Carosella, C., 2009. Alternative and complementary medicine for preventing and treating cardiovascular disease. Disease-a-Month 55, 121–192.

Gylling, H., Radhakrishnan, R., Miettinen, T.A., 1997. Reduction of serum cholesterol in postmenopausal women with previous myocardial infarction and cholesterol malabsorption induced by dietary sitostanol ester margarine: women and dietary sitostanol. Circulation 96, 4226–4231.

Heinemann, T., Axtmann, G., von Bergmann, K., 1993. Comparison of intestinal absorption of cholesterol with different plant sterols in man. European Journal of Clinical Investigation 23, 827–831.

Hernandez-Perera, O., Perez-Sala, D., Navarro-Antolin, J., et al., 1998. Effects of the 3-hydroxy-3-methylglutaryl-CoA reductase inhibitors, atorvastatin and simvastatin, on the expression of endothelin-1 and endothelial nitric oxide synthase in vascular endothelial cells. Journal of Clinical Investigation 101, 2711–2719.

Igel, M., Giesa, U., Lutjohann, D., von Bergmann, K., 2003. Comparison of the intestinal uptake of cholesterol, plant sterols, and stanols in mice. Journal of Lipid Research 44, 533–538.

Katan, M.B., Grundy, S.M., Jones, P., Law, M., Miettinen, T., Paoletti, R., 2003. Efficacy and safety of plant stanols and sterols in the management of blood cholesterol levels. Mayo Clinic Proceedings 78, 965–978.

Krum, H., Ashton, E., Reid, C., et al., 2007a. Double-blind, randomized, placebo-controlled study of high-dose HMG CoA reductase inhibitor therapy on ventricular remodeling, pro-inflammatory cytokines and neurohormonal parameters in patients with chronic systolic heart failure. Journal of Cardiac Failure 13, 1–7.

Krum, H., Latini, R., Maggioni, A.P., et al., 2007b. Statins and symptomatic chronic systolic heart failure: a post-hoc analysis of 5010 patients enrolled in Val-HeFT. International Journal of Cardiology 119, 48–53.

Lutjohann, D., Bjorkhem, I., Beil, U.F., von Bergmann, K., 1995. Sterol absorption and sterol balance in phytosterolemia evaluated by deuterium-labeled sterols: effect of sitostanol treatment. Journal of Lipid Research 36, 1763–1773.

Miettinen, T.A., Puska, P., Gylling, H., Vanhanen, H., Vartiainen, E., 1995. Reduction of serum cholesterol with sitostanol-ester margarine in a mildly hypercholesterolemic population. The New England Journal of Medicine 333, 1308–1312.

Molyneux, S.L., Florkowski, C.M., George, P.M., et al., 2008. Coenzyme Q10: an independent predictor of mortality in chronic heart failure. Journal of the American College of Cardiology 52, 1435–1441.

National Cholesterol Education Program (NCEP), 2001. Executive Summary of the Third Report of the National Cholesterol Education Program (NCEP) Expert Panel on Detection, Evaluation, and Treatment of High Blood Cholesterol in Adults (Adult Treatment Panel III). Journal of the American Medical Association 285, 2486–2497.

Noakes, M., Clifton, P., Ntanios, F., Shrapnel, W., Record, I., McInerney, J., 2002. An increase in dietary carotenoids when consuming plant sterols or stanols is effective in maintaining plasma carotenoid concentrations. American Journal of Clinical Nutrition 75, 79–86.

Patel, S.B., Salen, G., Hidaka, H., et al., 1998. Mapping a gene involved in regulating dietary cholesterol absorption. The sitosterolemia locus is found at chromosome 2p21. Journal of Clinical Investigation 102, 1041–1044.

Rosamond, W., Flegal, K., Furie, K., et al., 2008. Heart disease and stroke statistics – 2008 update: a report from the American Heart Association Statistics Committee and Stroke Statistics Subcommittee. Circulation 117, e25–146.

Salo, P., Wester, I., 2005. Low-fat formulations of plant stanols and sterols. The American Journal of Cardiology 96, 51D–54D.

Serebruany, V.L., 2008. Controlled rosuvastatin multinational trial in heart failure (the positive negative trial). The American Journal of Cardiology 101, 1808–1809.

Simons, L.A., 2002. Additive effect of plant sterol-ester margarine and cerivastatin in lowering low-density lipoprotein cholesterol in primary hypercholesterolemia. The American Journal of Cardiology 90, 737–740.

Spilburg, C.A., Goldberg, A.C., McGill, J.B., et al., 2003. Fat-free foods supplemented with soy stanol-lecithin powder reduce cholesterol absorption and LDL cholesterol. Journal of the American Dietetic Association 103, 577–581.

Sudhop, T., Gottwald, B.M., von Bergmann, K., 2002a. Serum plant sterols as a potential risk factor for coronary heart disease. Metabolism 51, 1519–1521.

Sudhop, T., Sahin, Y., Lindenthal, B., et al., 2002b. Comparison of the hepatic clearances of campesterol, sitosterol, and cholesterol in healthy subjects suggests that efflux transporters controlling intestinal sterol absorption also regulate biliary secretion. Gut 51, 860–863.

Tavazzi, L., Maggioni, A.P., Marchioli, R., et al., 2008. Effect of rosuvastatin in patients with chronic heart failure (the GISSI-HF trial): a randomised, double-blind, placebo-controlled trial. Lancet 372, 1231–1239.

Tousoulis, D., Antoniades, C., Bosinakou, E., et al., 2005. Effects of atorvastatin on reactive hyperemia and inflammatory process in patients with congestive heart failure. Atherosclerosis 178, 359–363.

Velavan, P., Huan Loh, P., Clark, A., Cleland, J.G., 2007. The cholesterol paradox in heart failure. Congestive Heart Failure 13, 336–341.

Weingartner, O., Lutjohann, D., Ji, S., et al., 2008. Vascular effects of diet supplementation with plant sterols. Journal of the American College of Cardiology 51, 1553–1561.

Weststrate, J.A., Meijer, G.W., 1998. Plant sterol-enriched margarines and reduction of plasma total- and LDL-cholesterol concentrations in normocholesterolaemic and mildly hypercholesterolaemic subjects. European Journal of Clinical Nutrition 52, 334–343.

CHAPTER 4

Bioactive Nutrients and Cardiovascular Disease

V. Juturu*,‡, J.J. Gormley†

*United Bio-Med Inc., Dobbs Ferry, NY, USA
†Gormley NPI Consulting, Riverdale, NY, USA
‡Avon Products, Inc., Suffern, NY

Coronary heart disease (CHD) accounts for the majority of cardiovascular disease (CVD) deaths in men and women. Strategies known to reduce the burden of CHD may have substantial benefits for the prevention of non-coronary atherosclerosis. CVD is an abnormal function of the heart or blood vessels. The abnormal function of the heart and blood vessels increases the risk for heart attack, heart failure, sudden death, stroke, and cardiac rhythm problems, thus resulting in decreased quality of life and decreased life expectancy. The causes of CVD range from structural defects to infection, inflammation, environment, and genetics. CVD is marked by or measured by many factors, including the following:

- Obesity
- Hypertension
- Dyslipidemia
- Impaired glucose tolerance
- Increase in inflammatory markers such as C-reactive protein (CRP)
- Cytokines
- Tumor necrosis factor alpha (TNFα)
- Interleukins 6 and 10 (IL-6 and IL-10)
- Changes in cell adhesion molecules
- Prothrombotic and fibrinolytic changes
- Increases in oxidative stress
- Endothelial dysfunction

The greater the number of reported risk factors the more likely will an individual be to develop heart disease. Some risk factors are modifiable such as diet and lifestyle. Improvements can help reduce major risk factors and reduce the risk of CHD. Other factors are non-modifiable, such as age and sex, and contribute to a higher risk score of CHD. The risk categories are based on guidelines established by the National Cholesterol Education Program (NIH NHLBI, 2004; Adult Treatment Panel, 2011):

- Highest risk: A risk score of more than 20% (history of heart disease and or diabetes).
- High risk: A risk score of 10–20% (two or more risk factors).

Bioactive Food as Dietary Interventions for Cardiovascular Disease
http://dx.doi.org/10.1016/B978-0-12-396485-4.00003-7

© 2013 Elsevier Inc.
All rights reserved.

- Moderate risk: A risk score below 10% (two or more risk factors).
- Low risk: One or no risk factors.

Growing evidence suggests that aggressive, comprehensive treatment for risk factors will improve survival and reduce recurring events. In addition, several interventional procedures will improve quality of life. This review will focus on the metabolic advantages of bioactive nutrients for the prevention of CVD.

1. BIOACTIVE NUTRIENTS

1.1 Nuts and Seeds

1.1.1 Omega-3 fatty acids

Nuts (e.g., walnuts) and vegetable oils (e.g., canola, soybean, flaxseed/linseed, and olive) contain alpha-linolenic acid. The polyunsaturated fatty acid compositions of different nuts and seeds are shown in Table 4.1. Dietary fish or fish oil supplements have been shown to lower triglycerides, reduce the risk of death, heart attacks, dangerous abnormal heart rhythms, and strokes in people with known CVD, and also slow the buildup of atherosclerotic plaques and lower blood pressure slightly.

A number of possible antiarrhythmic actions from long chain n-3 PUFA have been found in animal and laboratory studies, mainly on ventricular arrhythmias. Fish oil may prevent the development of atrial fibrillation in patients with symptomatic heart disease or prevent relapses of atrial fibrillation in patients with paroxysmal atrial fibrillation. It may also significantly reduce cardiac arrhythmias and heart rate variability (Archer et al., 1998). Several prospective controlled randomized studies have evaluated the use of omega-3 fatty acids (2.25–7.2 g/day) for preventing restenosis following coronary angioplasty produced neutral results. Overall, in one study restenosis was reduced by 13.9% (Gapinski et al., 1993).

Omega-3 fatty acids may reduce sudden death from heart disease (Kris-Etherton et al., 2002, 2003). Daily intake of omega-3 fatty acids for a mean duration of 37 months decreased all causes of mortality by 16% and the incidence of death due to MI by 24%. Mozaffarian et al. (2003) reported that trends for increased cardiac events were observed with increasing consumption of fried fish or fish sandwiches. Omega-3 fatty acids reduce platelet aggregation, including reactivity and adhesion, vasoconstriction, and enhanced fibrinolysis and reduce fibrin formation (Juturu, 2008). There is growing evidence that n-3 PUFA can directly or indirectly influence the induction of messenger RNA encoding cell surface molecules. There is convincing evidence that omega-3 fatty acids have beneficial effects on the prevention of cardiovascular risk complications.

1.1.2 Plant sterols and stanols, soy protein and isoflavones

Plant sterols and stanols are naturally present in small quantities in many fruits, vegetables, nuts, seeds, cereals, legumes, vegetable oils, and other plant sources. Phytosterols, which

Table 4.1 Polyunsaturated Fatty Acid Composition of Different Fishes, Nuts, and Seeds

	PUFA (g)			
Fish and nuts	n-6	n-3	EPA	DHA
Fish				
Salmon, Coho	0.089	0.089	0.491	1.385
Atlantic mackerel	0.219	0.159	0.898	1.401
Atlantic herring	0.130	0.103	0.709	0.862
Whitefish species	0.272	0.183	0.317	0.941
Haddock	0.009	0.002	0.059	0.126
Swordfish	0.029	0.186	0.108	0.531
Smelt, rainbow	0.045	0.049	0.275	0.418
Ocean perch	0.028	0.057	0.080	0.211
Flounder and sole species	0.008	0.008	0.093	0.106
Oyster, Eastern	0.028	0.044	0.188	0.203
Crab, blue	0.012	0.000	0.000	0.150
Lobster, Northern	0.004	0.000	0.090	0.108
Scallop species	0.053	0.000	0.283	0.890
Tuna, blue fin	3.543	0.498	0.473	0.509
Sardines, Atlantic	0.050	0.034	0.419	0.586
Salmon, pink	0.005	0.001	0.064	0.120
Cod, Atlantic	0.876	0.096	0.067	0.207
Cat fish, farmed	0.028	0.014	0.258	0.222
Shrimp	0.016	0.004	0.069	0.073
Nuts[a]				
Almonds	12.2	0.00	0.000	0.000
Brazil nuts	20.5	0.05	0.000	0.000
Cashew nuts	7.7	0.15	0.000	0.000
Hazelnuts	7.8	0.09	0.000	0.000
Macadamia nuts	1.3	0.21	0.000	0.000
Peanuts	15.6	0.00	0.000	0.000
Pecans	20.6	1.00	0.000	0.000
Pine nuts (dried)	33.2	0.16	0.000	0.000
Pistachios	13.2	0.25	0.000	0.000
Walnuts	38.1	9.08	0.000	0.000

Source: US Department of Agriculture Nutrient Database, http://www.nal.usda.gov/fnic/cgi-bin/nut_search.pl (accessed 08 March 2008).
[a] Data for raw nuts, except when specified. PUFA, polyunsaturated fatty acids; EPA, eicosapentaenoic acid; DHA, docosahexaenoic acid.

are found in all plant foods (the highest concentrations are found in unrefined plant oils, including vegetable, nut, and olive oils), are plant-derived stanols and sterols that are similar in structure and function to cholesterol. Table 4.2 provides the phytosterol content in different foods. Plant sterols or stanols are esterified by creating an ester bond between

Table 4.2 Total Phytosterol Content of Selected Foods

Food	Serving (g)	Phytosterols (mg)
Wheat germ	½ cup (57)	197
Corn oil	1 tablespoon (14)	102
Canola oil	1 tablespoon (14)	91
Peanuts	1 ounce (28)	62
Wheat bran	½ cup (29)	58
Almonds	1 ounce (28)	34
Brussels sprouts	½ cup (78)	34
Rye bread	2 slices (64)	33
Macadamia nuts	1 ounce (28)	33
Olive oil	1 tablespoon (14)	22
Take Control® spread	1 tablespoon (14)	1650 mg plant sterol esters (1000 mg free sterols)
Benecol® spread	1 tablespoon (14)	850 mg plant stanol esters (500 mg free stanols)

Source: US Department of Agriculture, Agricultural Research Service. USDA Nutrient Database for Standard Reference, Release 17, 2004.

a fatty acid and the sterol or stanol to make them more fat-soluble so they are easily incorporated into fat-containing foods such as margarines and salad dressings.

Plant sterols, stanols, esterified sterols or stanols, and mixtures are available both as supplemented foods (such as margarines or yogurts) and as dietary supplements (such as soft gels or tablets). Plant sterols and stanols have been incorporated into regular margarine, rapeseed oil (canola oil) margarine, rapeseed oil mayonnaise, reduced-fat spread and salad dressing, chocolate, butter, low-fat yogurt, reduced-fat spread, and beverages. Plant stanols are also available as a soft gel formulation. However, the efficacy is not well established. Scientific studies show that 1.3 g/day of plant sterol esters or 3.4 g/day of plant stanol esters in the diet are needed to show a significant cholesterol-lowering effect.

In order to qualify for the Food and Drug Administration (FDA) health claim, a food must contain at least 0.65 g of plant sterol esters per serving or at least 1.7 g of plant stanol esters per serving. The claim must specify that the daily dietary intake of plant sterol esters or plant stanol esters should be consumed in two servings, eaten at different times of the day with other foods (FDA, 1999). Dietary plant stanols and sterols have been found to inhibit the absorption of cholesterol in the small intestine by 50% and decrease LDL cholesterol by 14% (Spilburg et al., 2003). Stanols and sterols have been well tolerated in numerous clinical trials involving more than 1800 people, with doses up to 25 g/day. The significance of stanols and sterols on lipids suggests that 25 g/day of soy protein can be recommended to people with dyslipidemia and hypercholesterolemia (HC). The most frequently reported adverse events with plant stanols and sterols were gastrointestinal symptoms. No significant increase in liver enzymes was observed.

Table 4.3 Summary of the Potential Health Benefits of Bioactive Nutrients

Risk factors	Potential beneficial effects
Abnormal Lipid metabolism	↑ HDL-C
	↓ Postprandial lipemia; oxidation of LDL
Hypertension	↑ LDL-C
Endothelial-derived relaxation factor	Retards growth of atherosclerotic plaques
	↓ Arterial vasoconstrictor response
Arterial pressure	↓ Blood pressure
Microcirculation	Promotes nitric oxide induced endothelial relaxation
Glycemic control	↑ Increases dermal microcirculation and oxygen saturation
Hypercoagulation	↑ Postprandial insulin secretion
Thromboxane A_2	↓ Blood glucose
Prostacyclin	↓ Platelet aggregation, vasoconstriction, increases intracellular calcium ions
Tissue-plasminogen activator	↑ Prevents platelet aggregation, vasodilator, increases cyclic AMP
Fibrinogen	↑ Increases endogenous fibrinolysis
Red blood cell deformability	↓ Blood clotting factor
	↓ Decreases tendency to thrombosis and improves oxygen delivery to tissues
Platelet activating factor	Modulate cell adhesion molecules
Leukotriene B_4	↓ Activates platelets
Platelet-derived growth factor	↓ Chemoattractant and mitogen for smooth muscles and macrophages
Inflammation	
Oxygen free radicals	↓ Cellular damage, enhances LDL uptake via the scavenger pathway, stimulates arachidonic acid metabolism;
Lipid hydroperoxides	
Interleukin and tumor necrosis factor	↓ Plasma F2 isoprostane, IL-2 production, TNFα; IL-1 Beta, IL-4, IL-5; ↑ TGF beta
Obesity	Data not available
Microalbuminuria*	↓ Albumin excretion rate

Table 4.3 provides potential health benefits of bioactive ingredients and risk factors.

Other plant proteins, such as soy protein and isoflavones (e.g., genistein and daidzein) have been studied for their cholesterol-lowering effects in humans. The proposed improvements associated with these nutrients include increases in LDL receptor activity, increases in the synthesis and fecal excretion of bile acids, and a suppression of cholesterol absorption. An analysis of 41 trials found soy protein significantly reduced total and LDL cholesterol and increased HDL cholesterol (Reynolds et al., 2006). A number of cardioprotective benefits have been attributed to dietary isoflavones including a reduction in LDL cholesterol, an inhibition of proinflammatory cytokines, cell adhesion proteins and inducible NO production, potential reduction in the susceptibility of the LDL particle to oxidation, inhibition of platelet aggregation, and an improvement in vascular reactivity. Therefore, it is suggested that improvements in cholesterol levels may be helpful for people with HC.

A meta-analysis (Taku et al., 2007), soy isoflavones significantly decreased serum total cholesterol by 0.10 mmol/L (1.77%) and LDL cholesterol by 0.13 mmol/L (3.58%); no significant changes in HDL cholesterol and triacylglycerol were found. Isoflavone-depleted soy protein significantly decreased LDL cholesterol by 0.10 mmol/L (2.77%). Soy protein that contained enriched isoflavones significantly decreased LDL cholesterol by 0.18 mmol/L (4.98%) and significantly increased HDL cholesterol by 0.04 mmol/L (3%). In October 1999, the FDA approved a health claim for foods that contain 6.25 g of soy protein or more, allowing manufacturers to state that 25 g/day soy protein may reduce the risk of heart disease (U.S. Food and Drug Administration, 2009).

Further studies are recommended to evaluate the effect of stanols and soy protein on cardiac events, relative risk (RR) of CVD, and metabolic risk factors. Based on the current evidence, 25 g of soy protein or a food providing at least 0.65 g sterol ester or 1.7 g stanol esters per serving can be recommended to improve coronary risk lipids and lipoproteins. In addition, 30 min of aerobic exercise per day will also help increase HDL-cholesterol levels (FDA, 2010).

1.1.3 Cocoa

Cocoa is the dried and partially fermented fatty seed of the cacao tree. Cocoa powder is the dry powder made by grinding cocoa seeds and removing the cocoa butter from the dark, bitter cocoa solids. It may also refer to the combination of both cocoa powder and cocoa butter together. Cocoa powder is rich in polyphenols such as catechins and procyanidins. Cocoa, cocoa extracts, and purified cocoa flavanols and procyanidins exert strong antioxidant effects *in vitro*. Inhibition of LDL oxidation was reported within 2 h after the consumption of a flavanol-rich cocoa product (Kondo et al., 1996). Flavanol-rich cocoa and chocolate have the potential to augment an individual's antioxidant defense system; improvements in inflammation, platelet aggregation, and nitric oxide-mediated endothelial changes are additional factors that can be achieved by flavonols (Erdman et al., 2007). These nutrients have been shown to affect numerous intracellular signaling cascades and to influence the cardiovascular system by enhancing vascular function and decreasing platelet reactivity. Although short-term clinical trials have been reported on the beneficial effects of these nutrients, long-term, randomized, clinical trials are warranted.

In a double-blind study, 160 subjects who ingested either cocoa powder-containing low-polyphenolic compounds (placebo-cocoa group) or three levels of cocoa powder-containing high-polyphenolic compounds (13, 19.5, and 26 g/day for low-, middle-, and high-cocoa groups, respectively) for 4 weeks were examined. The test powders were consumed as a beverage after the addition of hot water, twice each day. A stratified analysis was performed on 131 subjects who had LDL cholesterol concentrations of ≥3.23 mmol/L at baseline. In these subjects, plasma LDL cholesterol, oxidized LDL, and apoB concentrations decreased, and the plasma HDL cholesterol concentration increased, relative to baseline in the low-, middle-, and high-cocoa groups (Baba et al., 2007). Brachial artery hyperemic blood flow increased significantly by 76% ($p < 0.05$ vs. baseline) after the 6-week cocoa intervention in the high-cocoa flavanols (CF) group (high-CF—446 mg of total flavanols), compared with 32% in the low-CF group ([low-CF—43 mg of total flavanols] $p =$ ns vs. baseline). The 2.4-fold increase in hyperemic blood flow with high-CF cocoa closely correlated ($r^2 = 0.8$) with a significant decrease (11%) in plasma levels of soluble vascular cell adhesion molecule-1 (Wang-Polagruto et al., 2006).

Wan et al. (2001) reported a randomized, two-period, crossover study in 23 healthy subjects fed two diets: an average American diet (AAD) controlled for fiber, caffeine, and theobromine and an AAD supplemented with 22 g cocoa powder and 16 g dark chocolate (CP-DC diet), providing approximately 466 mg procyanidins/day. LDL oxidation lag time was approximately 8% greater ($p = 0.01$) after the CP-DC diet than after the AAD. Serum total antioxidant capacity measured by oxygen radical absorbance capacity was approximately 4% greater ($p = 0.04$) after the CP-DC diet than after the AAD and was positively correlated with LDL oxidation lag time ($r = 0.32$, $p = 0.03$). HDL cholesterol was 4% greater after the CP-DC diet ($p = 0.02$) than after the AAD; however, LDL–HDL ratios were not significantly different. Twenty-four-hour urinary excretion of thromboxane B(2) and 6-keto-prostaglandin F(1) (alpha) and the ratio of the two compounds were not significantly different between the two diets.

Cocoa powder and dark chocolate may favorably affect CVD risk factors by reducing LDL oxidation susceptibility, and enhancing serum total antioxidant capacity and HDL-cholesterol concentrations, while improving endothelial function. The current studies suggest that 40–100 g of flavonoid-rich dark chocolate may decrease arterial hypertension. Dark chocolate induces coronary vasodilation, improves coronary vascular function, and decreases platelet adhesion 2 h after consumption. These changes reduce oxidative stress.

1.1.3.1 Safety

Consumption of polyphenols inhibits nonheme iron absorption and may lead to iron depletion in populations with marginal iron stores (Temme et al., 2002). Polyphenols may interact with certain pharmaceutical agents and enhance their biologic effects. Proanthocyanidins (condensed tannins) and ellagitannins have been considered anti-nutritional compounds, particularly in animal nutrition, because they are able to interact with proteins and inhibit several enzymes.

1.2 Oats

The common oat plant (*Avena sativa*) is a species of cereal grain grown for its seed, which is known by the same name, usually in the plural, unlike other grains. Oats are suitable for human consumption as oat meal and rolled oats. Eight clinical trials found that oat meal consumption for at least 4 weeks was associated with lower total cholesterol and LDL cholesterol (Kelly et al., 2007). Soluble fiber found in oats specifically helps to lower blood levels of small, dense LDL cholesterol that has been shown to increase the risk for heart attacks. Oats are a particularly good source of soluble fiber. Six grams of beta-glucan from oats and moderate physical activity improve lipid profile and can reduce the risk of cardiovascular events. A diet with added beta-glucan was well accepted and tolerated. Oat bran concentrate bread products improve glycemic, insulinemic, and lipidemic responses as well in diabetes. A daily dose of 50–70 g/day is suggested to meet the requirements to improve glycemic and lipidemic responses.

1.2.1 Psyllium

Psyllium husk comes from the crushed seeds of the *Plantago ovata* plant, an herb native to parts of Asia, the Mediterranean, and North Africa. Psyllium is very rich in soluble fiber. An analysis of eight clinical trials found that daily psyllium for at least 6 weeks lowered total cholesterol and LDL cholesterol compared to placebo (Anderson et al., 2000). In 1998, FDA approved the following health claim for psyllium: '3–12 g soluble fiber from psyllium seed husk when included as part of a diet low in saturated fat and cholesterol may reduce the risk of heart disease.'

1.2.2 Garlic

Garlic (*Allium sativum*) contains more than 200 chemical compounds. Some of the more important ones include volatile oil with sulfur-containing compounds (allicin, alliin, and ajoene) and enzymes (allinase, peroxidase, and myrosinase). The allyl contained in garlic is also found in several members of the onion family and is considered a valuable therapeutic compound. The allicins contained in garlic have a fibrinolytic activity that reduces platelet aggregation by inhibiting prostaglandin E_2. *A. sativum* has also exerted some effect on glucose tolerance for both hypo- and hyperglycemia by reducing insulin requirements to control blood sugar. The compounds contained in garlic have also demonstrated their ability to lower total serum cholesterol and triglyceride levels while elevating HDL levels. LDL synthesis is suppressed by garlic. B-vitamins, especially B-1 (thiamin), vitamin C, vitamin A, flavonoids, ascorbic acid, phosphorous, potassium, sulfur, selenium, calcium, magnesium, germanium, sodium, iron, manganese, and trace iodine, and essential amino acids are found in garlic.

An analysis of 10 trials found garlic to be effective at reducing total cholesterol, LDL, and triglycerides (Alder et al., 2003). A study by Gardner et al. (2007), reported that including raw garlic, when given at an approximate dose of a 4 g clove per day, 6 days/week for 6 months, had statistically or clinically significant effects on LDL cholesterol or other plasma lipid concentrations in adults with moderate HC. Dosages generally recommended in the literature for adults are 4 g (one to two cloves) of raw garlic per day, one 300 mg dried garlic powder tablet (standardized to 1.3% alliin or 0.6% allicin yield) two to three times per day, or 7.2 g of aged garlic extract per day. Further large clinical trials are required and its interaction with cholesterol-lowering drugs are encouraged before we recommend for CVD patients.

1.2.3 Policicosanol

Policosanol is a mixture of essential alcohols isolated from sugar cane wax (*Saccharum officinarum* L.) that consists of different components such as octacosanol (66%), hexacosanol (7%), triacontanol (12%), and eicosanol, tetracosanol, nonacosanol, dotriacontanol, tetratriacontanol, and heptacosanol (15%). It is not clear whether policosanol inhibits 3-hydroxyl-3 methyl glutaryl CoA reductase or increases receptor-mediated uptake of LDL cholesterol by the liver that may improve LDL metabolism (Menendez et al., 1994).

Cholesterol-lowering effects were observed in healthy volunteers, patients with type 2 HC, type 2 diabetes mellitus (type 2 DM) with HC, postmenopausal women with HC, and patients with combined HC and abnormal liver function tests (Castaño et al., 2004). Castaño et al. (2000) reported that after 24 weeks, 20 and 40 mg/day of policosanol significantly lowered LDL cholesterol by 27.4% and 28.1%, TC by 15.6% and 17.3%, and the LDL cholesterol/HDL cholesterol ratio by 37.2% and 36.5%, respectively. The ratio of TC/HDL cholesterol was lowered by 27.1% and 27.5%, while HDL cholesterol levels increased by 17.6% and 17.0%, respectively. A study by Mas et al. (2004) found that policosanol lowered LDL cholesterol (29.5%), TC (21.9%), TG (16.9%), and raised HDL cholesterol (12.4%) in older patients with type 2 DM. In addition, a few short-term studies indicated that the cholesterol-lowering effect of policosanol was better than that of statins such as simvastatin, pravastatin, lovastatin, probucol, or acipimox and had fewer side effects in patients with type 2 HC (Mas et al., 2004; Crespo et al., 1999; Castaño et al., 2000). Overall, policosanol has been well tolerated in numerous clinical trials in Cuban populations (more than 1200 people), with doses up to 40 mg/day. Policosanol has also been more effective in lipid lowering than other agents, with no significant effects on blood glucose, glycosylated hemoglobin $A1_C$, BP, abdominal obesity, or body weight. Further research is needed to determine the effects in other population groups including glycemic control, metabolic syndrome risk, RR of CVD, and cardiac events.

1.2.3.1 Safety

There are no studies available for policosanol interacting with other antiplatelet or anticoagulant drugs, such as clopidogrel, dalteparin, LMWH, heparin, and Coumadin®. The frequency of serious adverse events, mostly vascular, in policosanol patients (3.1%) was lower than in the placebo group (14.0%).

1.2.4 Tomatoes

Lycopene is a bright red carotenoid pigment, a phytochemical found in tomatoes and other red fruits. Lycopene is the most common carotenoid in the human body and is one of the most potent carotenoid antioxidants. A study of 31 subjects found 8 weeks of tomato extract significantly reduced systolic and diastolic BP (Engelhard et al., 2006). The Kuopio Ischaemic Heart Disease Risk Factor Study (Rissanen et al., 2001) showed that men in the lowest quartile of serum lycopene had more than a threefold risk of acute coronary event or stroke during a 5-year follow-up relative to higher concentrations. Intake of five or more servings of tomato sauce per week was significantly protective compared to tomato sauce eaten less than once per month. Because cooked tomato products, particularly those prepared with oil, are more readily absorbed, it appears that lycopene may be more available from such products than from fresh tomatoes. In CVD studies, 1243 g of 6% lycopene oleoresin capsules daily has been studied. Further studies are recommended to explore longer term lycopene supplementation and the incidence of cardiac events.

1.2.5 Onion

Garden onions, bulb onions, or shallots, *Allium cepa*, have been used as a heart tonic, blood purifier, antiseptic, digestive aid, sedative, and aphrodisiac. An onion a day will boost HDL level, lower BP by inhibiting platelet aggregation, and dissolve formed clots by stimulating the fibrinolytic system (Kawamoto et al., 2004). Research is very limited and it is difficult to extrapolate for prevention of CVD. Further long-term clinical trials are required to support the efficacy of ginger and onions on CVD risk factors.

1.2.6 Antioxidants

Antioxidants, found primarily in fruits and vegetables, nuts, and whole grains are substances that may protect cells against the effects of free radicals. Free radicals are molecules produced when the body breaks down food or by environmental exposures such as tobacco smoke and radiation. The Antioxidant Supplementation in Atherosclerosis Prevention study demonstrated that combined supplementation with reasonable doses of both vitamin E and slow-release vitamin C can retard the progression of common carotid atherosclerosis in men (Salonen et al., 2000). Antioxidants and CVD is controversial and inconclusive. Based on the current literature, it is difficult to support the efficacy of antioxidants for CVD risk factors. Few studies on long-term intervention are increasing the risk of CVD. Hence, long-term prevention clinical trials are required for antioxidants.

1.2.7 Other plants

Other plants such as brewer's yeast, buckwheat, broccoli and other related greens, okra, peas, fenugreek seeds, and sage have been found to help people with type 2 diabetes (de Munter et al., 2007). Most plant foods are rich in fiber, which is beneficial for helping control blood glucose levels. Some promising results on polyphenols suggest that it might be helpful to reduce cholesterol levels. However, long-term clinical trials are required and also the dose effective studies are encouraged.

1.3 Polyphenols and Dietary Flavonoids

Plant polyphenols, a large group of natural antioxidants found primarily in fruits and vegetables as flavonoids and phenolic acids, appear to have protective effects on heart disease (Lehtonen et al., 2011). Polyphenols have demonstrated several effects, including promoting scavenging of free radicals, regulating NO, decreasing leukocyte mobilization, inducing apoptosis, inhibiting cell proliferation and angiogenesis, and phytoestrogenic activity (Scalbert et al., 2005). Regular consumption of fruits and vegetables, which are rich in flavonoids, is associated to a reduction in cardiovascular events. The potential antiplatelet effect of flavonoids, focusing on the various platelet signaling pathways modulated by flavonoids, including oxidative stress, protein tyrosine phosphorylation, calcium mobilization, and nitric oxide pathway (El Haouari and Rosado 2011).

Flavonoids are a large family of polyphenolic compounds synthesized by plants. Dietary sources of flavonoids include tea, red wine, fruits, vegetables, and legumes. Dietary flavonoids found primarily in green tea and red wine (Hertog et al., 1997) may protect against CVD, but evidence is still conflicting.

1.3.1 Tea

Tea is the major source of flavonoids in Western populations and is the most widely consumed beverage in the world, second only to water. Tea polyphenols, known as catechins, usually account for 30–42% of the dry weight of the solids in brewed green tea. The four major catechins found in green tea are epigallocatechin gallate, epigallocatechin, epicatechin gallate, and epicatechin. Catechins can increase the antioxidant capacity of human plasma, which could help reduce CVD risk (Scalbert et al., 2005). The major components of black tea (the fermented product) are theaflavins (1–3% dry weight) and thearubigins (10–40% dry weight). It is not clear whether both green and black tea have similar beneficial effects on heart disease. More controlled clinical trials are required to show the risk reduction associated with tea. There is increasing evidence that flavonoids may have beneficial effects on endothelial control of thrombosis, inflammation, and vascular tone.

1.3.2 Coenzyme Q10

Coenzyme Q10 (CoQ10) a fat-soluble compound primarily synthesized by the body and also consumed in the diet, is a member of the ubiquinone family of compounds. Rich sources of dietary CoQ10 include meat, poultry, and fish. Other relatively rich sources include soybean and canola oils, and nuts. Fruits, vegetables, eggs, and dairy products are moderate sources of CoQ10 (Mattila et al., 2001). Most trials reported in the literature are small or not well designed. Additional research is needed to study the effects of CoQ10 on the quality of life, hospitalization and death rates, before recommendations can be made.

Table 4.4 Prevention Approaches for Reducing. Modifiable and Non-modifiable Cardiovascular Risk Factors
Modifiable Risk Factors

Diet and exercise	• Maintain ideal body weight.
	• Consume a well balanced nutritional diet and exercise regularly.
Abdominal obesity: BMI/WHR/visceral adiposity	• Reduce calories.
	• Exercise regularly.
	• Consume a high fiber diet.
	• Consume a low-fat diet.
	• No sodas/alcoholic beverages/soft drinks.
Dyslipidemia: Lipids and lipoproteins	• Reduce calories.
Small dense low-density lipoprotein (LDL)	• Lower saturated fatty acids.
Lipoprotein(a)[a]	• No trans-fatty acids.
Remnant lipoproteins	• Increase omega-3 fatty acids.
Apolipoproteins A1 and B	• Increase MUFA.
High-density lipoprotein subtypes	• Increase fruits, vegetables, and nuts.
Oxidized LDL	• Increase fiber.
	• Increase regular exercise.
	• Increase complex carbohydrates.
Glycemic Control: insulin resistance/impaired glucose tolerance	• Reduce calories.
	• Reduce simple sugars and carbohydrates.
	• Consume low glycemic diet.
	• Reduce total fat.
	• Increase dietary fiber.
	• Increase fruits and vegetables.
	• Increase MUFA.
	• Increase regular exercise.
	• Reduce sodas/soft drinks/alcoholic beverages.
Blood pressure and target organ damage/ endothelial function	• Reduce calories.
Heart	• Increase dietary fiber.
LVH	• Increase fruits and vegetables.
Angina/prior MI	• Reduce saturated fatty acids.
Prior coronary revascularization	• Increase MUFA.
Heart failure	• Reduce sodium and alcohol.
Brain	
Stroke or transient ischemic attack	
Dementia	
CKD	
Peripheral arterial disease	
Retinopathy	
Inflammatory markers	• Increase dietary fiber.
C-reactive protein	• Increase fruits and vegetables.

Continued

Table 4.4 Prevention Approaches for Reducing. Modifiable and Non-modifiable Cardiovascular Risk Factors—cont'd
Modifiable Risk Factors

Interleukins (e.g., IL-6)	• Reduce saturated fatty acids.
Serum amyloid A	• Increase MUFA.
Vascular and cellular adhesion molecules	• Increase omega-3 fatty acids.
Soluble CD40 ligand	
Leukocyte count	
Hemostasis/thrombosis markers	• Increase dietary fiber.
Fibrinogen	• Increase fruits and vegetables.
von Willebrand factor antigen	• Reduce saturated fatty acids.
Plasminogen activator inhibitor 1 (PAI-1)	
Tissue-plasminogen activator	• Increase MUFA.
Factors V, VII, and VIII	
D-dimer	
Fibrinopeptide A	
Prothrombin fragment 1+2	
Platelet-Related Factors	• Increase dietary fiber.
Platelet aggregation	• Increase fruits and vegetables.
Platelet activity	• Reduce saturated fatty acids.
Platelet size and volume	• Increase MUFA.
Smoking	• Do not smoke and avoid tobacco.
Stress	• Incorporate some type of exercise daily.
	• Eat a healthful diet rich in fruits, vegetables and whole grains.
	• Use alcohol only in moderation.
	• Create quiet time, meditate, pray, read, yoga and/or other relaxation techniques.
	• Use biofeedback to manage stress.
	• Use family, friends and fellow workers as support system. Talking about problems can help express feelings and reduce conflict.
Other factors	• Increase dietary fiber.
Homocysteine	• Increase fruits and vegetables.
Lipoprotein-associated phospholipase A(2)	• Reduce saturated fatty acids.
Microalbuminuria	• Increase MUFA.
Insulin resistance	• Increase folic acid and B complex vitamins.
PAI-1 genotype	
Angiotensin-converting enzyme genotype	
ApoE genotype	
Infectious agents: Cytomegalovirus, *Chlamydia pneumonia*, *Helicobacter pylori*, Herpes simplex virus	
Psychosocial factors	

Continued

Table 4.4 Prevention Approaches for Reducing. Modifiable and Non-modifiable Cardiovascular Risk Factors—cont'd
Modifiable Risk Factors

Non-modifiable risk factors	
Family history/genes	• Record medical history. • Regular screening of lipids, glucose and blood pressure. • Maintain body weight. • Increase regular physical exercise.
Age	• Regular screening of lipids, glucose and blood pressure. • Maintain body weight. • Increase regular physical exercise.
Sex: male/female	• Regular screening of lipids, glucose and blood pressure. • Maintain body weight • Increase regular physical exercise.

Source: Juturu, V., 2008, in press, Antioxidants and cardiovascular disease. Handbook of Nutrition in the Aged. In: Watson, R. (Ed.) fourth ed., Taylor and Francis.
CKD, chronic kidney disease; CVD, cardiovascular disease; GFR, glomerular filtration rate; HDL, high-density lipoprotein; LDL, low-density lipoprotein; LVH, left ventricular hypertrophy; MI, myocardial infarction; MUFA, monounsaturated fatty acids.
[a] Lipoprotein(a) [Lp(a)] consists of an LDL-like particle and the specific apolipoprotein(a) [apo(a)], which is covalently bound to the apoB of the LDL-like particle.

The National Kidney Foundation recommends drinking one glass of cranberry juice per day to prevent urinary tract infections. Further research is required to see the pathophysiological effects of cranberries and the phytochemical compounds present in cranberries on risk factors and for the prevention of CVD.

The American Heart Association guidelines are used to improve and enhance efforts to reduce CVD and provide preventive care for men and women with a broad range of cardiovascular risk. An expert panel developed the guidelines after reviewing randomized clinical trials or large cohort studies (>1000 subjects) of CVD risk-reducing interventions, meta-analyses, and end point studies that reported at least 10 cases of major clinical CVD end points. The common clinical recommendations are lifestyle interventions, individual risk factor interventions, and drug intervention. To improve the care of persons with or at risk for CVD, initial screening and assessment of CHD risk factors should be initiated in the primary care setting.

Preventive approaches for reducing CVD modifiable and non-modifiable risk factors are listed in Table 4.4. The estimated direct and indirect cost of CVD in the United States for 2007 was $431.8 billion. Counseling on lifestyle interventions, including smoking cessation, physical activity, a heart-healthy diet, and weight maintenance, is important for all people regardless of risk level, even if only to reinforce established healthy behaviors. Everyone should be encouraged to perform at least 30 min of moderate-intensity physical activity (e.g., brisk walking) every day to maintain or achieve a healthy weight, and to eat a diet low in saturated fat, cholesterol, trans-fatty acids, and sodium, and to include a variety of fruits, vegetables, whole grains, low-fat and nonfat dairy products, legumes, and fish in the diet.

REFERENCES

Adult Treatment Panel III, 2011. Detection, Evaluation, and Treatment of High Blood Cholesterol in Adults. Available from:http://www.nhlbi.nih.gov/guidelines/cholesterol/index.htm [accessed April 2011].

Alder, R., Lookinland, S., Berry, J.A., Williams, M.A., 2003. Systematic review of the effectiveness of garlic as an anti-hyperlipidemic agent. Journal of the American Academy of Nurse Practitioners 15 (3), 120–129.

Anderson, J.W., Allgood, L.D., Lawrence, A., et al., 2000. Cholesterol-lowering effects of psyllium intake adjunctive to diet therapy in men and women with hypercholesterolemia: meta-analysis of 8 controlled trials. American Journal of Clinical Nutrition 71 (2), 472–479.

Archer, S.L., Green, D., Chamberlain, M., 1998. Association of dietary fish and n-3 fatty acid intake with hemostatic factors in the coronary artery risk development in young adults (CARDIA) study. Arteriosclerosis, Thrombosis, and Vascular Biology 18 (7), 1119–1193.

Baba, S., Natsume, M., Yasuda, A., 2007. Plasma LDL and HDL cholesterol and oxidized LDL concentrations are altered in normo- and hypercholesterolemic humans after intake of different levels of cocoa powder. Journal of Nutrition 137 (6), 1436–1441.

Castaño, G., Más, R., Fernández, L., 2000. Effects of policosanol on postmenopausal women with type II hypercholesterolemia. Gynecological Endocrinology 14 (3), 187–195.

Castaño, G., Mas, R., Gámez, R., Fernández, J., et al., 2004. Concomitant use of policosanol and beta-blockers in older patients. International Journal of Clinical Pharmacology Research 24 (2–3), 65–77.

Crespo, N., Illnait, J., Más, R., 1999. Comparative study of the efficacy and tolerability of policosanol and lovastatin in patients with hypercholesterolemia and noninsulin dependent diabetes mellitus. International Journal of Clinical Pharmacology Research 19 (4), 117–127.

de Munter, J.S., Hu, F.B., Spiegelman, D., Franz, M., van Dam, R.M., 2007. Whole grain, bran, and germ intake and risk of type 2 diabetes: a prospective cohort study and systematic review. PLoS Medicine 4 (8), e261.

El Haouari, M., Rosado, J.A., 2011. Modulation of platelet function and signaling by flavonoids. Mini Reviews in Medicinal Chemistry 11 (2), 131–142.

Engelhard, Y.N., Gazer, B., Paran, E., 2006. Natural antioxidants from tomato extract reduce blood pressure in patients with grade-1 hypertension: a double-blind, placebo-controlled pilot study. American Heart Journal 151 (1), 100.

Erdman Jr., J.W., Balentine, D., Arab, L., et al., 2007. Flavonoids and heart health: proceedings of the ILSI North America Flavonoids Workshop, May 31-June 1, 2005, Washington, DC. Journal of Nutrition 137 (3 Suppl. 1), 718S–737S.

FDA, 1999. Food labeling: health claims: soy protein and coronary heart disease. Food and Drug Administration, HHS: final rule: soy protein and coronary heart disease. Fed Reg. 64, 57700–57733.

U.S. Food and Drug Administration, 2009. Guidance for Industry: A Food Labeling Guide (11, Appendix C: Health Claims). Available from:http://www.fda.gov/Food/GuidanceComplianceRegulatoryInformation/GuidanceDocuments/FoodLabelingNutrition/FoodLabelingGuide/ucm064919.htm [accessed April 2011].

U.S. Food and Drug Administration, 2010. Controlling Cholesterol with Statins [brochure]. Available from: http://www.fda.gov/downloads/forconsumers/consumerupdates/ucm048734.pdf [accessed April 2011].

Gapinski, J.P., VanRuiswyk, J.V., Heudebert, G.R., Schectman, G.S., 1993. Preventing restenosis with fish oils following coronary angioplasty: a meta-analysis 153 (13), 1595–1601.

Gardner, C.D., Lawson, L.D., Block, E., 2007. Effect of raw garlic vs commercial garlic supplements on plasma lipid concentrations in adults with moderate hypercholesterolemia: a randomized clinical trial. Archives of Internal Medicine 167 (4), 346–353.

Hertog, M.G., Feskens, E.J., Kromhout, D., 1997. Antioxidant flavonols and coronary heart disease risk. Lancet 349 (9053), 699.

Juturu, J., 2008. Omega-3 fatty acids and the cardiometabolic syndrome. Journal of the Cardiometabolic Syndrome 3 (4), 244–253.

Kawamoto, E., Sakai, Y., Okamura, Y., Yamamoto, Y., 2004. Effects of boiling on the antihypertensive and antioxidant activities of onion. J Nutr Sci Vitaminol (Tokyo) 50 (3), 171–176.

Kelly, S.A., Summerbell, C.D., Brynes, A., 2007. Wholegrain cereals for coronary heart disease. Cochrane Database of Systematic Reviews (2), CD005051.

Kondo, K., Hirano, R., Matsumoto, A., 1996. Inhibition of LDL oxidation by cocoa. Lancet 348 (9040), 1514.

Kris-Etherton, P.M., Harris, W.S., Appel, L.J., 2002. American Heart Association Nutrition Committee. Fish consumption, fish oil, omega-3 fatty acids, and cardiovascular disease. Circulation 106 (21), 2747–2757.

Kris-Etherton, P.M., Harris, W.S., Appel, L.J., 2003. AHA Nutrition Committee. Arteriosclerosis, Thrombosis, and Vascular Biology 23 (2), 151–152.

Lehtonen, H.M., Suomela, J.P., Tahvonen, R., 2011. Different berries and berry fractions have various but slightly positive effects on the associated variables of metabolic diseases on overweight and obese women. European Journal of Clinical Nutrition 65 (3), 394–401.

Mas, R., Castaño1, G., Fernández, J., et al., 2004. Long-term effects of policosanol on obese patients with type II hypercholesterolemia. Asia Pacific Journal of Clinical Nutrition 13 (Suppl.), S102.

Mattila, K., Ristola, M., Repo, H., Asikainen, S., Metsä-Ketelä, T., 2001. Neutrophil free oxygen radical production and blood total antioxidant capacity in patients with coronary heart disease using various medications. APMIS 109 (9), 618–624.

Menendez, R., Fernandez, S.I., Del Rio, A., 1994. Policosanol inhibits cholesterol biosynthesis and enhances low density lipoprotein processing in cultured human fibroblasts. Biological Research 27 (3–4), 199–203.

Mozaffarian, D., Lemaitre, R.N., Kuller, L.H., 2003. Cardiac benefits of fish consumption may depend on the type of fish meal consumed: the Cardiovascular Health Study. Circulation 107 (10), 1372–1377.

NIH Nation Heart Lung and Blood Institute. Third Report of the Expert Panel on. Available from: http://www.nhlbi.nih.gov/guidelines/cholesterol/atp3full.pdf

Reynolds, K., China, A., Lees, K.A., 2006. A meta-analysis of the effect of soy protein supplementation on serum lipids. The American Journal of Cardiology 98 (5), 633–640.

Rissanen, T.H., Voutilainen, S., Nyyssönen, K., 2001. Low serum lycopene concentration is associated with an excess incidence of acute coronary events and stroke: the Kuopio Ischaemic Heart Disease Risk Factor Study. British Journal of Nutrition 85 (6), 749–754.

Salonen, J.T., Nyyssönen, K., Salonen, R., 2000. Antioxidant Supplementation in Atherosclerosis Prevention (ASAP) study: a randomized trial of the effect of vitamins E and C on 3-year progression of carotid atherosclerosis. Journal of Internal Medicine 248 (5), 377–386.

Scalbert, A., Johnson, I.T., Saltmarsh, M., 2005. Polyphenols: antioxidants and beyond. American Journal of Clinical Nutrition 81 (Suppl. 1), 215S–217S.

Spilburg, C.A., Goldberg, A., McGill, J.B., 2003. Fat-free foods supplemented with soy stanol-lecithin powder reduce cholesterol absorption and LDL cholesterol. Journal of the American Dietetic Association 103 (5), 577–581.

Taku, K., Umegaki, K., Sato, Y., et al., 2007. Soy isoflavones lower serum total and LDL cholesterol in humans: a meta-analysis of 11 randomized controlled trials. American Journal of Clinical Nutrition 85 (4), 1148–1156.

Temme, E.H., Van Hoydonck, P.G., Schouten, E.G., Kesteloot, H., 2002. Effects of a plant sterol-enriched spread on serum lipids and lipoproteins in mildly hypercholesterolaemic subjects. Acta Cardiologica 57 (2), 111–115.

Wan, Y., Vinson, J.A., Etherton, T.D., et al., 2001. Effects of cocoa powder and dark chocolate on LDL oxidative susceptibility and prostaglandin concentrations in humans. American Journal of Clinical Nutrition 74 (5), 596–602.

Wang-Polagruto, J.F., Villablanca, A.C., Polagruto, J.A., et al., 2006. Chronic consumption of flavanol-rich cocoa improves endothelial function and decreases vascular cell adhesion molecule in hypercholesterolemic postmenopausal women. Journal of Cardiovascular Pharmacology 47 (Suppl. 2), S177–S186.

CHAPTER 5

Vitamins and Myocardial Infarction in Diabetics

T. Jaxa-Chamiec
Postgraduate Medical School, Grochowski Hospital, Warsaw, Poland

This article is dedicated to the Memory of My Grand Teacher Professor Leszek Ceremuzynski (1932-2009), the distinguished, long-serving Head of the Department of Cardiology in the Postgraduate Medical School in Warsaw.

ABBREVIATIONS

ACS Acute coronary syndrome
AMI Acute myocardial infarction
ATP Adenosine triphosphate
BH$_4$ Tetrahydrobiopterin
CVD Cardiovascular disease
DM Diabetes mellitus
DNA Deoxyribonucleic acid
eNOS Endothelial nitric oxide synthase
LDL Low–density lipoprotein
NADH Reduced forms of nicotinamide adenine dinucleotide
NFKB Nuclear factor kappa B
NO Nitric oxide
OS Oxidative stress
RI Reperfusion injury
RNS Reactive nitrogen species
ROS Reactive oxygen species
SOD Superoxide dismutase

1. INTRODUCTION

Cardiovascular disease (CVD) remains one of the major health problems of the modern world. Acute myocardial infarction (AMI), a dramatic manifestation of CVD, is the most common cause of premature death.

It is important to limit the area of myocardial damage and to prevent the development of dangerous ventricular tachyarrhythmias in order to improve the short- and long-term prognoses of patients suffering from AMI.

It is known that diabetes is an independent risk factor in the development of CVD, including myocardial infarction and sudden cardiac death. The coexistence of diabetes may impact negatively on the course and prognosis of CVD (Zuanetti et al., 1993).

Bioactive Food as Dietary Interventions for Cardiovascular Disease
http://dx.doi.org/10.1016/B978-0-12-396485-4.00004-9

© 2013 Elsevier Inc.
All rights reserved.

Reperfusion, mechanical or pharmacological, is the current method of choice for treating patients who suffer from AMI. This method has been reported to limit the area of myocardial damage and improve the prognosis (Van deWerf et al., 2003). However, opening of an occluded artery, which is the cause of infarction, may be associated with the development of reperfusion injury (RI). This may ultimately manifest itself as necrosis of cardiomyocytes and result in the irreversible impairment of myocardial function. RI, therefore, reduces the benefits that result from restoring the patency of a coronary vessel. The mechanism of RI has not been fully elucidated. RI is caused by a number of different processes such as oxidative stress (OS), which is associated with the overproduction of reactive oxygen species (ROS) and with the exhaustion of endogenous antioxidant enzyme systems. OS accompanies both AMI (Singal et al., 1998) and diabetes mellitus (DM) (Guzik et al., 2002). ROS play a key role in the progression of myocardial damage that develops during infarction-associated ischemia and reperfusion. In addition, ROS are also some of the more important factors responsible for endothelial dysfunction. It is believed that ROS also play an important role in the initiation and progression of combined pathophysiological processes in DM.

For a number of years, a search has been conducted for clinically effective methods of limiting OS in the belief that a reduction in both RI and endothelial dysfunction would result. Undoubtedly, knowledge gained in recent decades of such combined phenomena as myocardial stunning, hibernation, preconditioning, postconditioning, or no-reflow phenomenon, in which OS plays a significant role, provides the opportunity to develop a more effective therapeutic method.

In recent decades, vitamins were among numerous substances studied that have the potential of limiting OS and RI. Some vitamins, such as C, E, and carotenoids have antioxidant properties. Others, such as vitamins B6, B12, and folic acid, are involved in the metabolism of homocysteine, a factor that has been associated with an increased risk in the premature development of CVD.

The studies conducted in the previous 20 years showed that the administration of vitamins B6, B12, and folic acid, while significantly reducing homocysteine levels, fails to decrease the risk of myocardial infarction, cerebral stroke, thrombosis, peripheral artery atherosclerosis, or cardiovascular mortality (Albert et al., 2008).

The antioxidant efficacy of vitamins such as beta-carotene, provitamin A, and vitamin A and thus their ability to prevent CVD has been controversial for many years. Currently, the predominant opinion is that long-term supplementation with both beta-carotene and vitamin A not only fails to reduce the risk of CVD but also can even increase it (Bjelakovic et al., 2007). This finding is confirmed by a review of interventional studies in the Cochrane database.

It has been claimed that vitamins C and E reduce OS by a number of different mechanisms. It is important to note that while the beneficial antioxidant effects of these vitamins are well documented in experimental studies, a large number of randomized clinical trials returned mainly negative results. Moreover, these vitamins may act synergistically by a number of different mechanisms. Finally, it has been demonstrated that it is safe to administer vitamins C and E in adequately high doses.

The aim of this chapter is to present the views on the role of OS in the pathophysiology of ischemic and RI in patients suffering from AMI and in patients with coexistent DM and to show the potential benefits of adequate administration of antioxidant vitamins C and E in such patients.

2. PATIENTS WITH MYOCARDIAL INFARCTION AND DM ARE AT PARTICULAR RISK

DM is an acknowledged risk factor in the development of CVD, including cardiovascular pathologies such as myocardial infarction, sudden cardiac death, and heart failure. It is believed that almost 80% of hospitalizations for diabetic complications in the United States are associated with CVD. CVD is estimated to be the cause of death in 44% of type I DM and 52% of type II DM. It has been demonstrated that the coexistence of diabetes has a negative impact on the course and prognosis of patients with CVD.

Data published in recent years indicate that 1.5 million people in the United States are newly diagnosed diabetic sufferers. Among patients with acute coronary syndrome (ACS), 19–23% have previously been diagnosed with DM. Another 20–22% of patients are with DM diagnosed *de novo*, and those with glucose intolerance. Therefore, hyperglycemia occurs in almost half of the patients with ACS.

Patients with DM and AMI display poorer prognoses because of greater myocardial damage, more pronounced myocardial failure, and a more frequent incidence of dangerous, life-threatening ventricular arrhythmias. The mechanism by which hyperglycemia promotes both infarction-induced damage and electric instability has not been fully elucidated. It has been shown in experimental and observational studies that intense OS in hyperglycemic patients is one of the important processes responsible for a less favorable prognosis in myocardial infarction.

3. IMPORTANCE OF OS IN MYOCARDIAL INFARCTION

3.1 Ischemia, Reperfusion – OS – Myocardial Damage

In AMI, complicated disorders develop that impair myocardial perfusion and can cause both myocardial stunning and permanent damage. The disorders are the consequence of the development of ischemia following coronary vessel occlusion (Zuanetti et al., 1993) and reperfusion (Van deWerf et al., 2003) – that is, spontaneous or therapeutic patency restoration in the previously occluded vessel.

On the basis of experimental studies, it is estimated that RI can account for 30–50% of the final myocardial necrotic area (Yellon and Hausenloy, 2007). The mechanism of RI is complicated and is associated with mitochondrial function impairment, which may lead to a reduction in the energy sources of cardiomyocytes, damage to the cytoplasmic membrane, abrupt restoration of the physiological pH value, overloading of the cell with calcium, activation of neutrophils, thrombocytes, and the complement system causing intense inflammatory reactions and cell apoptosis, and also OS. OS is a condition characterized by an imbalance between excessive production of ROS and the endogenous antioxidant enzymatic system responsible for their removal.

The mitochondrial respiratory chain is one of the sources of ROS in the body. During the complete reduction of an oxygen molecule, intermediate products of varying toxicity are formed, including superoxide (O_2^-) and hydroxyl (OH^-) free radicals. These highly reactive compounds can destroy nucleic acids (DNA), proteins, carbohydrates, and lipids, leading to cell damage.

ROS play an important role during myocardial ischemia and hypoxia. They participate in the phenomena described as silent myocardial ischemia, myocardial stunning, or hibernation.

The lipid peroxidation of the cell membrane, which accompanies AMI, is an extremely important pathophysiological phenomenon. Lipid peroxidation is also a cause of tissue damage in many other pathological processes. It is believed that this mechanism plays a major role in endothelial dysfunction and development of atherosclerotic lesions and also, as demonstrated, leads to direct myocardial injury during ischemia and reperfusion.

There is much experimental and clinical evidence suggesting that acute local myocardial ischemia, resulting from coronary artery occlusion, leads to an increased amount of lipid peroxidation products both in the ischemic area and in 'healthy' muscle surrounding it (Herbaczyńska-Cedro and Gordon-Majszak, 1989). The effect of ROS is even more pronounced after patency restoration in the artery (Maxwell and Lip, 1997).

It has been proven that the initial minutes following restoration of blood flow to the previously ischemic area are critical for the future fate of cardiomyocytes. During this time, a characteristic reperfusion-induced hypercontraction of the muscle occurs, resulting, on the one hand, from overloading the cardiomyocytes with calcium ions and, on the other, from extremely low ATP (adenosine triphosphate) concentrations, which is the consequence of prolonged ischemia (Piper et al., 2004). ROS are directly involved in these processes. They also participate in complicated mechanisms leading to edema of cardiomyocytes and their further overloading with calcium ions following acidosis, which accompanies the ischemia.

Blood flow restoration leads to an increased accumulation of blood morphotic elements, including neutrophils that are responsible for RI. Neutrophils, in turn, release ROS, numerous proteases, and proinflammatory factors and may also cause embolization of microcirculation by interaction with the endothelium. It is also believed that neutrophils participate in the induction of apoptosis.

3.2 OS – Endothelial Dysfunction

The endothelium plays a key role in vascular wall biology and the maintenance of vessel patency. Numerous biologically active substances produced by both the endothelium and blood morphotic elements (platelets and leukocytes) are responsible for maintaining blood vessel patency. These compounds have antiatherosclerotic, antiinflammatory, antithrombotic, and antioxidant properties. Nitric oxide (NO) plays a key role in these processes. Endothelial dysfunction results in reduced NO bioavailability as a consequence of reduced NO production or increased rate of inactivation of NO.

ROS are the most important NO-inactivating factors. Free radicals include ROS as well as reactive nitrogen species – derivatives of NO. These include the extremely toxic peroxynitrite molecule. The role of NO in the propagation of both RI and endothelial dysfunction is complex. Depending on local concentration, NO can be toxic or protective. The cell-damaging character of NO becomes evident after ROS-induced transformation into peroxynitrite, while the protective effect is revealed through an increase in cellular cyclic guanosine monophosphate concentration and partial respiratory chain inhibition.

If sufficient quantities of ROS are not 'scavenged' by the endogenous antioxidant enzyme systems, the amount of available NO decreases. There is increased production of peroxynitrite, in turn leading to cell damage via activation of membrane lipid peroxidation or nitrosation of protein tyrosine residues. The effect of ROS on excessive NO degradation and also their direct damaging effects on cells were demonstrated in many pathological conditions with endothelial dysfunction, such as hypercholesterolemia, DM, or arterial hypertension. In ischemic heart disease, a very strong inverse correlation was found between ROS production in the vascular wall and NO bioavailability. That, in turn, was associated with a decrease in endothelial NO synthase (eNOS) activity, oxidation of tetrahydrobiopterin (BH_4), a cofactor important for NO production, and an increase in dihydrobiopterin, which has eNOS-inhibiting properties.

4. IMPORTANCE OF OS IN DM

Evidence is available from experimental and observational studies showing that DM is accompanied by intense OS. Intense OS can lead to diabetic cardiomyopathy and endothelial dysfunction. Hyperglycemia is the main reason for the development of complications in diabetics. Hyperglycemia accompanies both types of DM. Insufficient control of glycemia in DM patients increases the risk of death due to ischemic heart disease. The pathomechanisms connecting hyperglycemia and disturbances in vascular wall structure and function are not fully elucidated. However, it is already known that hyperglycemia is associated with excessive ROS production and that this may have a direct effect on vascular wall function. Hyperglycemia causes an intensification of glucose metabolism both in endothelial cells and in neutrophils, monocytes, and platelets with accompanying increases in ROS production. It has been demonstrated that hyperglycemia, accompanied by increased synthesis of pyruvates, which undergo further metabolism in mitochondria in the tricarboxylic acid cycle, leads to overproduction of reduced forms of nicotinamide adenine dinucleotide (NADH) and hydroquinone form of flavin adenine dinucleotide dinucleotides, the main energy carriers for ATP production and that this, in turn, leads to an increase in the amount of superoxide anions (O_2^-). It is also noteworthy that ROS production in hyperglycemia results in the oxidation of NADH to nicotinamide adenine dinucleotide in the polyol metabolic pathway. ROS production is also closely connected with glucose metabolism along the pentose and hexosamine pathways. The latter plays a particular role in the functioning of smooth muscle cells along the vascular wall. Glycation of superoxide dismutase (SOD), a biologically active free radical scavenger, also leads to an intensification of OS.

In addition to increased glycation of proteins, OS causes activation of protein kinase C and of the nuclear transcription factor (nuclear factor kappa B, NFKB), which is responsible, among others, for the development of inflammatory reactions. The effects of these disturbances include enhanced production of growth factors, collagen, endothelin-1, which displays strong vasoconstrictive effects, and also an increase in the expression of adhesion molecules. The synthesis of plasminogen activator inhibitor is also increased. This leads to an imbalance in the blood clotting and fibrinolysis systems. In addition, NO-dependent vasodilatation is impaired. The increased protein kinase C activity observed in DM leads to a reduction in NO bioavailability and to an inhibition in eNOS activity.

The activation of transcription factor NFKB leads to intense cytokine production, increased expression of adhesion molecules, and finally, intense cell apoptosis. It has also been shown that ROS exert a direct cytotoxic effect, leading to structural changes in the DNA. This can disturb endothelial proliferation and regeneration. Owing to OS, the amount of free Ca^{2+} in the cytosol may increase, while oxidation of protein cysteine residues causes inactivation of many defensive enzymes.

ROS-induced peroxidation of cell membrane lipids changes their functional and antigenic properties and also modifies the expression of receptors. This can lead to an accumulation of macrophages in the vascular wall, which may transform into foam cells after absorbing low-density lipoprotein (LDL) molecules that have been modified by the effect of ROS and nonenzymatic glycation. It has been demonstrated that the described processes accompanying endothelial dysfunction in diabetic patients are potentiated in cases of coexistence of other CVD risk factors such as hyperlipidemia, hypertension, obesity, or tobacco smoking.

5. ANTIOXIDANT EFFECT OF VITAMINS

Organisms have their own defense mechanisms against the adverse effects of ROS. These include SOD, catalase, and glutathione peroxidase. These specific scavengers eliminate free radicals by enzymatic reactions. It has been demonstrated that during myocardial infarction, the activity of endogenous antioxidant enzymes decreases. This phenomenon is probably due to the depletion of these enzymes during OS.

There also exist numerous exogenous compounds with nonenzymatic action, such as vitamin C (ascorbic acid) and vitamin E (tocopherol), which display antioxidant properties.

5.1 Vitamin C

Vitamin C, a water-soluble 6-carbon lactone, is present in both plants and animals. It is synthesized from glucose in the liver of most mammals with the exception of humans. The human body is deficient in the enzyme (L-gluconolactone oxidase) that is necessary for ascorbic acid synthesis. Vitamin C is essential for normal human functioning, and therefore, it must be supplied exogenously. The daily requirement of vitamin C in the adult human is 75–90 mg. This makes it possible to maintain a constant serum concentration of approximately 50–60 μmol l^{-1}.

Experimental and clinical trials demonstrate that ascorbic acid is a powerful reducing agent in the oxidation–reduction potential of cells. This constitutes the first line of defense against oxygen radicals in an aqueous environment. In serum and cytosol of cells, ascorbic acid prevents the peroxidation processes initiated by ROS. Vitamin C neutralizes ROS, which are produced as a consequence of neutrophil activation. In addition, vitamin C suppresses the release of peroxide anions from macrophages (Padayatty et al., 2003). Vitamin C, together with glutathione and other antioxidants, plays an important role in protecting mitochondrial structures. Ascorbic acid increases the amount of endogenous NO by increasing its synthesis and reducing its oxidation. Ascorbic acid also protects eNOS against the devastating effects of ROS.

It has been found in many studies that vitamin C exerts an arterial vasodilating effect. The mechanism of that effect is multifactorial. The most important is ascorbic acid-induced reduction in the concentration of ROS and that of oxidized LDLs, both of which are responsible for NO inactivation. It has been demonstrated that the protective effect of vitamin C on NO only takes place at adequately high doses of vitamin C, achievable when administered intravenously.

Vitamin C improves endothelial function in healthy and atherosclerotic vessels. Its beneficial effect was demonstrated in patients with coronary artery disease, hypertension, heart failure, and diabetes, both insulin dependent and insulin independent. It is also believed that ascorbic acid causes a reduction in thrombocyte aggregation and adhesion (Willkinson et al., 1999), while increasing blood fibrinolytic activity. Apart from its antioxidant effect, ascorbic acid acts by other important mechanisms. These include increasing the bioavailability of BH_4 and, consequently, increasing eNOS activity (d'Uscio et al., 2003). The most important mechanisms of action of vitamin C are shown in Table 5.1.

Table 5.1 Vitamin C – Some of the Mechanisms of Action

Vitamin C

- Directly reduces the level of free radicals and slows the process of LDL oxidation
- Increases the activity of tetrahydrobiopterin (BH$_4$) – an eNOS cofactor
- Regenerates vitamin E to its antioxidant state
- Increases the plasma NO pool from *S*-nitrosothiols
- Slows down NO oxidation to toxic peroxynitrite radicals
- Prevents glutathione degradation
- Inhibits leukocyte adhesion to endothelial cells
- Inhibits thrombocyte aggregation and activates fibrinolysis processes

5.2 Vitamin E

Vitamin E is present largely ($\sim$90%) in the alpha-tocopherol form. As in other tocopherols, it is an active lipophilic antioxidant, which interrupts the chain reactions that generate free radicals. The dextrorotatory (RRR) isomer (D–alpha-tocopherol) is the form of alpha-tocopherol that is naturally present in plants. This is the most active form of vitamin E, almost 1.5 times more potent than the synthetic racemic form commonly used (D,1–alpha-tocopherol). Because of its lipophilic nature, vitamin E requires fat in the diet for normal absorption. The recommended daily dose of vitamin E is 22.5 IU ($\sim$15 mg), which is easily achievable with a normal diet. This dose provides a normal serum concentration of approximately 15–40 μmol l^{-1}. As demonstrated in experimental and observational studies, alpha-tocopherol deficiencies are found in patients suffering from myocardial infarction or DM.

Experimental studies have shown that vitamin E displays antioxidant properties. As demonstrated, such properties depend on an adequately high dose and the correct form of the administered drug (Roberts et al., 2007). Alpha-tocopherol also modulates the enzymes associated with the cell membrane, which participate in the metabolism of arachidonic acid. These enzymes inhibit the proliferation of the cells of the vascular wall and in so doing are able to slow down the development of atherosclerotic lesions. The enzymes can also inhibit the activity of adhesion molecules, which exert a direct effect on the inflammatory reaction in the vascular wall. It has been demonstrated that in conditions of vitamin E deficiency, the sensitivity of tissues toward ROS increases, the oxidation of LDL cholesterol and the production of proinflammatory cytokines and chemokines are both intensified, blood platelets aggregation is increased, prostacyclin production is reduced, and the fibrinolysis process is slowed down. The main mechanisms of action of vitamin E are shown in Table 5.2.

5.3 Interaction of Vitamins C and E and Their Antioxidant Effect

Ascorbic acid and alpha-tocopherol exert synergistic effects. It has been demonstrated that in exerting its antioxidant effect, alpha-tocopherol is oxidized to a toxic tocopherol

Table 5.2 Vitamin E – Some of the Mechanisms of Action Reducing Endothelial Dysfunction and Oxidative Stress
Vitamin E

- Increases endogenous nitric oxide production
- Inhibits the process of LDL oxidation
- Slows down endothelial cell damage
- Inhibits the activity of intercellular adhesion molecules
- Reduces the amount of proinflammatory cytokines and chemokines
- Decreases smooth muscle cell proliferation
- Inhibits thrombocyte aggregation
- Increases prostacyclin production
- Decreases thromboxane A2 production
- Intensifies fibrinolysis

radical and is subsequently regenerated to its active antioxidant alpha-tocopherol form in the presence of vitamin C (Hamilton et al., 2000). The oxidized ascorbyl radicals thus produced can be reduced by glutathione and endogenous enzymes such as thioredoxin reductase (Figure 5.1).

5.4 Effect of Vitamins C and E in AMI Patients

The beneficial effects of antioxidant vitamins in CVD have been demonstrated in many experimental and epidemiological studies. However, such findings have not been confirmed in most clinical trials that have been published in recent years (Bjelakovic et al., 2007; Cook et al., 2007; Sesso et al., 2008). This was the reason for placing antioxidant vitamins in Class III of the guidelines of both the American Heart Association and the American College of Cardiology. It is, however, important to note that in these trials, the vitamins were administered on a long-term basis, for the prophylaxis of CVD.

On the other hand, the effect of antioxidant vitamins on the prognosis of patients with clinical conditions is poorly understood. Such patients are characterized by the development of a transient but extremely intense OS. AMI is, undoubtedly, such a condition.

Experimental studies demonstrate the beneficial effects of antioxidant vitamins in AMI. Several clinical papers, albeit small in number, seem to confirm this finding.

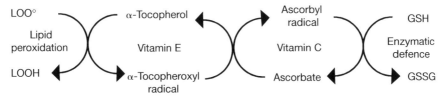

Figure 5.1 Proposed mechanism by which vitamin C restores vitamin E to its antioxidant state. LOO°, lipid peroxyl radical; LOOH, lipid hydroperoxide; GSH, glutathione; GSSG, glutathione disulfide.

In the era before revascularization treatment (only 15% of patients received thrombolytic treatment), Singh et al. (1996) demonstrated that the administration of antioxidants reduced the size of myocardial infarction and also decreased the incidence of complications. The authors' studies have also shown that the administration of vitamins C and E in patients with myocardial infarction (Bednarz et al., 2003; Chamiec et al., 1996; Herbaczyńska-Cedro et al., 1995) aided in limiting OS and reduced the predisposition to dangerous ventricular tachyarrhythmias. In the multicenter randomized double-blind MIVIT (myocardial infarction and vitamins) study (Jaxa-Chamiec et al., 2005), it is demonstrated that in patients with myocardial infarction, 85% of whom received fibrinolytic treatment, intravenous administration of vitamin C on the first day followed by oral administration of vitamin C together with vitamin E for 30 days significantly improved the clinical course of the disease. In the group treated with vitamins C and E, as compared to placebo, a significantly lower incidence of the main study endpoint was found. The study endpoint included in-hospital cardiac death, nonfatal ventricular fibrillation, ventricular tachycardia, or asystolia, and severe heart failure in the form of pulmonary edema or cardiogenic shock (55 [14%] vs. 75 [19%], OR 0.82 [95% CI, 0.68–1.00], $p=0.048$).

5.5 Effect of Vitamins C and E in Diabetic Patients

The synergistic effects of vitamins C and E were also demonstrated in DM patients. In studies designed to assess the influence of vitamins on the vascular system, it was found that the administration of vitamins C and E in DM patients had significant benefits. The administration of vitamin E 800 IU daily together with vitamin C 1000 mg daily led to a significant improvement of endothelium-dependent vasodilation in patients (Beckamn et al., 2003). The combination therapy of vitamins C and E also prevents endothelial damage, which is caused by hyperglycemia. The mechanism of action of antioxidant vitamins is due to the direct inactivation of free radicals, which are responsible for the breakdown of endothelial NO. It is also believed that the administration of vitamin C together with vitamin E in DM patients can decrease insulin resistance, and that this can improve the function of the endothelium.

5.6 Special Role of Vitamins C and E in Patients with Myocardial Infarction and DM Treated by Reperfusion

There is much evidence that the poorer prognosis in patients with myocardial infarction and DM can be associated with the degree of intensity of OS. In spite of the evidence demonstrating the benefits resulting from the administration of antioxidant treatment in diabetic patients with AMI, there are, as yet, no adequately powered, randomized trials assessing the effects of such treatments. Only in the retrospective analysis of the MIVIT study (Jaxa-Chamiec et al., 2009), the authors were able to demonstrate on a relatively small group of patients suffering from myocardial infarction and DM that coadministration of vitamins C and E exerts a beneficial effect on the prognosis. In this study, of 800 patients who suffered from AMI, 122 (15%) were diagnosed as sufferers of type I diabetes. Vitamin C was administered intravenously (1000 mg infusion in the first 12 h) followed by an oral administration of vitamin C together with an oral administration of vitamin E (600 mg daily) for 30 days. In DM patients receiving both vitamins C and E, a significant reduction was found in 30-day mortality due to cardiac reasons (5 [8%] vs. 14 [22%], OR 0.32 [95% CI, 0.11–0.93], $p=0.036$). No such effect of the vitamins on the prognosis was demonstrated in patients without DM (19 [6%] vs. 19 [6%], OR 0.97 [95% CI, 0.51–1.85], $p=0.94$) (Figure 5.2).

The currently used treatment for AMI by revascularization methods shows indisputable benefits related to the improvement of the prognosis. However, the complications due to RI remain a real challenge. Patients with DM or hyperglycemia display different reactions when subjected to typical treatments administered for AMI. For example, it has been demonstrated that both fibrinolytic therapy and treatment by means of percutaneous coronary intervention are less effective in these patients than in those without diabetes. RI manifestations, apart from predisposition to dangerous ventricular tachyarrhythmia or the so-called myocardial stunning, include the no-reflow phenomenon (Rezkalla and Kloner, 2002). It is believed that in each of these manifestations, an important role is played by intense OS. Matsumoto et al. (2004) demonstrated that no-reflow phenomenon, or regional disturbances of myocardial perfusion in the drainage area of the vessel with restored patency, is accompanied by not only an abrupt reduction

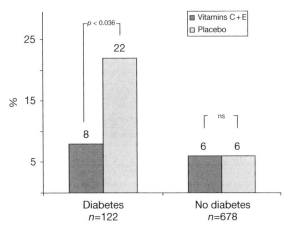

Figure 5.2 Vitamins C and E are effective in reducing 30-day mortality in myocardial infarction patients with diabetes mellitus. *Reproduced from Jaxa-Chamiec, T., Bednarz, B., Herbaczyńska-Cedro, K., Maciejewski, P., Ceremuzynski, L., 2009. Effects of vitamins C and E on outcome after acute myocardial infarction in diabetics: a retrospective, hypothesis-generating analysis from the MIVIT study. Cardiology 112, 219–223, with permission from S. Karger AG, Basel.*

in endogenous antioxidant enzymes such as glutathione peroxidase, SOD, or catalase but also a decrease in the serum level of antioxidant vitamins C and E.

Vitamins C and E, apart from their antioxidant effect on myocardial ischemic/RI, also play an important role in improving endothelial function. Endothelium plays a decisive role in regulating the tonus of the vascular wall, which, in turn, has a direct influence on myocardial perfusion. The main mechanism, as mentioned above, by which vitamins C and E improve endothelial function is by NO regeneration. Preventing endothelial damage caused by hyperglycemia is another beneficial effect of these antioxidants.

5.7 Mode of Administration of Vitamins C and E and Their Clinical Effectiveness

Several factors are important for antioxidant efficacy, that is, potential benefit resulting from administration of vitamins C and E in AMI and DM patients. First, there are significant premises justifying the administration of the vitamins together, since, as previously discussed, they exert synergistic effects. Importantly, ascorbic acid acts to regenerate alpha-tocopherol and thus promotes the antioxidant effect of vitamin E. Second, administration of vitamins C and E can bring potential benefits in clinical conditions, which are characterized by intense OS. Third, the antioxidant effect of the vitamins depends on the dose administered, which should be adequately high. It has been demonstrated (Hathcock et al., 2005; Roberts et al., 2007) that even daily doses of up to 3200 mg of vitamin E and 2000 mg of vitamin C are safe. Fourth, as demonstrated recently, the antioxidant effect of vitamin E is revealed in DM patients who display a specific genotype. In the population of Western countries, 36% of DM patients who have an Hp 2-2 genotype, are characterized by increased OS. In the retrospective analysis of the heart outcomes prevention evaluation study subgroup (Milman et al., 2008), it was demonstrated that vitamin E administration in patients with this genotype caused a significant reduction in the incidence of cardiovascular episodes. Finally, the route of vitamin administration is also important. Since vitamin E is lipophilic, the effect following its oral administration is delayed. Vitamin C, a hydrophilic compound, reaches its therapeutic level following oral administration very quickly and even within minutes following intravenous administration. The intravenous route of vitamin C administration during the first hours of AMI, as used in the previously discussed MIVIT study, seems particularly justified, since long-term oral administration of high doses results in a maximal serum level of approximately 100 μmol l^{-1} (further increases in the oral dose do not result in greater serum levels because of the clearance of the drug by the kidneys), but which is suboptimal for antioxidant action. On the other hand, it has been demonstrated that intravenous administration of vitamin C can result in tenfold greater serum concentration compared to oral therapy and only at that levels can its full antioxidant effect be realized (Jackson et al., 1998).

6. SUMMARY

The divergence between the results of experimental and epidemiological studies and the results of large prospective clinical trials of antioxidant vitamins C and E requires further investigation.

This, in turn, requires the planning of large randomized clinical trials in patient populations where OS is extremely intense. Such groups of patients include those with myocardial infarction and coexistent DM receiving reperfusion treatment. In such patients, the early administration of adequately high doses of antioxidant vitamins, including intravenously administered ascorbic acid, can bring significant benefits.

Until the results of such trials are known, forming a definitive opinion about the clinical usefulness of the antioxidant vitamins C and E may be the proverbial "throwing the baby out with the bath water" (Jialal and Devaraj, 2003).

REFERENCES

Albert, C.M., Cook, N.R., Ganiano, J.M., et al., 2008. Effect of folic acid and B vitamins on risk of cardiovascular events and total mortality among women at high risk of cardiovascular disease. Journal of the American Medical Association 299, 2027–2036.

Beckamn, J.A., Goldfine, A.B., Gordon, M.B., et al., 2003. Oral antioxidant therapy improves endothelial function in Type I, but not Type II diabetes mellitus. American Journal of Physiology – Heart and Circulatory Physiology 285, H2392–H2398.

Bednarz, B., Chamiec, T., Ceremużyński, L., 2003. Antioxidant vitamins decrease exercise-induced QT dispersion after myocardial infarction. Kardiologia Polska 58, 375–377.

Bjelakovic, G., Nikolova, D., Gluud, L.L., Simonetti, R.G., Gluud, C., 2007. Mortality in randomized trials of antioxidant supplements for primary and secondary prevention: systemic review and meta-analysis. Journal of the American Medical Association 297 (8), 842–857.

Chamiec, T., Herbaczyńska-Cedro, K., Ceremużyński, L., 1996. Effects of antioxidant vitamins C and E on signal-averaged electrocardiogram in acute myocardial infarction. American Journal of Cardiology 77, 237–241.

Cook, N.R., Albert, C.M., Gaziano, J.M., et al., 2007. A randomized factorial of vitamins C and E and beta carotene in the secondary prevention of cardiovascular events in women. Archives of Internal Medicine 167, 1610–1618.

d'Uscio, L.V., Milstien, S., Richardson, D., Smith, L., Katusic, Z.S., 2003. Long-term vitamin C treatment increases vascular tetrahydrobiopterin level and nitric oxide synthase activity. Circulation Research 92, 88–95.

Guzik, T.J., Mussa, S., Gastaldi, D., et al., 2002. Mechanisms of increased vascular superoxide production in human diabetes mellitus: role of NAD(P)H oxidase and endothelial nitric oxide synthase. Circulation 105, 1656–1662.

Hamilton, I.M., Gilmore, W.S., Benzie, I.F., Mulholland, C.W., Strain, J.J., 2000. Interaction between vitamins C and E in human subjects. British Journal of Nutrition 84, 261–267.

Hathcock, J.N., Azzi, A., Blumberg, J., et al., 2005. Vitamins E and C are safe across a broad range of intakes. American Journal of Clinical Nutrition 81, 736–745.

Herbaczyńska-Cedro, K., Gordon-Majszak, W., 1989. Evidence for increased lipid peroxidation in the non-ischemic portion of the heart with coronary occlusion. Cardiovascular Research 23, 596–599.

Herbaczyńska-Cedro, K., Kłosiewicz-Wąsek, B., Cedro, K., et al., 1995. Supplementation with vitamins C and E suppresses leukocyte oxygen free radical production in patients with myocardial infarction. European Heart Journal 16, 1044–1049.

Jackson, T.S., Xu, A., Vita, J.A., Keaney Jr., J.F., 1998. Ascorbate prevents the interaction of superoxide and nitric oxide only at very high physiological concentrations. Circulation Research 83, 916–922.

Jaxa-Chamiec, T., Bednarz, B., Herbaczyńska-Cedro, K., Maciejewski, P., Ceremuzynski, L., 2009. Effects of vitamins C and E on outcome after acute myocardial infarction in diabetics: a retrospective, hypothesis-generating analysis from the MIVIT study. Cardiology 112, 219–223.

Jaxa-Chamiec, T., Bednarz, B., Maciejewski, P., et al., 2005. Antioxidant effects of combined vitamins C and E in acute myocardial infartion. The randomized, double-blind, placebo controlled, multicenter pilot Myocardial Infarction and VITamins (MIVIT) trial. Kardiologia Polska 62, 344–349.

Jialal, I., Devaraj, S., 2003. Antioxidant and atherosclerosis. Don't throw out the baby with the bath water. Circulation 107, 926–928.

Matsumoto, H., Inoue, N., Takaoka, H., et al., 2004. Depletion of antioxidants is associated with no-reflow phenomenon in acute myocardial infarction. Clinical Cardiology 27, 466–470.

Maxwell, S.R., Lip, G.Y., 1997. Reperfusion injury: a review of the pathophysiology, clinical manifestations and therapeutic options. International Journal of Cardiology 58, 95–117.

Milman, U., Blum, S., Shapira, C., et al., 2008. Vitamin E supplementation reduces cardiovascular events in subgroup of middle-aged individuals with both type 2 diabetes mellitus and the haptoglobin 2-2 genotype. Arteriosclerosis, Thrombosis, and Vascular Biology 28, 341–347.

Padayatty, S.J., Katz, A., Wang, Y., et al., 2003. Vitamin C as an antioxidant: evaluation of its role in disease prevention. Journal of the American College of Nutrition 22, 18–35.

Piper, H.M., Abdallah, Y., Schäfer, C., 2004. The first minutes of reperfusion: a window of opportunity for cardioprotection. Cardiovascular Research 61, 365–371.

Rezkalla, S.H., Kloner, R.A., 2002. No-reflow phenomenon. Circulation 105, 656–662.

Roberts 2nd, L.J., Oates, J.A., Linton, M.F., et al., 2007. The relationship between dose of vitamin E and suppression of oxidative stress in humans. Free Radical Biology and Medicine 43, 1388–1393.

Sesso, H.D., Buring, J.E., Christen, W.G., et al., 2008. Vitamins E and C in the prevention of cardiovascular disease in men. The Physician' Health Study II randomized controlled trial. Journal of the American Medical Association 300, 2123–2133.

Singal, P.K., Khaper, N., Palace, V., Kumar, D., 1998. The role of oxidative stress in the genesis of heart disease. Cardiovascular Research 40, 426–432.

Singh, R.B., Niaz, M.A., Rastogi, S.S., Rastogi, S., 1996. Usefulness of antioxidant vitamins in suspected acute myocardial infarction (the Indian experiment of infarct survival-3). American Journal of Cardiology 77, 232–236.

Van deWerf, F., Ardissino, D., Betriu, A., et al., 2003. Management of acute myocardial infarction in patients presenting with ST-segment elevation. European Heart Journal 24, 28–66.

Willkinson, I.B., Megson, I.L., MacCallum, H., et al., 1999. Oral vitamin C reduces arterial stiffness and platelet aggregation in humans. Journal of Cardiovascular Pharmacology 34, 690–693.

Yellon, D.M., Hausenloy, D.J., 2007. Myocardial reperfusion injury. New England Journal of Medicine 357, 1121–1135.

Zuanetti, G., Latini, R., Maggioni, A.P., Santoro, L., Franzosi, M.G., 1993. Influence of diabetes on mortality in acute myocardial infarction: data from the GISSI-2 study. Journal of the American College of Cardiology 22, 1788–1794.

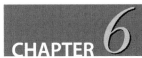

CHAPTER *6*

Cardioprotective Nutrients

R. Jaffe

Fellow, Health Studies Collegium, Ashburn, VA, USA

A range of foods and bioavailable supplements are now available that provide better outcomes and clinically significant leverage in managing the pathophysiology of cardiovascular disease. Targeted supplementation, in combination with individualized diet therapy, are included as are mental and physical exercises aimed at evoking healing responses in proportion to documented risk reductions.

1. INTRODUCTION

Careful risk assessment of the individual utilizing conventional medical guidelines is the first step in quantifying the needs of the patient. Although the following cardioprotective nutrients provide valuable clinical tools, high-risk patients may require pharmaceutical intervention individually or in combination with nutrients.

2. CARDIOPROTECTIVE NUTRIENTS

The beneficial biochemical effects of cardioprotective nutrients include antioxidant protection and repair stimulating anti-inflammatory properties. Immune regulation, endothelial cell protection, cell membrane stabilization, methylation epigenetic support, and healthier blood lipids are among the results (Table 6.1).

2.1 Antioxidant Vitamins and Polyphenolics

Antioxidant nutrients are central in any cardioprotective protocol. Sufficient levels of antioxidants from diet can help to prevent or delay the occurrence of pathological changes associated with oxidative stress. Antioxidants include ascorbate, flavonoids, mixed natural carotenoids, B complex and mixed natural tocopherols, minerals and cofactors such as coenzyme Q_{10} (Giugliano, 2000).

2.1.1 Ascorbate (vitamin C) and cardiovascular health

The role of vitamin C or ascorbate in defending the immune system is recognized. However, the question of which form of ascorbate to recommend (buffered ascorbate or ascorbic acid) has been less clear.

One of the cardioprotective strategies of the Alkaline Way paradigm is the reduction of metabolic acidosis with an alkaline diet and sufficient, available buffering minerals

Bioactive Food as Dietary Interventions for Cardiovascular Disease
http://dx.doi.org/10.1016/B978-0-12-396485-4.00005-0
© 2013 Elsevier Inc.
All rights reserved.

Table 6.1 Cardiovascular Diseases: Nutrients to Address Primary Causes and Secondary Consequences

Beneficial nutrients from foods and supplements	Comorbidity

Nutrients from food
  Prebiotic fiber from grains, grasses, tubers, and pulses
  Probiotic mixed flora from fermented foods
  G, G, O, B, E*
  Green tea: ECGC*
Vitamins and flavonoids
  Ascorbate
  Quercetin dihydrate, soluble OPC, resveratrol, curcumin
Amino acid cofactor
  Carnitine fumarate
  Taurine
  NAC
Minerals
  Calcium
  Magnesium
  Potassium
  Trace minerals
Fatty acids
  Omega 3s
  Omega 6s
Cofactors
  CoQ_{10}
Bioactive components of food
  Policosanols
  Red Rice Yeast – (certified as traditional and authentic)
  Plant sterols
  Tocotrienols
Botanicals
  Hawthorne, Pine tea, bilberry, rosehips, equisetum
	• Hypertension
	• Glucose regulation
	• Lipid levels – cholesterol
	• Homocysteine levels
	• Inflammation
	• Free radicals
	• (Endothelial health, plaque risk)

EAA, essential amino acids; GGOBE, ginger, garlic, onions, brassica sprouts, and eggs; NAC, *N*-acetyl cysteine; B complex, vitamins include B_1, B_2, B_3, B_6, B_{12}, folates (B_7); PABA, Para Amino Benzoic Acid; ECGC, epigallocatechin gallate; SAMe *S*-adenosylmethionine; SeMet selenomethionine; carotenoids: alpha and beta-carotene, cryptoxanthine, lycopene, and xeaxanthine.

(Souto et al., 2011). The links between renal acid load and cardiovascular risk factors were evaluated (Murakami et al., 2007) in a population of more than 1100 female participants, aged 18–22. This study evaluated potential acid load due to diet, including dietary protein, phosphorus, potassium, calcium, and magnesium intake and also tracked the ratio of protein to potassium. The data showed that more acidic diets were associated with elevated hypertension, higher total and LDL cholesterol, and increased body-mass index and waist circumference, all primary markers of cardiovascular risk. The findings are especially notable given the young age of the participants.

With the aim of balancing metabolic acidity, a vitamin C source that is fully reduced with buffering minerals such as potassium, calcium, magnesium, and zinc can be more helpful in neutralizing excess cell acids. Adequate amounts of buffered ascorbate are able to provide rest to the body's immune system and boost hormonal and neurochemical function. Additionally, buffered ascorbate functions as a steroid-sparing agent, a detoxifying agent, and an electron donor to enhance cell energy. Ascorbate is uniquely able to donate an electron and restore ATP-generating capacity to the mitochondria of the cell, thus increasing its energy output.

Low ascorbate levels are associated with all aspects of cardiovascular disease (CVD) (Loria et al., 2000). Ascorbate deficiencies adversely influence endothelial functions, smooth muscle cell proliferation, thrombosis, and plaque ruptures. A shortage of antioxidants in the diet promotes coronary heart disease (CHD) through the accumulation of oxidized LDL in macrophages initiating plaque formation. In that light, it is prudent to incorporate adequate buffered ascorbate in a cardiovascular health protocol. How much ascorbate one needs is dependent on how rapidly this vital nutrient is being consumed. Ascorbate calibration provides a practical solution – a method that each individual can use to determine how much ascorbate he/she requires at any given point in time. When ascorbate demands increase, with infections, high stress, or allergic conditions, ascorbate calibration (cleanse) is repeated on a weekly basis until stable ascorbate need is met (Figure 6.1).

2.1.2 Flavonoids: Quercetin dihydrate and OPC flavonoids

The proanthocyanidins (oligomeric proanthocyanidins or OPC) are naturally occurring antioxidants widely available in plant sources, including fruits, vegetables, nuts, seeds, flowers, and bark. Grape seed extract is one the most potent source of OPC, and has demonstrated excellent protection against myocardial ischemia-reperfusion injury and myocardial infarction. In addition, grape seed extract supplementation to high fat diets has been shown to normalize body weight, support epididymal tissue, normalize lipid concentrations, and improve carnitine levels by controlling lipid metabolism. Coupled with quercetin dihydrate, it makes for a formulation that is one of the best in this category.

2.1.3 B complex vitamins

The full range of B complex vitamins affects a tremendously broad range of biochemical processes in the body. Of particular relevance to cardiovascular function and protection is their role in methylation chemistry, insulin sensitivity, lipid regulation, energy production, free radical management, and inflammatory processes.

2.1.3.1 Folate, vitamin B6, and vitamin B12

Naturally occurring in whole, unprocessed foods, B vitamins have been closely linked to cardiovascular health status. Folate, vitamin B6, and vitamin B12 are essential in the

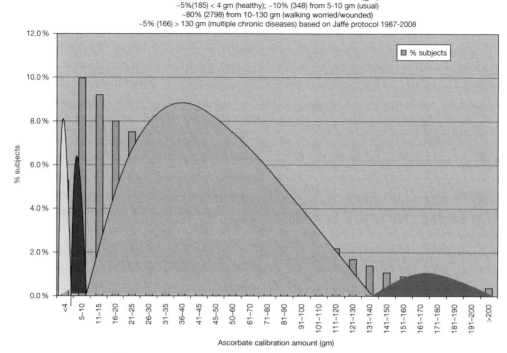

Figure 6.1 Amount of ascorbate needed to achieve calibrated individual need.

conversion of homocysteine into methionine, and without these B vitamins, this conversion process becomes inefficient and homocysteine levels rise. Research has shown that excessive amounts of homocysteine can damage blood vessels, increasing the risk of cardiovascular disease, stroke, and hypertension. Conversely, these risks are reduced among people with higher intakes of folate, those who use multivitamin supplements, and those with higher levels of serum folate (He et al., 2004; Ishihara et al., 2008).

2.1.3.2 Niacin
Niacin assists in vasodilation, enabling improved blood circulation. Additionally, because niacin lowers LDL cholesterol levels, it helps prevent plaque build-up. The result is improved blood flow that reduces the risk of heart attack or stroke. Recent research has demonstrated greater safety and efficacy of niacin supplementation in comparison with certain cardiovascular medications in lowering blood lipids.

2.1.3.3 Pantothenic acid
Pantothenic acid is vital to the healthy production, transport, and breakdown of lipids and in significant amounts helps weight loss. Pantothenic acid supplementation facilitates complete catabolism of fatty acids without the formation of ketone bodies (Leung, 1995).

2.1.4 Carotenoids

Carotenoids are especially important for their antioxidant roles in cardiovascular health. Found in fruits and vegetables, the most abundant carotenoids in the diet are beta-carotene, lycopene, lutein, beta-cryptoxanthin, zeaxanthin, and astaxanthin. In terms of supplementation, natural and mixed carotenoids have been found superior to synthetic single carotenoids. Studies have shown that synthetic beta-carotene does not protect against heart disease (Hennekens et al., 1996). There is a strong association between dietary sources of lycopene and reduced risk of heart attacks. Lutein and zeaxanthin (in the xanthophyll family of carotenoids) have been found to inhibit the thickening of carotid artery walls and to reduce arterial inflammation, combating LDL-induced migration of monocytes to human artery cell walls (Dwyer et al., 2011). Changes in carotid intima-media thickness (IMT), considered a measure of atherosclerotic cardiovascular disease, are also significantly inversely associated with lutein and zeaxanthin levels.

2.1.5 Vitamin D3

Individuals with vitamin D deficiency have increased incidence of CVD. CVD risk is also higher in areas of increased geographic latitude and during the winter months' lack of sunshine (Holick, 2007). These associations are numerous and well documented. Vitamin D deficiency can lead to secondary hyperparathyroidism. Studies have shown CVD risk lined with high parathyroid hormone levels (Lee et al., 2008). In addition, vitamin D deficiency increases systemic inflammation, confirmed by elevated levels of C-reactive protein and interleukin-10. Another vital connection between vitamin D and CVD is the link with metabolic syndrome and diabetes, which significantly increase the risk of heart disease. Increased body fat results in sequestration of vitamin D in adipose tissue, thus lowering serum vitamin D concentrations and, ultimately, leading to insulin resistance and metabolic syndrome. Adequate vitamin D levels are required for healthy insulin secretion. We suggest 25-OH vitamin D levels of 50–80 ng/ml as the healthier target values.

2.1.6 Vitamin E

Naturally occurring vitamin E exists in eight chemical forms (alpha-, beta-, gamma-, and delta-tocopherol and alpha-, beta-, gamma-, and delta-tocotrienol) that have varying levels of biological benefit to specific parts of the body. Vitamin E particularly gamma tocopherol has effects on immune function, and has been found to decrease platelet aggregation. *In vitro* studies have shown that vitamin E in all its forms inhibits oxidation of low-density lipoprotein (LDL) cholesterol. Vitamin E also appears to prevent the formation of blood clots that can provoke heart attacks or venous thromboembolism (Glynn et al., 2007). As in the case of carotenoids, mixed natural tocopherols are the form of vitamin E that have been shown to provide safer and more effective results. We use only the mixed natural forms of nutrients. For vitamins E, this means 800–3600 I.U per day, sufficient to quench oxidized HDL/LDL. We never use d-alpha tocopherol succinate or acetate as these are less safe and less effective forms of vitamin E with high toxicity profiles.

2.2 Intermediates and Cofactors

2.2.1 Alpha lipoic acid

As another powerful antioxidant, alpha lipoic acid plays an enormous role in diabetes and associated complications, particularly cardiovascular health. Oral treatment with 800 mg per day for 4 months has supported short-term improvement of cardiac autonomic dysfunction in Type 2 diabetes (Ziegler and Gries, 1997). Increased oxidative stress and inflammation causally contribute to CVDs and increasing age usually exacerbates this issue. Alpha lipoic acid supplementation has been shown to ameliorate these effects (Li et al., 2010). We suggest optimized ascorbate intake as the more clinically effective way to recycle, restore, and enhance alpha lipoic acid levels.

2.2.2 Coenzyme Q10

CoQ_{10} has been found to increase energy production in the heart, improving the heart muscle's ability to contract and lowering blood pressure. CoQ_{10} has been shown to be highly concentrated in heart muscle cells, reflecting their high energy requirements. Conversely, congestive heart failure from a wide variety of causes has been strongly correlated with low blood and tissue levels of CoQ_{10}. Reflecting a dose–response relationship, the severity of heart failure has been found to correlate with the severity of CoQ_{10} deficiency. Deficiency of CoQ_{10} is easily treated with micellized CoQ_{10} supplements (in a suspension of rice bran oil), which is documented to slow the progression of heart failure.

The production of CoQ_{10} is known to reduce with age and with dietary deprivations, such as the lack of healthy fats. Patients with other conditions associated with reduced energy levels in the body, such as depression and chronic fatigue syndrome, have shown significantly depleted CoQ_{10} levels (Maes et al., 2009). Medications such as statin drugs can reduce CoQ_{10} production by as much as 50%. It, therefore, makes sense for anyone on statin medication to supplement with CoQ_{10} for natural, safe cardiac support (Langsjoen, et al., 2005). Individuals who want to maintain cardiovascular health with advancing years might require 30–300 mg per day. Those who want to achieve repletion might need 100–1,200 mg per day for a period of 1 or 2 months until CoQ_{10} levels have been increased and the health of the health of the cell mitochondria has been effectively restored. Intake can then be reduced to a maintenance level of 60–300 mg per day.

2.2.3 Omega-3 Fatty Acids

One of the key issues in omega-3 supplementation is the bioavailability of the source. When using flaxseeds, it is important to note that the alpha-linoleic acid content must be converted to EPA and DHA in order to be used by the body. The metabolic steps in this conversion are frequently incomplete, dependent on deviations in individual epigenetics, genetics, metabolism, and age (Bloedon et al., 2003). As with any nutrient, the efficiency of metabolism is individual.

Flax cannot be relied upon as a consistent, clinically effective source of omega-3, because consumption of flax oil or flaxseed products does not predictably result in increased physiologic levels of EPA or DHA. Fish oil, which contains both EPA and DHA, provides a more reliable source of those nutrients. The EPA and DHA in fish oil are already in a bioavailable form. A Canadian study (which evaluated daily supplementation with ground flaxseeds) reported significant changes in plasma ALA in younger subjects (aged 18–29) with a decrease in triglycerides. However, subjects aged 49–69 did not achieve statistically significant levels of ALA, nor were there changes in their triglyceride levels (Patenaude et al., 2009). We suggest EPA/DHA in the 2–9 g/day range, sufficient to bring blood pressure and vascular compliance to their healthier levels.

2.2.4 Omega-3 fatty acids from fish oil

A comparative animal study evaluated the effects of omega-3 fatty acids from both flax oil and fish oil on arrhythmogenic cardiomyopathy in boxer dogs. Initially, the incidence of arrhythmia averaged 543 episodes per day. After 6 weeks of supplementation, the median for animals receiving fish oil supplements was reduced to 162 episodes daily (a reduction of ~70%), but no change was observed in the flax oil group or the controls. This suggests that EPA/DHA sources are more effective than ALA as Omega-3 sources.

2.2.5 Omega-3 fatty acids from flax

Despite the conversion issues, flax can make a significant contribution to nutrition. In another study of flax, the most significant improvement noted was a 23.7% reduction in markers of insulin resistance after 10 weeks and also 15% lower Lp(a) (Bloedon et al., 2003). Dosage reported was 30 g daily (two tablespoons). However, no sustained reductions were noted in inflammation, oxidative stress, or LDL cholesterol. This suggests that flax fiber may be helpful aside from its Omega-3 and Omega-6 essential fat content.

2.3 Minerals and Trace Minerals

Impaired insulin–glucose metabolism is the central underlying biochemical error in CVD. As in diabetes, assessment for mineral status and repletion of deficiencies can be critically important. Foremost among the minerals are chromium and magnesium for better sugar metabolism, although deficiencies of other trace minerals can also complicate recovery.

2.3.1 Magnesium and choline citrate

The minerals that buffer the cells are principally magnesium and potassium (Quamme and de Rouffignac, 2000). Magnesium is the fourth most abundant cation in the body, and its vital functions are extensive. Magnesium activates hundreds of cellular enzymes. Adequate magnesium avoids or mitigates atherosclerosis, hypertension, coronary spasm, cardiac irritability, arrhythmias, preeclampsia of pregnancy, pain syndromes, headaches, restless leg syndrome, hypokalemia, hypocalcemia, and muscle irritability and spasm (Jaffe and Brown, 2000). The majority of the body's magnesium ($\sim$60%) is found in the bones and $\sim$40% in cells. Ionized magnesium is in dynamic equilibrium with intracellular, bioactive magnesium. Consequently, the measurement of ionized magnesium is a more predictive measure of intracellular, functional magnesium status than total Mg, RBC Mg, or serum Mg.

In supplementation, enhanced magnesium uptake is observed when choline citrate and ionized, soluble magnesium salts are taken at the same time. Only the choline citrate form is effective. Choline bitartrate does not enhance magnesium uptake. Choline builds acetylcholine, a relaxing neurotransmitter, providing cholinergic bile salts and improving the production and solubility of bile. This citrate form alkalinizes and energizes mitochondrial ATP energy production. A sustained increase in plasma-ionized magnesium has been observed after concurrent administration of choline citrate.

The preferred combination of active magnesium salts is magnesium as glycinate, citrate, and ascorbate. Sustained increase in ionized magnesium is observed over a 4-week

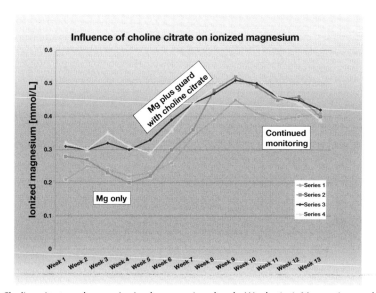

Figure 6.2 Choline citrate enhances ionized magnesium levels. Weeks 1–4: Magnesium only. Weeks 5–8: Magnesium salts with concurrent choline citrate. Weeks 9–12: Continued monitoring with only magnesium.

period in subjects previously found to be refractory to or blocked in magnesium uptake. When choline citrate and ionized magnesium are taken together, a neutral 'nano' size droplet is formed that is readily absorbed through the neutral pores of the intestinal enterocytes. This form of supplementation becomes important when the calcium, magnesium ATPase enzyme system is inhibited, preventing the usual uptake of magnesium and calcium (Jaffe and Brown, 2000) (Figure 6.2).

2.3.2 Selenomethionine

Selenium is a trace mineral with potent antioxidant effects, and selenomethinine has been found to be the safer, more bioactive form. Selenium supplementation increases the ratio of HDL to LDL cholesterol and inhibits platelet aggregation. Overall benefits to the cardiovascular system stem from antioxidant effects of selenium in the production of glutathione peroxidase. Due to this function, selenomethionine also has an important role in autoimmune thyroiditis, prostate cancer prevention, and the treatment of autoimmune conditions, such as rheumatoid arthritis, eczema, and psoriasis. Deficiency of selenium and also vitamin E has been shown to increase markers of free radical damage.

2.4 Amino Acids

2.4.1 Glutamine and Arginine

L-Arginine is a precursor to nitric oxide, which relaxes endothelial cells and helps regulate blood pressure. Clinically, L-arginine supplementation improves large artery elasticity index (LAEI) in patients with multiple cardiovascular risk factors. This improvement is associated with a decrease in systolic blood pressure and peripheral vascular resistance, as well as a decrease in aldosterone levels reducing the risk of hypertension (Guttman et al., 2010). Arginine also improves systemic and pulmonary hemodynamics, aiding in the treatment of diastolic heart failure (Orea-Tejeda et al., 2010). Glutamine, another conditionally essential amino acid, has found its place as a cardioprotective agent especially in patients with ischemic heart disease (IHD) patients. In addition, along with Omega-3 fatty acids, it has a positive effect on oxidative metabolism, lipolysis, and inflammation.

2.4.2 S-adenosylmethionine and methionine

S-adenosylmethionine (SAMe) is a natural mood stabilizer formed by adenylation (the modification of the amino acid methionine by SAMe synthase). SAMe is a primary methyl donor in virtually all known biological methylations, playing an important role in detoxification. Once a SAMe molecule loses its methyl group, it breaks down to form homocysteine. However, with adequate vitamin B12, B6, folate, and trimethylglycine (TMG, betaine), the body can convert homocysteine to glutathione or remethylate it to methionine. This role in homocysteine metabolism is an important link with cardiovascular health. An association between hyperlipidemia and hyperhomocysteinemia (HHCY) has been suggested. This link is clinically important in management of vascular risk factors. Hypomethylation associated with HHCY is responsible for lipid accumulation in tissues. Decreased methyl groups will impair the synthesis of phosphatidylcholine, a major phospholipid required for very low-density lipoprotein (VLDL) assembly and homeostasis (Obeid and Herrman, 2009).

2.4.3 Carnitine fumarate and GABA

Carnitine is an amino acid required for the vital transport of fatty acids in the process of energy metabolism. Cardiovascular health is supported by enhanced fat burning in the heart muscle, significantly lowering LDL cholesterol and triglycerides, while raising HDL levels (Elisaf et al., 1998). Carnitine helps to keep coronary arteries clear and can lower blood pressure in those with hypertension. Studies have shown that carnitine supplementation can considerably improve the health of cardiac cells even at an advanced phase when valve replacement is being seriously considered (Xiang et al., 2005).

For adequate cardiac support, a good formulation of carnitine should include at least 500 mg of L-carnitine derived from an alkaline and energy-enhancing source such as carnitine fumarate, found in medium chain triglycerides (MCTs). This supports the delivery of carnitine to the body through 'micellization' or nano droplet formation. Since MCTs also tend to provide a sense of satiety, they tend to enhance weight management.

The addition of a calming neurotransmitter such as GABA (gamma amino butyric acid) can achieve the changes in neuronal activity, that support effective weight loss. In addition to functions as a calming neurotransmitter essential for brain metabolism, GABA *decreases* neuron excitation and prevents over-firing of brain neurons, thereby reducing anxiety and stress levels. In some cases, the addition of kelp extract to this type of formulation not only helps detoxify but also gives the required thyroid hormone support that is synergistic with weight management.

2.5 Food Constituents and Botanicals

Food constituents and botanicals can play a surprisingly important role in CVD management. For example, more than 300 clinical trials have confirmed the importance of dietary fiber in health and disease prevention. Adjusting the diet to include larger quantities of these familiar foods is a practical, accessible aspect of a dietary intervention program (Table 6.2).

2.5.1 Prebiotic fiber

A diet high in soluble-type dietary fiber has been found to decrease the risk of CVD, while lowering total and LDL cholesterol levels and aiding in the control of glucose levels. Studies have confirmed that an optimal low-cholesterol, low-fat diet, which includes high levels of soluble dietary fiber, can reduce blood cholesterol significantly more than the same diet with a lower fiber content. The prebiotic nature of dietary fiber increases bacteria growth in the intestines necessary for complete digestion and optimum nutrient absorption (Jenkins et al., 1999; Parnell and Reimer, 2010).

Table 6.2 Cardiovascular diseases: Nutrients in relation to primary cause and secondary consequence risk

	Hypertension, CAD, PAD, ASHD	Glucose regulation/insulin resistance	Lipid status	Homocysteine detox status	Free radical status	Inflammation repair deficit	Hypercoagulation, stroke, heart attack
Diet	Prebiotic fiber Green and herbal tea Water Alkaline, mineral-rich foods Substitutes for reactive foods and meds	Choose based on glycemic load and individual food sensitivities	Healthy fat (uncontaminated and unoxidized) with omega 3 dominance recommended <20% of calories	Avoid black tea Prebiotic fiber Green and herbal tea Water Alkaline, mineral-rich foods Substitutes for reactive foods and meds	Prebiotic fiber Green and herbal tea Water Alkaline, mineral-rich foods Substitutes for reactive foods and meds	Avoid simple carbs and processed sugar, as well as reactive foods and meds that are acidifying and proinflammatory	Prebiotic fiber Green and herbal tea Water Alkaline, mineral-rich foods Substitutes for reactive foods and meds
Food nutrients	Prebiotic fiber Low glycemic load meals GGOBE Green tea/ECGC	Prebiotic fiber Low glycemic load meals Flax, sesame, or hemp seeds	Prebiotic fiber Low glycemic load meals GGOBE Green tea/ECGC	Prebiotic fiber Low glycemic load meals GGOBE Green tea/ECGC	GGOBE Green tea/ECGC Flax, sesame, or hemp seeds	Prebiotic fiber Low glycemic load meals GGOBE Green tea/ECGC	Prebiotic fiber Low glycemic load meals GGOBE Green tea/ECGC
Vitamins and polyphenolics	Ascorbate Quercetin dihydrate Flavonoids	Ascorbate Quercetin dihydrate Flavonoids	Ascorbate Quercetin dihydrate flavonoids and	B6, B12, folates TMG (B15) DMG	Ascorbate Quercetin dihydrate Vitamins E +	Ascorbate Quercetin dihydrate Flavonoids and	Ascorbate Quercetin dihydrate flavonoids and

Continued

Table 6.2 Cardiovascular diseases: Nutrients in relation to primary cause and secondary consequence risk—cont'd

	Hypertension, CAD, PAD, ASHD	Glucose regulation/ insulin resistance	Lipid status	Homocysteine detox status	Free radical status	Inflammation repair deficit	Hypercoagulation, stroke, heart attack
	and LMW OPC flavonols B complex vitamins Carotenoids Vitamin D$_3$ Vitamins E + SeMet	and LMW OPC flavonols B complex vitamins Carotenoids Vitamin D$_3$ Vitamins E + SeMet	LMW OPC flavonols B complex vitamins Carotenoids Vitamin D$_3$ Vitamins E + SeMet		SeMet Selenomethionine	LMW OPC flavonols B complex vitamins Carotenoids Vitamin D$_3$ Vitamins E + SeMet	flavonols B complex vitamins Carotenoids Vitamin D$_3$ Vitamins E + SeMet
Amino acids	Taurine Alpha lipoic acid EAAs, NAC	Taurine Alpha lipoate EAAs	Aminos Carnitine fumarate	SAMe and glycine/ MgAsp/ methionine	Carnitine fumarate Taurine Cysteine, NAC Glutamine PAK	EAAs Glutamine PAK	Carnitine fumarate Taurine Alpha lipoic acid Cysteine, NAC
Minerals	Calcium, magnesium, potassium, zinc	Calcium, Magnesium, potassium, vanadium, zinc	Magnesium	Magnesium, potassium	Magnesium, potassium	Magnesium	Magnesium, potassium
Fatty acids	EPA/DHA GLA	EPA/DHA CLA	EPA/DHA CLA	Phosphtidyl- serine	EPA/DHA	EPA/DHA CLA	EPA/DHAGLAs
Intermediates	CoQ_{10}	CoQ_{10}	CoQ_{10}		CoQ_{10}	CoQ_{10}	CoQ_{10}
Bioactive components of foods	Tocotrienols Polycosanols Plant sterols	Tocotrienols Polycosanols Plant sterols Red rice yeast	Tocotrienols Polycosanols Plant sterols	Tocotrienols Polycosanols Plant sterols	Tocotrienols Polycosanols Plant sterols	Tocotrienols Polycosanols Plant sterols Red rice yeast	Tocotrienols Polycosanols Plant sterols

Botanicals				
Hawthorne	French lilac	Hawthorne	Hawthorne	Hawthorne
Pine tea	Bitter melon/	Alginates		
Bilberry	Marah			
Rosehips	Huckleberry/			
Equisetum	bilberry			
	Agnus castus			
	Phosphatides			
	Banaba			
	(corosolate)			
	Gymnema			
	sylvestre			

2.5.2 Catechins in green tea

Catechins, the major polyphenolic compounds in green tea, exert vascular protective effects through several mechanisms, including antioxidative, anti-hypertensive, anti-inflammatory, anti-proliferative, anti-thrombogenic, and lipid-lowering effects (Babu and Liu, 2008). Catechins are also critically involved in the suppression of proinflammatory signaling pathways and have proved to be potent agents for the treatment and prevention of inflammation-related CVDs (Suzuki et al., 2009) (Figure 6.3).

2.5.3 GGOBE (Ginger, Garlic, Onions, Brassica, and Eggs)

The anti-inflammatory properties of ginger have been known and valued for centuries. During the past 25 years, scientific research has substantiated these benefits. Ginger's inhibitory effects on prostaglandin biosynthesis were shown in the early 1970s and have been replicated several times. Found to be as effective as over-the-counter medication, ginger demonstrates a better therapeutic profile with fewer side effects than non-steroidal anti-inflammatory drugs (NSAIDs) (Grzanna et al., 2005). Gingerols calm inflammation by inhibiting prostaglandin release (of cyclooxygenase-1 and cyclooxygenase-2) and possibly by reducing levels of arachidonic acid (5-lipoxygenase) produced by imbalances in the body's fatty acid levels. Ginger can help lower elevated blood pressure, one of the major risk factors for stroke and CHD, and dosages of 5 g or more have demonstrated significant anti-platelet activity in human trials.

Garlic and onions contain a number of sulfides that can lower blood lipids and reduce blood pressure. Onions are also natural anti-clotting agents since they possess substances with fibrinolytic activity that can suppress platelet clumping and break down the products of coagulation. The anti-clotting effect of onions also closely correlates with their sulfur content (Amagase et al., 2001).

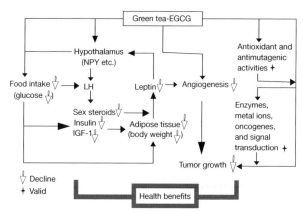

Figure 6.3 Beneficial effects of active constituents in green tea.

Sulfur-rich vegetables such as cauliflower and broccoli are rich in lignans (estrogen-like chemicals that serve as antioxidants) and in aromatic polyphenolic plant compounds. A lignan-rich diet has demonstrated benefits in decreasing risk of CVD as well as certain cancers due to the toxin-binding effects of insoluble fiber. Further, GGOBE foods (ginger, garlic, onions, brassica sprouts, and eggs) are antioxidant rich and repair promoting, and, thus, anti-inflammatory in action (Vanharanta et al., 2002).

3. CONCLUSION

An approach based on *Physiology First* employs functional understanding of biological systems to enhance heart and vascular health. This approach rethinks cardiovascular health from a functional, integrative, comprehensive, holistic, and systems-dynamics perspective. The goal is to apply low-cost, low-risk clinical strategies that remove obstacles to recovery, providing better care and better outcomes. These integrative strategies are a synthesis of classic wisdom and evidence-based advanced insights into individual needs for protective nutrients and other health-promoting factors, including physical and mental exercise, meaningful work, and a tolerable environment. The Alkaline Way of integrative health care management described here provides safer and more effective outcome results in cardiovascular risks. While we await results of larger trials using the above approach, we are confident that these benefits can be applied individually today.

REFERENCES

Amagase, H., Petesch, B.L., Matsuura, H., et al., 2001. Intake of garlic and its bioactive components. The Journal of Nutrition 131, 955S–976S.

Babu, P.V., Liu, D., 2008. Green tea catechins and cardiovascular health: An update. Current Medicinal Chemistry 15, 1840–1850.

Bloedon, L.T., Balikai, S., Chittams, J., et al., 2003. Flaxseed and cardiovascular risk factors: Results from a double blind, randomized, controlled clinical trial. Journal of the American College of Nutrition 27, 65–74.

Dwyer, J.H., Navab, M., Dwyer, K.M., et al., 2011. Oxygenated carotenoid lutein and progression of early atherosclerosis: The Los Angeles Atherosclerosis Study. Circulation 103, 2922–2927.

Elisaf, M., Bairaktari, E., Katopodis, K., et al., 1998. Effect of L-carnitine supplementation on lipid parameters in hemodialysis patients. American Journal of Nephrology 18 (5), 416–421.

Giugliano, D., 2000. Dietary antioxidants for cardiovascular prevention. Nutrition, Metabolism, and Cardiovascular Diseases 10, 38–44.

Glynn, R.J., Ridker, P.M., Goldhaber, S.Z., Zee, R.Y., Buring, J.E., 2007. Effects of random allocation to vitamin E supplementation on the occurrence of venous thromboembolism: Report from the women's health study. Circulation 116, 1497–1503.

Grzanna, R., Lindmark, L., Frondoza, C.G., 2005. Ginger: An herbal medicinal product with broad anti-inflammatory actions. Journal of Medicinal Food 8, 125–132.

Guttman, H., Zimlichman, R., Boaz, M., Matas, Z., Shargorodsky, M.J., 2010. Effect of long-term L-arginine supplementation on arterial compliance and metabolic parameters in patients with multiple cardiovascular risk factors: Randomized, placebo-controlled study. Journal of Cardiovascular Pharmacology [Epub ahead of print].

He, K., Merchant, A., Rimm, E.B., et al., 2004. Folate, vitamin B6, and B12 intakes in relation to risk of stroke among men. Stroke 35, 169–174.

Hennekens, C.H., Buring, J.E., Manson, J.E., et al., 1996. Lack of effect of long-term supplementation with beta carotene on the incidence of malignant neoplasms and cardiovascular disease. The New England Journal of Medicine 334, 1145–1149.

Holick, M.F., 2007. Vitamin D deficiency. The New England Journal of Medicine 357, 266–281.

Ishihara, J., Iso, H., Inoue, M., et al., 2008. Intake of folate, vitamin B6, and vitamin B12 and the risk of CHD: The Japan Public Health Center-Based Prospective Study Cohort I. Journal of the American College of Nutrition 27, 127–136.

Jaffe, R., Brown, S.E., 2000. Acid-alkaline balance and its effect on bone health. International Journal of Integrative Medicine 2, 7–18.

Jenkins, D.J., Kendall, C.W., Vuksan, V., 1999. Inulin, oligofructose, and intestinal function. Journal of Nutrition 129, 1431S–1433S.

Langsjoen, P.H., Langsjoen, J.O., Langsjoen, A.M., Lucas, L.A., 2005. Treatment of statin adverse effects with supplemental coenzyme Q10 and statin drug discontinuation. BioFactors 25, 147–152.

Lee, J.H., O'Keefe, J.H., Bell, D., et al., 2008. Vitamin D deficiency: An important, common, and easily treatable cardiovascular risk factor? Journal of the American College of Cardiology 52, 1949–1952.

Leung, L.H., 1995. Pantothenic acid as a weight-reducing agent: Fasting without hunger, weakness and ketosis. Medical Hypotheses 44, 403–405.

Li, L., Smith, A., Hagen, T.M., Frei, B., 2010. Vascular oxidative stress and inflammation increase with age: Ameliorating effects of alpha-lipoic acid supplementation. Annals of the New York Academy of Sciences 1203, 151–159.

Loria, C.M., Klag, M.J., Caulfield, L.E., Whelton, P.K., 2000. Vitamin C status and mortality in US adults. The American Journal of Clinical Nutrition 72, 139–145.

Maes, M., Mihaylova, I., Kubera, M., et al., 2009. Lower plasma coenzyme Q10 in depression: A marker for treatment resistance and chronic fatigue in depression and a risk factor to cardiovascular disorder in that illness. Neuroendocrinology Letters 30, 462–469.

Murakami, K., Sasaki, S., Okubo, H., et al., 2007. Dietary fiber intake, dietary glycemic index and load, and body mass index: A cross-sectional study of 3931 Japanese women aged 18–20 years. European Journal of Clinical Nutrition 61, 986–995.

Obeid, R., Herrmann, W., 2009. Homocysteine and lipids: S-adenosyl methionine as a key intermediate. FEBS Letters 583 (8), 1215–1225.

Orea-Tejeda, A., Orozco-Gutiérrez, J.J., Castillo-Martínez, L., et al., 2010. The effect of L-arginine and citrulline on endothelial function in patients in heart failure with preserved ejection fraction. Cardiology Journal 17, 464–470.

Parnell, J.A., Reimer, R.A., 2010. Effect of prebiotic fibre supplementation on hepatic gene expression and serum lipids: A dose-response study in JCR: LA-cp rats. British Journal of Nutrition 103, 1577–1584.

Patenaude, A., Rodriguez-Leyva, D., Edel, A.L., et al., 2009. Bioavailability of alpha-linolenic acid from flaxseed diets as a function of the age of the subject. European Journal of Clinical Nutrition 63, 1123–1129.

Quamme, G.A., de Rouffignac, C., 2000. Epithelial magnesium transport and regulation by the kidney. Frontiers in Bioscience 5, D694–D711.

Souto, G., Donapetry, C., Calviño, J., Adeva, M.M., 2011. Metabolic acidosis-induced insulin resistance and cardiovascular risk. Metabolic Syndrome and Related Disorders 9 (4), 247–253.

Suzuki, J., Isobe, M., Morishita, R., Nagai, R., 2009. Tea polyphenols regulate key mediators on inflammatory cardiovascular diseases. Mediators of Inflammation, article ID 494928.

Vanharanta, M., Voutilainen, S., Nurmi, T., et al., 2002. Association between low serum enterolactone and increased plasma F2-isoprostanes, a measure of lipid peroxidation. Atherosclerosis 160, 465–469.

Xiang, D., Sun, Z., Xia, J., et al., 2005. Effect of L-carnitine on cardiomyocyte apoptosis and cardiac function in patients undergoing heart valve replacement operation. Journal of Huazhong University of Science and Technology 25, 501–504.

Ziegler, D., Gries, F.A., 1997. Alpha-lipoic acid in the treatment of diabetic peripheral and cardiac autonomic neuropathy. Diabetes 46 (Suppl. 2), S62–S66.

RELEVANT WEBSITES

www.Healthstudiescollegium.org
www.ELISAACT.com
www.PERQUE.com
www.PERQUEWheyGuard.com
www.ncbi.nlm.nih.gov/pubmed

CHAPTER 7

Fruit and Vegetable Consumption and Risk of Noncommunicable Diseases

P. Mirmiran, F. Hosseini-Esfahani, F. Azizi

Nutrition and Endocrine Research Center, Research Institute for Endocrine Sciences, Shahid Beheshti University of Medical Sciences, Tehran, Iran

ABBREVIATIONS

ACS Acute coronary syndrome
CVD Cardiovascular disease
CHD Coronary heart disease
FAO Food and Agriculture Organization
FV Fruits and vegetables
MetS Metabolic syndrome
RCTs Randomized clinical trials
WHO World Health Organization

1. INTRODUCTION

Lifestyle practices can have a marked impact on the prevention of chronic disease and diet remains the cornerstone of prevention strategies. Consumption of sufficient amounts of fruits and vegetables (FV) is recommended as part of a healthy diet. In epidemiological studies, FV intake has been associated with decreased mortality from a variety of health outcomes including obesity, hypertension, metabolic syndrome (MetS), and cardiovascular disease (CVD) risk factors. A higher consumption of FV has also been associated with a lower risk of coronary heart disease (CHD), stroke, diabetes, and some cancers. It is estimated that up to 2.6 million deaths per year are attributable to inadequate consumption of FV worldwide, and increasing FV consumption to $600\,g\,day^{-1}$ could reduce the burden of CHD by 31% (He et al., 2007). Adherence to a Mediterranean-style diet, rich in FV, legumes, and nuts, affords protection from degenerative diseases such as cardiovascular disorders and cancers (Ortega, 2006). Generally, nutritional advice given in the context of foods or dietary patterns is often easier to comprehend and use, than that available on the nutrients contained within them (He et al., 2007; de Kok et al., 2008).

Several mechanisms may explain the possible protective qualities of FV, such as reducing oxidative stress and inflammatory markers, lowering blood pressure, increasing insulin sensitivity, and improving homeostasis regulation, for which the protective

© 2013 Elsevier Inc.
All rights reserved.
121

constituents, such as potassium, magnesium, folate, vitamins, fiber, and other phyto-chemical compounds, may be responsible. Differences in the nutrient and phytochemical contents of FV could lead to differences in health outcomes; thus the groupings for fruits, such as citrus fruits, apples, fruit juices, and for vegetables, such as cruciferous, green leafy, root vegetables, onions, and sprouts, have been of particular interest in epidemiological studies (He et al., 2007; de Kok et al., 2008). Investigations of dietary components may help to shed more light on the intricate mechanisms behind the benefits of foods or dietary patterns.

The aim of this review is to discuss the association of FV and risk factors of CVD, with a focus on overall FV intake and the dietary patterns provided in well-designed clinical trials, cohort, case–control, and cross-sectional studies.

2. FV AND CVD

CVD is one of the most common causes of morbidity and mortality in different communities. According to World Health Organization (WHO) estimates, by 2020, chronic diseases, notably CVD, will account for approximately three quarters of all deaths worldwide—71% and 75% of all deaths due to ischemic heart disease and stroke, respectively, will occur in developing countries (World Health Organization, 2003a). The rapid rise in CHD burden in most of the low- and middle-income countries is due to socioeconomic changes, increase in lifespan, and acquisition of lifestyle-related risk factors. Primary prevention of CHD is, therefore, now a major public health priority and an increase in the consumption of FV has been advocated for the prevention of CHD (World Health Organization, 2003b).

Twelve cohort studies from North America, Northern Europe, and Japan reported the effect of FV intake and CVD events. A significant inverse relationship between FV intake and CVD events was observed in some of these studies (Dauchet et al., 2009). A prospective study in men, aged 50–59 years, who were recruited in France and Northern Ireland, reported that high FV intake was associated with a lower risk of CVD in male smokers (Dauchet et al., 2010). The pooled relative risks for CVD were 0.89 and 0.94 for increments of one serving per day of green leafy vegetables and vitamin-C rich FV, respectively, in the Health Professionals' Follow-up study and the Nurses' Health Study. Participants, eating at least five servings of FV daily, had a 28% lower risk of CVD than participants eating fewer than 1.5 servings per day. Fruit intakes were associated with a greater reduction in CVD risk than vegetables (Hung et al., 2004).

Dauchet et al. (2006) reviewed the evidence from nine cohort studies (from the United States and Finland) for a relationship between FV consumption and the occurrence of CHD. The clinical end points of CHD were fatal and nonfatal CHD and CHD-related mortality. In a random effect model, the pooled relative risk of

CHD for each additional portion of FV per day was 0.96 (4% reduction) and for each increment of one portion per day of fruits was 0.93 (7% reduction). The association between vegetable intake and CHD risk was heterogeneous, depending on the outcomes. He et al. (2007) reported in a meta-analysis of 13 cohort studies (nine from the United States and four from Europe) and found that increased consumption of FV was related to risk reduction of CHD. Compared with those consuming less than three servings of FV per day, individuals with more than five servings per day had an approximately 17% reduction in CHD risk; individuals with three to five servings per day had a smaller and borderline significant reduction in CHD risk (7% reduction). A pooled analysis of the Health Professionals Follow-up Study and the Nurses' Health Study (NHS) showed a decrease in risk of CHD event risk with an additional serving of either fruits (relative risk (RR) 0.94) or vegetables (RR 0.95). Other cohort studies failed to show any statistically significant effect of FV intake on reducing the risk of ischemic coronary events; however, in some of these studies, a trend toward a beneficial effect of FV intake was observed (Dauchet et al., 2009).

The relationship between FV intake and CHD-related deaths has been reported in ten cohort studies. The RR for mortality was 0.74 with no evidence of heterogeneity in three studies (Dauchet et al., 2006). Only one study showed a significant inverse relationship between intakes of fruits and berries and CHD-related deaths (Dauchet et al., 2009).

The risk reduction estimates from cohort studies are less impressive than those of case–control studies but one large, international, standardized case–control study (INTERHEART Study), which enrolled 15 152 cases of acute MI and 14 820 controls from 262 centers in 52 countries, showed that individuals who ate FV everyday had a reduction of 30% (95% CI: 21–38%) in MI risk, compared with those who did not. Several other case–control studies have generally observed a stronger association between FV intake and CHD compared to meta-analyses of cohort studies; however, potential selection bias, recall bias, and bias due to changes in diet and lifestyle following CHD events cannot be ruled out in these studies.

A pooled analysis of cohort studies suggested that dietary fiber is inversely associated with the risk of CHD in both men and women (27% reduction in risk for coronary mortality for each $10 \, \text{g day}^{-1}$ increment in total dietary fiber). Although cereal and fruit fiber had strong inverse associations with CHD risk, no such associations were observed for vegetable fiber (Pereira et al., 2004).

There has been little support for an inverse association between vegetable fiber intake and risk of CHD. One possible explanation for this finding is the nutrient-poor high-glycemic load nature of common starchy and heavily processed vegetables such as corn and peas. Dietary glycemic load has been shown to substantially increase the risk of CHD and type 2 diabetes mellitus. Therefore, any beneficial effects of vegetable fiber may be countered by some adverse effects of starchy vegetables. More attention needs to be given, both in research and public health strategies/recommendations, to the types of foods being studied and recommended (Alinia et al., 2009).

There is limited evidence of outcomes from long-term randomized trials examining the role of FV alone in the primary prevention of CHD. Clinical randomized trials show that increasing FV intake, along with other diet and lifestyle changes, can significantly reduce the risk of CHD. The Lyon Diet Heart study has shown a reduction in CHD risk in subjects following the Mediterranean diet in the secondary prevention setting. The traditional Mediterranean diet emphasizes a high intake of fruits, vegetables, bread, other forms of cereals, potatoes, beans, nuts, and seeds. This diet includes olive oil as a major fat source and dairy products, fish, and poultry, which are consumed in low to moderate amounts (Kris-Etherton et al., 2001). The Diet and Reinfarction Trial II recommendations, which aimed at promoting increased consumption of FV, fiber, and orange juice, showed no effect on cardiac deaths in patients with angina pectoris. However, the small difference in FV intake, of 20 g day^{-1} between the study and control groups, might well have contributed to lack of significance.

The success of these studies relies on compliance of the participants for the duration of the study, which can be of several years. The difficulties in long-term modification of FV intake on the basis of nutritional advice alone should be taken into account in implementing and interpreting these studies (Dauchet et al., 2009).

2.1 FV and Acute Coronary Syndrome

The association between FV intake and specific FV grouping in relation to acute coronary syndrome (ACS) (the composite of unstable angina pectosis, myocardial infarction cardiac arrest) was investigated in the prospective Danish Diet, Cancer and Health Cohort Study in Denmark. An inverse association (borderline significant) between apple intake, the major contributor to fruits intake in this study, for both men and women was observed during 7.7 years of follow-up, which might be because of the cholesterol-lowering effect of apple. Phytochemicals, catechin and epicatechin, and apple polyphenols, were found to lower total and LDL cholesterol and increase HDL cholesterol in intervention studies. Total fruit intake also indicated a protective association with ACS. A higher risk (4%) was seen among women with increased fruit juice intake. In the NHS II, increasing juice intake was associated with higher weight gain, which is also a risk factor for coronary diseases (Hansen et al., 2010).

2.2 FV and Stroke

Stroke is the third leading cause of death and the leading cause of long-term disability worldwide (World Health Organization, 2003a). Primary prevention of stroke is a major health priority and an increase in the consumption of FV has been advocated for this reason. The pooled analyses of eight cohort studies from the USA, Europe, and Japan showed that individuals who have three to five servings of FV and those with more than five servings per day, respectively, have 11% and 26% reduction in the risk of stroke compared with individuals who have less than three FV servings per day. The pooled analysis showed that for the highest category of intake, while fruits as well as vegetables both had a significant protective effect against stroke, the association was only significant for fruits in the middle category. There is no evidence from long-term randomized trials assessing the effect of FV intake on stroke risk. An important point is whether different types of FV have an equal protective effect; documented data on this issue is scarce (He et al., 2006)

The specific components present in FV might induce their protective effect on stroke. Potassium, with its inhibitory effect on free radical formation, vascular smooth muscle proliferation, arterial thrombosis, macrophage adherence to vascular wall and vascular lesions, could have a direct effect on stroke independent of its effect on blood pressure. Dietary folate is a determinant of homocysteine level and dietary fiber might also contribute to the reduction of stroke by lowering blood pressure and cholesterol. Long-term interventional studies of vitamin C, vitamin E, and betacarotene reveal no beneficial effects from FV on total stroke incidence or mortality. However, antioxidants have been shown to reduce atherosclerosis, mainly by lowering the amount of oxidized LDL available to be incorporated into lesions. These results provide strong support for recommendations on consuming more than five FV servings per day (He et al., 2006).

There are several limitations associated with meta-analyses of cohort studies assessing the relationship of FV intake with CVD events. Although meta-analyses report relative risk as an indication of a protective effect of FV, they also show substantial inter-study heterogeneity, explained possibly by methodological issues or publication bias. Since most studies were conducted in North America and a few in Europe and Japan, the results reflect the association in these regions and not necessarily those from other parts of the world where dietary habits and backgrounds may differ substantially. Individuals who eat more FV are likely to have healthier lifestyles, shown to reduce the risk of CHD. Social and behavioral factors, such as lower rates of smoking, lower salt and saturated fat intakes, higher levels of physical activity, and decreased chances of being overweight, cannot always be measured precisely, and often their confounding effects might not be appropriately captured and controlled in statistical analyses. The observation of a favorable association between FV consumption and CHD risk does not necessarily indicate causality. However, the adjustment of major confounding factors in the studies included in meta-analyses is reported to reduce the potential bias that might occur because of other dietary and lifestyle factors.

In conclusion, based on cohort and case–control studies, FV intake can reduce the risk of incidence and mortality of CVD. Further investigations should focus on the proportion of different types of FV in reducing CVD risk.

3. FV AND DIABETES MELLITUS

The worldwide burden of type 2 diabetes has increased rapidly along with an increase in obesity. The most recent estimate for the worldwide prevalence of diabetes in 2000 was 171 million, a figure believed to increase to at least 366 million by the year 2030 (World Health Organization, 2003a). FV consumption may play a protective role in the development of type 2 diabetes. The meta-analysis of five cohort studies of FV intake and the risk of type 2 diabetes from the USA and Finland, however, found that the consumption of FV is not associated with a substantial reduction in the risk of type 2 diabetes. The pooled relative risk of type 2 diabetes for consuming five or more servings of FV per day, for consuming three or more daily serving of fruits, and for consuming three or more daily servings of vegetables were 0.96, 1.01, and 0.97, respectively (Hamer and Chida, 2007; Dauchet et al., 2009). In the large prospective cohort of middle-aged American women, the role of all FV, specific groups of FV, and fruit juice consumption in the development of diabetes was examined. Overall FV intake was not associated with change in the development of type 2 diabetes. Intake of fruit juices was positively associated with incidence of type 2 diabetes, whereas intake of whole fruits and green leafy vegetables showed an inverse association (Bazzano et al., 2008). In the large population-based prospective study of middle-aged women in Shanghai, China, where consumption of vegetables, especially green leafy vegetables, is high and dietary patterns are quite different from western societies, the effect of the intake of specific subgroups of vegetables and fruits was examined, and it was found that both green and yellow vegetables were inversely associated with the risk of type 2 diabetes, while neither BMI nor WHR modified the effect of vegetable intake on the risk of type 2 diabetes. Fruit intake and type 2 diabetes were not associated (Villegas et al., 2008).

Randomized prevention trials have demonstrated the effectiveness of complex life-style interventions (including promotion of FV intake, physical activity, and body weight reduction) on reducing the risk of diabetes. Given the complexity of lifestyle interventions, it is difficult to estimate the effect of FV intake on risk reduction of diabetes, independent of other dietary and lifestyle changes. Nutrition trials have not shown the association of FV intake or estimated fiber intake with the risk of diabetes or levels of glycemia and insulin sensitivity.

The discrepancies between studies could be explained by confounding factors, including educational level, social condition, physical activity, and by the possible antagonistic effects of sugars, fiber, and antioxidants in FV. The potential healthy lifestyle bias, such as exercise, not smoking, reduced intake of saturated fat, maintaining a healthy weight, and reducing adiposity, that is accompanied with consuming FV and may contribute to a beneficial effect, make it very difficult to determine the exact benefit of FV on the risk of type 2 diabetes.

The mechanisms by which vegetables affect glucose tolerance have not been clearly defined. These could include high antioxidants, fiber and magnesium content, or the low glycemic index and low energy density in vegetables. In particular, green leafy vegetables may supply magnesium, which has been inversely related to the development of type 2 diabetes. In another study, the inverse association between vegetables intake and type 2 diabetes persisted after adjustment for vitamin C, vitamin E, carotene, and fiber intake, and further adjustment for magnesium intake did not alter the association; so the beneficial effects of vegetables intake on the risk of type 2 diabetes cannot be explained entirely by antioxidant vitamins, magnesium, or fiber intake. Vegetables also contain other compounds, such as phytates, lignan, and isoflavones, that might have an additive or synergistic effect on lowering the risk of type 2 diabetes (Villegas et al., 2008).

Although fruit juices may have antioxidant activity, they lack fiber and other phytochemicals, are less satiating, and tend to have high sugar content. The rapid delivery of a large sugar load and fructose may be an important mechanism by which fruit juices contribute to the development of diabetes and insulin-resistance syndrome. Fruit juices have higher glycemic load, which might contribute to the development of diabetes (Bazzano et al., 2008). A positive association between fruit juice intake and the hazard of diabetes indicated that the recommendation of dietary guidelines that 100% fruit juices be considered a serving of the fruit group should be implemented with caution. It is further recommended to replace some sugar-free fruit nectars with pulp in them in an effort to provide healthier options with nutrients, fiber, and phytochemicals.

In conclusion, cohort and clinical trials studies published to date do not provide clear evidence that consumption of FV reduces the risk of type 2 diabetes and some cohort studies have produced conflicting results. Differences in the nutrient content of FVs by group could lead to differences in health effects. Specific groups of FV, such as green leafy vegetables and whole fruits, may be important in reducing the risk of type 2 diabetes. This is noteworthy that the majority of studies examining FV intake were drawn from cohorts of participants in the United States. Given that those with western cultures are largely over-nourished, the high and increasing incidence of obesity may overwhelm any specific nutrient effects. Underreporting of usual dietary intake, which is most common in obese persons (Mirmiran et al., 2006), is one of the important sources of bias in nutrition research. Further evidence from other cultures and populations is required.

Table 7.1 summarizes the pooled relative risks for the association of FV intake and noncommunicable diseases, based on meta-analysis studies.

4. FV AND METS

MetS is a clustering of metabolic risk factors, including abdominal obesity, dysfunctional glucose metabolism, atherogenic dyslipidemia, and elevated blood pressure. Patients with

Table 7.1 Summary of Relative Risk for the Association of Fruits and Vegetables (FV) Intake and Noncommunicable Disease Based on Meta-Analysis Studies

Diseases or risk factors	Men	Women	Both	Region	No. of cohort studies
Coronary Heart Disease (Mente et al., 2009)				The United States & Europe	
Vegetables	0.79 (0.65–0.94)	0.81 (0.60–1.02)	0.68 (0.38–0.99)		9
Fruits	0.79 (0.49–1.09)	0.81 (0.53–1.09)	0.84 (0.68–1.00)		10
FV	0.75 (0.58–0.92)	0.74 (0.50–0.99)	0.81 (0.72–0.90)		7
(Pereira et al., 2004)				United States & Europe	10
Fruit fiber (per 10 g day^{-1} increments)			0.84 (0.70–0.99)		
Vegetable fiber (per 10 g day^{-1} increments)			1.00 (0.88–1.03)		
(He et al., 2007)				United States & Europe	12
FV, 3–5 servings per day	0.90 (0.82–0.98)	0.76 (0.55–1.05)	0.93 (0.86–1.00)		
FV, >5 servings per day	0.84 (0.78–0.90)	0.76 (0.64–0.90)	0.83 (0.77–0.89)		
Fruits, 3–5 servings per day			0.90 (0.83–0.98)		
Fruits, >5 servings per day			0.87 (0.80–0.95)		
Vegetables, 3–5 servings per day			0.92 (0.87–0.97)		
Vegetables, >5 servings per day			0.84 (0.76–0.92)		
(Dauchet et al., 2006)				United States & Europe	9
FV (per 1 portion per day increments)			0.96 (0.93–0.99)		
Fruit (per 1 portion per day increments)			0.93 (0.89–0.96)		
Vegetables (per 1 portion per day increments)			0.89 (0.83–0.95)		

Continued

Table 7.1 Summary of Relative Risk for the Association of Fruits and Vegetables (FV) Intake and Noncommunicable Disease Based on Meta-Analysis Studies—cont'd

Diseases or risk factors	Sex			Region	No. of cohort studies
	Men	Women	Both		
Fatal and Nonfatal MI					4
FV (per 1 portion per day increments)			0.95 (0.92–0.99)		
Coronary heart disease mortality					3
FV (per 1 portion per day increments)			0.74 (0.75–0.84)		
Cardiovascular disease (Hung et al., 2004)				United States	2
FV (per 5 servings per day increments)			0.88 (0.81–0.95)		
Fruits (per 5 servings per day increments)			0.87 (0.80–0.94)		
Vegetables (per 5 servings per day increments)			0.93 (0.86–1.00)		
Stroke (He et al., 2006)				United States, Europe, & Asia	8
FV, 3–5 servings per day	0.83 (0.77–0.89)	0.95 (0.88–1.04)	0.89 (0.83–0.97)		
FV, >5 servings per day	0.71 (0.63–0.80)	0.76 (0.69–0.83)	0.74 (0.69–0.79)		
Fruit, 3–5 servings per day			0.89 (0.82–0.98)		
Fruit, >5 servings per day			0.72 (0.66–0.79)		
Vegetables, 3–5 servings per day			0.93 (0.82–1.06)		
Vegetables, >5 servings per day			0.81 (0.72–0.90)		
Diabetes (Hamer and Chida, 2007)				United States & Europe	5
≥5 servings per day, FV			0.96 (0.79–1.17)		
≥3 servings per day, Vegetables			0.97 (0.86–1.10)		

Continued

Table 7.1 Summary of Relative Risk for the Association of Fruits and Vegetables (FV) Intake and Noncommunicable Disease Based on Meta-Analysis Studies—cont'd

Diseases or risk factors	Sex			Region	No. of cohort studies
	Men	Women	Both		
≥3 servings per day, Fruit Cancer			1.01 (0.88–1.15)		
(Hung et al., 2004)				United States	2
FV (per 5 servings per day increments)			1.00 (0.95–1.05)		
Fruits (per 5 servings per day increments)			1.01 (0.95–1.06)		
Vegetables (per 5 servings per day increments)			0.99 (0.95–1.04)		
Major chronic disease (Hung et al., 2004)				United States	2
FV (per 5 servings per day increments)			0.96 (0.92–1.00)		
Fruits (per 5 servings per day increments)			0.97 (0.93–1.01)		
Vegetables (per 5 servings per day increments)			0.97 (0.93–1.01)		

this syndrome have an increased risk of morbidity and mortality because of CVD, CHD, and diabetes. Identifying the effect of FV on MetS risk factors or components may be important in determining the possible causal relationship between FV and CHD, CVD, and diabetes risk. Studies of these end points are, therefore, more relevant than other biological experiments in assessing cause-and-effect relationships.

Dietary patterns with a frequent intake of raw and salad vegetables, both summer and winter fruits, fish, pasta, and rice and a low intake of fried foods, sausages, fried fish, and potatoes have been negatively correlated with many components of the MetS, including central obesity, fasting plasma glucose, and triglycerides, and were positively correlated with HDL cholesterol. In the third National Health and Nutrition Examination Survey (NHANES III), participants with the MetS were found to have significantly lower consumption of FV than those without the MetS. In the ATTICA study, adherence to a Mediterranean-style dietary pattern was associated with a 20% lower risk of having the MetS, irrespective of many confounding variables, including age, sex, physical activity, lipid profile, and blood pressure. However, epidemiological evidence suggests a lower prevalence of MetS in individuals with dietary patterns rich in FV, whole grains, dairy products, and unsaturated fats. The interaction of dietary components offers protection against MetS (Giugliano et al., 2008). In the Tehran Lipid and Glucose Study (Azizi et al., 2009), higher intakes of FV were associated with lower concentrations of total and low-density lipoprotein cholesterol and with the risk of CVD per se in a dose–response manner (Mirmiran et al., 2009).

In a randomized controlled outpatient trial, in an Iranian population, the prevalence of MetS decreased by 35% in the Dietary Approach to Stop Hypertension (DASH) diet group compared with the control diet (Azadbakht et al., 2005). The other dietary intervention study explored possible mechanisms underlying a randomly assigned 180 patients ($n = 99$ men and 81 women) with MetS to either a Mediterranean-style diet (an increase in daily consumption of whole grains, vegetables, fruits, nuts, and olive oil) or a cardiac-prudent diet with a fat intake of <30% of total calories. Only 40 patients in the intervention group still had MetS after 2 years compared with 78 patients who consumed the control diet; thus, there was a 48% net reduction in the prevalence of the MetS (Esposito et al., 2004).

In conclusion, epidemiological studies have documented that adherence to dietary patterns rich in FV, similar to those of the Mediterranean-style diet, may exert positive effects on almost all components of the MetS.

5. FV AND HYPERTENSION

Consumption of FV has been shown to be associated with decreased blood pressure under controlled conditions, particularly in hypertensive individuals (Dauchet et al., 2009). A randomized controlled trial investigated the effect of 6-month primary care intervention to increase FV consumption in a general healthy population with a wide range of eating habits. The results showed that FV intake raised plasma concentrations of α-carotene, lycopene, β-cryptoxanthin, and ascorbic acid and significant decrease in blood pressure (4.0 mmHg systolic and 1.5 mmHg diastolic). This fall in blood pressure is expected to produce small clinical effects, but would substantially reduce CVD at the population level. A reduction of 2 mmHg in diastolic blood pressure results in a decrease of about 17% in the incidence of hypertension, 6% in the risk of CHD, and 15% in the risk of stroke and transient ischemic attack (John et al., 2002).

There is a significant dose–response relationship between FV consumption and endothelium-dependent vasodilatation, with an extra daily portion improving the maximum forearm blood flow response to acetylcholine by ~6%, a finding that links an achievable dietary goal with improvement in a vascular measure of known prognostic value. It also provides evidence that eating just one extra portion of FV a day has potential benefits (McCall DO, 2009) and it implicates important public health recommendations to eat 4–13 servings of FV daily, based on the 2005 dietary guidelines for Americans (USDA, 2010).

The specific components present in FV that reduce blood pressure have not been fully characterized. Flavonoids, the major class of polyphenolics, are abundant in FV. Flavonoids may account for some of the health-promoting effects of FV based on their antioxidant effect. Some foods are particularly rich in flavonoids, such as tea, wine, onions, apples, or dark chocolate, which have established beneficial cardiovascular effects. Flavonoids, and especially quercetin, chemically interact with reactive oxygen species and exert inhibitory activity against a diverse variety of enzymes, ion channels, and transcription factors (Perez-Vizcaino et al., 2009).

Recently, oxidative stress has been proposed as the cause of hypertension. An imbalance in superoxide and nitric oxide production may account for reduced vasodilation, which in turn can favor the development of hypertension. The supplementation of antioxidants, particularly in the form of fresh FV, reduces blood pressure, supporting a role for free radicals in hypertension (Ceriello, 2008).

In conclusion, findings of observational population-based studies and clinical trials support the hypothesis that FV consumption can affect blood pressure regulation. Additional studies are needed to validate these findings in long term.

6. FV AND OBESITY

Overweight and obesity are considered to be among the most challenging and steadily increasing public health concerns worldwide. Strategies to effectively reduce and maintain a healthy body weight are urgently required. A number of observational and interventional studies have investigated the possible association between FV intake and body weight. In an ambulatory setting, promoting FV consumption showed no substantial effect on body weight or BMI; however, these studies did not specifically target overweight or obese individuals. Other studies have shown that decreased fat intake combined with increased FV intake results in greater weight loss when compared with low-fat diets. Accumulating evidence indicates that the combination of increased FV intake, together with other dietary recommendations, might promote satiety and weight loss in overweight individuals (Dauchet et al., 2009). In another review article, the emphasis was given to the role of fruits alone on the risk of developing overweight and obesity (Alinia et al., 2009). Fruits are typically more consumed at occasions than vegetables as they can be obtained in various physical forms, such as fresh, dried, canned, and pureed, making them convenient as between-meal snacks, potentially substituting more energy-dense snacks. Fruits are frequently consumed raw, whereas vegetables are often prepared by addition of fatty substances, which diminishes the low-energy-dense characteristics of vegetables.

Most cross-sectional and prospective studies found an inverse association between fruits intake and body weight. In two interventional studies, increased fruits intake (an addition of approximately one and a half to three pieces of fruits per day) significantly decreased mean body weight with about 0.84–1.6 kg. One interventional study did not find a significant difference in body weight reduction between a high-fruit diet and a low-fruit diet group, although only the high-fruit diet group significantly reduced their waist circumferences. Results of predominant studies, regardless of study types, suggest that fruit intake is inversely associated with body weight, but these studies did not precisely satisfy the conclusive aim of assessing the role of fruits intake on body weight (Alinia et al., 2009).

FV are low in fat and have high water and indigestible fiber content, soluble dietary fibers, in particular; increasing FV intake, therefore, lowers the energy density of meals. According to some short-term studies, food intake is seemingly regulated by the weight of the food ingested, rather than by its energy content. When consuming low-energy-dense foods, satiation may occur relatively early and the feeling of satiety may persist for a relatively long period. Hence, substitution of high-energy-dense foods with low-energy-dense foods, such as FV, could potentially decrease the total energy intake. In the generally energy-abundant diets, replacing energy-dense foods with FV could help to decrease calorie intake and, therefore, eventually body weight (Dauchet et al., 2009; Alinia et al., 2009). Soluble dietary fibers, abundant in FV, reportedly also decrease total energy intake and can consequently cause body weight reduction. This may be due partly to a dilution of the diet energy density and partly a delay in gastric emptying of ingested food. Hence, the feeling of satiation and satiety increases, causing a reduction in the total energy intake; in addition, soluble dietary fibers form a gel-like environment in the small intestine, resulting partly in decreased activity of the enzymes involved in the digestion of fat, protein, and carbohydrates and partly in the capture and subsequent loss of these energy-yielding macronutrients, resulting in overall lowered energy absorption. The gel-like environment in the small intestine and the subsequent slow digestion of the nutrients may also presumably prolong the contact of the nutrients with receptors in the small intestine, potentially causing the release of putative satiety peptides. Such effects have been shown to decrease insulin secretion and improve glucose control. A pooled analysis of cohort studies found inverse associations for both types of fiber. The relative risks were stronger for soluble fiber, reaching 0.46 for risk of coronary mortality per each 10 g day^{-1} increment (Pereira et al., 2004). Another aspect of dietary fibers in relation to satiety is that they decrease the glycemic index of foods. Foods with low glycemic index generate small and sustained elevation in postprandial blood glucose concentrations, which may be associated with long-term satiety (Alinia et al., 2009).

Fructose, the main sugar in fruits, has a relatively low glycemic index, producing a slow increase in postprandial blood glucose followed by a possible increase in satiety. The slow absorption may also increase satiety as a result of extended contact time with the gastrointestinal receptors that produce satiety signals. Another factor that may connect fructose to satiety involves incomplete absorption of fructose with subsequent hyperosmolar environment in the colon. This results in attraction of fluids into the gut lumen, causing a feeling of indisposition and lost interest in further food consumption.

In conclusion, most studies found that consuming low-energy-dense foods such as FV decreased the risk of overweight and obesity, which might be due to low glycemic index, high water and indigestible fiber content. Most of these studies also failed to report other variables that could affect the relationship between fruits consumption and body weight, i.e., physical form of the fruits, ways of preparation of fruits, and what is classified as the fruits category (fruit juices, canned or dried fruits, etc.). Promotion of increased FV consumption in the general population may form part of the strategies designed to handle the increasing global challenge of overweight and obesity (Alinia et al., 2009).

7. FV AND BONE MINERAL STATUS

Osteoporosis is a major public health problem around the world. The deterioration in bone mass and microarchitecture associated with the disease, leads to greater risk of fragility fracture, disability, and premature mortality. Nutrition is an important modifiable factor in the development and maintenance of bone mass and adequate dietary calcium intake and vitamin D status have long been recognized as factors in maintaining bone health. Other dietary components, such as magnesium, zinc, copper, iron, fluoride, and vitamins A, C, and K, are required for normal bone metabolism, nutrients, which occur together in foods. The results of the Data collected from three different studies including five cohorts on adolescent boys and girls, young women, and older men and women, aged 16–83 years, showed that higher FV intakes may have a positive effect on bone mineral status in adolescent boys and girls and older women, especially at the spine and femoral neck. Higher intakes of FV were associated with other diet and lifestyle characteristics that may have an overall beneficial effect on bone health (Prynne et al., 2006). A dietary acid load, such as the western dietary pattern, appears to have a detrimental effect on bone health indices. FV intake may balance the excess acidity by providing potassium (Wynn et al., 2010).

In conclusion, FV intake has the potential role to prevent osteoporosis in an easy and cost-effective way.

8. FV AND CANCER

Despite the enormous amount of research and rapid developments seen during the past decade, cancer continues to be one of the leading causes of death in the world. Cancer has a complex etiology, and many factors, both environmental and genetic, contribute to it. Of the environmental factors, the link between diet and cancer risk

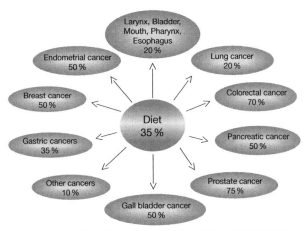

Figure 7.1 Cancer deaths (%) linked to diet as reported by Willett WC, 2000 (Anand et al., 2008, with permission).

has long been recognized. It is estimated that 30–40% of cancer-related incidents (over 20% by increased FV intakes) are preventable by consuming a healthy diet (Figure 7.1) (Ruhul Amin et al., 2009). The contribution of dietary factors/elements to cancer deaths varies a great deal, according to the type of cancer. A large set of published meta-analyses of cohort and case–control studies indicated limited but significant evidence for a cancer preventive effect associated with the consumption of FV for sites that included the mouth and pharynx, esophagus, stomach, colon–rectum, larynx, lung, ovary, bladder, and kidney but with inadequate evidence for other sites; statistically significant odds ratios, as low as 0.5, were found (Ware, 2009).

The high incidence of cancers and the related mortality and lack of effective treatment have spurred extensive research on dietary phytochemicals. It is generally accepted that the consumption of FV may reduce the risk of human cancers. Several cell culture and animal studies have addressed the cancer preventive effects of the active components derived from FV.

In this section, an attempt is made to introduce and discuss the preventive properties of FV on some cancers and the phytochemicals included, focusing on some epidemiological and preclinical studies.

8.1 FV and Endometrial Cancer

Endometrial cancer accounts for about 4% of all cancers in women worldwide. Among known risk factors for endometrial cancer, there is a strong evidence of relationship between obesity and this cancer, particularly for older women. In part of this relationship, there has been growing interest in the role that dietary factors may play on risk of endometrial cancer. The possible protective role of FV on endometrial cancer risk was reported in the World Cancer Research Fund/American Institute for Cancer Research (WCRF/AICR) 1997. The meta-analysis based on a limited number of published case–control studies suggests an inverse association between FV consumption and endometrial cancer risk. The random effects pooled OR among ten case–control studies, comparing high vs low intakes of total vegetables as a group was 0.71. Among the eight case–control studies for which it was possible to derive a quantitative estimate of consumption, the random effect pooled OR was 0.9, for a difference of 100 g day^{-1} of vegetables intake. This inverse association seemed to hold for cruciferous vegetables, the only subgroup of vegetables for which there were enough studies to warrant meta-analysis.

Many compounds in plant foods have been found to be potent modulators of the cytochrome P450 (CYP) monooxygenases in vitro and in animal models; certain CYP enzymes that metabolize phytochemicals also contribute to the inactivation of endogenous steroid hormones. Cruciferous vegetables, which include broccoli sprouts, kale, and cabbage, contain glucosinolates; certain hydrolysis products of glucosinolates, including indoles and isothiocyanates, have shown anticarcinogenic properties. Isothiocyanates and indoles may inhibit tumorigenesis, in part, from their ability to influence phase I and II biotransformation enzymes, thus influencing several processes related to chemical carcinogenesis, such as the metabolism and carcinogen binding to DNA. Glutathione S-transferase (GST) is a phase I enzyme involved in conjugation of xenobiotics. In an intervention study of botanically defined diets, GST responses were more pronounced in women than in men (Bandera et al., 2007).

The suggestion that intake of vegetables may decrease risk of endometrial cancer risk is generally plausible. Nonstarchy vegetables, including green-leafy and deep-yellow varieties, contain vitamins, minerals, dietary fiber, carotenoids, flavonoids, and allium compounds that may influence cancer risk through their antioxidant activity, modulation of detoxification enzymes, stimulation of the immune system, and modulation of steroid hormone concentration and hormone metabolism. More cohort studies are needed to evaluate these associations as well as their role in certain population subgroups. In addition, harmonization of the vegetable group is needed for defining and analyzing this group to compare results in different populations.

8.2 FV and Bladder Cancer

Bladder cancer presents a substantial challenge to public health. Accumulating evidence from epidemiologic studies and clinical trials indicates that dietary components may substantially alter the natural history of bladder cancer; evidence suggests that diet modifications may prevent incidence of bladder cancer or reduce the risk of recurrence or progression. Some prospective clinical trials, although none large enough, promising dietary agents for prevention of incident or recurrent bladder cancer, include selenium, carrots, cruciferous vegetables, and fruits. In the Health Professional's Follow-Up Study and the Netherlands Cohort Study, participants in the highest quartile of cruciferous vegetable intake compared with those in the lowest quartile, had a 51% and 25% reduced risk of urothelial cancer respectively. Three additional case–control and one cohort analysis have also shown inverse associations with the risk of bladder cancer although a cohort study of Swedish women demonstrated no association. A recent systematic review of published reports, based on four case–control analyses, two meta-analyses, and two cohort studies, determined that fruit intake is associated with a moderate reduction in bladder cancer risk. Although less information on individual fruit items, apples, citrus, and tomatoes are found to be potentially beneficial. Cruciferous vegetables are believed to exert anticarcinogenic effects against urothelial cancer through isothiocyanates-mediated activation of these enzymatic pathways. An increased risk of urothelial carcinoma has been demonstrated in individuals with GST and quinolonone oxidoreductase 1 (NQ01) genotypes associated with null or suboptimal phenotypes.

These data should serve primarily as a guide to researchers to design future clinical trials to promote healthy lifestyle interventions based on diet change, specifically by increasing FV intakes among patients with bladder cancer (Silberstein and Parsons, 2010).

8.3 FV and Breast Cancer

Breast cancer is one of the most common cancers among women in several countries. The role of diet on the risk of breast cancer is of great interest as a potentially modifiable risk factor. Six prospective cohort studies have considered the relationship between FV consumption and the incidence of breast cancer; of these, three were limited to postmenopausal women. The only significant association was reported from the NHS, which reported an inverse association for regular consumption of five or more vegetables per day and premenopausal breast cancer incidence, as compared to consuming less than two vegetables per day (RR $= 0.64$; 95% CI, 0.43–0.95). In a meta-analysis including five cohorts and 2608 cases, an RR of 0.73 (95% CI, 0.64–0.83) for breast cancer was found to be associated with high vegetable consumption. However, a pooled analysis of data from eight prospective cohorts, including 7377 cases, resulted in an RR $= 0.96$ (95% CI, 0.89–1.04) for vegetable consumption and an RR $= 0.93$ (95% CI, 0.86–1.00) for FV consumption comparing the women in the highest versus the lowest category of intakes. FV consumption may prevent breast cancer through their antioxidants, fiber, and other nutrients (Michels et al., 2007).

Pierce clarified the role of dietary pattern on prognosis in breast cancer survivors. There is no convincing evidence that changing dietary pattern (increasing FV, whole grain products, low-fat dairy and poultry, fiber and fish consumption) following breast cancer diagnosis will improve prognosis for most women with early stage breast cancer. However, it would appear to be important for some subgroups, and further investigation of mechanisms for such selective action is needed (Pierce, 2009).

To date, current data from prospective epidemiologic studies conducted on diet and breast cancer, reveals no association that is consistent, strong, and statistically significant. Most studies on diet and breast cancer have been conducted in industrialized countries, primarily North America, Europe, and Japan, and considering the substantial variation in diet across industrialized and developing countries and the role of diet for breast cancer risk in developing countries has been less explored. Also the human breast may be most susceptible to dietary influences during early life, in particular, before puberty and current data available do not allow inferences about the role of diet before or during puberty and the risk of breast cancer (Michels et al., 2007). It is possible that a protective effect of foods such as FV on breast cancer risk is countered by a harmful effect of food residues such as pesticides. Furthermore, there is insufficient data on the association of more restrictive dietary patterns such as organic foods, whole foods, raw foods, or a vegan diet with breast cancer incidence.

8.4 FV and Gastric Cancer

In 2000, gastric cancer was the second most frequent cause of cancer death worldwide and the fourth most common cancer. There are geographic and ethnic differences in the worldwide incidence of gastric cancer and its trends for each population with time. Almost two-thirds of these new cases occurred in developing countries. The incidence patterns observed among immigrants change according to where they live. These factors indicate the progression of cancer, being modulated by environmental exposures, including dietary factors. The association between FV intake and risk for gastric cancer has been evaluated extensively in observational epidemiologic studies, which generally suggest an inverse association, particularly for raw and allium vegetables and citrus fruits. In 2005, a meta-analysis showed that this inverse association is stronger for fruits than for vegetables; it was however, weaker in cohort studies than in case–control studies. This meta-analysis showed that design options might play a key role in the observed magnitude or the direction of the association between FV intake and gastric cancer (Liu and Russell, 2008). The summary relative risks of gastric cancer were 0.82 for fruits, being stronger for follow-up periods of ≥ 10 year (RR $= 0.66$); for vegetables, the RR was 0.88, based on all incidence studies and 0.71 when considering only those with longer follow-ups (Lunet et al., 2005). The results from the European Prospective Investigation into Cancer and Nutrition (EPIC) cohort study, conducted on 521 457 men and women living in ten European countries, showed no significant association between consumption of fresh fruits, total vegetables, or specific groups of vegetables and the risk of gastric cancer, regardless of anatomic site; however, a nonsignificant inverse association was observed for citrus fruits, onion, and garlic, and risk for gastric cardiac cancer only (Liu and Russell, 2008).

Thus consumption of FV, particularly fruits, is most probably protective against gastric cancer; however, it remains unknown that which of the constituents in FV play a more significant role in the prevention of gastric cancer. FV are rich sources of vitamin C. Relatively consistent epidemiological evidence and biological plausibility are documented indicating that dietary or supplemental vitamin C intake may decrease the risk of gastric cancer. Vitamin C acts as an antioxidant and can quench reactive oxygen species produced in the gastric environment; it is also known to inhibit production of carcinogenic N-nitroso compound in the stomach. A possible relation between *Helicobacter pylori* infection and ascorbic acid is under investigation, as some research has indicated that high-dose vitamin C is effective in inhibiting *H. pylori* infection. Hence, dietary modification to increase intake of FV, particularly vitamin C-rich foods, represents one of the effective, practical, and low-cost means of preventing gastric cancer (Tsugane and Sasazuki, 2007; Liu and Russell, 2008).

8.5 FV and Colorectal Cancer

Colorectal cancer is one of the most prevalent cancers worldwide. Relationships between nutrition and colorectal cancer have long been hypothesized. It has been shown that the risk of colorectal cancer is decreased by adherence to healthy nutrition-related behaviors. However, the particular effect of the consumption of each type of food on colorectal cancer risk remains questionable. Fifteen studies assessed the relationship between total vegetables consumption and colorectal cancer risk; 12 failed to find any significant linkage, whereas two studies found an inverse relationship to be confirmed and only in one study, this association was found in women, but not in men. The overall findings concerning the protective/deleterious effect of the consumption of selected vegetables/legumes are rather conflicting. Fourteen studies reported data on fruit consumption and colorectal cancer risk; no significant relationship was found in 11 studies, two reported an inverse relationship in women, whereas one showed a positive association in women, but not in men. As for vegetable consumption, data available indicate that increased fruit consumption per se may only slightly reduce the risk of colorectal cancer. Six studies assessed the effect of the combined consumption of FV. Three studies on colon and rectal cancer risk found little or no effect of the individual consumption of vegetables or fruits, whereas their combined consumption decreased colon cancer risk or mortality, specifically in women, but not in men. Taken together, those findings suggest that the relationship between vegetable consumption and colorectal cancer risk is relatively low. Conversely, the combined consumption of FV might be of interest. Cruciferous vegetables might be related to an increased risk, whereas other types of vegetables per se appear to exert little or no effect (Marques-Vidal, 2006).

8.6 FV and Prostate Health

The prostate, a major male accessory gland, is a potential source of serious disorders affecting the health and quality of life in older men. The long preclinical phase (latency) of prostate cancer implies that environmental factors, such as diet and nutrition, may significantly influence progression of this malignancy at various stages of the male life cycle. There is inconsistency in the epidemiological studies trying to correlate the intake of FV with prostate cancer incidence and mortality, depending on the investigated population, the methods of estimating the dietary intake, and the statistical evaluation of accumulated data. In the prospective study of seven European countries, 130 544 men were included, of whom 1104 cases were registered after the 5-year baseline intake estimate. The highest median consumption of FV in Spain and Sweden coincided with a low incidence of prostate cancer. Prospective data from the National Health and Nutrition Examination Survey Epidemiological Follow-up Study cohorts showed that prostate cancer risk was not associated with FV intake, but intermediate intake of FV tended to increase the risk of prostate cancer (RR = 1.5). Dietary intervention by intensive counseling to consume a low-fat, high FV (increased FV intake by 2.25 servings per day compared to control group diet) failed to slow the increase of serum PSA concentrations in healthy subjects over time in the Polyp Prevention Trial. However, quite the opposite relationship is indicated by many between prostate cancer and plant-based diets, which included large amounts of FV. The high levels of FV intake in India produced a very low OR for developing prostate cancer (OR = 0.4). Most possibly the studies conducted in Western societies are limited to relatively low levels of intake, which fail to reach an optimal range and are, therefore, inconclusive.

FVs rich in carotenoids have processed antioxidant properties. Carotenoids are well absorbed by the human intestinal epithelium and accumulate in many tissues, including the prostate, where they may exert anticancer effects. Multiethnic case–control studies in United States and Canada and another in China identified that while yellow-orange and red FV intakes were inversely associated with the risk of prostate cancer, individual vegetables, i.e., corn, carrots, tomato, watermelon, pumpkin, spinach, and citrus were especially effective. The growing popularity of tomato products in the diet causes lycopene to be a predominant carotenoid in serum and prompted many researchers to study its possible interaction with prostate cancer. Tomato sauce, a good source of bioavailable lycopene, was associated with a greater reduction in prostate cancer risk than the calculated lycopene intake from all sources. A lycopene-augmented diet may increase tumor necrosis rates by downregulation of genes involved in inflammatory signaling (IGF-1 and IL-6), generation of reactive oxygen species, and androgen expression. Lycopene may increase apoptosis and decrease proliferation by arresting the cell cycle of various human prostate cell lines. Also, allium vegetables (onions, garlic, leeks) seem to significantly decrease prostate cancer mortality worldwide, possibly because of their organosulfur compounds, which inhibit growth of human cancer cells in vitro, including prostate cancer cell lines. In a large data set from Italian case–control studies, the multivariate ORs for prostate cancer were 0.29 and 0.81, respectively, for the highest categories of onion and garlic consumption compared with the lowest. Another group of protective vegetables are the cruciferae (cabbage, broccoli, cauliflower, brussels sprouts), which were inversely related to prostate cancer risk in case–control studies. Cruciferous vegetables contain isothiocyanate compounds, with sulforaphane being the most predominant and widely investigated in cancer research. It is reported to inhibit the growth of DU-145 prostate cancer cells in vitro by retarding cell cycle progression and activation of apoptosis. Hot chili peppers, containing a potent irritant capsaicin, have a profound inhibiting effect on the growth of prostate cancer cell lines in vitro, arresting the cell cycle, inducing apoptosis, and blocking dihydrotestosterone-induced PSA production. Recently, pomegranate juice was reported to slow the PSA rise in prostate cancer patients after surgery or radiotherapy, indicating possibly the modulation of disease progression; daily pomegranate juice consumption for 9 months decreased serum lipid peroxidation in these patients, and their serum had increased apoptotic and antiproliferative effects on prostate cancer cell line (LNCaP) in vitro. The presence and synergistic action of many agents in plant food may have a considerable preventive effect on the development and progression of prostate diseases (Stacewicz-Sapuntzakis et al., 2008).

9. PREVENTION OF NONCOMMUNICABLE DISEASE BY FV INTAKE

9.1 Dietary Chemopreventive Agents

Chemo prevention, by definition, is a means of noncommunicable disease control by which the occurrence of the diseases can be entirely prevented, slowed down, or reversed by the administration of one or more naturally occurring and/or synthetic agents. The concept of dietary chemoprevention is gaining increasing attention because it is a cost-effective alternative to cancer treatment. The protective effect of colorful FVs is believed to rely on their potential multiple anticancer components and cytoprotectants, such as vitamins, minerals, and numerous antioxidants and phytochemicals. Various epidemiological and preclinical findings and results of several early clinical studies are continually identifying individual and combinations of phytochemicals and antioxidants of FVs that selectively target precancerous and cancer cells. The evidence for specific vegetables, and indeed phytochemicals, is less convincing and the best simple advice that can be given is to recommend as much variety as possible. Its action may be both multifactorial and synergistic, vastly increasing the difficulty of eventually achieving significant mechanistic understanding (Ruhul Amin et al., 2009). A growing number of in vitro and in vivo studies indicate that combinations of dietary chemopreventive agents (phytochemicals) can sometimes act synergistically, which may explain why some food items or diets may show cancer preventive effects, though it cannot be explained on the basis of individual bioactive ingredients (de Kok et al., 2008). These phytochemicals are safe and usually target multiple cell-signaling pathways. The key challenge to researchers is how best to use this information for effective cancer prevention in populations with different cancer risks. Moreover, low potency and poor bioavailability of dietary agents pose further challenges to scientists. The introduction of synthetic analogs of natural compounds may be a solution for these potency and bioavailability limitations. (Ruhul Amin et al., 2009).

Since drug-associated toxicity remains a significant barrier for currently available chemotherapeutic and chemopreventive drugs, using natural compounds (which have better safety profiles) as adjuvant therapy with current chemotherapeutic agents may help to mitigate drug-associated toxicities. Major phytochemicals identified from FV include carotenoids, polyphenols, flavonoids, quercetin, vitamins, resveratrol, silymarin, organosulfur compounds, and sulforaphane (Anand et al., 2008). Sources, mechanism of action, and synergistic interactions with other drugs of chemopreventives in FV are summarized in Table 7.2 (Ruhul Amin et al., 2009).

9.2 Carotenoids

Carotenoids are the pigments responsible for the yellow to red color of some FVs; the most common are lycopene, lutein, α-carotene, β-carotene, β-cryptoxanthin, and zeaxanthin. Lycopene is present in fruits, including watermelon, apricots, pink guava, grapefruits, rosehip, and tomatoes. A wide variety of processed tomato-based products accounts for more than 85% of dietary lycopene (Anand et al., 2008). Various natural carotenoids present in FV were reported to have anti–inflammatory and anticarcinogenic activity. A number of in vitro studies have shown that lycopene can protect native LDL from oxidation and can suppress cholesterol synthesis (Ignarro et al., 2007).

One of the most interesting aspects of the potential link between carotenoid consumption and chemoprevention is that lycopene shows a greater bioavailability from processed tomato products (e.g., paste, puree, sauce) than from the raw vegetables and that addition of olive oil further promotes absorption. The traditional Mediterranean habit of consuming processed, cooked tomato products (e.g., over pasta or pizza) might thus add value to the health-promoting properties of tomato (Gomez-Romero et al., 2007).

9.3 Flavonoids

Polyphenolic compounds were divided into various classes on the basis of their molecular structure, with flavonoids being one of the main groups. Many studies dealing with flavonoids have focused on their antioxidant properties through scavenging of free radicals, but a number of reports in different cell lines, animal models, and human epidemiological trials have pointed out an association between consumption of FV and certain beverages and the reduced risk of chronic diseases, including cancer (Ramos, 2007; Ignarro et al., 2007). Flavonoids are potent bioactive molecules that possess anticarcinogenic effects since they can interfere with the initiation, development, and progression of cancer by the modulation of cellular proliferation, differentiation,

Table 7.2 Sources, Mechanism of Action, and Synergistic Interactions with Other Drugs of Certain Chemopreventives in Fruits and Vegetables

Agent	Natural source	Mechanism of action	Organ site	Synergistic interaction
Pomegranate (Ruhul Amin et al., 2009)	*Punica granatum* (pomegranate fruit, pomegranate juice, pomegranate seed and seed oil)	Antioxidant, antiproliferation (growth inhibition, cell cycle disruption and apoptosis), antiangiogenesis, *anti-inflammatory*	Prostate, skin, breast, lung, colon, oral, leukemia	
Carotenoids				
Lycopene (Ruhul Amin et al., 2009)	Tomatoes, guava, rosehip, watermelon, papaya, apricot and pink grapefruit; most abundant in red tomatoes and processed tomato products	Antioxidant, antiproliferation (growth inhibition, cell cycle arrest, apoptosis), antiangiogenesis, *anti-inflammatory* immunomodulator	Prostate, lung, breast, gastric, liver, pancreas, colorectal, head and neck, skin	Genistein, adriamycin, cisplatin
Flavonoids	Epidermis of leaves and the skin of fruits			
Quercetin (Anand et al., 2008)	Onions, apples	Antioxidant, anti-inflammation, antiproliferation, apoptosis	Colon and Lung cancer	
Indol-3-carbinol (Anand et al., 2008)	Cabbage, broccoli, Brussels sprout, cauliflower, daikon artichoke	Modulation of several nuclear transcription factors, Induction of phase 1 and 2 enzymes that metabolize carcinogens, including estrogens		
Luteolin (Ruhul Amin et al., 2009)	Artichoke, broccoli, celery, cabbage, spinach, green pepper, pomegranate leaves, peppermint, tamarind, and cauliflower	Anti-inflammation, antiallergy, antiproliferation (G1 and G2/M arrest, apoptosis), antioxidant, prooxidant	Ovarian, gastric, liver, colon, breast, oral, esophageal adenocarcinoma, prostate, lung, nasopharyngeal, cervix, leukemia, skin, and pancreatic	Cisplatin, doxorubicin, TRAIL, TNF-_

Continued

Table 7.2 Sources, Mechanism of Action, and Synergistic Interactions with Other Drugs of Certain Chemopreventives in Fruits and Vegetables—cont'd

Agent	Natural source	Mechanism of action	Organ site	Synergistic interaction
Resveratrol (Ruhul Amin et al., 2009)	Red wine, grapes (mainly in the skin), mulberries, peanuts, vines, pines	Antioxidant, antiproliferation (cell cycle arrest and apoptosis), antiangiogenesis, anti-inflammatory	Ovarian, breast, prostate, liver, uterine, leukemia, lung, gastric	EGCG, indole-3-carbinol, vitamin E analogue, methylseleninic acid, quercetin, genistein, TRAIL, cisplatin, doxorubicin, ellagic acid, platinum compounds, FU, paclitaxel
Lupeol (Ruhul Amin et al., 2009)	Mango, olive, fig, strawberry, red grapes	Antioxidant, antimutagenesis, anti-inflammatory, antiproliferation, cell cycle arrest, apoptosis, induction of differentiation	Skin, lung, leukemia, pancreas, prostate, colon, liver, head, and neck	Cisplatin
Sulforaphane, isothiothiocyanate (Anand et al., 2008)	Cruciferous vegetables such as broccoli	Inhibition of phase 1 enzymes, induction of phase 2 enzymes to detoxify carcinogens, cell-cycle arrest, induction of apoptosis, inhibition of histone deacetylase, modulation of the MAPK pathway, inhibition of NF-κB, and production of ROS.		

Diallyldisulfide (Anand et al., 2008)	Garlic	Inhibits the growth and proliferation of a number of cancer cell lines, scavenging of radicals; increasing gluathione levels; increasing the activities of enzymes such as glutathione S-transferase and catalase; inhibiting cytochrome p4502E1 and DNA repair mechanisms; and preventing chromosomal damage	Colon, breast, glioblastoma, melanoma, and neuroblastoma
Capsaicin (Anand et al., 2008)	Red chili	Antioxidant, anti-inflammatory, and antitumor, inhibit platelet aggregation and suppress calcium-ionophore–stimulated proinflammatory responses, interaction with xenobiotic metabolizing enzymes	

apoptosis, angiogenesis, and metastasis. Moreover, it has been shown that flavonoids induce apoptosis. However, because of the complexity and interrelationships of transduction pathways, the mechanisms for inducing the apoptosis of these polyphenols may overlap with other signaling cascades; thus, programmed cell death can be promoted through the modulation of different proteins in other pathways that can contribute to cell death. More studies are needed to clearly understand the mechanisms of the action of flavonoids as modulators of cell apoptosis, which is crucial for the evaluation of their potential as anticancer agents (Ramos, 2007). Quercetin is a major dietary flavonoid, found in a broad range of FV and beverages such as apple, tea, and wine (Russo, 2007).

Anthocyans are flavanols that occur in the diet at relatively high concentrations and confer bright red or blue coloration on berries and other FV. The limited epidemiological data available report their potential anticarcinogenicity. In a cohort of elderly individuals, who consumed large amounts of strawberries, the odds ratio for developing cancer at any site was 0.3, compared to subjects, who refrained from high berry consumption. Consumption of colored FV has also been associated with a reduced risk of human breast cancer and colorectal polyp recurrence. Anthocyan-containing foodstuffs have been linked with a decreased risk of CHD. They have been shown to possess beneficial effects in several parts of the organism, including the central nervous system and the eye, and have been suspected to account, at least in part, for the "French paradox," i.e., the decreased risk of CVD despite a high-fat diet in individuals living in France. (Cooke et al., 2005).

The soluble polyphenol content of pomegranate juice varies between 0.2% and 1.0%, depending on variety, and includes mainly anthocyanins, catechins, ellagic tannins, and gallic and ellagic acids. The antioxidant level in pomegranate juice was found to be higher than in other natural juices such as blueberry, cranberry, and orange as well as in red wine. In clinical trials, pomegranate juice induced decline in blood pressure, reduced common carotid intima-media thickness, and LDL oxidation. Pomegranate juice and its by products may improve the redox status of arterial cells. Daily consumption of pomegranate juice by diabetic patients resulted in antioxidative effects on serum and macrophages and improved stress-induced myocardial ischemia in patients who have CHD. Recent studies suggest that pomegranate juice can exert these beneficial effects on CHD and atherogenesis by enhancing eNOS bioactivity (Ignarro et al., 2007). A double-blind, placebo-controlled randomized clinical trial (RCT) investigating 51 hyperlipidemic subjects found that administration of pomegranate seed oil for 4 weeks in hyperlipidemic subjects had favorable effects on lipid profiles including the TAG, TAG:HDL-C and the cholesterol:HDL-C ratios in the pomegranate seed oil group, as compared to the placebo group (Mirmiran et al., 2010).

Consumption of polyphenols contained in purple grapes, grape seed extract, and grape-based products had beneficial effects on endothelial function in patients with CHD and in the general population in the fight against cancer (Kaur et al., 2009; Ignarro et al., 2007).

Resveratrol increased its importance as a cancer preventive agent when it was initially documented in scientific literature as a cardiovascular protective agent, able to explain the "French paradox." In fact, the molecule inhibits platelet aggregation, prevents LDL oxidation by means of its antioxidant properties, and exerts a vasorelaxing effect on the animal model. After that, resveratrol became synonymous with naturally occurred molecules, possessing chemopreventive activities. Finally, and more recently, resveratrol showed potential antiaging properties as well (Russo, 2007).

To summarize, FVs are rich in nutrients as well as phytochemicals. Some of the individual phytochemical properties against diseases were well characterized, and many new phytochemicals, not yet identified, and their characteristics and potential preventive properties against cancer are being discovered.

9.4 Implications to Increase FV Intake

Studies indicate that FV can prevent noncommunicable disease as part of a healthy diet and lifestyle. The statistics available from the Food and Agriculture Organization (FAO) suggest that most populations are not meeting currently recommended levels of FV in all age groups, which is why effective methods to promote healthy eating and to increase FV are urgently needed (World Health Organization, 2003b). Previous reviews of literature suggest that a majority of intervention studies are successful in promoting FV intake at least for a short time. However, the long-term effects of intervention are generally observed among adult individuals with high risk of disease. In healthy adult populations, increases in FV consumption ranged from about 0.1 to 1.4 servings per day. Self-efficacy, social support, and knowledge were found as predictors of adult FV intake. Weaker evidence was found for variables, including barriers, intentions, attitudes/beliefs, stages of change, and autonomous motivation (Shaikh, 2008).

Evidence shows that a diet high in FV and a healthy diet during childhood have many beneficial effects on health outcomes throughout childhood into adulthood. Studies have also shown that dietary habits and preferences for foods are established in childhood and track through into adulthood. Therefore, it is important to know the factors that influence the dietary habits of children to implement long-term changes in their consumption. The Avon longitudinal study of parents and children found that in primary school children, consumption of FV appears to be influenced by parental rules and vice versa. Parents' action could influence this (Jones et al., 2010), and more work is definitely needed on how to increase FV intake, and the use of future interventions, aimed at encouraging parents to be positive role models by targeting parental intake and creating a supportive home environment, by encouraging their children to consume more FV and by increasing availability of FV. There were also positive associations between parental occupational status and adolescent fruit consumption and between parental education and adolescent FV consumption. For adolescents, indicators of family circumstances (e.g., parental education) should be used to identify target groups for interventions aimed at promoting healthy eating (Pearson et al., 2009).

The high cost, time demands, and need for trained staff required for intervention studies might not seem to be applicable and feasible for whole populations aimed at motivating healthy lifestyles, especially in developing countries. Printed individually, customized information and computer-based information appear to be reasonable alternatives to face-to-face interviews, which are difficult and expensive. Data available show that computer-tailored nutrition education is more effective than general information in motivating people to make dietary changes, providing respondents with individualized feedback about their dietary behaviors.

In developing countries, FV promotion may focus on consumption of adequate nutrients or improving methods to prepare FV dishes to conserve nutrients, rather than just increasing FV consumption and very few studies have used community-based interventions for primary prevention of noncommunicable diseases (NCD) in these countries. Although some countries now suffer from the double burden of under- and overnutrition, known to be associated with nutrition transition. Several programs have been initiated but without any evaluation of effectiveness, particularly in developing countries (Pomerleau et al., 2005). The Tehran Lipid and Glucose Study (TLGS) has provided a unique opportunity to address this issue, through a large-scale community-based prospective trial on a representative sample of residents of District 13 of Tehran. Interventions were aimed at lifestyle modification through primary preventions for NCD by improving nutrition and dietary pattern, increasing physical activity levels, and reducing cigarette smoking. The lifestyle modification program was effective in reducing major modifiable diabetes risk factors, had a favorable effect on weight reduction in overweight and obese individuals, and resulted in a 65% reduction in the incidence of diabetes in men and women in the first follow-up survey after approximately 3 years (Harati et al., 2010).

There is a need to better understand the factors influencing FV intake, including economic, social, and environmental factors that influence food availability and the ability of an individual to make healthy choices, and the barriers encountered in making changes (Pomerleau et al., 2005). Also presenting nutrient profile models help consumers identify foods that provide optimal nutrition at an affordable cost (Drewnowski, 2010).

10. CONCLUSION

A variety of observational (cross-sectional, cohort, and case–control) studies have addressed the hypothesis of relation between changes in FV intake and CVD. However, evidence supporting this hypothesis by RCTs is scanty and the extent of the quantitative association is uncertain. Among dietary patterns, only the Mediterranean dietary pattern, rich in FV, has been shown to be related to risk factors of CVD by RCTs. The general consensus from the evidence currently available is that higher intakes of FV are beneficial in preventing risk factors of CVD; therefore, FV should be eaten as part of a balanced diet, as a source of vitamins, minerals, fibers, and phytochemicals. The results of these studies support the current dietary recommendations to encourage FV consumption of five or more servings per day. If this were achieved, there would be a large reduction in morbidity and mortality of certain CVD. Helping people to adhere to these recommendations and to substitute harmful foods with FV might reduce CVD risk factors and related events and provide a basis for implementation of much needed public health recommendations.

The effects of FV intake in prevention of noncommunicable disease is frequently associated with particular social, cultural, and lifestyle characteristics. These confounders are not adequately controlled in observational studies; therefore, conclusion of a causal relationship between FV intake and CVD prevention following these types of studies is hardly justified. Confirmation of this causal association needs further evidence from nutritional prevention trials and clinical interventions on CVD. Also further evidence from other cohorts in a variety of culture, including populations in developing countries, is required. More research is needed to examine the biological mechanisms behind these associations.

REFERENCES

Alinia, S., Hels, O., Tetens, I., 2009. The potential association between fruit intake and body weight-a review'. Obesity Reviews 10 (6), 639–647.

Anand, P., Kunnumakara, A.B., Sundaram, C., et al., 2008. Cancer is a preventable disease that requires major lifestyle changes. Pharmaceutical Research 25 (9), 2097–2116.

Azadbakht, L., Mirmiran, P., Esmaillzadeh, A., et al., 2005. Beneficial effects of a dietary approaches to stop hypertension eating plan on features of the metabolic syndrome. Diabetes Care 28, 2823–2831.

Azizi, F., Ghanbarian, A., Momenan, A.A., et al., 2009. Prevention of non-communicable disease in a population in nutrition transition: tehran lipid and glucose study phase II. Trials 10 (5).

Bandera, E.V., Kushi, L.H., Moore, D.F., et al., 2007. Fruits and vegetables and endometrial cancer risk: a systematic literature review and meta-analysis. Nutrition and Cancer 58 (1), 6–21.

Bazzano, L.A., Li, T.Y., Joshipura, K.J., et al., 2008. Intake of fruit, vegetables, and fruit juices and risk of diabetes in women. Diabetes Care 31 (7), 1311–1317.

Ceriello, A., 2008. Possible role of oxidative stress in the pathogenesis of hypertension. Diabetes Care 31 (Suppl 2), S181–S184.

Cooke, D., Steward, W.P., Gescher, A.J., et al., 2005. Anthocyans from fruits and vegetables-does bright colour signal cancer chemopreventive activity? European Journal of Cancer 41 (13), 1931–1940.

Dauchet, L., Amouyel, P., Hercberg, S., et al., 2006. Fruit and vegetable consumption and risk of coronary heart disease: a meta-analysis of cohort studies. The Journal of Nutrition 136, 2588–2593.

Dauchet, L., Amouyel, P., Dallongeville, J., 2009. Fruits, vegetables and coronary heart disease. Nature Reviews Cardiology 6, 599–608.

Dauchet, L., Montaye, M., Ruidavets, J.B., et al., 2010. Association between the frequency of fruit and vegetable consumption and cardiovascular disease in male smokers and non-smokers. European Journal of Clinical Nutrition 64, 578–586 advance online publication 31 March 2010.

de Kok, T.M., van Breda, S.G., Manson, M.M., 2008. 'Mechanisms of combined action of different chemopreventive dietary compounds: a review. European Journal of Nutrition 47 (Suppl. 2), 51–59.

Drewnowski, A., 2010. The Nutrient Rich Foods Index helps to identify healthy, affordable foods. The American Journal of Clinical Nutrition 91 (4), 1095S–1101S.

Esposito, K., Marfella, R., Ciotola, M., et al., 2004. Effect of a mediterranean-style diet on endothelial dysfunction and markers of vascular inflammation in the metabolic syndrome: a randomized trial. JAMA: The Journal of the American Medical Association 292, 1440–1446.

Giugliano, D., Ceriello, A., Esposito, K., 2008. Are there specific treatments for the metabolic syndrome? The American Journal of Clinical Nutrition 87 (1), 8–11.

Gomez-Romero, M., Arraez-Roman, D., Segura-Carretero, A., et al., 2007. Analytical determination of antioxidants in tomato: typical components of the Mediterranean diet. Journal of Separation Science 30, 452–461.

Hamer, M., Chida, Y., 2007. Intake of fruit, vegetables, and antioxidants and risk of type 2 diabetes: systematic review and meta-analysis. Journal of Hypertension 25 (12), 2361–2369.

Hansen, L., Dragsted, L.O., Olsen, A., et al., 2010. Fruit and vegetable intake and risk of acute coronary syndrome. The British Journal of Nutrition 24, 1–8.

Harati, H., Hadaegh, F., Momenan, A.A., et al., 2010. Reduction in incidence of type 2 diabetes by lifestyle intervention in a middle eastern community. American Journal of Preventive Medicine 38, 628–636. e1002E.

He, F.J., Nowson, C.A., MacGregor, G.A., 2006. Fruit and vegetable consumption and stroke: meta-analysis of cohort studies. Lancet 28 (367), 320–326.

He, F.J., Nowson, C.A., Lucas, M., et al., 2007. Increased consumption of fruit and vegetables is related to a reduced risk of coronary heart disease: meta-analysis of cohort studies. Journal of Human Hypertension 21, 717–728.

Hung, H.C., Joshipura, K.J., Jiang, R., et al., 2004. Fruit and vegetable intake and risk of major chronic disease. JNCI 96 (21), 1577–1584.

Ignarro, L.J., Balestrieri, M.L., Napoli, C., 2007. Nutrition, physical activity, and cardiovascular disease: an update. Cardiovascular Research 73, 326–340.

John, J.H., Ziebland, S., Yudkin, P., et al., 2002. Effects of fruit and vegetable consumption on plasma antioxidant concentrations and blood pressure: a randomised controlled trial. Lancet 359 (9322), 1969–1974.

Jones, L.R., Steer, C.D., Rogers, I.S., 2010. Influences on child fruit and vegetable intake: sociodemographic, parental and child factors in a longitudinal cohort study. Public Health Nutrition 3, 1–9.

Kaur, M., Agarwal, C., Agarwal, R., 2009. Anticancer and cancer chemopreventive potential of grape seed extract and other grape-based products. The Journal of Nutrition 139, 1806S–1812S.

Kris-Etherton, P., Eckel, R.H., Howard, B.V., et al., 2001. Lyon Diet Heart Study: benefits of a Mediterranean-Style, National Cholesterol Education Program/American Heart Association Step I dietary pattern on cardiovascular disease. Circulation 103, 1823–1825.

Liu, C., Russell, R.M., 2008. Nutrition and gastric cancer risk: an update. Nutrition Reviews 66 (5), 237–249.

Lunet, N., Lacerda-Vieira, A., Barros, H., 2005. Fruit and vegetables consumption and gastric cancer: a systematic review and meta-analysis of cohort studies. Nutrition and Cancer 53 (1), 1–10.

Marques-Vidal, P., Ravasco, P., Ermelinda Camilo, M., 2006. Foodstuffs and colorectal cancer risk: A review. Clinical Nutrition 25, 14–36.

McCall, D.O., McGartland, C.P., McKinley, M.C., et al., 2009. Dietary intake of fruits and vegetables improves microvascular function in hypertensive subjects in a dose-dependent manner. Circulation 119, 2153–2160.

Mente, A., Koning, L., Shannon, H.S., Anand, S.S., 2009. A systematic review of the evidence supporting a causal link between dietary factors and coronary heart disease. Archives of Internal Medicine 169 (7), 659–669.

Michels, K.B., Mohllajee, A.P., Roset-Bahmanyar, E., et al., 2007. Diet and breast cancer: a review of the prospective observational studies. Cancer 109 (12 Suppl), 2712–2749.

Mirmiran, P., Esmaillzadeh, A., Azizi, F., 2006. Diet composition and body mass index in Tehranian adults. Asia Pacific Journal of Clinical Nutrition 15 (2), 224–230.

Mirmiran, P., Noori, N., Beheshti Zavareh, M., Azizi, F., 2009. Fruit and vegetable consumption and risk factors for cardiovascular disease. Metabolism 58, 460–468.

Mirmiran, P., Fazeli, M.R., Asghari, G., Shafiee, A., Azizi, F., 2010. Effect of pomegranate seed oil on hyperlipidaemic subjects: a double-blind placebo-controlled clinical trial. British Journal of Nutrition 104, 402–406.

Ortega, R.M., 2006. Importance of functional foods in the Mediterranean diet. Public Health Nutrition 9 (8A), 1136–1140.

Pearson, N., Biddle, S.J., Gorely, T., 2009. Family correlates of fruit and vegetable consumption in children and adolescents: a systematic review. Public Health Nutrition 12 (2), 267–283.

Pereira, M.A., O'Reilly, E., Augustsson, K., et al., 2004. Dietary fiber and risk of coronary heart disease: a pooled analysis of cohort studies. Archives of Internal Medicine 164 (4), 370–376.

Perez-Vizcaino, F., Duarte, J., Jimenez, R., et al., 2009. Antihypertensive effects of the flavonoid quercetin. Pharmacological Reports 61 (1), 67–75.

Pierce, J.P., 2009. Diet and breast cancer prognosis: making sense of the Women's Healthy Eating and Living and Women's Intervention Nutrition Study trials. Curr Opin Obstet Gynecol 21, 86–91.

Pomerleau, J., Lock, K., Knai, C., et al., 2005. Interventions designed to increase adult fruit and vegetable intake can be effective: a systematic review of the literature. The Journal of Nutrition 135, 2486–2495.

Prynne, C.J., Mishra, G.D., O'Connell, M.A., et al., 2006. Fruit and vegetable intakes and bone mineral status: a cross-sectional study in 5 age and sex cohorts. The American Journal of Clinical Nutrition 83 (6), 1420–1428.

Ramos, S., 2007. Effects of dietary flavonoids on apoptotic pathways related to cancer chemoprevention. The Journal of Nutritional Biochemistry 18, 427–442.

Resnicow, K., Davis, R.E., Zhang, G., et al., 2008. Tailoring a fruit and vegetable intervention on novel motivational constructs: results of a randomized study. Annals of Behavioral Medicine 35, 159–169.

Ruhul Amin, A.R.M., Kucuk, O., Khuri, F.R., et al., 2009. Perspectives for cancer prevention with natural compounds. Journal of Clinical Oncology 27 (16), 2712–2725.

Russo, G.L., 2007. Ins and outs of dietary phytochemicals in cancer chemoprevention. Biochemical pharmacololgy 7 (4), 533–544.

Silberstein, J.L., Parsons, J.K., 2010. Evidence-based Principles of Bladder Cancer and Diet. Urology 75 (2), 340–346.

Stacewicz-Sapuntzakis, M., Borthakur, G., Burns, J.L., 2008. Correlations of dietary patterns with prostate health. Molecular Nutrition & Food Research 52, 114–130.

Tsugane, S., Sasazuki, S., 2007. Diet and the risk of gastric cancer: review of epidemiological evidence. Gastric Cancer 10 (2), 75–83.

USDA, 'Dietary Guidelines for Americans', 2010. 7th ed. US Department of Agriculture and Department of Health and Human Services, 2010, Washington, DC: US. Government.

Villegas, R., Shu, X.O., Gao, Y.T., et al., 2008. Vegetable but Not Fruit Consumption Reduces the Risk of Type 2 Diabetes in Chinese Women. The Journal of Nutrition 138, 574–580.

Ware, W.R., 2009. Nutrition and the Prevention and Treatment of Cancer: association of Cytochrome P450 CYP1B1 With the Role of Fruit and Fruit Extracts. Integrative Cancer Therapies 8 (1), 22–28.

World Health Organization, 2003a. Global burden of disease 2002: deaths by age, sex and cause for the year 2002. Geneva, Switzerland.

World Health Organization, 2003b. Diet, nutrition and the prevention of chronic disease, Technical Report Series 916, Geneva.

Wynn, E., Krieg, M.A., Lanham-New, S.A., et al., 2010. Conference on Over- and undernutrition: challenges and approaches' Postgraduate Symposium Positive influence of nutritional alkalinity on bone healthProceedings of the Nutrition Society 69, 166–173.

RELEVANT WEBSITES

http://www.who.int/hpr/NPH/fruit_and_vegetables/fruit_and_vegetable_report.pdf [26 April 2010] – WHO Fruit and Vegetable Promotion Initiative – report of the meeting, Geneva, 25–27 August 2003. World Health Organization 2003.

www.vfpck.org/ – Vegetable and Fruit Promotion Council, Keralam (VFPCK).

www.hpb.gov.sg – Health Promotion Board - Harness the Goodness of Fruit and Vegetables.

www.dhhs.nh.gov/DHHS/NHP/fruitsandveggies.htm – Nutrition & Health Promotion-Fruits and Veggies.

http://www.who.int/dietphysicalactivity/fruit/en/index.html – Promoting fruit and vegetable consumption around the world.

www.hsph.harvard.edu – Vegetables and Fruits - What Should You Eat?

www.cdc.gov/mmwr/preview/mmwrhtml/mm5610a2.htm – Fruit and Vegetable Consumption Among Adults –– United States, 2005.

http://www.fao.org/english/newsroom/focus/2003/fruitveg1.htm – Increasing fruit and vegetable consumption becomes a global priority.

http://www.ers.usda.gov/publications/aib792/aib792-2/ – U.S. Fruit and Vegetable Consumption: Who, What, Where, and How Much.

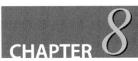

CHAPTER 8

Diet and Homocysteinemia
A Role in Cardiovascular Disease?

Y. Kumar*, A. Bhatia[†]
*Chhuttani Medical Centre, Chandigarh, India
[†]PGIMER, Chandigarh, India

ABBREVIATIONS

5-methylTHF 5-methyltetrahydrofolate
CBS Cystathione β-synthase
CVD Cardiovascular disease
fHcy Fasting homocysteine
GNMT Glycine *N*-methyltransferase
HCA Homocysteinemia
Hcy Homocysteine
LDL Lipoproteins
MI Myocardial infarction
MLT Methionine loading test
MS Methionine synthase
MTHFR Methylene-tetrahydrofolate reductase
NO Nitric oxide
PLP Pyrodoxal-5'-phosphate
PUFA Polyunsaturated fatty acid
RDA Recommended dietary allowance
ROS Reactive oxygen species
SAH *S*-adenosylhomocysteine
SAM *S*-adenosylmethionine
tHcy Total homocysteine
THF Tetrahydrofolate
Vitamin B$_{12}$ Cobalamin
Vitamin B$_6$ Pyridoxine

1. INTRODUCTION

Cardiovascular disease (CVD) is the leading cause of death worldwide accounting for 30% of the total deaths globally. It has been predicted that by the year 2020, the coronary artery disease (CAD) by itself will be the leading cause of mortality worldwide (Murray and Lopez, 1997). Earlier, most of the morbidity and mortalities due to CVD were reported from developed countries of Europe and America, but in recent years a

Bioactive Food as Dietary Interventions for Cardiovascular Disease
http://dx.doi.org/10.1016/B978-0-12-396485-4.00007-4

© 2013 Elsevier Inc.
All rights reserved.

rapid increase has been noted in developing countries as well. This is attributed to control of infections and parasitic and nutritional disorders, which has allowed most of the population to reach the age where CVD manifests itself. Accompanying changes in lifestyle and diet have further contributed to this problem. In fact, unhealthy diet and physical inactivity are now claimed to be responsible for 80% of cases of CVD in these countries (World health report, 2003). Increased intake of fat particularly saturated fatty acids, sugars, and salts and reduced intake of fruits and vegetables can lead to overweight/obesity, hyperlipidemia, hypertension, and diabetes mellitus, which are considered to be traditional risk factors for CVD. There are 15–20% cases of CVD, especially the younger patients, that do not have these traditional risk factors. This suggests involvement of factors besides the conventional ones in CVD (Smith, 2006). Recently, homocysteinemia (HCA), an elevation of the plasma concentration of homocysteine (Hcy), has emerged as an independent risk factor for CVD. Like other factors, that is, hyperlipidemia, HCA is also influenced by lifestyle and diet. A moderate elevation of Hcy may often be caused by low nutritional intake of vitamins, obesity, lack of physical exercise, stress, smoking, and high alcohol and coffee consumption. Since the dietary factors have emerged as one of the major players in the development of CVD, suitable modifications in the diet could help curb the rising trends of CVD. The chapter briefly summarizes the current knowledge on Hcy and important dietary factors contributing to HCA. The pathogenic role of HCA in the causation of CVD, dietary changes important in the prevention of HCA and current concepts about association of HCA and CVD have also been discussed.

2. HOMOCYSTEINE

2.1 Biochemistry

In 1932, Butz and Du Vigneaud obtained Hcy by treating methionine with strong sulfuric acid and proved that it is a thiol (an organosulfur compound) containing amino acid (Butz and du Vigneaud, 1932). Chemically it is known as (2S)-2-amino-4-sulfanylbutanoic acid ($C_4H_9NO_2S$). Human plasma contains both its reduced and oxidized forms (Jacobsen, 1998). The disulfide or oxidized form is nonprotein-bound Hcy and called homocystine. Disulfide forms also exist with cysteine and with proteins containing reactive cysteine residues (protein-bound Hcy). The latter oxidized forms are referred to as mixed disulfides. The sulfhydryl or reduced form is called Hcy and is bound to proteins by a disulfide bond. The oxidized forms of Hcy usually comprise 98–99% of total Hcy (tHcy) in human plasma, 80–90% of which is protein bound. Total plasma Hcy, therefore, is the sum total of all forms of Hcy that exist in plasma or serum (Figure 8.1).

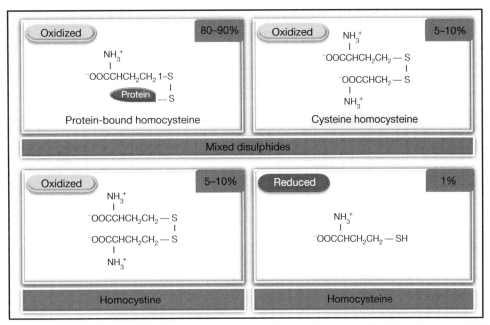

Figure 8.1 Various forms of homocysteine present in human blood. *Modified from Jacobsen, D.W., 1998. Homocysteine and vitamins in cardiovascular disease. Clinical Chemistry 44, 1833–1843.*

2.2 Metabolism

Hcy is either totally absent or present in very small quantities in various commonly consumed foods of plant origin like cereals, pulses, fruits, and vegetables. Most of it is derived indirectly when dietary methionine is metabolized. Once formed, the fate of Hcy depends on two pathways: remethylation and transsulfuration (Figure 8.2). The initial step in this process is demethylation in which there is activation of methionine by adenosine triphosphate and adenylation by methionine *S*-adenosyltransferase. This leads to the formation of *S*-adenosylmethionine (SAM). SAM so formed then donates its methyl group to a variety of acceptors, that is, phosphotidylethanolamine, guanidinoacetate, nucleic acids (DNA, RNA), neurotransmitters (dopamine, etc.), proteins (myelin, etc.), phospholipids, or hormones and forms *S*-adenosylhomocysteine (SAH). The latter is hydrolyzed to adenosine and Hcy. The resulting Hcy is either catabolized into cystathionine or remethylated into methionine. Remethylation is catalyzed by methionine synthase (MS), also known as methyltetrahydrofolate homocysteine methyltransferase (MTR). This enzymatic reaction requires 5-methyltetrahydrofolate (5-methylTHF) as a methyl donor and cobalamin (vitamin B_{12}) as cofactor. Formation of 5-methylTHF (circulating form of folic acid) depends on the enzyme 5,10-methylenetetrahydrofolatereductase (MTHFR), which catalyzes the reduction of 5,10-methylene tetrahydrofolate obtained from tetrahydrofolate (THF). The methyl group of 5-methylTHF is synthesized *de novo* when a carbon unit is transferred from a carbon

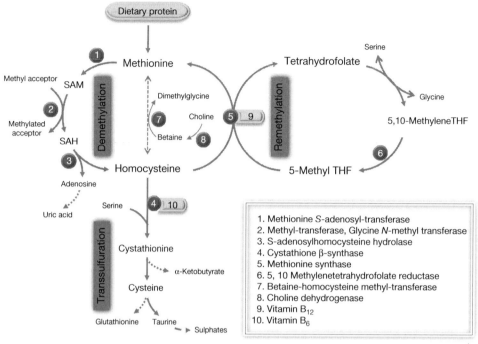

Figure 8.2 The metabolic pathway of homocysteine.

source, such as serine or glycine, to THF producing 5, 10-methyleneTHF, which is subsequently reduced by MTHFR. Thus this pathway needs folic acid and vitamin B_{12} as essential components. An alternative remethylation of Hcy to methionine, which is independent of these vitamins, may also take place using betaine as methyl donor and catalyzed by betaine-homocysteine–methyltransferase. This reaction uses preformed methyl groups because betaine is derived from choline, which in part is supplemented in diet and partly synthesized through successive methylations of phosphatidylethanolamine.

When in excess, the majority of Hcy is catabolized by the transsulfuration pathway where it condenses with serine to form cystathionine. The enzyme required for this route is cystathione β-synthase (CBS), which needs pyridoxine (vitamin B_6). Cystathionine is hydrolyzed to form cysteine and α-ketobutyrate. Excess cysteine is oxidized to taurine and inorganic sulfates or excreted in the urine. Thus, in addition to the synthesis of cysteine, this transsulfuration pathway effectively catabolizes excess Hcy, which is not required for methyl transfer and delivers sulfates for the synthesis of heparin, heparin sulfate, dermatan sulfate, and chondroitin sulfate.

2.2.1 Factors Regulating Hcy Metabolism

Metabolism of Hcy molecules is nutritionally regulated. Methionine, folic acid, vitamin B_{12}, and vitamin B_6 are major dietary components affecting Hcy metabolism (Figure 8.3).

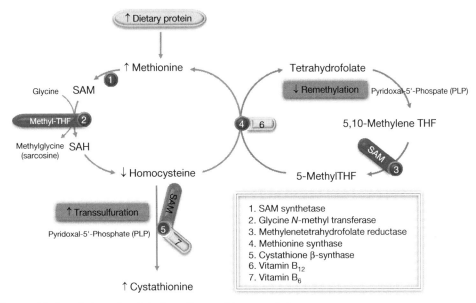

Figure 8.3 Regulation of metabolic pathway of homocysteine.

2.2.1.1 *S*-Adenosyl Methionine

The coordination between transsulfuration and remethylation depends on the amount of methionine in the diet. SAM, a derivative of methionine, plays an important role in this mechanism. In the liver, changes in intracellular methionine affect the rate of SAM synthesis. When dietary intake of methionine-rich animal proteins is high, methionine *S*-adenosyltransferase rapidly converts the incoming methionine to SAM. SAM inhibits MTHFR, thereby reducing conversion of THF into 5-methyl THF (an inhibitor of GNMT). This increases glycine *N*-methyltransferase (GNMT) enzyme activity leading to more production of SAH. Raised SAM also activates CBS, thus increasing the rate of Hcy catabolism. In this way, Hcy transsulfuration is promoted over remethylation, consistent with the reduced need for *de novo* methionine synthesis owing to the high dietary supply of methionine.

Conversely, when the dietary methionine supply is low, SAM concentration is insufficient for the inhibition of MTHFR. This increases 5-methylTHF production, which inhibits GNMT (thereby production of SAM), and an increase in the availability of substrate (5-methylTHF) for Hcy remethylation. In such a condition, remethylation is favored over transsulfuration also because the concentration of SAM is too low to activate the CBS enzyme. This process is consistent with the increased need for *de novo* methionine synthesis attributed to the low dietary input of methionine (Selhub, 1999).

2.2.1.2 Folic Acid

Folic acid supplies 5-methylTHF necessary for the cellular remethylation of Hcy into methionine. 5-methylTHF maintains optimum tissue levels of SAM when there is a restricted exogenous methyl group supply from methionine and choline. Depletion of the folate stores leads to decreased synthesis of methionine by remethylation. Low levels of 5-methylTHF also allow GNMT to be fully active, which reduces SAM levels and increases Hcy levels. Hence, both transsulfuration and remethylation pathways get affected and result in accumulation and cellular effluxes of Hcy causing increase in circulating Hcy levels.

2.2.1.3 Vitamin B_{12}

Vitamin B_{12} is required by the MS, which converts excess of Hcy back into methionine. If a person does not have an adequate supply of vitamin B_{12}, then Hcy is not converted to methionine and the net result is an increase in Hcy.

2.2.1.4 Vitamin B_6

In the transsulfuration, vitamin B_6 is required for the conversion of Hcy into cysteine. Two enzymes CBS, which catalyzes the condensation of Hcy with serine to form cystathionine, and cystathionase, which catalyzes the hydrolysis of cystathionine to cysteine and α-ketobutyrate, are dependent on this vitamin. Therefore, its suboptimal levels may also be associated with elevated Hcy concentrations.

3. HOMOCYSTEINEMIA

The normal reference range for plasma tHcy is usually defined as the 2.5th to 97.5th percentile interval for presumably healthy people. HCA by definition is the presence of an abnormally elevated concentration of tHcy in serum or plasma. A person is supposed to have HCA if there is increase in fasting plasma Hcy (fHcy), an increased plasma tHcy 6 h after a methionine loading test (MLT), or both (Refsum et al., 1998). HCA has been classified by several researchers. Among the earlier studies, Kang and coworkers classified HCA in relation to plasma Hcy concentrations. They defined HCA as severe if concentrations were higher than 100 $\mu mol\, l^{-1}$, intermediate between 30 and 100 $\mu mol\, l^{-1}$, moderate for concentrations 15–30 $\mu mol\, l^{-1}$, and a reference tHcy range as 5–15 $\mu mol\, l^{-1}$ (Kang et al., 1992). On the basis of the gradually increasing relative CVD risk, in a multicenter case–control study, the European Concerted Action Project defined elevated tHcy for levels $\geq 12\,\mu mol\, l^{-1}$ for fHcy and $\geq 38\,\mu mol\, l^{-1}$ after MLT (Graham et al., 1997). As a treatment goal strategy, later on, the Nutrition Committee of the American Heart Association proposed $<10\,\mu mol\, l^{-1}$ as a reasonable fHcy diagnostic cutoff value and treatment goal for subjects at increased risk of CVD (Fokkema et al., 2001). From diagnostic and therapeutic points of view, HCA may be categorized as mild, moderate, and severe (with plasma tHcy 10–30, 31–100, and $>100\,\mu mol\, l^{-1}$, respectively).

3.1 Causes of HCA

Prevalence of HCA ranges from 5% in the general population (McCully, 1996) to 13–47% in patients with symptomatic vascular disease (Malinow et al., 1998). The actual prevalence, however, may be much more, especially in younger population with or without CVD (Kumar et al., 2009). The reasons for such variation are multifactorial, and include genetic, nutritional, and lifestyle factors (Table 8.1). Broadly, HCA may be categorized as genetic or acquired; the former is common in younger population while the latter may be more important in older people.

3.1.1 Primary or Genetic HCA

In primary HCA, there is either deficiency or reduced activity of the enzymes involved in Hcy metabolism because of certain mutations. A common cause that is associated with moderate-to-severe HCA is genetic deficiency of CBS. It is an autosomal recessive disorder usually seen in young patients who have moderate-to-severe HCA and homocystinuria (excrete Hcy in their urine). They may also develop other abnormalities such as dislocation of lens, skeletal deformities, mental retardation, and premature atherosclerosis.

Another more common and extensively studied genetic abnormality is MTHFR gene polymorphism. More than 18 mutations are known for the enzyme MTHFR,

Table 8.1 Causes of Homocysteinemia

Severe HCA (tHcy > 100 μmol l^{-1})
Homozygosity for CBS defects
Homozygosity for MTHFR defects
Defective vitamin B_{12} utilization
Severe deficiency of vitamin B_{12}
Moderate HCA (tHcy 31–100 μmol l^{-1})
Moderate deficiency of vitamin B_{12}
Severe deficiency of folic acid
Renal failure
Mild HCA (tHcy 10–30 μmol l^{-1})
Heterozygosity for CBS defects
Heterozygosity for MTHFR defects
MTR gene mutation
Mild deficiency of vitamin B and folic acid
Tobacco, coffee, or alcohol consumption
Clinical disorders (renal impairment, hepatic impairment, hypothyroidism, diabetes mellitus, systemic lupus erythematosus, psoriasis)
Organ transplantation
Malignancies (carcinoma of breast or ovary, acute lymphoblastic leukemia)
Medications (folate, vitamins B_{12} and B_6 antagonists, antiepileptic drugs, nicotine, metformin, thiazide diuretics, colestipol, L-dopa, aminothiols, and methotrexate).

the most common being C677T polymorphism (C to T substitution at position 677 of the MTHFR gene, which results in an alanine to valine amino acid substitution in the protein) and A1298C missense mutation. Its overall prevalence ranges from as low as <1% in African countries to as high as up to 62% in a few Americans (Schneider et al., 1998). The C677T leads to a thermolabile form of MTHFR with reduced activity (30% decrease in enzyme activity in heterozygotes and a 60% decrease in homozygotes). Homozygotes for C677T are prone to develop mild-to-moderate HCA, while the majority of heterozygotes are either normal or have mild increase in Hcy levels. The homozygosity for A1298C reduces MTHFR activity and has been reported to be a risk factor for neural tube defects, but it is rarely associated with significantly increased plasma Hcy levels. Another comparatively less common defect is the mutations in the MTR gene, which encodes MS (uses cobalamin as cofactor and converts Hcy to methionine). This leads to methylcobalamin deficiency and is characterized by HCA, homocystinuria, and hypomethioninemia.

3.1.2 Secondary or Acquired HCA

3.1.2.1 Diet

Dietary deficiencies of folic acid, vitamin B_{12}, and vitamin B_6 occurring either singly or in combination are the most common causes of secondary HCA, especially in elderly persons.

3.1.2.2 Demographic factors

HCA is more common in whites than in black and elderly males. The variation may partly be because of the differences in vitamin status, influence of sex hormones, creatine/creatinine synthesis, and muscle mass.

3.1.2.3 Lifestyle

Smoking and caffeinated coffee consumption cause a shift of the distribution towards higher tHcy values, whereas physical activity is associated with low levels. Chronic, high alcohol consumption is also associated with HCA, possibly through its effect on vitamin status.

3.1.2.4 Clinical conditions and drugs

HCA may be seen in renal failure, diabetes, hypothyroidism, and in certain malignancies and drugs, especially those affecting the vitamins related to Hcy metabolism, that is, folic acid, vitamin B_{12} and B_6 antagonists.

3.2 Detection of HCA

The most important diagnostic test for HCA is to measure tHcy after overnight fasting and with oral ingestion of 0.1 g of L-methionine per kilogram of body weight. tHcy is then measured 4–6 h after methionine load. MLT increases the sensitivity of detecting occult vitamin B_6 deficiency and obligate heterozygotes for CBS deficiency (Van Cott and Lapasota, 1998). Commonly used methods for the estimation of tHcy include chromatographic methods (high performance liquid chromatography, or gas chromatography with mass spectrometry), immunoassays, and enzyme cycling method.

Other tests used in the workup of HCA include assessment of RBC and serum folate, vitamin B_{12} and vitamin B_6 levels, and screening for mutations in the genes encoding the enzymes involved in Hcy metabolism. In order to associate the genetic polymorphisms in MTHFR and CBS, genotypes are monitored by either restriction fragment length polymorphism techniques or polymerase chain reaction assays. For determining the severity of CVD risk, levels of C-reactive protein, fibrinogen, plasma viscosity, and leukocytes are also assessed sometimes either by immunoassays or colorimetric measurements.

3.3 Homocysteinemia and Cardiovascular Disease

Biomedical significance of Hcy was recognized years after its discovery when in 1962, children with mental retardation, accelerated growth, and propensity to thrombosis of arteries and veins were found to have HCA with homocysteinuria (Gerritsen et al., 1962). McCully studied the histopathology of vessels in such patients and showed smooth muscle proliferation in the vessel wall, progressive arterial stenosis, and hemostatic changes, which he suggested were responsible for premature arteriosclerosis, thromboembolism and recurrent cardiovascular events, and proposed atherogenic potential of Hcy (McCully, 1969). Until the 1990s, his 'homocysteine hypothesis' had emerged as a potential risk factor for CVD and Hcy became notorious as 'the cholesterol of the 1990s.' This led to pouring of numerous cross sectional, retrospective case–control and prospective studies on the association between diet, HCA, and CVD. In 1995, Boushey et al. published a meta-analysis data from approximately 2500 patients, which indicated a linear relationship between elevated plasma Hcy levels and risk of CVD (Boushey et al., 1995). This was supported by another meta-analysis, which included all prospective studies and large retrospective studies published after the meta-analysis by Boushey et al. described above. It showed an association between moderate elevation of plasma or serum Hcy and increased risk of CVD, independent of other risk factors (Eikelboom et al., 1999). A meta-analysis has also found that for every $2.5\ \mu mol\ l^{-1}$ increase in plasma Hcy, the risk of myocardial infarction (MI) increases by about 10% and the risk of stroke increases by about 20% (Homocysteine Studies Collaboration, 2002).

3.4 Mechanism of Hcy-Induced CVDs

Functionally intact endothelium exerts potent antiatherothrombotic effects and Hcy causes endothelial injury (Welch and Loscalzo, 1998). When added to plasma, Hcy reduces activity of glutathione peroxidase and undergoes auto-oxidation, which is accompanied by the generation of free radicals or reactive oxygen species (ROS), such as hydrogen peroxide or superoxide anion. These free radicals along with reduced activity of glutathione peroxidase impair endothelial activity and react with nitric oxide (NO), an endothelium-derived vascular relaxing factor. This leads to the formation of highly reactive peroxynitrite resulting in the diminution of bioavailability of NO. NO is a strong endogenous vasodilator, inhibits platelet aggregation, leukocytes proliferation, and migration. It also restricts expression of adhesion molecules and the production of superoxide anions. Decreased NO together with reduced endothelial synthesis of prostacyclin promotes platelet activation and aggregation. Elevated Hcy levels induce expression of several chemokines and adhesion molecules by endothelial cells that lead to increased recruitment and adhesion of circulating inflammatory cells. ROS initiates peroxidation of low-density lipoproteins (LDL) and the oxidized LDL is then rapidly taken up by the monocyte-derived macrophages, which migrate into the subendothelial space and become lipid-laden foam cells. This further stimulates a vascular proinflammatory response leading to the expression of adhesion molecules, chemotactic proteins, and growth factors and causes intimal smooth muscle proliferation and deposition of extracellular matrix. All these events are thought to play an important role in the pathogenesis of early atherosclerotic lesions and their progression. Hcy also promotes thrombosis by activating endothelium-dependent prothrombotic mechanisms, such as induction of tissue factor expression, increase in activity of coagulant factors XII, V, and von Willebrand factor, thrombomodulin expression, and inhibition of tissue plasminogen activator (Figure 8.4).

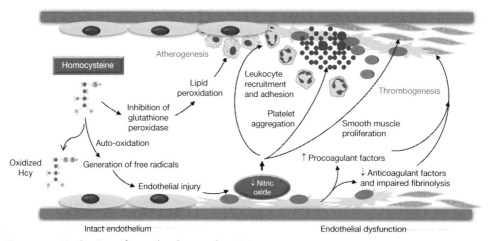

Figure 8.4 Mechanism of vascular damage by HCA.

3.5 Diet, its Bioactive Components and Effects on HCA

3.5.1 Dietary Habits

Dietary habits play an important role in the regulation of HCA, and upto two thirds of all HCA may be attributable to dietary deficiencies of folic acid or one or more B vitamins (Selhub et al., 1993). In vegetarians (people who thrive on plant products and abstain from animal flesh or byproducts, but may include eggs and dairy products), intake of folic acid generally meets the recommended dietary allowance (RDA). Despite this fact, its deficiency may occur as only half of the folate obtained from vegetarian diet is absorbed and available for various metabolic functions. Besides poor absorption, prolonged cooking in large amounts of water also destroys the absorbable folate (Omenn et al., 1998).

Vitamin B_{12} is essentially absent from plant foods but present in small amounts in dairy products and meat. Dietary intake of vitamin B_{12} in vegetarians therefore is low unless they consume large amounts of dairy products and eggs or regularly consume fortified foods (especially meat analogs, soya milks, yeast extracts, and breakfast cereals) or take vitamin supplements. In this respect, the lacto-ovovegetarian (a vegetarian who does not eat animal flesh of any kind, but is willing to consume dairy and egg products) diet is the most permissive and the vegan (a vegetarian who consumes no animal products at all) diet is the most restrictive. Although nonvegetarian food provides many important nutrients, including magnesium and zinc, which are absorbed better than that obtained from vegetarian diet, it is low in vitamins except vitamin B_{12}.

Vitamin B_6, besides having a role in Hcy metabolism, is involved in polyunsaturated fatty acid (PUFA) metabolism too. Adequate pyridoxine intake is important particularly when PUFA dietary level is high. In fact, adequate vitamin B_6 intake could ensure the normal long-chain fatty acid biosynthesis and the reduction of the risk linked to HCA.

Vegetarians have a high intake of folate and similar intake of vitamin B_6 as compared with nonvegetarian population but still as a consequence of vitamin B_{12} deficiency might develop HCA. Similarly, nonvegetarians may develop HCA due to their diet being low in folate and vitamin B_6. Therefore, a balanced diet including food both from plant and animal origin may be most efficient in regulating the Hcy levels.

Among other dietary components, riboflavin (vitamin B_2), antioxidants, that is, vitamins A, D, E, and C, trace elements like magnesium, selenium, copper, zinc, and trimethylglycine (betaine) have also been shown to reduce Hcy levels. These compounds protect against the harmful effects of free radicals originating from the oxidation of Hcy and lipid peroxidation.

Interaction of these dietary components with genetic factors (i.e., deficiency of CBS, MTHFR, MS) is important in the development of HCA. Genetic mutations if accompanied with nutritional deficiencies, especially of vitamins, may manifest HCA. For example, raised tHcy concentrations have been found to be related to homozygous MTHFR C677T, especially in the presence of low folate concentrations, and higher folate intake is required to bring down the Hcy levels in such cases (Dedoussis et al., 2004). In addition to all of this, a methionine-rich diet or acute methionine load also causes Hcy to be exported from the cells, leading to increased plasma Hcy levels.

3.5.2 Dietary Modifications

To control HCA, current dietary guidelines recommend increased consumption of fruits, vegetables, along with low-fat dairy products (often milk consumed with breakfast cereals), if other forms of animal products are not consumed. Only a balanced diet can provide the optimal amount of required nutrients; that is, for adults an RDA of folic acid, vitamin B_{12}, and vitamin B_6 is 400, 6, and 2 μg, respectively (US Department of Health and Human Services, 1995). Subjects using fruits and vegetables in their diet regularly along with vegetable oils, drinking low-fat or skimmed milk, avoiding cream, and consuming fish or fish-oil supplements have been found to have lower tHcy concentrations. Various fruits that are considered to be a good source of folic acid and vitamins are dried apricots, peanuts, figs, apple, pear, kiwi, papaya, orange, raspberries, blueberries, strawberries, grapes, pineapple, and melon. Vegetables rich in folic acid and vitamin B are lettuce, endive, avocado, sunflower seeds, spinach, broccoli, brussels sprouts, beans, tomatoes, and cooked lentils. A list of vitamin-rich fruits and vegetables is given in Table 8.2 (US Department of Agriculture, Agricultural Research Service, 2009).

3.5.3 Vitamin Supplementation/Food Fortification

Vitamin supplements or fortified foods may be used when the diet does not provide enough or dietary measures fail to bring down Hcy levels especially in those with moderate HCA. Vitamin supplementation may be needed for homocysteinemic patients who are vegans and nonvegetarians, who have a deficiency of folate or vitamin B_{12}. In a meta-analysis by Boushey et al., nine of the 11 intervention studies showed reduction of Hcy and normalization of serum folate after isolated supplementation of folic acid (>400 μg day^{-1}). The authors also highlighted that besides dietary measures, vitamin supplementation and fortification could have a greater impact on the prevention of HCA (Boushey et al., 1995). In another meta-analysis with 12 randomized studies and 1114 individuals, it was found that the supplementation of folic acid with vitamin B_{12} potentialized the reduction of Hcy in 7% of the cases. Vitamin B_6 at a dose of 250 mg day^{-1} or above was able to reduce Hcy levels and when combined with betaine and folic acid could even normalize the Hcy levels in these patients (Homocysteine Lowering Trialists' Collaboration, 1998). Hcy reduction is greatest in subjects who are homozygous for the thermolabile MTHFR mutation when compared with heterozygous and normozygous subjects. Other therapeutic options that have been used are trimethylglycine, choline, inositol, zinc, and SAM in varying doses.

Table 8.2 Rich Sources of Folate, Vitamin B$_{12}$, and Vitamin B$_6$

Food	Content
Folic acid	*(in μg per 100 g)*
Grilled chicken liver	560
Soy flour	303
Grilled bovine liver	253
Cooked beans	149
Cooked spinach	73
Raw broccoli	71
Oat flour	52
Wheat bran	44
Cooked egg	44
Orange	30
Raw cabbage	29
White bread	25
Banana	20
Raw tomato	15
Cooked potato	9
Vitamin B$_{12}$	*(in μg per 100 g)*
Roasted bovine liver	70.5
Roasted chicken liver	16.8
Roasted fish	2.8
Beef	2.4
Mozzarella-type cheese	2.2
Cooked shrimp	1.8
Cooked egg	1.3
Whole cow milk	0.4
Vitamin B$_6$	*(in mg per 100 g)*
Grilled bovine liver	1.00
Grilled chicken liver	0.87
Banana	0.36
Wheat bran	0.34
Oleaginous foods	0.27
Cooked potato	0.26
Avocado	0.25
Cooked broccoli	0.20
Oat flour	0.16
Cooked bean	0.06

In addition to dietary modifications and vitamin supplementation, other measures that can effectively reduce Hcy levels are weight reduction, low intake of saturated fat, tea and coffee, avoidance of alcohol, managing stress levels, regular exercise, and cessation of cigarette smoking.

3.6 Diet, HCA, and CVD Risk: Current Scenario

Studies of the past two decades have been claiming an association between HCA and CVD and proposed that up to 10% of cardiovascular events could be prevented by lowering Hcy in patients with HCA. Folic acid and vitamin B therapy from supplements and fortified foods were also shown to reduce Hcy levels and long-term total mortality rate due to CVD (Voutilainen et al., 2004). The optimistic thought of this causal association of HCA and CVD and the promising role of vitamin-lowering therapy, however, have been let down by the recent major prospective studies and clinical trials, that is, VISP (vitamin intervention for stroke prevention), NORVIT (Norwegian vitamin trial), HOPE-2 (Heart Outcomes Prevention Evaluation-2), and SEARCH (Study of Effectiveness of Additional Reduction in Cholesterol and Hcy) trials.

The VISP, a large-scale randomized interventional trial, investigated the lowering of Hcy with high- and low-dose vitamin B formulation in 3680 patients with ischemic stroke. Compared with the low doses, treatment with high dose had no significant effect on recurrent stroke, coronary events, or deaths (Toole et al., 2004).

NORVIT recruited 3749 patients from Norway testing the hypotheses that long-term (median follow-up of 40 months) treatment with vitamin B would lower the incidence of MI, stroke, and sudden cardiac death in patients with acute MI. Plasma Hcy levels decreased by about 27% in patients taking folic acid (whether or not they were also taking vitamin B_6) compared with vitamin B_6 and placebo treated patients; however, a significant relative increase was noted in the primary end point by 22% and nonfatal MI by 30% (Bønaa et al., 2006).

The HOPE-2, a randomized, double-blind trial, recruited 5522 patients. These patients were aged 55 years or more and had a history of vascular disease or diabetes. The patients were randomized to receive a combined pill containing 2.5 mg of folic acid, 50 mg of vitamin B_6, and 1 mg of vitamin B_{12} or placebo daily for an average of 5 years. The primary outcome was a composite of death from cardiovascular causes, MI, and stroke. Mean Hcy levels decreased by 0.3 mg l^{-1} among those receiving the active treatment, while a slight increase was seen in the placebo group. Despite this effective Hcy lowering, no significant effect was seen on the primary outcome or the individual components except for a 25% reduction in stroke (Lonn et al., 2006).

SEARCH, a large, prospective, randomized, placebo-controlled, long-term (7 years) trial, included 12 064 MI survivors who were randomized to either 20 or 80 mg of simvastatin daily for the more versus less LDL lowering comparison and to folic acid 2 mg plus vitamin B_{12} 1 mg day^{-1} or placebo for the Hcy lowering comparison for a total of 7 years. On analysis of Hcy lowering effect, there were 1537 major vascular events in the folic acid/vitamin B_{12} arm versus 1493 in the placebo arm. The results suggested that Hcy lowering does not affect the risk of vascular events and is not beneficial for preventing CVD (SEARCH Study Collaborative Group, 2007).

In view of these results, it is quite plausible that the relationship between HCA and CVD is indirect and is confounded by other factors (e.g., deficiencies of folate, vitamin B_{12}, or vitamin B_6) that influence both Hcy levels and CVD risk.

4. FUTURE PERSPECTIVES

The existing data suggest that Hcy exerts a detrimental effect on vascular wall and moderate/severe HCA may be associated with thromboembolic events. It is however unclear whether a causal relationship exists between HCA and CVD risk, or if Hcy is related to other confounding CVD risk factors or is just a disease marker. Although vitamin supplementation with folic acid B_{12} and B_6 reduces/lowers Hcy concentration, recent clinical trials have failed to establish their beneficial effects in CVD. Therefore, routine screening for HCA and prescribing vitamins to lower Hcy are unwarranted except in high-risk individuals (i.e., those with a history of premature CVD, or those thought to be at high risk because other risk factors are present). Several large-scale studies totaling nearly 50 000 subjects are still underway in the United States, Canada, and Europe – WENBIT (the Western Norway B-vitamin Intervention Trial), PACIFIC (Prevention with a Combined Inhibitor and Folate in Coronary Heart Disease) trial, VITATOPS (Vitamins to Prevent Stroke) trial, and others. One will have to await the results from these trial data before finally confirming or refuting the Hcy hypothesis in atherothrombotic vascular disease. Till unequivocal evidence on benefit of vitamin supplementation is apparent, an intake of low-fat diet rich in vitamins and antioxidants together with regular exercise and avoidance of alcohol and smoking appears to be the best strategy for reducing CVD risk associated with HCA.

REFERENCES

Bønaa, K.H., Njølstad, I., Ueland, P.M., et al., 2006. NORVIT Trial Investigators. Homocysteine lowering and cardiovascular events after acute myocardial infarction. The New England Journal of Medicine 354, 1578–1588.

Boushey, C.J., Beresford, S.A.A., Omenn, G.S., Motulsky, A.G., 1995. A quantitative assessment of plasma homocysteine as a risk factor for vascular disease: probable benefits of increasing folic acid intake. Journal of the American Medical Association 274, 1049–1057.

Butz, L.W., du Vigneaud, V., 1932. The formation of a homologue of cystine by the decomposition of methionine with sulfuric acid. Journal of Biological Chemistry 99, 135–142.

Dedoussis, G.V., Panagiotakos, D.B., Chrysohoou, C., et al., 2004. Effect of interaction between adherence to a Mediterranean diet and the methylenetetrahydrofolate reductase 677C3T mutation on homocysteine concentrations in healthy adults: the ATTICA Study. The American Journal of Clinical Nutrition 80, 849–854.

Eikelboom, J.E., Lonn, E., Genest, J., Hankey, G., Yusuf, S., 1999. Homocysteine and cardiovascular disease. A critical review of the epidemiological evidence. Annals of Internal Medicine 131, 363–375.

Fokkema, M.R., Weijer, J.M., Dijck-Brouwer, D.A.J., Doormaal, J.J., Muskiet, F.A.J., 2001. Influence of vitamin-optimized plasma homocysteine cutoff values on the prevalence of hyperhomocysteinemia in healthy adults. Clinical Chemistry 47, 1001–1007.

Gerritsen, T., Vaughn, J.G., Waisman, H.A., 1962. The identification of homocysteine in the urine. Biochemical and Biophysical Research Communications 9, 493–496.

Graham, I.M., Daly, L.E., Refsum, H.M., et al., 1997. Plasma homocysteine as a risk factor for vascular disease. The European Concerted Action Project. Journal of the American Medical Association 277, 1775–1781.

Homocysteine Lowering Trialists' Collaboration, 1998. Lowering blood homocysteine with Folic acid based supplements: meta-analysis of randomized trials. BMJ 316, 894–898.

Homocysteine Studies Collaboration, 2002. Homocysteine and risk of ischemic heart disease and stroke: a meta-analysis. Journal of the American Medical Association 288, 2015–2022.

Jacobsen, D.W., 1998. Homocysteine and vitamins in cardiovascular disease. Clinical Chemistry 44, 1833–1843.

Kang, S.S., Wong, P.W.K., Malinow, M.R., 1992. Hyperhomocyst(e)inemia as a risk factor for occlusive vascular disease. Annual Review of Nutrition 12, 279–298.

Kumar, Y., Das, R., Garewal, G., Bali, H.K., 2009. High prevalence of hyperhomocysteinemia in young population of North India – a potential risk factor for coronary artery disease? Thrombosis Research 123, 800–802.

Lonn, E., Yusuf, S., Arnold, M.J., et al., 2006. Heart Outcomes Prevention Evaluation (HOPE) 2 Investigators. Homocysteine lowering with folic acid and B vitamins in vascular disease. The New England Journal of Medicine 354, 1567–1577.

Malinow, M.R., Duell, P.B., Hess, D.L., et al., 1998. Reduction of plasma homocysteine levels by breakfast cereal fortified with folic acid in patients with coronary heart disease. The New England Journal of Medicine 338, 1009–1015.

McCully, K.S., 1969. Vascular pathology of homocysteinemia: implications for the pathogenesis of arteriosclerosis. The American Journal of Pathology 56, 111–128.

McCully, K.S., 1996. Homocysteine and vascular disease. Nature Medicine 2, 386–389.

Murray, C.J.L., Lopez, A.D., 1997. Alternative projections of mortality and disability by cause 1990–2020: Global Burden of Disease Study. Lancet 349, 1498–1504.

Omenn, G.S., Beresford, S.A.A., Motulsky, A.G., 1998. Preventing coronary heart disease: B vitamins and homocysteine. Circulation 97, 421–424.

Refsum, H., Ueland, P.M., Nygard, O., Vollset, S.E., 1998. Homocysteine and cardiovascular disease. Annual Review of Medicine 49, 31–62.

Schneider, J.A., Rees, D.C., Liu, Y., Clegg, J.B., 1998. Worldwide distribution of a common methylenetetrahydrofolate reductase mutation. The American Journal of Human Genetics 62, 1258–1260.

SEARCH Study Collaborative Group, Bowman, L., Armitage, J., et al., 2007. Study of the effectiveness of additional reductions in cholesterol and homocysteine (SEARCH): characteristics of a randomized trial among 12064 myocardial infarction survivors. American Heart Journal 154, 815–823.

Selhub, J., 1999. Homocysteine metabolism. Annual Review of Nutrition 19, 217–246.

Selhub, J., Jacques, P.F., Wilson, P.W.F., Rush, D., Rosenberg, I.H., 1993. Vitamin status and intake as primary determinants of homocysteinemia in an elderly population. Journal of the American Medical Association 270, 2693–2698.

Smith, S.C., 2006. Current and future directions of cardiovascular risk prediction. The American Journal of Cardiology 97 (2A), 28A–32A.

The World Health Report, 2003. Global Health: Today's Challenges. World Health Organization, Geneva.

Toole, J.F., Malinow, M.R., Chambless, L.E., et al., 2004. Lowering homocysteine in patients with ischemic stroke to prevent recurrent stroke, myocardial infarction, and death: the Vitamin Intervention for Stroke Prevention (VISP) randomized controlled trial. Journal of the American Medical Association 291, 565–575.

U.S. Department of Agriculture, Agricultural Research Service. 2009. USDA National Nutrient Database for Standard Reference, Release 22. Nutrient Data Laboratory Home Page, http://www.ars.usda.gov/ba/bhnrc/ndl.

US Department of Health and Human Services, 1995. Nutrition and Your Health: Dietary Guidelines for Americans, fourth ed. US Government Printing Office, Washington, DC.

Van Cott, E.M., Lapasota, M., 1998. Laboratory evaluation of hypercoagulable states. Hematology/Oncology Clinics of North America 12, 1141–1166.

Voutilainen, S., Virtanen, J.K., Rissanen, T.H., et al., 2004. Serum folate and homocysteine and the incidence of acute coronary events: the Kuopio Ischaemic Heart Disease Risk Factor Study. The American Journal of Clinical Nutrition 80, 317–323.

Welch, G.N., Loscalzo, J., 1998. Homocysteine and atherothrombosis. The New England Journal of Medicine 338, 1042–1049.

CHAPTER 9

Phytosterols and Cardiovascular Disease

D.S. MacKay, P.J.H. Jones
University of Manitoba, Winnipeg, Manitoba, Canada

ABBREVIATIONS

APOE Apolipoprotein E
CHD Coronary heart disease
CVD Cardiovascular disease
LDL Low-density lipoprotein
MetS Metabolic syndrome
T2DM Type 2 diabetes mellitus
VLDL Very low-density lipoproteins

1. INTRODUCTION

Phytosterols, which encompass plant sterols and stanols, are steroid compounds similar to cholesterol which occur naturally in plants and vary only in carbon side chain and/or presence or absence of a double bond. Stanols are saturated sterols, having no double bonds in the sterol ring structure. More than 200 phytosterols and similar compounds have been identified (Akihisa et al., 1991); the most common dietary sourced phytosterols are β–sitosterol, campesterol, and stigmasterol (Figure 9.1; Jones and AbuMweis, 2009). The ability of phytosterols to lower cholesterol in humans was first demonstrated in 1953 (Pollak, 1953). Phytosterols were subsequently marketed under the name Cytellin as a treatment for elevated cholesterol from 1954 to 1982 (Jones, 2007). The more contemporary use of phytosterols in functional foods began with the introduction of plant stanol ester margarines to the Finnish market in 1995.

Plant sterols and stanols have demonstrated equal ability to lower low-density lipoprotein (LDL) cholesterol in head to head comparisons (Hallikainen et al., 2000a; O'Neill et al., 2004; Vanstone et al., 2002) and in meta-analyses (Demonty et al., 2009; Katan et al., 2003). However, plant sterol and stanols differ significantly in terms of intestinal efficiency of absorption. Plant sterols are absorbed in the range of 4–15% depending on the structure, whereas stanols are absorbed at approximately 1%. This difference in absorption is reflected in higher circulating sterol as compared to stanol levels. Plant sterol

Bioactive Food as Dietary Interventions for Cardiovascular Disease
http://dx.doi.org/10.1016/B978-0-12-396485-4.00008-6

© 2013 Elsevier Inc.
All rights reserved.

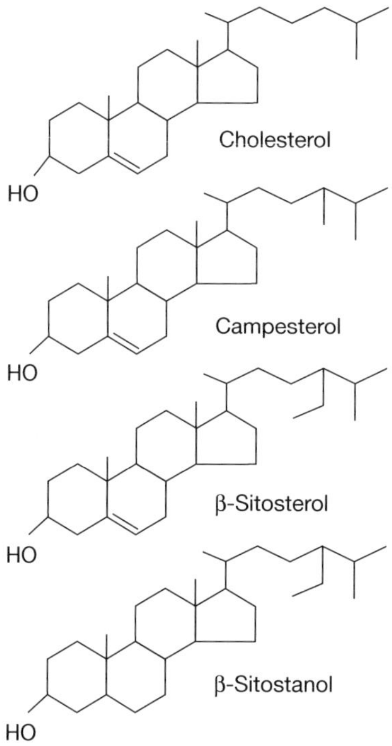

Figure 9.1 Chemical structures of cholesterol, campesterol, and β-sitostanol

consumption increases plant sterol levels in the plasma while not significantly affecting circulating plant stanol level, whereas plant stanol supplementation increases plant stanol levels in the plasma but decreases plant sterol levels by reducing their absorption, along with that of cholesterol.

Cardiovascular disease (CVD) is the leading cause of death accounting for 12.2% of deaths worldwide. The economic impact of CVD is very large and expected to grow as the mean population ages. In the United States alone, the total direct costs of CVD were estimated at $273 billion in 2010 and are expected to triple to $818 billion dollars by 2030 (Heidenreich et al., 2011). The indirect costs of lost productivity due to illness or death were estimated at an additional $172 million in 2010. Clearly, a prevention strategy is required to reduce the incidence of CVD and its economic burden, not to mention the incalculable cost in human suffering related to CVD's associated morbidity and mortality.

Since introduction as a functional food ingredient in margarines during the mid-1990s, plant sterols have been added to numerous other matrices, including dairy and nondairy beverages, yogurts, baked goods and deli meats (Abumweis et al., 2008). These phytosterol containing functional foods have been repeatedly shown to successfully lower total and LDL–cholesterol values in numerous clinical trials

(Abumweis et al., 2008; Katan et al., 2003; Musa-Veloso et al., 2011). A dose of 2–3 g day^{-1} of phytosterols is recommended for optimal LDL-cholesterol lowering. While larger doses of phytosterols up to 8–9 g day^{-1} have been well tolerated, the LDL-cholesterol lowering effect may be attenuated (Demonty et al., 2009). As LDL-cholesterol lowering is still the number one therapeutic target for CVD risk reduction and treatment (NCEP, 2002), phytosterols are a valuable adjunct to lifestyle and pharmaceutical intervention in prevention and treatment of CVD. The implications of phytosterol intake and plasma levels will be discussed as they relate to CVD risk, prevention and treatment.

2. PHYTOSTEROLS IN THE DIET

The evidence for supplemental use of phytosterols can be found in ancestral human diets, which contained much higher intakes of phytosterols in the grams per day range, and would have had a functional impact on cholesterol absorption and circulating cholesterol levels (Jenkins et al., 2003). However, the level of phytosterols in the diet has decreased as humans moved from foraging through the agricultural and industrial ages, into the diet seen today. In modern diets, the phytosterol content ranges from 170 to 360 mg day^{-1}, depending on eating habits and geographic region (de Vries et al., 1997). These naturally occurring levels of phytosterols in many foods have been shown to measurably reduce cholesterol absorption, and may be a confounding factor in dietary trials evaluating health benefits of different fatty acids, where phytosterol-rich vegetable fatty acid sources may be compared to animals' sources without phytosterols (Ostlund, 2007). Dietary choices such as veganism can significantly increase naturally occurring dietary phytosterol levels, which in turn can be predicted to reduce cholesterol levels (Racette et al., 2009).

3. PLASMA PHYTOSTEROLS AND CVD

Phytosterols are not produced in humans, therefore, levels in blood are entirely of dietary origin. Phytosterol levels have been shown to vary greatly within and between different populations. The underlying factors which contribute to the variability have been reviewed and different analytical methods were found to be most responsible for the variation in circulating phytosterol levels reported in the literature (Chan et al., 2006). Genetic factors, gender, and the presence or absence of diabetes and metabolic syndrome (MetS) were all also found to have a larger impact on plasma plant sterol levels than plant sterol intake itself. These findings suggest that while the average levels of plasma plant sterols found across different populations may correlate with the populations' plant sterol intake, differences seen between individuals are more likely due to biological factors such as genetics.

Phytosterolemia is a rare autosomal recessive genetic disorder that results in an inability to effectively clear absorbed plant sterols from the blood. The disorder results in a 50–100-fold increase in plant sterol levels and is associated with rapid development of coronary atherosclerosis. Myocardial infarctions and deaths have been attributed to phytosterolemia in individuals as young as 5 years of age (Wang et al., 2004). The cause of phytosterolemia has been linked to mutations in the ABCG5/G8 proteins which are responsible for pumping plant sterols out of enterocytes and hepatocytes into the lumen and bile ducts, respectively.

Due to the link between phytoserolemia and CVD, plant sterol levels in nonphytosterolemics have been examined in relation to CVD risk, yielding mixed results. Plant sterol levels in the blood have been shown to be positively, negatively, or unassociated with CVD risk depending on the human study population investigated. Glueck et al., (1991) suggested that elevated plant sterol levels may be associated with increased CVD risk because campesterol and total plant sterol levels correlated positively with cholesterol levels, and in the top quintile of the 3472 hypercholesterolemic patients high campesterol was associated with increased personal or familial coronary heart disease (CHD). Sudhop et al., (2002) also concluded that plant sterol levels may exist as an additional risk factor for CVD after finding a positive relationship between β-sitosterol and campesterol levels and a family history of CHD. These findings are in contrast to those of Fassbender et al., (2008) who found that plant sterol levels were lower in individuals with CHD from the Longitudinal Aging Study Amsterdam, and that elevated β-sitosterol levels were associated with a significant reduced risk of CHD. Pinedo et al., (2007) also found a reduced CVD odds ratio for individuals in the highest sitosterol tertile, suggesting that plant sterols in the physiological range found in the EPIC-norfolk population are not aversely related to CVD.

These mixed results from epidemiological trials are further complicated by the fact that phytosterol levels reflect cholesterol absorption in individuals. This relationship between phytosterols and cholesterol absorption was first introduced by Tilvis and Miettinen (1986) who demonstrated that phytosterol levels, when normalized to circulating cholesterol levels, correlated positively with cholesterol absorption measured using a radio-isotopic method. This finding has led to the conclusion that elevated cholesterol absorption, rather than elevated phytosterols themselves, are associated with increased CVD risk (Rajaratnam et al., 2000; Silbernagel et al., 2010). It has, subsequently, been demonstrated that precursors to cholesterol, such as desmosterol and lathosterol, correlate positively with cholesterol synthesis. Changes in phytosterol to cholesterol ratios and cholesterol precursor to cholesterol ratios are now often used in clinical and epidemiological trials to access cholesterol metabolism. This ratio approach of accessing cholesterol absorption, however, cannot be used to access the impact of phytosterols because supplementation with phytosterols causes their plasma levels to rise, which would be perceived as an increase in cholesterol absorption, when in fact phytosterols decrease cholesterol absorption (Vanstone and Jones, 2004).

4. PHYTOSTEROL MECHANISM OF ACTION

Phytosterols are thought to work as competitive inhibitors of cholesterol absorption (Katan et al., 2003). Phytosterols compete with dietary and biliary cholesterol in the intestinal lumen for incorporation into the mixed micelles, which are the spherical collections of hydrophobic molecules, surrounded by surfactants such as bile salts and phospholipids, which form in the aqueous lumen. These micelles associate with the enterocytes which line the intestinal tract and are the site from which cholesterol, fatty acids, and other hydrophobic compounds such as fat soluble vitamins are absorbed (Narushima et al., 2008). Cholesterol is thought to be absorbed into the enterocytes by a process which requires the NPC1L1 transporter; it is this process at which phytosterols are thought to exert their competitive inhibition. Once inside the enterocyte, phytosterols are preferential pumped back out into the lumen by the ABGC5/G8 transporter system. Phytosterols that do get incorporated into chylomicrons in the enterocytes and enter the circulation are transported out in the liver to the bile by the same ABGC5/G8 system. Phytosterol consumption has been repeatedly shown to reduce cholesterol absorption in numerous studies using stable isotope tracer methods to measure absorption (Ostlund et al., 2003; Rideout et al., 2009) .

5. PHYSICAL FACTORS AFFECTING PHYTOSTEROL LDL LOWERING

The cardiovascular benefit of phytosterol supplementation is its demonstrated ability to lower LDL-cholesterol levels (Abumweis et al., 2008; Demonty et al., 2009; Katan et al., 2003; Musa-Veloso et al., 2011). However, the effectiveness of phytosterol supplementation may be affected by numerous factors such as physical form, dose, frequency, and matrix. The physical form of phytosterol used in supplementation can affect LDL lowering. Unesterified (free) and esterified phytosterols have both been shown to similarly affect plasma lipoproteins (Demonty et al., 2009), however, esterified phytosterols are preferred, especially for stanols because of the low solubility of the free form which can reduce efficacy (Denke, 1995; Thompson and Grundy, 2005). Esterified forms of phytosterols have much higher lipid solubility than free phytosterols and are much easier to incorporate in food products such as margarine. A dose–response relationship in LDL-cholesterol lowering by phytosterol supplementation has been demonstrated (Hallikainen et al., 2000b) and reported in meta-analyses (Demonty et al., 2009; Musa-Veloso et al., 2011). The dose–response of both plant sterols and stanols has been shown to equally affect plasma lipoproteins over recommended dose ranges. However, it has been suggested that the theoretical maximal LDL-cholesterol reduction for plant stanols is higher than that of plant sterols (Musa-Veloso et al., 2011). This theoretical maximum LDL-cholesterol lowering is at doses ($>4\,\mathrm{g\,day^{-1}}$) much higher than the currently recommended guidelines for supplementation and requires further validation as only limited studies have been conducted in this range. The frequency of phytosterol supplementation has also been shown to influence the extent of LDL-cholesterol lowering. In a trial comparing 1.8 g day^{-1} of plant sterols supplemented at breakfast to 1.8 d/day of plant sterols divided equally across three daily meals, only the three times per day supplementation reduced LDL cholesterol compared to control (AbuMweis et al., 2009). A tendency ($p = 0.054$) toward reduced efficacy of single versus multiple daily intakes of phytosterols has also been seen in a recent meta-analysis by Demonty et al. (2009). This type of supplemental a phytosterol matrix has a substantial effect on its LDL-cholesterol lowering. Phytosterols incorporated in margarines, mayonnaise, salad dressing, milk, and yogurt were more effective in lowering LDL cholesterol than other supplemental food matrices such a orange juice, nonfat beverages, and cereals bars (Abumweis et al., 2008), suggesting that food matrix is important in achieving maximal LDL lowering.

6. BIOLOGICAL FACTORS AFFECTING RESPONSE TO PHYTOSTEROLS

Within studies the LDL lowering in response to phytosterols between individuals can be very large, and an individual's response to phytosterols is repeatable across multiple supplementation periods. Because the environmental factors discussed above are controlled within a trial this variability in response to phytosterol supplementation suggests that genetic factors may influence response. Apolipoprotein E (APOE) is a lipoprotein that is found in triglyceride-rich chylomicrons and very low-density lipoproteins (VLDLs). The APOE gene has three major isoforms E2, E3, and E4, which have been shown to be associated with the response to phytosterols. In a randomized, double blind, study of 217 hypercholesterolemic adults, only individuals with the E2 and E3 isoforms responded to phytosterol supplementation with lowered total and LDL cholesterol, suggesting that phytosterols may not work for individuals with the E4 isoform (Sanchez-Muniz et al., 2009). The CYP7A1 gene codes for 7α-hydroxylase, an enzyme involved in the synthesis of bile acid from cholesterol. Variation at the -204 A > C promoter region of the CYP7A1 gene has been shown to have an association with response to phytosterols. Individuals possessing the CA or CC allele at -204 of the CYP7A1 gene manifested higher mean reductions in total circulating cholesterol levels (-0.34 compared to -0.10 mmol l^{-1} for AA carriers) in response to phytosterol supplementation (De Castro-Oros et al., 2010). The C variant of the at -204 in the CYP7A1 gene was associated with increased bile acid synthesis and increased feedback elevation in cholesterol synthesis in response to phytosterols. These studies strongly demonstrate that genetic factors can have a significant impact on response to phytosterols and account for much of the variability seen between individuals in phytosterol trials.

7. PHYTOSTEROLS AND PHARMACEUTICAL CHOLESTEROL LOWERING THERAPIES

Currently, statins are the most widely prescribed pharmaceutical in the world (Wang et al., 2004). Statins work by reducing endogenous cholesterol synthesis via inhibition of the key HMG-CoA reductase enzyme. Phytosterols reduce cholesterol levels by competing with cholesterol absorption in the gut, a mechanism which is complementary to that of statins. Both plant sterol and stanol consumption reduced LDL cholesterol by 0.34 mmol l^{-1} on average when supplemented at 2.5 g day^{-1} in individuals on statin treatment, with no differences seen in LDL lowering between sterol or stanol interventions (De Jong et al., 2008). These results were supported in a meta-analysis by Scholle et al., (2009) showing that phytosterol therapy further reduces cholesterol levels by 9.18–17.34% in current statin users. The type or dose of statin being taken does not appear to affect phytosterols' LDL-cholesterol lowering efficacy. Phytosterols have also been shown to be effective in combination with fibrate drugs. In participants on a low cholesterol STEP 1 diet, phytosterols reduced total and LDL cholesterol by 8.5 and 11.1%, respectively, in individuals taking fibrate drugs compared to 5.5 and 7.7% in those not receiving fibrate treatment. (Gupta et al., 2011). These data suggest that phytosterols are a viable adjunct to statin and fibrate therapies, current statin users may benefit more from phytosterol supplementation than increasing their current statin dose, especially with regard to potential side-effects associated with statin use (Katan et al., 2003).

8. PHYTOSTEROLS, METS, AND DIABETES

MetS and type 2 diabetes mellitus (T2DM) are both strong risk factors for the development of CVD. The insulin resistance associated with MetS and T2DM drives increased cholesterol synthesis and lowers cholesterol absorption compared to individuals with normal insulin sensitivity, although this change in cholesterol metabolism does not seem to impair the effectiveness of phytosterol supplementation (Baker et al., 2009). In 108 individuals with MetS who were randomly assigned to consume yogurt beverages containing 4 g day^{-1} phytosterols or yogurt beverages without phytosterols for 2 months, total cholesterol, LDL cholesterol, and triglycerides were significantly reduced in the phytosterol group (Sialvera et al., 2011). In a meta-analysis of phytosterol supplementation in individuals with T2DM, total and LDL cholesterol were significantly reduced in response to phytosterol supplementation (Baker et al., 2009). These results suggest a role for phytosterol supplementation in the treatment for the dyslipidemia that is associated with MetS and T2DM.

9. PHYTOSTEROLS AND TRIGLYCERIDE LOWERING

Elevated triglyceride levels have been established as an important risk marker for CVD (Malloy and Kane, 2001). Growing evidence points to phytosterol supplementation reducing circulating total and LDL cholesterol, as well as triglyceride levels, making PS even more attractive in the treatment and prevention of CVD. Triglycerides were found to be reduced by 14% in individual supplementing 1.6 g day^{-1} of plant sterols in a fermented milk beverage for 6 weeks (Plana et al., 2008). The triglyceride lowering effects of phytosterols have been shown to be more pronounced in individuals with elevated baseline triglycerides (Theuwissen et al., 2009). The proposed mechanism behind the triglyceride lowering effect of phytosterols was believed to be due to a reduction in triglyceride-rich VLDL particle produced by the liver (Plat and Mensink, 2009). The ability of phytosterols to lower triglyceride levels, especially in individuals with elevated triglycerides, offers a further reduction in a CVD risk factor in addition to their reliable LDL lowering.

10. PHYTOSTEROLS AND CVD RISK REDUCTION

Although long-term trials have yet to be carried out targeting demonstration of a reduction in hard cardiovascular endpoints in response to phytosterol supplementation, phytosterols do have a positive impact on multiple risk markers for CVD. The LDL lowering of phytosterols is well established and growing evidence that phytosterols lower triglyceride levels makes them an attractive tool in the treatment and prevention of CVD, especially due to their minimal side-effects. The direct CVD risk reduction of incorporating supplemental phytosterols in the 2 g day^{-1} range has been estimated at 25% (Law, 2000), a level of decrease greater than that realized through a reduced intake of saturated fat.

11. CONCLUSION

Phytosterols offer an easy, safe, and effective nutritional supplement that reduces total and LDL cholesterol and in some cases triglycerides; all risk factors for CVD. Functional foods with phytosterols can be effectively added to other dietary and lifestyle modifications, as well as statin use, in most dyslipidemic individuals to achieve additional lipid lowering. Phytosterols are also effective in lowering total and LDL cholesterol in dyslipidemic individuals with MetS and T2DM who have an elevated risk of CVD. Research into the genetic factors which affect an individual's response to phytosterols must be continued to help optimize their use in personalized health strategies.

12. SUMMARY POINTS

1. Phytosterols are safe and naturally occurring in the diet, particularly in foods rich in plant-based fats and oils.

2. Supplemental phytosterols lower total and LDL–cholesterol levels. This reduction in cholesterol is due to lower cholesterol absorption.

3. Phytosterol supplementation can be effectively combined with statin and fibrate therapy to further lower cholesterol levels and can help to achieve cholesterol goals without increasing statin doses.

4. Phytosterol supplementation effectively reduces established CVD risk factors.

GLOSSARY

Isoform One of any different type of the same protein arising from variation in nucleotide sequence or splicing.

Functional food A food with health benefits or disease prevention beyond its basic nutritive value.

Hydrophobic Lacking an affinity for water.

Phytosterolemia A lipid metabolic disorder resulting in the accumulation of phytosterols.

Micelles Spherical collections of hydrophobic molecules surrounded by surfactants which form in the aqueous environments.

Insulin resistance A physiological condition where the glucose lowering response to insulin is reduced.

REFERENCES

Abumweis, S.S., Barake, R., Jones, P.J., 2008. Plant sterols/stanols as cholesterol lowering agents: a meta-analysis of randomized controlled trials. Food Nutr Res 52.

Abumweis, S.S., Vanstone, C.A., Lichtenstein, A.H., Jones, P.J., 2009. Plant sterol consumption frequency affects plasma lipid levels and cholesterol kinetics in humans. European Journal of Clinical Nutrition 63, 747–755.

Akihisa, T., Kokke, W., Tamura, T., 1991. Naturally occurring sterols and related compounds from plants. In: Patterson, G.W., Nes, W.D. (Eds.), Physiology and Biochemistry of Sterols. American Oil Chemists' Society, Champaign, IL.

Baker, W.L., Baker, E.L., Coleman, C.I., 2009. The effect of plant sterols or stanols on lipid parameters in patients with type 2 diabetes: a meta-analysis. Diabetes Research and Clinical Practice 84, e33–e37.

Chan, Y.M., Varady, K.A., Lin, Y., et al., 2006. Plasma concentrations of plant sterols: physiology and relationship with coronary heart disease. Nutrition Reviews 64, 385–402.

Clifton, P.M., Noakes, M., Sullivan, D., et al., 2004. Cholesterol-lowering effects of plant sterol esters differ in milk, yoghurt, bread and cereal. European Journal of Clinical Nutrition 58, 503–509.

De Castro-Oros, I., Pampin, S., Cofan, M., et al., 2010. Promoter variant −204A > C of the cholesterol 7alpha-hydroxylase gene: Association with response to plant sterols in humans and increased transcriptional activity in transfected HepG2 cells. Clinical Nutrition 30, 239–246.

de Jong, A., Plat, J., Bast, A., et al., 2008. Effects of plant sterol and stanol ester consumption on lipid metabolism, antioxidant status and markers of oxidative stress, endothelial function and low-grade inflammation in patients on current statin treatment. European Journal of Clinical Nutrition 62, 263–273.

de Vries, J.H.M., Jansen, A., Kromhout, D., et al., 1997. The fatty acid and sterol content of food composites of middle-aged men in seven countries. Journal of Food Composition and Analysis 10, 115–141.

Demonty, I., Ras, R.T., van der Knaap, H.C., et al., 2009. Continuous dose-response relationship of the LDL-cholesterol-lowering effect of phytosterol intake. The Journal of Nutrition 139, 271–284.

Denke, M.A., 1995. Lack of efficacy of low-dose sitostanol therapy as an adjunct to a cholesterol-lowering diet in men with moderate hypercholesterolemia. The American Journal of Clinical Nutrition 61, 392–396.

Fassbender, K., Lutjohann, D., Dik, M.G., et al., 2008. Moderately elevated plant sterol levels are associated with reduced cardiovascular risk – the LASA study. Atherosclerosis 196, 283–288.

Glueck, C.J., Speirs, J., Tracy, T., et al., 1991. Relationships of serum plant sterols (phytosterols) and cholesterol in 595 hypercholesterolemic subjects, and familial aggregation of phytosterols, cholesterol, and premature coronary heart disease in hyperphytosterolemic probands and their first-degree relatives. Metabolism 40, 842–848.

Gupta, A.K., Savopoulos, C.G., Ahuja, J., Hatzitolios, A.I., 2011. Role of phytosterols in lipid-lowering: current perspectives. QJM: Monthly Journal of the Association of Physicians 104, 301–308.

Hallikainen, M.A., Sarkkinen, E.S., Gylling, H., Erkkila, A.T., Uusitupa, M.I., 2000. Comparison of the effects of plant sterol ester and plant stanol ester-enriched margarines in lowering serum cholesterol concentrations in hypercholesterolaemic subjects on a low-fat diet. European Journal of Clinical Nutrition 54, 715–725.

Hallikainen, M.A., Sarkkinen, E.S., Uusitupa, M.I., 2000. Plant stanol esters affect serum cholesterol concentrations of hypercholesterolemic men and women in a dose-dependent manner. The Journal of Nutrition 130, 767–776.

Heidenreich, P.A., Trogdon, J.G., Khavjou, O.A., et al., 2011. Forecasting the future of cardiovascular disease in the United States: a policy statement from the American Heart Association. Circulation 123, 933–944.

Jenkins, D.J., Kendall, C.W., Marchie, A., et al., 2003. The Garden of Eden – plant based diets, the genetic drive to conserve cholesterol and its implications for heart disease in the 21st century. Comparative Biochemistry and Physiology. Part A, Molecular & Integrative Physiology 136, 141–151.

Jones, P.J., 2007. Ingestion of phytosterols is not potentially hazardous. The Journal of Nutrition 137, 2485 author reply 2486.

Jones, P.J., Abumweis, S.S., 2009. Phytosterols as functional food ingredients: linkages to cardiovascular disease and cancer. Current Opinion in Clinical Nutrition and Metabolic Care 12, 147–151.

Katan, M.B., Grundy, S.M., Jones, P., et al., 2003. Efficacy and safety of plant stanols and sterols in the management of blood cholesterol levels. Mayo Clinic Proceedings 78, 965–978.

Law, M., 2000. Plant sterol and stanol margarines and health. BMJ 320, 861–864.

Malloy, M.J., Kane, J.P., 2001. A risk factor for atherosclerosis: triglyceride-rich lipoproteins. Advances in Internal Medicine 47, 111–136.

Musa-Veloso, K., Poon, T.H., Elliot, J.A., Chung, C., 2011. A comparison of the LDL-cholesterol lowering efficacy of plant stanols and plant sterols over a continuous dose range: results of a meta-analysis of randomized, placebo-controlled trials. Prostaglandins, Leukotrienes, and Essential Fatty Acids 85, 9–28.

Narushima, K., Takada, T., Yamanashi, Y., Suzuki, H., 2008. Niemann-pick C1-like 1 mediates alpha-tocopherol transport. Molecular Pharmacology 74, 42–49.

NCEP, 2002. Third Report of the National Cholesterol Education Program (NCEP) Expert Panel on Detection, Evaluation, and Treatment of High Blood Cholesterol in Adults (Adult Treatment Panel III) final report. Circulation 106, 3143–3421.

O'Neill, F.H., Brynes, A., Mandeno, R., et al., 2004. Comparison of the effects of dietary plant sterol and stanol esters on lipid metabolism. Nutrition, Metabolism, and Cardiovascular Diseases 14, 133–142.

Ostlund Jr., R.E., 2007. Phytosterols, cholesterol absorption and healthy diets. Lipids 42, 41–45.

Ostlund Jr., R.E., Racette, S.B., Stenson, W.F., 2003. Inhibition of cholesterol absorption by phytosterol-replete wheat germ compared with phytosterol-depleted wheat germ. The American Journal of Clinical Nutrition 77, 1385–1389.

Pinedo, S., Vissers, M.N., von Bergmann, K., et al., 2007. Plasma levels of plant sterols and the risk of coronary artery disease: the prospective EPIC-Norfolk Population Study. Journal of Lipid Research 48, 139–144.

Plana, N., Nicolle, C., Ferre, R., et al., 2008. Plant sterol-enriched fermented milk enhances the attainment of LDL-cholesterol goal in hypercholesterolemic subjects. European Journal of Nutrition 47, 32–39.

Plat, J., Mensink, R.P., 2009. Plant stanol esters lower serum triacylglycerol concentrations via a reduced hepatic VLDL-1 production. Lipids 44, 1149–1153.

Pollak, O.J., 1953. Reduction of blood cholesterol in man. Circulation 7, 702–706.

Racette, S.B., Spearie, C.A., Phillips, K.M., et al., 2009. Phytosterol-deficient and high-phytosterol diets developed for controlled feeding studies. Journal of the American Dietetic Association 109, 2043–2051.

Rajaratnam, R.A., Gylling, H., Miettinen, T.A., 2000. Independent association of serum squalene and noncholesterol sterols with coronary artery disease in postmenopausal women. Journal of the American College of Cardiology 35, 1185–1191.

Rideout, T.C., Chan, Y.M., Harding, S.V., Jones, P.J., 2009. Low and moderate-fat plant sterol fortified soymilk in modulation of plasma lipids and cholesterol kinetics in subjects with normal to high cholesterol concentrations: report on two randomized crossover studies. Lipids in Health and Disease 8, 45.

Sanchez-Muniz, F.J., Maki, K.C., Schaefer, E.J., Ordovas, J.M., 2009. Serum lipid and antioxidant responses in hypercholesterolemic men and women receiving plant sterol esters vary by apolipoprotein E genotype. The Journal of Nutrition 139, 13–19.

Scholle, J.M., Baker, W.L., Talati, R., Coleman, C.I., 2009. The effect of adding plant sterols or stanols to statin therapy in hypercholesterolemic patients: systematic review and meta-analysis. Journal of the American College of Nutrition 28, 517–524.

Sialvera, T.E., Pounis, G.D., Koutelidakis, A.E., et al., 2011. Phytosterols supplementation decreases plasma small and dense LDL levels in metabolic syndrome patients on a westernized type diet. Nutrition, Metabolism, and Cardiovascular Diseases.

Silbernagel, G., Fauler, G., Hoffmann, M.M., et al., 2010. The associations of cholesterol metabolism and plasma plant sterols with all-cause and cardiovascular mortality. Journal of Lipid Research 51, 2384–2393.

Sudhop, T., Gottwald, B.M., von Bergmann, K., 2002. Serum plant sterols as a potential risk factor for coronary heart disease. Metabolism 51, 1519–1521.

Theuwissen, E., Plat, J., van der Kallen, C.J., van Greevenbroek, M.M., Mensink, R.P., 2009. Plant stanol supplementation decreases serum triacylglycerols in subjects with overt hypertriglyceridemia. Lipids 44, 1131–1140.

Thompson, G.R., Grundy, S.M., 2005. History and development of plant sterol and stanol esters for cholesterol-lowering purposes. The American Journal of Cardiology 96, 3D–9D.

Tilvis, R.S., Miettinen, T.A., 1986. Serum plant sterols and their relation to cholesterol absorption. The American Journal of Clinical Nutrition 43, 92–97.

Vanstone, C.A., Jones, P.J., 2004. Limitations of plasma plant sterols as indicators of cholesterol absorption. The American Journal of Clinical Nutrition 79, 340–341.

Vanstone, C.A., Raeini-Sarjaz, M., Parsons, W.E., Jones, P.J., 2002. Unesterified plant sterols and stanols lower LDL-cholesterol concentrations equivalently in hypercholesterolemic persons. The American Journal of Clinical Nutrition 76, 1272–1278.

Wang, J., Joy, T., Mymin, D., Frohlich, J., Hegele, R.A., 2004. Phenotypic heterogeneity of sitosterolemia. Journal of Lipid Research 45, 2361–2367.

CHAPTER 10

Taurine Effects on Arterial Pressure Control

S. Roysommuti*, J.M. Wyss[†]
*Khon Kaen University, Khon Kaen, Thailand
[†]University of Alabama at Birmingham, Birmingham, AL, USA

ABBREVIATIONS

ANP Atrial natriuretic peptide
BNP Brain natriuretic peptide
GABA Gamma–aminobutyric acid
OVLT Organum vasculosum laminar terminalis
RVLM Rostral ventrolateral medulla
Tau–Cl Taurine chloramine
TauT Taurine transporter
TauTKO TauT knockout

Taurine, 2-aminoethanesulfonic acid, is the most abundant intracellular free amino acid present in mammalian tissues, and taurine in brain, kidneys, heart, and blood vessels appears to be particularly important to cardiovascular control. Taurine has been reported to protect against many cardiovascular disorders, especially hypertension and cardiac ischemia, and it plays a role in cardiovascular control throughout life, that is, from perinatal to aged life. The present chapter reviews the interplay of taurine on the arterial pressure control mechanism and its therapeutic action on some cardiovascular disorders.

1. AN OVERVIEW OF ARTERIAL PRESSURE CONTROL

To understand the role of taurine in cardiovascular control, it is necessary to first review the major physiological mechanisms that regulate blood flow. The cardiovascular system provides blood flow to all organs, but it gives priority to organs that are most vital to maintaining life, that is, heart and brain. Generally, blood flow to each tissue is determined by the arterial–venous pressure gradient (the driving force) and tissue vascular resistance. The heart circulates blood to both systemic and pulmonary beds, with tissue blood flow being dependent on cardiac output, arterial pressure, total peripheral resistance, and venous return. Among these parameters, the arterial pressure is well regulated within a narrow range by adjusting other parameters. While these functions lay the template for blood flow, the differential and dynamic blood flow requirements

Bioactive Food as Dietary Interventions for Cardiovascular Disease
http://dx.doi.org/10.1016/B978-0-12-396485-4.00009-8

© 2013 Elsevier Inc.
All rights reserved.

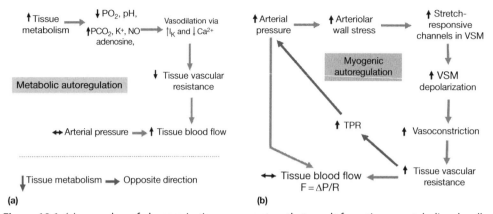

Figure 10.1 (a) a number of changes in tissue parameters that result from tissue metabolism locally regulate tissue blood flow, leading to the ability of tissue to regulate blood flow dynamically, that is, metabolic autoregulation (I_K=potassium outward current, NO=nitric oxide). (b) myogenic autoregulation of blood flow is regulated by a sequence of changes in parameters related to vascular wall stress to regulate tissue blood flow in response to acute increases in arterial pressure (F=tissue blood flow, ΔP=arterial-venous pressure gradient across a tissue, R=tissue vascular resistance, TPR=total peripheral resistance, VSM=vascular smooth muscle).

of each tissue are met by a variety of local control mechanisms, particularly metabolic- and myogenic-dependent phenomenon (Figure 10.1).

Arterial pressure is regulated by a complex interplay of the nervous system, hormones, cardiac contraction, vascular impedance, and renal function. In addition, several factors including genetics, diet, internal and external environment, race, gender, behaviors, maternal–child interaction, and socioeconomic status dictate an individual's cardiovascular function (Figure 10.2). Cardiovascular nuclei in the brainstem integrate the brain's ongoing regulation of blood pressure with feedback from baroreceptors, chemoreceptors, and other sensory inputs, and thereby control the heart, blood vessel, and kidney function via the autonomic nervous system and circulating hormones, thus regulating cardiac output by changes in stroke volume and heart rate while regulating blood vessels by adjusting their diameter (peripheral resistance). In addition, the nervous system regulates renal function, thereby adjusting the kidney's ability to regulate blood volume through pressure-diuretic/natriuretic mechanisms. While blood volume is a major determinant of venous pressure, venous return, and cardiac output, this renal/blood volume mechanism is best suited for long-term arterial pressure regulation since it needs considerable time to adjust the water and electrolyte input and output balance.

The cardiovascular brainstem center is a very complex neural network, involving several brain areas and peripheral input signals (Figure 10.3). Although the hypothalamus and brainstem play a crucial role in adjusting the final neuronal output to

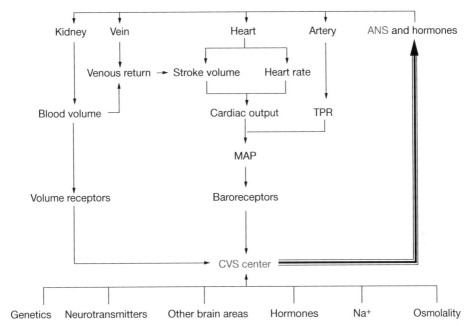

Figure 10.2 Many diverse components are integrated together to regulate arterial pressure and cardiac function (ANS=autonomic nervous system, CVS=cardiovascular system, MAP=mean arterial pressure, TPR=total peripheral resistance).

the cardiovascular system, they do so by integrating information from the cerebral cortex, limbic system, reticular formation, and other brain areas, with the final neural output to the target organs being controlled mainly by the neurons in the rostral ventro-lateral medulla (RVLM) (Campos et al., 2008; Carlson et al., 2001). The hypothalamus controls the secretion of pituitary hormones, particularly antidiuretic hormone and corticotrophin-releasing hormone. Abnormalities of these hypothalamic nuclei and re-lated areas have been reported to contribute to hypertension and heart diseases.

2. PHYSIOLOGY OF TAURINE

Taurine (2-aminoethanesulfonic acid; $C_2H_7NO_3S$) is a sulfur-containing β–amino acid (i.e., amino sulfonic acid) first discovered and isolated from ox bile in 1827. Taurine is present in all mammalian tissues, and its levels in most tissues are in micromoles per gram wet tissue weight. Taurine is the most abundant free amino acid in several mammalian tissues, including heart, kidney, and blood vessels (Huxtable, 1992). It makes up more than 50% of the total free amino acid pool in the heart, with an intracellular concentration

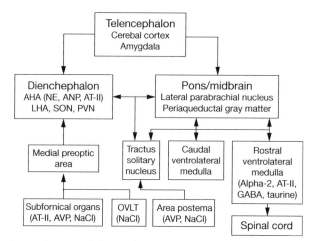

Figure 10.3 Central organization of the cardiovascular control system in the brain (AHA, anterior hypothalamic area; LHA, lateral hypothalamic area; OVLT, organum vasculosum of lamina terminalis; PVN, paraventricular nucleus; SON, supraoptic nucleus; alpha-2, alpha-adrenergic receptor subtype 2; ANP, atrial natriuretic peptide; AT-II, angiotensin II; AVP, arginine vasopressin; GABA, gamma-aminobutyric acid; NE, norepinephrine).

of about 6–35 mM. Although taurine is a nonessential amino acid that does not incorporate into proteins, it is involved in a number of important physiological processes throughout life, from prenatal development to old age.

Mammalian cells appear to synthesize taurine via the following five synthetic pathways:

(a) Methionine→cysteine→cysteine sulfinic acid→hypotaurine→taurine
(b) Methionine→cysteine→cysteine sulfinic acid→cysteic acid→taurine
(c) Cysteamine→cystamine→intermediates→hypotaurine→taurine
(d) Sulfate→sulfite→intermediates→cysteic acid→taurine
(e) Cystine→cystine disulfoxide→cystamine disulfoxide→hypotaurine→taurine

In adults, taurine can be synthesized in hepatocytes from cysteine and methionine with the aid of pyridoxine or pyridoxal-5′-phosphate (the active coenzyme form of vitamin B_6). If cysteine or B_6 is insufficient in the individual, an external source is necessary, thus allowing taurine to be considered as a 'conditional' essential amino acid. Biochemists have also classified taurine as a conditional essential amino acid since it is essential for the fetuses and newborns, due to their limited ability to synthesize protein (Sturman, 1993). Fetuses receive taurine mainly via placenta and maternal milk, and therefore, taurine supplies for fetuses and neonates are occasionally limited due to insufficient maternal delivery, especially in mothers who are vegetarians, malnourished, or receiving an imbalanced diet.

A number of species including cats and humans have very modest ability to synthesize taurine, and thus, they rely on dietary sources of taurine, which is particularly abundant in oysters, mussels, bovine bile, and human breast milk. It has been added to a number of food products, most prominently infant formulas, to make them more like human milk (note that cow's milk is deficient of taurine). Taurine is also used in a wide variety of functional drinks, ranging from 'smart drinks' in Europe to 'energy tonics' in Asia, and it is often used in conjunction with caffeine. In Asia, especially Japan and Korea, it is used to treat and prevent some disorders, including alcoholism, and to delay aging.

3. TAURINE AND PERINATAL DEVELOPMENT

Taurine is a vital substance that ensures proper maturation of the young. As a key organic osmolyte, membrane stabilizer, and antioxidant, taurine facilitates cellular function from the first stages of embryonic development. Generally, cell division involves changes in cell number and cell volume, and fetal growth and development are retarded in pregnant women consuming diets that are deficient in protein. Taurine deficits may play a major role in many of these cases. The human fetus requires taurine for all tissue development but is able to synthesize it only in a limited amount (Sturman, 1993). Many children diagnosed with minimal cerebral dysfunction display disturbances in the metabolism of amino acids including taurine, perhaps in part due to the dose–dependent tropic effect of taurine on the human fetal brain cell proliferation and differentiation. The protective action of taurine against hypoxia may also prevent perinatal asphyxia, the leading cause of cerebral palsy. During development, taurine is also critical to the production of normal function in fetal beta cell in the islets of Langerhans.

A number of chronic conditions in developing children may result from or be exacerbated by abnormalities in taurine concentrations. In neonatal cardiomyocytes, taurine functions as an organic osmolyte (Schaffer et al., 2010). When taurine is absent, these cardiac cells reduce in size and change in shape and configuration. This adaptation of the cell's shape and size to protect against tonicity demonstrates the critical role of taurine in the regulation of osmotic balance. In obese children, taurine supplementation improves some liver enzyme levels, independent of the success or failure of weight control measures. It is also beneficial as an adjunct therapy in fatty liver associated with simple obesity.

4. TAURINE AND THE HEART

Taurine supplementation is one of the several therapeutic interventions that have been reported to prevent or decrease cardiac dysfunction (Schaffer et al., 2010). Taurine makes up more than 50% of the total free amino acid pool in the heart, with an intracellular concentration of about 6–35 mM. It has a positive inotropic effect on the myocardium and appears to exert its cytoprotection by reducing oxidation and apoptosis and by improving osmoregulation, membrane stabilization, and intracellular calcium flux regulation. Plasma taurine increases in patients with acute myocardial ischemia and may be markedly elevated following more severe infarction (Oriyanhan et al., 2005). The taurine source appears to be primarily from the myocardium. The blood taurine concentration in these patients increases for up to 3 days after infarct, paralleling the increased creatine kinase levels. The increased taurine appears to protect cardiac function from ischemic damage. Taurine also inhibits the sympathetic nerve activity in many conditions, and it may retard the rise in sympathetic nerve activity during ischemia and postcardiac reperfusion and thus protect the heart from adverse effects of sympathetic nerve hyperactivity.

Arrhythmias in the ischemic heart may be induced by abnormal extracellular cardiac calcium concentrations. Both low and high concentrations of calcium can adversely affect the number of beating cells, the beating rate, and the number of arrhythmic cells. Taurine supplementation has been reported to attenuate this cardiomyocyte response to varying calcium concentrations (Schaffer et al., 2010), and its effect is very specific since analogs (including glycine) are not effective substitutes. Both the incidence of premature beats and tachycardias of the ventricles are significantly decreased by taurine treatment.

Taurine protects the heart from oxidative stress and postischemic injury and reduces lipoperoxidation (free radical damage). In patients undergoing coronary artery bypasses, pretreatment with taurine protects heart cell mitochondria from damage. Taurine's ability to scavenge free radicals is significantly cardioprotective, and its administration to individuals recovering from ischemia improves heart rate control. Both lactate (a marker of ischemic challenge) and glutathione (a marker of oxidative stress) concentrations can be attenuated in patients with ischemia by taurine administration. ATP levels (denoting cellular energy production) are also suppressed in ischemia and increased by taurine.

Taurine decreases malondialdehyde levels in anoxic guinea pig hearts, reaching concentrations up to 50 mM in leukocytes during cardiac arrest, and it is tissue protective in many models of oxidant-induced injury. One potential mechanism underlying this effect is that taurine reacts with hypochlorous acid (HOCl) produced by the myeloperoxidase (MPO) pathway, resulting in the more stable but less toxic taurine chloramine (Tau-Cl) (Schuller-Levis and Park, 2004). Recent molecular studies indicate that taurine is a constituent of several biological macromolecules. Two novel taurine-containing modified uridines have been found in both human and bovine mitochondria. By oxidation of methionine, Tau-Cl inhibits the activation of nuclear factor-kappa B, a potent signal transducer for inflammatory cytokines. In addition, taurine may prevent ischemia-induced apoptosis in cardiomyocytes through Akt-mediated caspase-9 inactivation. Akt is both necessary and sufficient to inhibit apoptosis, and taurine is an activator of Akt action. Thus, it is likely that the beneficial effects of taurine in the treatment of heart failure relate, in part, to suppression of ischemia-induced cellular responses.

In animal models of cardiac ischemia and reperfusion, cardiac injury markers increase in perinatal taurine-depleted animals consuming a high (compared to normal) level of dietary sugar, suggesting increased myocardial damage in these animals (Kulthinee et al., 2010). These large increases also suggest that a combination of high sugar intake and perinatal taurine depletion has synergistic effects on ischemia/reperfusion-induced myocardial damage. Elevated troponin T and N-terminal prohormone brain natriuretic peptide confirm significant ventricular injury in these animals compared to all controls. In contrast to perinatal taurine depletion, perinatal taurine supplementation appears to lessen the effects of myocardial injury.

Taurine transporters (TauT) on the cell membrane play a crucial role in regulating taurine balance and cell volume in mammalian cells (Ito et al., 2010; Warskulat et al., 2007). TauT knockout (TauTKO) mice have been used to explore long-term effects of taurine deficiency. In the heart, TauTKO mice display ventricular remodeling, characterized by reductions in ventricular wall thickness and cardiac atrophy accompanied by smaller cardiomyocytes. Compared to wild-type mice, TauTKO mice display decreased cardiac output and increased expression of cardiac failure (fetal) marker genes, including atrial natriuretic peptide (ANP), brain natriuretic peptide (BNP), and beta-MHC. These mice also display ultrastructural damage of myofilaments and mitochondria. α-Actin type 1 mRNA levels are reduced by 70% in the heart of young and older TauTKO mice compared to wild-type controls, and the hearts of TauTKO mice switch from α-actin 1 to α-actin 2 expression. In addition, the hearts of TauTKO mice demonstrate upregulated mRNA biomarkers for pressure overload and hypertension, for example, ANP ($+848\%$), BNP ($+90\%$), cardiac ankyrin repeat protein ($+118\%$), and procollagen 1a1, 1a2, and 3a1 ($+ >40\%$). The TauTKO mice also have dilated cardiomyopathy, similar to that in taurine-depleted cats, and cardiac dysfunction is an age-dependent manner, that is, its severity increases with age. The absence of TauT also has age-dependent adverse effects on visual, auditory, olfactory, liver, and renal functions. In TauTKO mice, taurine supplementation improves or attenuates cardiac dysfunction with advancing age. Thus, the TauTKO mice have been useful in demonstrating aspects of the physiology and pathophysiology of taurine.

5. TAURINE AND THE AUTONOMIC NERVOUS SYSTEM

Taurine plays many physiological roles in the central nervous system, acting as everything from a cellular osmolyte to a neurotransmitter/neuromodulator (Wu and Prentice, 2010). Intracerebroventricular taurine injection decreases peripheral sympathetic nervous system activity, arterial pressure, and heart rate. Similar results are observed when taurine is injected into organum vasculosum laminar terminalis (OVLT) or RVLM. It is uncertain whether taurine acts directly via its specific receptor or indirectly via its other physiologic functions, for example, osmolytic and antioxidative properties.

Two subtypes of taurine receptors have pharmacological properties similar to gamma-aminobutyric acid (GABA) and glycine receptors in the mammalian central nervous system (Oja and Saransaari, 2007). These receptors may be modulated by extracellular Mg^{2+}.

Taurine plays an important role in cell volume regulation and appears to activate osmosensitive neurons in the brain, thereby increasing sympathoinhibition. Furthermore, taurine concentrates in cells, and changes in cell volume and osmolarity due to fluctuations in intracellular taurine concentration may alter ionic balance in neurons and thereby alter neural activity. Taurine may also act directly on neurons by receptor activation and thereby modulate autonomic nervous system activity. *In vitro* studies indicate that taurine inhibits calcium influx at nerve terminals, decreases norepinephrine release, and increases norepinephrine degradation, perhaps due to taurine-induced decreased norepinephrine reuptake (Hano et al., 2009). Taurine action on its receptor is reported to presynaptically inhibit norepinephrine release. Although taurine inhibits norepinephrine release from peripheral sympathetic nerves *in vitro*, intravenous taurine injection does not appear to produce a similar effect, suggesting that most of its effects are central. However, acute taurine administration decreases heart rate and arterial pressure in young students, suggesting the need for further studies of its peripheral effect.

6. PERINATAL TAURINE AND ARTERIAL PRESSURE CONTROL

Diets high in taurine prevent or attenuate hypertension in several animal models, including spontaneously hypertensive rats, sugar-induced hypertension, and renal hypertension. However, taurine's beneficial effects on arterial pressure appear to be specific for salt-sensitive (but not salt-resistant) models of hypertension. Several mechanisms have been reported to underlie the antihypertensive effects of perinatal taurine, including decreasing sympathetic nerve activity, increased antioxidant activity, and increasing renal pressure-natriuresis. Epidemiologic studies indicate that high dietary consumption of taurine (e.g., from fish) is related to low incidences of hypertension and other cardiovascular diseases that are related to overactivity of sympathetic nervous system (Oja and Saransaari, 2007; Yamori et al., 2010a,b). Renal norepinephrine excretion and heart rate variability studies have supported this hypothesis.

The perinatal environment has long-term effects on adult organ function and diseases. This is known as the Baker hypothesis or perinatal origin of adult diseases (Morley, 2006). We have reported that perinatal taurine depletion by oral beta-alanine administration alters autonomic nervous system control of arterial pressure in adult Sprague Dawley rats (Roysommuti et al., 2009b,c). Both sympathetic and parasympathetic nerve activities are depressed in these animals; however, arterial pressure and heart rate are relatively normal. Baroreflex sensitivity control of heart rate or renal sympathetic nerve activity is also blunted by perinatal taurine depletion. Surprisingly, postweaning glucose supplementation reverses these abnormalities and increases sympathetic nerve activity but exacerbates baroreflex sensitivity abnormalities. Furthermore, the supplementation is not associated with insulin resistance or diabetes mellitus, and it slightly increases arterial pressure (but not heart rate). Moreover, the angiotensin-converting enzyme inhibitor, captopril, abolishes the heightened sympathetic nerve activity, suggesting that renin–angiotensin system overactivity contributes to this phenomenon (Thaeomor et al., 2010).

The renin–angiotensin system, sympathetic nerve activity, insulin resistance, and hyperinsulinemia interact in a complex manner to elevate arterial pressure. Sympathetic nerve activity stimulates renin release from juxtaglomerular cells of the kidney, and renin activates a cascade reaction to produce angiotensin II, that is, activating the renin–angiotensin system. Angiotensin II can centrally stimulate sympathetic nerve activity and directly alter norepinephrine release at nerve terminals (Figure 10.3). Both the angiotensin II and sympathetic nerve activity can contribute to insulin resistance and subsequently hyperinsulinemia, and in turn, further elevate sympathetic nerve activity. The independent contribution of the renin–angiotensin system and sympathetic nerve overactivity to kidney dysregulation and/or hypertension following perinatal taurine depletion and high sugar diets remains unclear.

While taurine can decrease abnormally high sympathetic nerve activity, it has little effect on resting sympathetic nerve activity in healthy subjects. To date, no data explain how perinatal taurine exposure can affect the autonomic nervous system in adult life, irrespective of adult taurine exposure. Since high sugar intake heightens sympathetic nerve activity in adult rats that were perinatally depleted of taurine, perinatal taurine depletion does not appear to have an irreversible effect on this parameter. TauT play a key role in regulating taurine balance and cell taurine content, but alterations in TauT have not been examined in taurine-depleted or taurine-supplemented animals. Taurine is necessary for brain growth and development. Neural reorganization might underline some of the adult alteration of the autonomic nervous system function that results from perinatal taurine deficit or excess, but again this has not been tested.

Several lines of evidence have reported that compared with wild-type controls, TauTKO mice decrease taurine levels in skeletal and heart muscle by about 98%; in brain, kidney, plasma, and retina by 80–90%; and in liver by about 70% (Warskulat et al., 2007). These animals display many disorders similar to those with perinatal taurine depletion. In the central nervous system, TauTKO mice exhibit several phenotypic changes (Sergeeva et al., 2007). Reduced brain taurine levels are associated with increased GABA(A), kainate, and AMPA receptor densities in the molecular layer of the hippocampal dentate gyrus and in the cerebellum. Disinhibition of striatal network activity is also observed in TauTKO mice, and this can be corrected by taurine supplementation. Modification of GABA(A) (but not glycine receptors) may underlie this disinhibition (Molchanova et al., 2007).

7. ADULT TAURINE EXPOSURE AND HYPERTENSION

Dietary taurine inhibits or attenuates the development of hypertension in deoxycorticos-terone acetate and salt treated rats (DOCA-salt rats). The effect is dose dependent; 3% (compared to 1%) taurine in drinking water produces greater hypotensive effects. Taurine acts in the central nervous system to produce this antihypertensive effect (Gupta et al., 2005; Militante and Lombardini, 2002). When injected into the cerebrospinal fluid of animals, taurine, glycine, GABA, L(α)-alanine, and L-serine all lower arterial pressure acutely in this model, with the greatest effect being that of taurine. Oral taurine treatment is also an effective antihypertensive regimen in humans. These findings have been validated in separate double-blind placebo-controlled studies. In contrast, taurine produces no effects on arterial pressure in normotensive subjects.

8. TAURINE AND THE KIDNEY

Long-term arterial pressure control is largely dependent on renal pressure-diuretic/natriuretic mechanisms. Under normal conditions, the kidneys will excrete sufficient water and sodium to maintain arterial pressure at a normotensive level. Thus, many chronic forms of hypertension cannot be sustained without compromised renal function. Taurine influences renal excretory function from early life through death. Renal function is impaired in the aged and is inversely correlated to a reduction in renal taurine content. Diets high in taurine attenuate renal damage with age and improve renal function in many diseases, including hypertension, nephrotic syndrome, and renal failure (Chesney et al., 2010; Cruz et al., 2000). Taurine-deficient neonatal kittens show renal developmental abnormalities, and the regulation of the taurine transporter gene appears to be critical in mammalian species. TauTKO mice display renal taurine loss and subsequently, hypotaurinemia and impaired ability to lower urine osmolality to increased urinary water excretion (Huang et al., 2006). The latter defect likely results from a role of taurine in the suppression of vasopressin release, but intrarenal effects may also play a role.

Taurine supplementation could prevent age-related renal damage. While perinatal taurine depletion impairs renal function in adult rats, perinatal taurine supplementation increases renal sodium excretion following an acute saline load (Roysommuti et al., 2009a). Tubular sodium reabsorption also decreases in these animals. However, their renal blood flows are decreased by the perinatal taurine supplementation, rather than the perinatal depletion, consistent with a rise in renal vascular resistance. In addition, renal potassium excretion is less affected by perinatal taurine excess or deficit (Roysommuti et al., 2010b). Although both prenatal and postnatal taurine exposures are critical to adult renal function, prenatal rather than postnatal exposure is more effective (Roysommuti et al., 2010a). High carbohydrate intake can induce renal

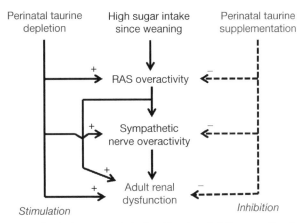

Figure 10.4 A high sugar diet induces renal dysfunction in adult Sprague Dawley rats via the renin–angiotensin system (RAS) overactivity, the condition that is exacerbated by perinatal taurine depletion but prevented by perinatal taurine supplementation. It is note worthy that perinatal taurine exposure with or without the high sugar diet might alter renal function via local taurine action.

dysfunction before insulin resistance and hypertension via the renin–angiotensin system in mature rats (Roysommuti et al., 2002). With perinatal taurine excess or deficit, the effect of a high sugar diet on renal dysfunction is complicated; some parameters are improved, while others are exacerbated.

There are at least three possible mechanisms that could alter renal function due to perinatal taurine exposure in combination with a high sugar intake in adult offspring (Figure 10.4). First, they could induce renin–angiotensin system overactivity, which could directly impair renal function. Second, renin–angiotensin system overactivity or the effect of taurine on the nervous system could alter sympathetic nerve activity, thereby altering renal function directly. Third, renal function may be altered by local taurine actions in the kidney.

9. SUMMARY

Taurine, the major free amino acid in all mammalian cells, plays many physiological roles in arterial pressure and renal regulation. Research indicates that the taurine influences the contributions of the heart, nervous system, blood vessels, and the kidney in their contribution to arterial pressure regulation. Taurine's effects on these functions extend from fetal to the elderly life, but the greatest effects appear to be due to perinatal taurine exposure. Hypertension and other cardiovascular diseases can be reduced or prevented by diets high in taurine content. Furthermore, taurine's interaction with high sugar intake and other pressor factors appears to provide clues to the mechanisms by which taurine alters cardiovascular and renal functions. Finally, taurine appears to act via several mechanisms, including direct effects on brain regulation of the sympathetic nervous system, antioxidant actions, direct modifications of renal function, and alterations in renin–angiotensin regulation.

REFERENCES

Campos, R.R., Carillo, B.A., Oliveira-Sales, E.B., et al., 2008. Role of the caudal pressor area in the regulation of sympathetic vasomotor tone. Brazilian Journal of Medical and Biological Research 41 (7), 557–562.

Carlson, S.H., Roysomutti, S., Peng, N., Wyss, J.M., 2001. The role of the central nervous system in NaCl-sensitive hypertension in spontaneously hypertensive rats. American Journal of Hypertension 14 (6 Pt 2), 155S–162S.

Chesney, R.W., Han, X., Patters, A.B., 2010. Taurine and the renal system. Journal of Biomedical Science 17 (Suppl. 1), S4.

Cruz, C.I., Ruiz-Torres, P., del Moral, R.G., Rodriguez-Puyol, M., Rodriguez-Puyol, D., 2000. Age-related progressive renal fibrosis in rats and its prevention with ACE inhibitors and taurine. American Journal of Physiology. Renal Physiology 278 (1), F122–F129.

Gupta, R.C., Win, T., Bittner, S., 2005. Taurine analogues: a new class of therapeutics: retrospect and prospects. Current Medicinal Chemistry 12 (17), 2021–2039.

Hano, T., Kasano, M., Tomari, H., Iwane, N., 2009. Taurine suppresses pressor response through the inhibition of sympathetic nerve activity and the improvement in baro-reflex sensitivity of spontaneously hypertensive rats. Advances in Experimental Medicine and Biology 643, 57–63.

Huang, D.Y., Boini, K.M., Lang, P.A., et al., 2006. Impaired ability to increase water excretion in mice lacking the taurine transporter gene TAUT. Pflügers Archiv 451 (5), 668–677.

Huxtable, R.J., 1992. Physiological actions of taurine. Physiological Reviews 72 (1), 101–163.

Ito, T., Oishi, S., Takai, M., et al., 2010. Cardiac and skeletal muscle abnormality in taurine transporter-knockout mice. Journal of Biomedical Science 17 (Suppl. 1), S20.

Kulthinee, S., Wyss, J.M., Jirakulsomchok, D., Roysommuti, S., 2010. High sugar intake exacerbates cardiac reperfusion injury in perinatal taurine-depleted adult rats. Journal of Biomedical Science 17 (1), S22.

Militante, J.D., Lombardini, J.B., 2002. Treatment of hypertension with oral taurine: experimental and clinical studies. Amino Acids 23 (4), 381–393.

Molchanova, S.M., Oja, S.S., Saransaari, P., 2007. Effect of taurine on the concentrations of glutamate, GABA, glutamine and alanine in the rat striatum and hippocampus. Proceedings of the Western Pharmacology Society 50, 95–97.

Morley, R., 2006. Fetal origins of adult disease. Seminars in Fetal and Neonatal Medicine 11 (2), 73–78.

Oja, S.S., Saransaari, P., 2007. Pharmacology of taurine. Proceedings of the Western Pharmacology Society 50, 8–15.

Oriyanhan, W., Yamazaki, K., Miwa, S., Takaba, K., Ikeda, T., Komeda, M., 2005. Taurine prevents myocardial ischemia/reperfusion-induced oxidative stress and apoptosis in prolonged hypothermic rat heart preservation. Heart and Vessels 20 (6), 278–285.

Roysommuti, S., Khongnakha, T., Jirakulsomchok, D., Wyss, J.M., 2002. Excess dietary glucose alters renal function before increasing arterial pressure and inducing insulin resistance. American Journal of Hypertension 15 (9), 773–779.

Roysommuti, S., Lerdweeraphon, W., Malila, P., Jirakulsomchok, D., Wyss, J.M., 2009a. Perinatal taurine alters arterial pressure control and renal function in adult offspring. Advances in Experimental Medicine and Biology 643, 145–156.

Roysommuti, S., Suwanich, A., Jirakulsomchok, D., Wyss, J.M., 2009b. Perinatal taurine depletion increases susceptibility to adult sugar-induced hypertension in rats. Advances in Experimental Medicine and Biology 643, 123–133.

Roysommuti, S., Suwanich, A., Lerdweeraphon, W., Thaeomor, A., Jirakulsomchok, D., Wyss, J.M., 2009c. Sex dependent effects of perinatal taurine exposure on the arterial pressure control in adult offspring. Advances in Experimental Medicine and Biology 643, 135–144.

Roysommuti, S., Malila, P., Jirakulsomchok, D., Wyss, J.M., 2010a. Adult renal function is modified by perinatal taurine status in conscious male rats. Journal of Biomedical Science 17 (Suppl. 1), S31.

Roysommuti, S., Malila, P., Lerdweeraphon, W., Jirakulsomchok, D., Wyss, J.M., 2010b. Perinatal taurine exposure alters renal potassium excretion mechanisms in adult conscious rats. Journal of Biomedical Science 17 (Suppl. 1), S29.

Schaffer, S.W., Jong, C.J., Ramila, K.C., Azuma, J., 2010. Physiological roles of taurine in heart and muscle. Journal of Biomedical Science 17 (Suppl. 1), S2.

Schuller-Levis, G.B., Park, E., 2004. Taurine and its chloramine: modulators of immunity. Neurochemical Research 29 (1), 117–126.

Sergeeva, O.A., Fleischer, W., Chepkova, A.N., et al., 2007. GABAA-receptor modification in taurine transporter knockout mice causes striatal disinhibition. The Journal of Physiology 585 (Pt 2), 539–548.

Sturman, J.A., 1993. Taurine in development. Physiological Reviews 73 (1), 119–147.

Thaeomor, A., Wyss, J.M., Jirakulsomchok, D., Roysommuti, S., 2010. High sugar intake via the renin–angiotensin system blunts the baroreceptor reflex in adult rats that were perinatally depleted of taurine. Journal of Biomedical Science 17 (Suppl. 1), S30.

Warskulat, U., Heller-Stilb, B., Oermann, E., et al., 2007. Phenotype of the taurine transporter knockout mouse. Methods in Enzymology 428, 439–458.

Wu, J.Y., Prentice, H., 2010. Role of taurine in the central nervous system. Journal of Biomedical Science 17 (Suppl. 1), S1.

Yamori, Y., Taguchi, T., Hamada, A., Kunimasa, K., Mori, H., Mori, M., 2010a. Taurine in health and diseases: consistent evidence from experimental and epidemiological studies. Journal of Biomedical Science 17 (Suppl. 1), S6.

Yamori, Y., Taguchi, T., Mori, H., Mori, M., 2010b. Low cardiovascular risks in the middle aged males and females excreting greater 24-hour urinary taurine and magnesium in 41 WHO-CARDIAC study populations in the world. Journal of Biomedical Science 17 (Suppl. 1), S21.

CHAPTER 11

Fish Consumption and Risk of Cardiovascular Disease – Part 1

C.-M. Kastorini*,†, H.J. Milionis*, J.A. Goudevenos*, D.B. Panagiotakos†
*University of Ioannina, Ioannina, Greece
†Harokopio University, Athens, Greece

ABBREVIATIONS

CVD Cardiovascular disease
DHA Docosahexaenoic acid
EPA Eicosapentaenoic acid

1. INTRODUCTION

Cardiovascular disease (CVD) is the leading cause of morbidity and mortality worldwide, influencing significantly quality of life and posing an important economic burden (AHA, 2008). It is estimated that in 2008, 7.3 million people died of coronary heart disease and 6.2 million of stroke, while according to the World Health Organization (WHO) estimates, the number of CVD events is expected to increase further, partly due to the demographic changes. Thus, prevention of CVD is considered of major public health importance.

Fish consumption is an integral part of a healthy diet, as it is an excellent source of protein, the essential omega-3 fatty acids, and certain micronutrients. Fish is one of the best dietary sources of the omega-3 polyunsaturated fatty acids and especially eicosapentaenoic acid (EPA) and docosahexaenoic acid (DHA), which are associated with several beneficial roles for human health. Furthermore, fish consumption provides vitamin D and other vitamins and minerals, such as phosphorus and calcium, as well as trace elements such as selenium and iodine.

The beneficial relationship between fish consumption and reduced risk of CVD is not new. Almost 30 years ago, reports in arctic Greenland on a small population of Eskimos (Bang et al., 1980) as well as on inhabitants of the Japanese island of Okinawa, both consuming high amounts of marine animals, were the first to indicate such a relationship. In addition, a large number of observational studies have suggested the beneficial effects of fish intake on all-cause mortality, coronary heart disease mortality, coronary heart disease, heart failure, and ischemic stroke (He et al., 2004; Konig et al., 2005; Mozaffarian and Rimm, 2006; Whelton et al., 2004).

Bioactive Food as Dietary Interventions for Cardiovascular Disease
http://dx.doi.org/10.1016/B978-0-12-396485-4.00010-4

© 2013 Elsevier Inc.
All rights reserved.

2. ALL-CAUSE MORTALITY

Fish consumption has a beneficial effect regarding all-cause mortality. According to the results of an ecological study across 36 countries, fish consumption was associated with a reduced risk from all-cause, ischaemic heart disease, and stroke mortalities (Zhang et al., 1999). A meta-analysis of 15 randomized clinical trials showed that modest fish consumption of 1–2 servings per week and especially fish rich in the omega-3 fatty acids, EPA, and DHA was associated with a 17% (95% CI: 0–32%) reduction in total mortality (Mozaffarian and Rimm, 2006).

According to the US Physicians' Health Study, conducted in 20 551 US male physicians and after 11 years of follow-up, men who consumed fish at least one time per week had reduced risk of total mortality and sudden cardiac death, compared with men who consumed fish less than one time per month (Albert et al., 1998).

The NHANES I Epidemiologic Follow-up study, with 8825 participants, followed for a mean time of 18.8 years, showed that white men consuming fish once a week had an age-adjusted risk of noncardiovascular death only about three quarters than those who never consumed fish, while no further benefit was observed regarding fish consumption of more than one time per week, as far as coronary heart disease incidence or mortality were concerned (Gillum et al., 2000).

Results from the Chicago Western Electric Study, conducted in 1822 men, followed for 30 years, showed that the age-adjusted rates of all-cause mortality were lowest for the men with the highest consumption of fish, with a trend toward lower rates with higher levels of consumption (Daviglus et al., 1997).

A Finnish study conducted in 6410 fishermen and their wives ($n = 4260$), followed for 12 years, showed that fishermen had 22% (95% CI: 0.73–0.82) lower mortality from all causes, while their wives had 16% (95% CI: 0.76–0.93) lower all-cause mortality, compared with the general population (Turunen et al., 2008).

A prospective cohort study from Finland following 415 patients with coronary artery disease for 5 years showed a reduction in all-cause mortality for patients who consumed more than 57 g fish per day, compared with rare consumption (RR = 0.37, 95% CI: 0.14–1.00) (Erkkila et al., 2003).

In addition, according to the randomized controlled trial, Diet And Reinfarction Trial (DART), focusing on the secondary prevention of coronary heart disease with 2033 male participants, over the 2-year follow-up, a 29% reduction in all-cause mortality was observed in male myocardial infarction survivors, who were advised to increase their intake of fatty fish from 200 to 400 g per week. Nevertheless, this observation was attenuated during the more recent follow-ups – beyond 10 years, due to an excess of deaths not attributed to coronary heart disease (Burr et al., 1994; Ness et al., 2002).

However, according to a cohort study of 4513 men and 3984 women, no associations were observed between fish consumption and all-cause mortality, possibly because of the frequent consumption of fish in open sandwiches with butter and mayonnaise or pan-fried and served with a butter sauce in Denmark (Osler et al., 2003).

3. CORONARY HEART DISEASE MORTALITY

Fish consumption of at least one time per week is suggested to have a protective effect on coronary heart disease mortality. According to a meta-analysis of 13 cohorts from 11 prospective studies, eating fish one to three times per month was associated with 15% lower risk, one time per week with 24%, two to four times per week with 23%, and more than five times per week with 38% lower risk. A dose–response relation was observed, as an increment of 20 g per day of fish intake could lower coronary heart disease mortality rates by 7% (p for trend $= 0.03$). The association was more apparent for studies with a follow-up period of longer than 12 years (He et al., 2004). In addition, a meta-analysis of 19 observational studies, 14 cohort and 5 case-control, showed that fish consumption versus little to no fish consumption was associated with a 10% reduction in total coronary heart disease ($RR = 0.86$, 95% CI: 0.81–0.92) and an approximately 20% reduction in the risk of fatal coronary heart disease ($RR = 0.83$, 95% CI: 0.76–0.90) (Whelton et al., 2004). A third meta-analysis showed that modest fish consumption of one to two servings per week, and especially fish rich in the omega-3 fatty acids, EPA, and DHA, was associated with a 36% (95% CI: 20–50%) reduction of coronary death (Mozaffarian and Rimm, 2006).

Another study, evaluating the impact of fish consumption on coronary heart disease risk, suggested a decrease of 17% in the risk of coronary heart disease mortality, compared with consumption of fish less than one serving per month. Furthermore, each additional serving per week was associated with a further reduction in this risk of 3.9% (Konig et al., 2005).

In addition, according to the Nurses' Health Study, including 84 688 female nurses, with a 16-year follow-up, an inverse association was observed between fish and omega-3 fatty acids intake and coronary heart disease mortality. Compared with women eating fish less than one time per month, the risk of coronary heart disease death was 21%, 29%, 31%, and 34% lower for fish consumption of one to three times per month, one time per week, two to four times per week, and more than five times per week, respectively (Hu et al., 2002).

Results from a prospective study of three European cohorts from the Seven Countries Study, including 1088 Finnish, 1097 Italian, and 553 Dutch men, showed that fatty fish consumption compared to lean fish consumption was associated with a 34% (95% CI: 0.49–0.90) reduction in 20-year coronary heart disease mortality, whereas no association was found between total fish or lean fish consumption and coronary heart disease death (Oomen et al., 2000).

The Chicago Western Electric Study, conducted in 1822 men, followed for 30 years, showed that consumption of 35 g of fish per day was inversely associated with death from coronary heart disease, especially nonsudden death from myocardial infarction. In particular, men consuming more than 35 g of fish per day had a 42% lower rate of death from myocardial infarction than the nonconsumers. In addition, the age-adjusted rates of death from myocardial infarction, coronary heart disease, and CVD were lowest for the men with the highest consumption of fish (Daviglus et al., 1997).

Furthermore, 18 244 middle-aged or older men in Shanghai, China, followed up for 12 years, who consumed more than 200 g of fish or shellfish per week had a 59% (95% CI: 0.22–0.78) reduction of fatal acute myocardial infarction compared with men consuming less than 50 g per week and approximately a 20% reduction in total mortality (RR = 0.79, 95% CI: 0.69–0.91) (Yuan et al., 2001).

According to the Zutphen study, conducted in 1373 men who were followed up for 30 years, long-term fish consumption of 22 g per day – corresponding to one to two servings per week – was associated with 27% (95% CI: 0.47–1.13) lower coronary heart disease mortality risk, while fatty fish consumption of 7 g daily lowered sudden coronary death risk by 54% (95% CI: 0.27–0.78) (Streppel et al., 2008).

A Finnish study conducted in 6410 fishermen and their wives ($n = 6420$), followed up for 12 years, showed that fishermen had 27% (95% CI: 0.65–0.81) and their wives 35% (95% CI: 0.50–0.83) lower ischaemic heart disease mortality, compared with the general population (Turunen et al., 2008). Results from the Cardiovascular Health Study following 3910 participants over 65 years of age, for a mean time of 9.3 years, indicated that the type of fish may also influence this relationship, as consumption of broiled or baked fish three or more times per week was associated with 49% (95% CI: 0.31–0.83) lower risk of total ischaemic heart disease mortality and 58% (95% CI: 0.21–0.84) of arrhythmic ischaemic heart disease death but not nonfatal myocardial infarction, compared with consumption less than once per month (Mozaffarian et al., 2003).

The protective effect of a small amount of fish consumption in relation to coronary heart disease mortality observed in middle-aged people seems to be also present in the elderly. According to a study in 272 elderly people, followed up for 17 years, fish eaters had a 49% lower risk of coronary heart disease compared with non-fish eaters (Kromhout et al., 1995). A recent prospective study of 21 342 participants followed up for 9–14 years showed that participants in the top quartile of EPA and DHA consumption had a 49% (95% CI: 6–73%) lower risk of fatal coronary heart disease and a 62% (95% CI: 23–81%) lower risk of fatal myocardial infarction, compared with the lowest quartile (de Goede et al., 2010).

Nevertheless, a number of studies showed no associations between coronary heart disease mortality for subjects consuming fish regularly. The Health Professionals' Follow-up Study (44 895 participants, 6 years follow-up) (Ascherio et al., 1995) and the US Physicians' Health Study (20 551 participants, 11 years follow-up)

(Albert et al., 1998) showed insignificant associations regarding fish intake and risk of total cardiovascular mortality or any fatal coronary disease, including sudden and nonsudden cardiac death, total or nonfatal myocardial infarction, coronary artery bypass grafting, or angioplasty. In addition, according to the Seven Countries Study, conducted in 12763 middle-aged men, despite the observation of an inverse association between fish consumption and 25-year mortality from coronary heart disease across several populations, after taking into account the confounding effects of saturated fatty acids, flavonoids, and smoking, the association was not significant anymore (Kromhout et al., 1996).

4. CORONARY HEART DISEASE PREVENTION

Consumption of fish is also suggested to beneficially influence coronary heart disease development. According to a quantitative analysis of fish consumption and coronary heart disease, low fish intake has been associated with risk reductions in nonfatal myocardial infarction risk by 27%; however, additional fish consumption did not further improve the results (Konig et al., 2005).

In the Nurses' Health Study, in 84 688 females, and after 16 years of follow-up, higher consumption of fish was associated with lower risk of coronary heart disease, in particular 21% lower risk for fish consumption of one to three times per month to 34% for fish intake of five or more times per week (Hu et al., 2002).

The Danish follow-up study including 57 053 participants, followed up for a mean period of 7.6 years, showed that men consuming fatty fish had 33% (95% CI: 0.53–0.85) lower risk of an acute coronary syndrome. No associations were observed for women, or regarding lean fish consumption (Bjerregaard et al., 2010).

The Japan Public Health Center-Based (JPHC) Study Cohort I, conducted in 41 578 middle-aged men and women, with a follow-up of 10 years, showed that high fish intake, eight times per week, was associated with lower risk of coronary heart disease and more specifically, myocardial infarction and nonfatal coronary heart disease, compared with fish intake of one time per week (Iso et al., 2006).

It should be mentioned that a J-shape association between fish consumption and coronary risk has been proposed by a case–control study of 848 patients and 1078 controls. In addition, compared with rare consumption, moderate consumption of fish, less than 150 g per week, was associated with 38% lower odds of developing an acute coronary syndrome ($p < 0.05$) (Panagiotakos et al., 2005).

Fish consumption and the omega-3 polyunsaturated fatty acids intake were inversely associated with nonfatal acute myocardial infarction according to a case–control study conducted in Italy with 507 patients and 478 controls; compared to those eating fish less than one time per week, participants eating fish less than two times per week had an OR of 0.80 (95% CI: 0.56–1.13) and those eating fish twice or more per week had an OR of 0.68 (95% CI: 0.47–0.98) (Tavani et al., 2001).

Some studies have shown insignificant or opposite results regarding fish consumption and coronary heart disease. According to a cohort study of 4513 men and 3984 women, no associations were observed between fish consumption and all-cause mortality or incident coronary heart disease in the population as a whole. However, frequent consumption of fish was associated with a beneficial effect regarding those at high risk for coronary heart disease. A possible explanation for the above observations could be the type of the preparation method, as in Denmark, fish is often consumed on open sandwiches with butter and mayonnaise or pan-fried and served with a butter sauce (Osler et al., 2003).

A prospective study with 1752 male participants from rural Sweden followed up for 12 years showed that consumption of fish at least twice per week showed no associations with the development of coronary heart disease (Holmberg et al., 2009). Moreover, a case–control study conducted in Japan, in 660 cases with first myocardial infarction and 1277 controls, an inverse trend between fish consumption and likelihood of developing a nonfatal myocardial infarction was observed, in both genders; however, it was not significant (Sasazuki, 2001).

The EURAMIC (European Multicenter Case–control Study on Antioxidants, Myocardial Infarction and Breast Cancer) Study, a large case–control study, conducted in eight countries, including 639 cases and 700 controls, showed no evidence of a protective effect of adipose tissue DHA, a measure of long-term fish consumption, on the risk of developing myocardial infarction (Guallar et al., 1999). Finally, a randomized controlled trial of 3114 men under 70 years of age with stable angina pectoris showed that patients advised to eat fatty fish twice a week had an increased risk of coronary heart disease after 3–9 years of follow up. Total mortality increased by 15% (95% CI: 0.96–1.36), coronary deaths by 26% (95% CI: 1.00–1.58), and sudden cardiac death by 54% (95% CI: 1.06–2.23) in the fish advice group (Burr et al., 2003).

REFERENCES

AHA, 2008. Heart and Stroke Statistical Update. American Heart Association, Dallas, TX.

Albert, C.M., Hennekens, C.H., O'Donnell, C.J., et al., 1998. Fish consumption and risk of sudden cardiac death. JAMA: The Journal of the American Medical Association 279, 23–28.

Ascherio, A., Rimm, E.B., Stampfer, M.J., Giovannucci, E.L., Willett, W.C., 1995. Dietary intake of marine n-3 fatty acids, fish intake, and the risk of coronary disease among men. The New England Journal of Medicine 332, 977–982.

Bang, H.O., Dyerberg, J., Sinclair, H.M., 1980. The composition of the Eskimo food in north western Greenland. American Journal of Clinical Nutrition 33, 2657–2661.

Bjerregaard, L.J., Joensen, A.M., Dethlefsen, C., et al., 2010. Fish intake and acute coronary syndrome. European Heart Journal 31, 29–34.

Burr, M.L., Sweetham, P.M., Fehily, A.M., 1994. Diet and reinfarction. European Heart Journal 15, 1152–1153.

Burr, M.L., Ashfield-Watt, P.A., Dunstan, F.D., et al., 2003. Lack of benefit of dietary advice to men with angina: results of a controlled trial. European Journal of Clinical Nutrition 57, 193–200.

Daviglus, M.L., Stamler, J., Orencia, A.J., et al., 1997. Fish consumption and the 30-year risk of fatal myocardial infarction. The New England Journal of Medicine 336, 1046–1053.

de Goede, J., Geleijnse, J.M., Boer, J.M., Kromhout, D., Verschuren, W.M., 2010. Marine (n-3) fatty acids, fish consumption, and the 10-year risk of fatal and nonfatal coronary heart disease in a large population of Dutch adults with low fish intake. Journal of Nutrition 140, 1023–1028.

Erkkila, A.T., Lehto, S., Pyorala, K., Uusitupa, M.I., 2003. n-3 Fatty acids and 5-y risks of death and cardiovascular disease events in patients with coronary artery disease. American Journal of Clinical Nutrition 78, 65–71.

Gillum, R.F., Mussolino, M., Madans, J.H., 2000. The relation between fish consumption, death from all causes, and incidence of coronary heart disease. The NHANES I Epidemiologic Follow-up Study. Journal of Clinical Epidemiology 53, 237–244.

Guallar, E., Aro, A., Jimenez, F.J., et al., 1999. Omega-3 fatty acids in adipose tissue and risk of myocardial infarction: the EURAMIC study. Arteriosclerosis, Thrombosis, and Vascular Biology 19, 1111–1118.

He, K., Song, Y., Daviglus, M.L., et al., 2004. Accumulated evidence on fish consumption and coronary heart disease mortality: a meta-analysis of cohort studies. Circulation 109, 2705–2711.

Holmberg, S., Thelin, A., Stiernstrom, E.L., 2009. Food choices and coronary heart disease: a population based cohort study of rural Swedish men with 12 years of follow-up. International Journal of Environmental Research and Public Health 6, 2626–2638.

Hu, F.B., Bronner, L., Willett, W.C., et al., 2002. Fish and omega-3 fatty acid intake and risk of coronary heart disease in women. JAMA: The Journal of the American Medical Association 287, 1815–1821.

Iso, H., Kobayashi, M., Ishihara, J., et al., 2006. Intake of fish and n3 fatty acids and risk of coronary heart disease among Japanese: The Japan Public Health Center-Based (JPHC) Study Cohort I. Circulation 113, 195–202.

Konig, A., Bouzan, C., Cohen, J.T., et al., 2005. A quantitative analysis of fish consumption and coronary heart disease mortality. American Journal of Preventive Medicine 29, 335–346.

Kromhout, D., Feskens, E.J., Bowles, C.H., 1995. The protective effect of a small amount of fish on coronary heart disease mortality in an elderly population. International Journal of Epidemiology 24, 340–345.

Kromhout, D., Bloemberg, B.P., Feskens, E.J., et al., 1996. Alcohol, fish, fibre and antioxidant vitamins intake do not explain population differences in coronary heart disease mortality. International Journal of Epidemiology 25, 753–759.

Mozaffarian, D., Rimm, E.B., 2006. Fish intake, contaminants, and human health: evaluating the risks and the benefits. JAMA: The Journal of the American Medical Association 296, 1885–1899.

Mozaffarian, D., Lemaitre, R.N., Kuller, L.H., et al., 2003. Cardiac benefits of fish consumption may depend on the type of fish meal consumed: the Cardiovascular Health Study. Circulation 107, 1372–1377.

Ness, A.R., Hughes, J., Elwood, P.C., et al., 2002. The long-term effect of dietary advice in men with coronary disease: follow-up of the Diet and Reinfarction trial (DART). European Journal of Clinical Nutrition 56, 512–518.

Oomen, C.M., Feskens, E.J., Rasanen, L., et al., 2000. Fish consumption and coronary heart disease mortality in Finland, Italy, and The Netherlands. American Journal of Epidemiology 151, 999–1006.

Osler, M., Andreasen, A.H., Hoidrup, S., 2003. No inverse association between fish consumption and risk of death from all-causes, and incidence of coronary heart disease in middle-aged, Danish adults. Journal of Clinical Epidemiology 56, 274–279.

Panagiotakos, D.B., Pitsavos, C., Zampelas, A., et al., 2005. Fish consumption and the risk of developing acute coronary syndromes: the CARDIO2000 study. International Journal of Cardiology 102, 403–409.

Sasazuki, S., 2001. Case–control study of nonfatal myocardial infarction in relation to selected foods in Japanese men and women. Japanese Circulation Journal 65, 200–206.

Streppel, M.T., Ocke, M.C., Boshuizen, H.C., Kok, F.J., Kromhout, D., 2008. Long-term fish consumption and n-3 fatty acid intake in relation to (sudden) coronary heart disease death: the Zutphen study. European Heart Journal 29, 2024–2030.

Tavani, A., Pelucchi, C., Negri, E., Bertuzzi, M., La Vecchia, C., 2001. n-3 Polyunsaturated fatty acids, fish, and nonfatal acute myocardial infarction. Circulation 104, 2269–2272.

Turunen, A.W., Verkasalo, P.K., Kiviranta, H., et al., 2008. Mortality in a cohort with high fish consumption. International Journal of Epidemiology 37, 1008–1017.

Whelton, S.P., He, J., Whelton, P.K., Muntner, P., 2004. Meta-analysis of observational studies on fish intake and coronary heart disease. The American Journal of Cardiology 93, 1119–1123.

Yuan, J.M., Ross, R.K., Gao, Y.T., Yu, M.C., 2001. Fish and shellfish consumption in relation to death from myocardial infarction among men in Shanghai, China. American Journal of Epidemiology 154, 809–816.

Zhang, J., Sasaki, S., Amano, K., Kesteloot, H., 1999. Fish consumption and mortality from all causes, ischemic heart disease, and stroke: an ecological study. Preventive Medicine 28, 520–529.

RELEVANT WEBSITES

http://www.eatright.org/ – American Dietetic Association.
http://www.efsa.europa.eu/ – European Food Safety Authority.
http://www.heart.org – American Heart Association.
http://www.mhlw.go.jp/english/index.html – Ministry of Health, Labor and Welfare of Japan.
http://www.nutrition.org.uk/ – British Nutrition Foundation.
http://www.who.int/en/ – World Health Organization.

CHAPTER 12

Fish Consumption and Risk of Cardiovascular Disease – Part 2

C.-M. Kastorini*,†, H.J. Milionis*, J.A. Goudevenos*, D.B. Panagiotakos†
*University of Ioannina, Ioannina, Greece
†Harokopio University, Athens, Greece

ABBREVIATIONS

CVD Cardiovascular disease
DHA Docosahexaenoic acid
EPA Eicosapentaenoic acid
LVSD Left ventricular systolic dysfunction

1. HEART FAILURE – LEFT VENTRICULAR SYSTOLIC DYSFUNCTION

Fish consumption is suggested to have a protective effect against left ventricular systolic dysfunction (LVSD) and heart failure. A population-based prospective study of 39 367 Swedish middle-aged men followed for 6 years showed that consumption of fatty fish once a week was associated with a 12% (95% CI: 0.68–1.13) lower risk of heart failure. Higher fish intake was not associated with any additional benefit; fish consumption two times per week was associated with a 1% lower risk and more than three times per week with a 3% lower risk (Levitan et al., 2009).

The Rotterdam Study, a prospective cohort study with 11.4 years of follow-up of 5299 subjects, showed that fish consumption of more than 20 g day^{-1} was associated with a 4% (95% CI: 0.78–1.18) lower risk of heart failure, compared with no fish intake (Dijkstra et al., 2009). According to a prospective cohort study of 4738 participants with a 12-year follow-up period, consumption of tuna or other boiled or baked fish one to two times per week was associated with a 20% (95% CI: 0.64–0.99) lower risk and consumption more than three times per week with a 30% lower risk, compared with consumption less than once a month, while fried fish consumption was associated with an increased risk of congestive heart failure (Mozaffarian et al., 2005a).

A recent study including 934 participants showed that moderate fish consumption was associated with a 53% (95% CI: 0.22–0.97) lower likelihood of developing LVSD after an acute coronary event, compared with no/rare consumption, after adjustment for various confounding factors (Kastorini et al., 2010).

Bioactive Food as Dietary Interventions for Cardiovascular Disease
http://dx.doi.org/10.1016/B978-0-12-396485-4.00037-2

© 2013 Elsevier Inc.
All rights reserved.

Nevertheless, according to the Atherosclerosis Risk in Community prospective study conducted in 14 153 participants with a 13-year follow-up, fish consumption was not associated with the risk of developing heart failure (Nettleton et al., 2008). According to the Cardiovascular Health Study with 5888 elderly participants, consumption of fried fish was associated with abnormal levels of markers indicating LVSD, including reduced left ventricular ejection fraction (Mozaffarian et al., 2006). Additionally, consumption of fried fish or fish sandwiches more than once a week was associated with a 42% higher risk of heart failure, compared with consumption less than once a month (Mozaffarian et al., 2005a).

2. STROKE PREVENTION

Strokes are classified into two main categories: ischemic and hemorrhagic. Ischemic strokes result from atherosclerosis of the carotid and cerebral arteries, and they are caused by blockage of arteries leading to the brain and interruption of the blood supply. Hemorrhagic strokes result from a ruptured blood vessel, which bleeds into the surrounding brain tissue (Bouzan et al., 2005). Studies examining the relationship between fish consumption and stroke show conflicting results, as some studies show a beneficial effect (Bouzan et al., 2005; He et al., 2002, 2004; Iso et al., 2001; Keli et al., 1994; Mozaffarian et al., 2005b), while others suggest that high fish consumption is associated with an increased risk of stroke (Caicoya, 2002; Orencia et al., 1996). It should also be mentioned that most studies focus on total stroke risk, meaning that the results could differ if a type-specific stroke analysis was performed (Kris-Etherton et al., 2002).

The majority of studies indicate a protective effect of fish consumption. Even consumption of one portion of fish per week could be beneficial in stroke development (Keli et al., 1994), especially ischemic stroke (Bouzan et al., 2005). The results of a meta-analysis of eight prospective cohort studies suggested an inverse association between fish consumption and risk of stroke, particularly ischemic stroke, even though a strong dose–response relationship was not observed. Compared with those who consume fish less than once a month, those who consume fish one to three times per month have a 9% lower risk (95% CI: 0.79–1.06); consumption once a week provided a 13% lower risk (95% CI: 0.77–0.98); two to four times per week, an 18% lower risk (95% CI: 0.72–0.94); and more than five times per week, a 31% lower risk (95% CI: 0.54–0.88) (He et al., 2004).

The results of another meta-analysis of five prospective and one case–control studies showed that any fish consumption was associated with a 12% decreased stroke risk compared with no fish consumption (Bouzan et al., 2005).

The Nurses' Health Study examining 79 839 women after 14 years of follow-up showed that consumption of fish two to four times per week, compared with less than once a month, was associated with a 52% (95% CI: 0.21–1.06) reduced risk of total stroke and a 51% (95% CI: 0.26–0.93) reduced risk of thrombotic infarction, primarily among women who did not take aspirin regularly. No excess risk of hemorrhagic stroke was found for more frequent fish consumption (Iso et al., 2001). Similarly, the Health Professionals' Follow-Up Study, a large prospective study among 43 671 male health-care professionals followed for 12 years, showed that men who consumed fish more than one to three times per month had a 40% (95% CI: 0.35–0.95) lower risk of ischemic stroke compared with those who ate fish less often. However, more frequent fish intake was not associated with a greater protective effect. Additionally, fish consumption was not associated with the risk of hemorrhagic stroke (He et al., 2002).

A study conducted in 4775 elderly individuals followed for 12 years showed that tuna or other fish consumption one to four times per week was associated with a 27% (95% CI: 0.55–0.98) lower risk of ischemic stroke and more than five times per week with a 30% (95% CI: 0.50–0.99) lower risk, compared with consumption of less than once a month. Insignificant associations were observed regarding hemorrhagic stroke (Mozaffarian et al., 2005b).

According to the Zutphen Study, conducted in 552 men with a 15-year follow-up, participants who consumed more than 20 g of fish per day in 1970 had a 51% lower risk of stroke compared with those who consumed less fish (Keli et al., 1994). A case–control study with 536 patients, matched to up to five control subjects, showed that consumption of fish more than two times per month was associated with a reduced likelihood of a first-ever stroke and primary intracerebral hemorrhage (Jamrozik et al., 1994).

However, some studies failed to show significant associations between fish consumption and incidence of stroke. In the EPIC-Norfolk prospective population study, with 24 312 participants who were followed up for 8.5 years, inconsistent results regarding fish consumption and stroke were found, and only in women, fatty fish consumption was associated with a 31% (95% CI: 0.51–0.94) lower risk of stroke (Myint et al., 2006). According to the Physicians' Health Study, which followed 21 185 U.S. men for 4 years, fish consumption of more than five servings per week was not associated with a lower risk of fatal and nonfatal stroke, compared with consumption of less than one serving per week (Morris et al., 1995).

A study investigating 3654 participants showed that participants consuming fish at least once a week had 43% (95% CI: 0.35–0.93) lower 10-year stroke-related mortality, compared with less frequent fish consumption. Nonetheless, the long-term protective effects on stroke mortality associated with eating fish were attenuated after incorporating the adjustment for retinal vessel diameters (Kaushik et al., 2008).

It should also be mentioned that some studies showed an increased risk of stroke for subjects eating high amounts of fish. However, the type of fish consumed or the way of preparation could have influenced the relationship between fish consumption and stroke development. The Finish Mobile Clinic Health Examination Survey, conducted in 3958 men and women, who were followed for 28 years, did not show any significant associations between fish intake and cerebrovascular disease; however, it showed that salted fish consumption was associated with 98% (95% CI: 1.02–3.84) higher risk of intracerebral hemorrhage (Montonen et al., 2009).

According to the Chicago Western Electric Study, with 2107 male participants, after 30 years of follow-up, subjects consuming 35 g of fish per day, the highest level of fish, had 34% (95% CI: 0.53–3.41) higher risk of stroke mortality than men consuming <17 g of fish per day (Orencia et al., 1996).

Results of a case–control study, including 440 stroke cases and 473 controls, indicated that participants in the highest quintile of consumption, 46 g of fish per day, had 95% (95% CI: 1.14–3.33) higher likelihood of stroke compared with those in the lowest quintile of fish consumption, 11 g day^{-1}. The risk of cerebral infarction also increased with higher consumption of fish (Caicoya, 2002).

Finally, fried fish or fish sandwich consumption was positively associated with total stroke and ischemic stroke risk. In particular, fried fish or fish sandwich consumption more than once a week was associated with a 44% (95% CI: 1.12–1.85) higher risk of ischemic stroke compared with consumption less than once a month (Mozaffarian et al., 2005b). Nevertheless, even if some studies show that fish intake may increase the risk of ischemic stroke, reductions in fish consumption should not be recommended.

Gender and race might also play a role regarding the relationship between stroke risk and fish intake. These differences could reflect different dietary patterns and type of fish consumed, as well as preparation methods (Myint et al., 2006). Fish intake has different effects on stroke risk in men and women. In particular, fish intake was associated with an increased risk of ischemic stroke only in men (OR = 1.24, 95% CI: 1.01–1.51 per meal per week), but the effect appears to be small compared with the protective effect on myocardial infarction. For women, a nonsignificant decrease in stroke risk was observed (Wennberg et al., 2007). In addition, according to the National Health and Nutrition Examination Survey (NHANES) I Epidemiologic Follow-up Study with an average follow-up of 12 years, white women who consumed fish more than once a week had a 45% (95% CI: 0.32–0.93) lower risk of stroke incidence compared with women who never consumed fish. On the contrary, insignificant associations were observed regarding white men. In both black women and men, however, any fish consumption compared with rare consumption was significantly associated with lower risk of stroke (Gillum et al., 1996).

Regarding the type of stroke, high fish intake has been suggested to have adverse effects on the risk of hemorrhagic stroke, following observations of high incidence of hemorrhage in Eskimos, a population consuming large amounts of fish, in accordance with biological evidence (He et al., 2004; Mozaffarian et al., 2005b); however, more recent studies do not verify these results (He et al., 2002; Iso et al., 2001; Skerrett and Hennekens, 2003). According to a meta-analysis of eight prospective cohort studies, insignificant associations were observed between fish intake and hemorrhagic stroke.

This result may be explained by the fact that hemorrhagic strokes represent a modest proportion of all strokes and because the other benefits of fish intake balance the risk of hemorrhage caused by high fish consumption (He et al., 2004).

3. PATHOPHYSIOLOGICAL MECHANISMS

The protective effects of fish are mainly attributed to the long-chain polyunsaturated omega-3 fatty acids, eicosapentaenoic acid (EPA), and docosahexaenoic acid (DHA), found in higher quantities in fatty fish and reported to influence several cardiovascular risk factors (Mozaffarian and Rimm, 2006). The content of omega-3 polyunsaturated fatty acid concentrations varies between fish species and depends on the location and the season of capture, even in the same species. However, besides omega-3 fatty acids, other components present in fish might also contribute to the beneficial effects of fish consumption.

3.1 Cardiovascular Disease Risk Factors

Long-term fish consumption has a beneficial effect on cardiac health, as it is associated with a protective action against the most common cardiovascular disease risk factors: hypertension, hypercholesterolemia, and impaired glucose metabolism (Das, 2000; Kris-Etherton et al., 2002; Mozaffarian and Rimm, 2006). Furthermore, the beneficial effect of omega-3 fatty acids on triglyceride levels is well known, and they are prescribed in the treatment of hypertriglyceridemia (Kris-Etherton et al., 2002).

4. METHODOLOGICAL PROBLEMS

It is important to mention that some methodological problems occur when examining the effects of fish consumption on cardiovascular health. Variations in the assessing of fish intake, differences in overall dietary patterns between populations; consumption of different types of fish, fatty or lean fish; potential contamination of fish by toxic heavy metals; reverse causality (as people become more aware of the protective effects of fish consumption regarding cardiovascular health), as well as differences in the methods used to validate and classify endpoints or differences in risk levels among different populations.

First of all, focusing on the types of fish consumed, intake of fatty fish, such as salmon, herring, and sardines, is associated with a lower risk than intake of lean fish, such as cod, catfish, or halibut (Mozaffarian and Rimm, 2006). Regarding the type of fish meal consumed and the preparation method, fried fish or fish sandwich consumption from fast-food restaurants is associated with a trend of increased risk of total ischemic heart disease mortality, arrhythmic ischemic heart disease death, or nonfatal myocardial infarction, as well as heart failure and stroke (Mozaffarian et al., 2005a,b, 2006), possibly because of the lower omega-3 PUFA content of these products, which are prepared mostly from lean fish. Additionally, frying is associated with the presence of trans-fatty acids because of the use of partially hydrogenated oils and the presence of lipid oxidation products. However, it is also possible that other lifestyle factors affect this relationship (Mozaffarian and Rimm, 2006).

5. FISH CONTAMINANTS

Fish and shellfish are good sources of omega-3 fatty acids; however, they also supply the human diet with highly toxic chemicals (Mahaffey, 2004; Mahaffey et al., 2008), mainly heavy metals (methylmercury, arsenic, cadmium, lead, etc.) and organohalogenated compounds (polychlorinated dioxins, furans, and biphenyls, various brominated flame retardants, various organochlorine insecticides, etc.), which have well-known adverse effects on human health (Mozaffarian and Rimm, 2006; Park and Mozaffarian, 2010).

5.1 Methylmercury

Mercury is a reactive heavy metal, which cycles from rainwater into lakes and oceans. There it is converted by microbial activity into organic methylmercury. Methylmercury, in contrast to inorganic mercury, is easily absorbed and actively transported into tissues, and it can accumulate in the body if consumed at a greater rate than it is excreted. Mercury is suggested to negatively influence human health, affecting the immune, cardiovascular, and reproductive systems, while at high doses it acts as a neurotoxic agent.

Results of studies investigating the role of methylmercury are conflicting. A recent meta-analysis showed insignificant associations between mercury exposure and cardiovascular disease risk, when comparing the highest and lowest categories of exposure. Therefore, in humans, the evidence regarding the effect of methylmercury on cardiovascular health is still inconclusive and further investigation is warranted (Park and Mozaffarian, 2010). However, a possible suggestion of the above findings is that the methylmercury present in fish may attenuate the benefits of fish consumption to at least some degree. Therefore, it is possible that fish consumption would be associated with an even lower cardiovascular risk if methylmercury were not present (Mozaffarian and Rimm, 2006).

Mechanisms by which mercury is thought to increase the risk of cardiovascular disease include the reduction of antioxidative capacity, promotion of free radical stress and lipid peroxidation in cell membranes and lipoproteins, promotion of blood coagulation, inhibition of endothelial cell formation and migration, as well as effects on apoptosis and inflammatory responses (Mozaffarian and Rimm, 2006).

Methylmercury in fish meat is bound to muscle proteins. As a result, skimming, trimming of fish, or cooking does not significantly reduce its concentration (Kris-Etherton et al., 2002; Sidhu, 2003). Larger and longer-living predatory fish, such as swordfish, tile-fish tuna, orange roughy, and shark, have higher tissue concentrations of mercury, while smaller or shorter-living species that are not predatory have very low concentrations (Mozaffarian and Rimm, 2006).

5.2 Polychlorinated Biphenyls

Polychlorinated biphenyls, dibenzo-*p*-dioxins, and dibenzo-furans are toxic and persistent environmental synthetic pollutants (Mozaffarian and Rimm, 2006), mainly associated with cancer risk. Carcinogenic compounds present in fish are TCDD (2,3,7,8-tetrachlorodibenzo-*p*-dioxin), classified as a group I carcinogen, dichlorodiphenyltrichloroethane, dieldrin, and heptachlor (Mozaffarian and Rimm, 2006). Adverse effects of these compounds include immunotoxicity, reproductive toxicity, endocrine disruption, developmental neurotoxicity, and increased risk of diabetes (Mozaffarian and Rimm, 2006).

As these compounds are lipophilic, high levels are found in fatty fish compared with lean fish, while no differences are observed between farmed and wild-caught fish. It is important to mention that removing the skin and fatty areas, belly, back, and dark side meat, as well as trimming the fat from fish bodies before cooking, reduces the levels of these contaminants in the fish. Also certain cooking procedures, such as using grills in cooking or cooking the fish on a rack to allow the fat to drain, minimize their concentrations (Kris-Etherton et al., 2002).

6. DIETARY GUIDELINES

The majority of national and international organizations, for the primary prevention of coronary heart disease, suggest consumption of fish at least two servings per week, mainly from fatty fish (Table 12.1). According to the Scientific Statement of the American Heart Association, fish and seafood are potential sources of various environmental contaminants, such as methylmercury and polychlorinated biphenyls and, therefore, consumers should be aware of the possible health risks of eating fish (Kris-Etherton et al., 2002). Fish with higher mercury concentrations should be consumed in smaller quantities. Therefore, consumers should be aware of the fish species that are low in mercury and rich sources of omega-3 fatty acids, as well as other fish species highly contaminated with mercury, while being poor sources of omega-3 fatty acids. A new approach regarding fish consumption recommendations taking into account the risks and benefits focuses on the frequency of consumption of fish species according to their omega-3 fatty acid and methylmercury contents. Fish species rich in omega-3 fatty acids and low in methylmercury, such as salmon, herring, and trout, have a beneficial effect on human health. Other species such as flounder and canned light tuna are associated with a small net

Table 12.1 Dietary Recommendations for Omega-3 Fatty Acids and Fish Consumption – General Population

Organization	Fish	Omega-3 fatty acids
World		
World Health Organization (FAO/WHO, 2003)	One to two servings of fish per week	Each serving 200–500 mg EPA and DHA
USA		
American Dietetic Association Dieticians of Canada (Kris-Etherton et al., 2007)	Two servings of fatty fish per week	500 mg day^{-1}
American Diabetes Association (Bantle et al., 2008)	Two servings of fish per week (excluding commercially fried fish and fillets)	–
American Heart Association (Kris-Etherton et al., 2002; Lichtenstein et al., 2006)	Two servings of fish per week (preferably fatty)	–
Europe		
European Food Safety Agency (EFSA Panel on Dietetic Products, 2010)	–	250 mg day^{-1}
United Kingdom Specific Advisory Committee on Nutrition (2004)	At least two portions of fish per week, one of which should be oily	450 mg EPA and DHA per day
British Nutrition Foundation	One to two portions of oily fish per week	2–3 g of the very long-chain omega-3 fatty acids, 1.5 g EPA and DHA per week
Asia		
Ministry of Health, Labor and Welfare of Japan	–	Adults: 2.0–2.9 g total omega-3 depending on age and sex

Source: EFSA Panel on Dietetic Products, Nutrition, and Allergies (NDA), 2010. Scientific Opinion on Dietary Reference Values for fats, including saturated fatty acids, polyunsaturated fatty acids, monounsaturated fatty acids, trans fatty acids, and cholesterol. EFSA Journal 8 (3), 1461. Available online: http://www.efsa.europa.eu. Joint report of the Scientific Advisory Committee on Nutrition (SACN) and the Committee on Toxicity (COT) on the consumption of fish (2004). Advice on fish consumption: benefits and risks. British Nutrition Foundation. Conference held on 1 December 1999 to draw attention to the briefing paper on 'n-3 Fatty acids and Health'. Japanese Nutritional Requirement – Dietary Reference Intakes: Policy-Making Committee (Chairperson: Mr. Heizo Tanaka, Former Board Chairman of National Institute of Health and Nutrition). Announced October, 2004 and valid from 2005 to 2010 (for 5 years).

benefit, while species such as canned white tuna and halibut carry a small net risk. Finally, because of their high methylmercury content, fish such as swordfish and shark are associated with an increased risk (Ginsberg and Toal, 2009). Especially for individuals who consume more than five servings per week, limitation of the intake of species highest in methylmercury levels is necessary.

However, it is important to know that although many species of fish are rich sources of the omega-3 fatty acids and have lower methylmercury concentrations, these species may not be consistently low in other organic contaminants, such as dioxins and polychlorinated biphenyls. With the present knowledge regarding dioxin and polychlorinated biphenyl intake, potential carcinogenic or other adverse effects are possibly outweighed by the protective effects of fish intake (Mozaffarian and Rimm, 2006).

7. CONCLUSION

Fish consumption is an important part of a healthy diet. When consumed in moderation and when a variety of species is selected, its beneficial effects outweigh the possible risks. For this reason, consumers should be aware of the fish species that both are rich in omega-3 polyunsaturated fatty acids and have low methylmercury concentrations.

REFERENCES

Bantle, J.P., Wylie-Rosett, J., Albright, A.L., et al., 2008. Nutrition recommendations and interventions for diabetes: a position statement of the American Diabetes Association. Diabetes Care 31 (Suppl 1), S61–S78.

Bouzan, C., Cohen, J.T., Connor, W.E., et al., 2005. A quantitative analysis of fish consumption and stroke risk. American Journal of Preventive Medicine 29, 347–352.

Caicoya, M., 2002. Fish consumption and stroke: a community case–control study in Asturias, Spain. Neuroepidemiology 21, 107–114.

Das, U.N., 2000. Beneficial effect(s) of n-3 fatty acids in cardiovascular diseases: but, why and how? Prostaglandins, Leukotrienes, and Essential Fatty Acids 63, 351–362.

De Lorgeril, M., Salen, P., 2002. Fish and n-3 fatty acids for the prevention and treatment of coronary heart disease: nutrition is not pharmacology. American Journal of Medicine 112, 316–319.

Dijkstra, S.C., Brouwer, I.A., van Rooij, F.J., et al., 2009. Intake of very long chain n-3 fatty acids from fish and the incidence of heart failure: the Rotterdam Study. European Journal of Heart Failure 11, 922–928.

FAO/WHO, 2003. Technical Report. Diet, nutrition, and the prevention of chronic diseases. Geneva, Switzerland: World Health Organization.

Gillum, R.F., Mussolino, M.E., Madans, J.H., 1996. The relationship between fish consumption and stroke incidence. The NHANES I Epidemiologic Follow-up Study (National Health and Nutrition Examination Survey). Archives of Internal Medicine 156, 537–542.

Ginsberg, G.L., Toal, B.F., 2009. Quantitative approach for incorporating methylmercury risks and omega-3 fatty acid benefits in developing species-specific fish consumption advice. Environmental Health Perspectives 117, 267–275.

He, K., Rimm, E.B., Merchant, A., et al., 2002. Fish consumption and risk of stroke in men. The Journal of the American Medical Association 288, 3130–3136.

He, K., Song, Y., Daviglus, M.L., et al., 2004. Fish consumption and incidence of stroke: a meta-analysis of cohort studies. Stroke 35, 1538–1542.

Iso, H., Rexrode, K.M., Stampfer, M.J., et al., 2001. Intake of fish and omega-3 fatty acids and risk of stroke in women. The Journal of the American Medical Association 285, 304–312.

Jamrozik, K., Broadhurst, R.J., Anderson, C.S., Stewart-Wynne, E.G., 1994. The role of lifestyle factors in the etiology of stroke. A population-based case–control study in Perth, Western Australia. Stroke 25, 51–59.

Kastorini, C.M., Chrysohoou, C., Aggelopoulos, P., et al., 2010. Moderate fish consumption is associated with lower likelihood of developing left ventricular systolic dysfunction in acute coronary syndrome patients. Journal of Food Science 75, H24–H29.

Kaushik, S., Wang, J.J., Flood, V., et al., 2008. Frequency of fish consumption, retinal microvascular signs, and vascular mortality. Microcirculation 15, 27–36.

Keli, S.O., Feskens, E.J., Kromhout, D., 1994. Fish consumption and risk of stroke. The Zutphen Study. Stroke 25, 328–332.

Kris-Etherton, P.M., Harris, W.S., Appel, L.J., 2002. Fish consumption, fish oil, omega-3 fatty acids, and cardiovascular disease. Circulation 106, 2747–2757.

Kris-Etherton, P.M., Innis, S., American Dietetic, Association, and Dietitians of Canada, 2007. Position of the American Dietetic Association and Dietitians of Canada: dietary fatty acids. Journal of American Dietetic Association 107, 1599–1611.

Levitan, E.B., Wolk, A., Mittleman, M.A., 2009. Fish consumption, marine omega-3 fatty acids, and incidence of heart failure: a population-based prospective study of middle-aged and elderly men. European Heart Journal 30, 1495–1500.

Lichtenstein, A.H., Appel, L.J., Brands, M., et al., 2006. Diet and lifestyle recommendations revision 2006: a scientific statement from the American Heart Association Nutrition Committee. Circulation 114, 82–96.

Mahaffey, K.R., 2004. Fish and shellfish as dietary sources of methylmercury and the omega-3 fatty acids, eicosahexaenoic acid and docosahexaenoic acid: risks and benefits. Environmental Research 95, 414–428.

Mahaffey, K.R., Clickner, R.P., Jeffries, R.A., 2008. Methylmercury and omega-3 fatty acids: co-occurrence of dietary sources with emphasis on fish and shellfish. Environmental Research 107, 20–29.

Montonen, J., Jarvinen, R., Reunanen, A., Knekt, P., 2009. Fish consumption and the incidence of cerebrovascular disease. British Journal of Nutrition 102, 750–756.

Morris, M.C., Manson, J.E., Rosner, B., Buring, J.E., Willett, W.C., Hennekens, C.H., 1995. Fish consumption and cardiovascular disease in the physicians' health study: a prospective study. American Journal of Epidemiology 142, 166–175.

Mozaffarian, D., Bryson, C.L., Lemaitre, R.N., Burke, G.L., Siscovick, D.S., 2005a. Fish intake and risk of incident heart failure. Journal of the American College of Cardiology 45, 2015–2021.

Mozaffarian, D., Longstreth Jr., W.T., Lemaitre, R.N., et al., 2005b. Fish consumption and stroke risk in elderly individuals: the cardiovascular health study. Archives of Internal Medicine 165, 200–206.

Mozaffarian, D., Gottdiener, J.S., Siscovick, D.S., 2006. Intake of tuna or other broiled or baked fish versus fried fish and cardiac structure, function, and hemodynamics. The American Journal of Cardiology 97, 216–222.

Mozaffarian, D., Rimm, E.B., 2006. Fish intake, contaminants, and human health: evaluating the risks and the benefits. The Journal of the American Medical Association 296, 1885–1899.

Myint, P.K., Welch, A.A., Bingham, S.A., et al., 2006. Habitual fish consumption and risk of incident stroke: the European Prospective Investigation into Cancer (EPIC)-Norfolk prospective population study. Public Health Nutrition 9, 882–888.

Nettleton, J.A., Steffen, L.M., Loehr, L.R., Rosamond, W.D., Folsom, A.R., 2008. Incident heart failure is associated with lower whole-grain intake and greater high-fat dairy and egg intake in the Atherosclerosis Risk in Communities (ARIC) study. Journal of American Dietetic Association 108, 1881–1887.

Orencia, A.J., Daviglus, M.L., Dyer, A.R., Shekelle, R.B., Stamler, J., 1996. Fish consumption and stroke in men: 30-year findings of the Chicago Western Electric Study. Stroke 27, 204–209.

Park, K., Mozaffarian, D., 2010. Omega-3 fatty acids, mercury, and selenium in fish, and the risk of cardiovascular diseases. Current Atherosclerosis Reports 12, 414–422.

Sidhu, K.S., 2003. Health benefits and potential risks related to consumption of fish or fish oil. Regulatory Toxicology and Pharmacology 38, 336–344.

Skerrett, P.J., Hennekens, C.H., 2003. Consumption of fish and fish oils and decreased risk of stroke. Preventive Cardiology 6, 38–41.

Wennberg, M., Bergdahl, I.A., Stegmayr, B., et al., 2007. Fish intake, mercury, long-chain n-3 polyunsaturated fatty acids and risk of stroke in northern Sweden. British Journal of Nutrition 98, 1038–1045.

RELEVANT WEBSITES

http://www.eatright.org/ – American Dietetic Association.
http://www.efsa.europa.eu/ – European Food Safety Authority.
http://www.heart.org – American Heart Association.
http://www.mhlw.go.jp/english/index.html – Ministry of Health, Labor and Welfare of Japan.
http://www.nutrition.org.uk/ – British Nutrition Foundation.
http://www.who.int/en/ – World Health Organization.

CHAPTER 13

Quercetin and Its Metabolites in Heart Health

S. Hrelia, C. Angeloni
University of Bologna, Bologna, Italy

1. QUERCETIN: CHEMISTRY AND BIOAVAILABILITY

Quercetin (3,5,7,3′,4′-pentahydroxyflavone) (Figure 13.1) is a typical flavonol-type flavonoid. Quercetin is the most abundant of the flavonoids and forms the backbone for many other flavonoids. Flavonoids are characterized by two benzene rings that are connected by an oxygen-containing pyrene ring. The three rings are planar, and the molecule is quite polarized. This structure is characterized by three intermolecular hydrogen bonds: one between the hydroxyl groups in ring B and two with the carbonyl group. Quercetin possesses all the structural elements characteristic of an antioxidant: an ortho-dihydroxy or catechol group in ring B, a 2,3-double bond, and the 3- and 5-OH groups with the 4-oxo group. Within the flavonoid family, quercetin is one of the most potent scavengers of reactive oxygen species including superoxide and reactive nitrogen species such as nitric oxide. Quercetin occurs in a variety of human foods such as apples, red onions, grapes, berries, citrus fruits, cherries, broccoli, tea, capers, and lovage. Dietary quercetin is mostly present as glycoside form such as rutin (quercetin rutinoside), in which one or more sugar groups are bound to phenolic groups by glycosidic linkage. The water solubility of quercetin increases with increasing number of sugar groups.

The numerous evidences on the potential beneficial effects of quercetin on human health have recently led to the development of high-dose quercetin nutraceutical preparations. However, a major concern has been the low oral bioavailability of quercetin and most other flavonoids. Early studies on quercetin bioavailability suggested that only quercetin without a sugar group was taken up in the gastrointestinal tract by passive diffusion because of the hydrophilic character of its glycosides. However, many studies demonstrated that the absorption of quercetin is considerably enhanced by its conjugation with a sugar group. Absorption of flavonoid glycosides requires either hydrolysis of the L–glucoside or a specific active transport mechanism. Various mammalian L–glucosidases are present in the small intestine, and all of them, with the exception of lactase-phlorizin hydrolase (LPH), act intracellularly and would require transport of the intact (iso)flavonoid glycoside if they were to play a role in the metabolism of these compounds. LPH, however, is present on the luminal side of the brush border in the small intestine and can

Bioactive Food as Dietary Interventions for Cardiovascular Disease
http://dx.doi.org/10.1016/B978-0-12-396485-4.00011-6

© 2013 Elsevier Inc.
All rights reserved.

217

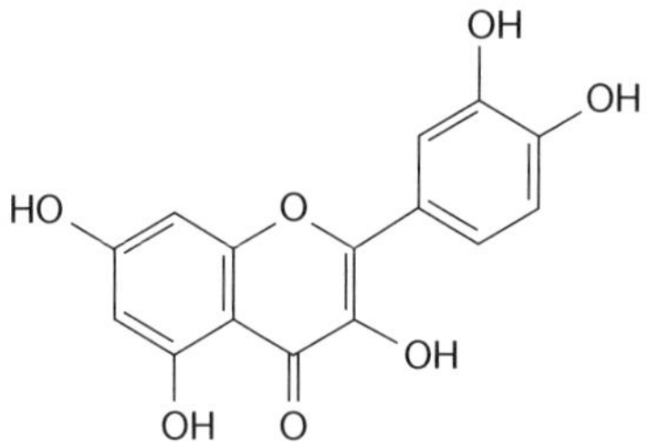

Figure 13.1 Structural formula of quercetin.

act on dietary glycosides before absorption. The released aglycone may then enter the epithelial cells by passive diffusion as a result of its increased lipophilicity and its proximity to the cellular membrane. An alternative site of hydrolysis is a cytosolic β–glucosidase (CBG) within the epithelial cells. In order for CBG-mediated hydrolysis to occur, the polar glucosides must be transported into the epithelial cells, possibly with the involvement of the active sodium-dependent glucose transporter SGLT1. However, a recent investigation, in which SGLT1 was expressed in *Xenopus laevis* oocytes, indicated that SLGT1 does not transport flavonoids and that glycosylated flavonoids, and some aglycones, have the capability to inhibit the glucose transporter (Kottra and Daniel, 2007). After absorption, quercetin becomes metabolized in the small intestine, colon, liver, and kidney. In the absorptive cells of the intestinal epithelium, quercetin may be O-methylated, primarily resulting in the formation of 3′-O-methylquercetin (isorhamnetin) and to a smaller extent, 4′-O-methylquercetin (tamaraxetin), sulfated, or glucuronidated at one of the hydroxyl groups. Subsequently, the resulting derivatives and any unmetabolized quercetin are released into the circulation via the hepatic portal vein. In the liver, quercetin and its derivatives are further subjected to conjugation, leading to the formation of sulfate and/or glucuronide derivatives. In addition, the catechol-O-methyltransferase enzymes of the liver and kidneys may also participate in further methylation of quercetin or its derivatives. Flavonoids and their metabolites not absorbed in the small intestine will be subjected to the action of the colonic microflora, resulting in the production of phenolic acids and hydroxycinnamates. These can be absorbed and ultimately excreted in urine in substantial quantities that, in most instances, are well in excess of the flavonoid metabolites that entered the circulatory system via the small intestine.

Normally, human quercetin plasma concentrations are in the low nanomolar range, but after quercetin intake, they may reach the high nanomolar or low micromolar range. A recent study demonstrated that low to moderate oral dose of quercetin (50, 100, or 150 mg per day) for 2 weeks increased plasma quercetin concentrations dose dependently in healthy individuals. The highest supplementation of 150 mg per day increased plasma quercetin concentrations over 570%, with a median concentration of 0.38 μM and a maximal concentration observed at 1.3 μM (Egert et al., 2008). Moreover, we demonstrated that a single dose of 600 g of unpeeled apples is able to increase plasma antioxidant level with a maximum at 3 h after ingestion in healthy human subjects (Maffei et al., 2007). Regarding the tissue distribution, quercetin mainly concentrates in lungs, testes, kidneys, thymus, heart, and liver, with the highest concentrations of quercetin and its methylated derivatives detected in the pulmonary tissue.

2. CARDIOVASCULAR DISEASE AND QUERCETIN

Cardiovascular disease is a broad term used to describe a range of diseases that affect heart and blood vessels. While the term technically refers to any disease that affects the cardiovascular system such as infection, inflammation, vascular relaxation, platelet aggregation, hypertension, and cardiac hypertrophy, however, in developed countries, the main underlying problem is atherosclerosis.

The major preventable risk factors for cardiovascular disease are tobacco smoking, high blood pressure, high blood cholesterol, insufficient physical activity, overweight and obesity, poor nutrition, and diabetes. Most cardiovascular diseases reflect chronic conditions that develop or persist over a long period of time. However, sometimes, the outcome of cardiovascular disease could be acute events such as heart attacks that occur suddenly when a vessel supplying blood to the heart becomes blocked. Many studies have investigated the role of quercetin in preventing cardiovascular disease, and interestingly, it has been shown that quercetin has multiple effects in counteracting the different diseases that affect heart and blood vessels.

2.1 Atherosclerosis

Atherosclerosis is a multifactorial disease characterized by the intimal accumulation of smooth muscle cells, macrophages, T lymphocytes, lipids, and extracellular matrix components over many years. Oxidative stress, inflammation, serum lipid profile alteration, and endothelial dysfunction are associated with the pathogenesis of atherosclerosis.

Dietary consumption of low doses of quercetin leads to attenuation in the development of the atherosclerotic lesion in ApoE-deficient mice (Loke et al., 2010). The positive effect of quercetin against atherosclerosis is due to its ability to counteract several processes involved in disease progression, such as endothelial dysfunction, oxidative stress, and inflammation. Quercetin inhibits the crucial steps in the development of atherosclerosis including the aortic fatty streak formation, the oxidation of LDL, and the LDL-induced cytotoxicity. Interestingly, quercetin metabolites specifically accumulate in human atherosclerotic lesions but not in the normal aorta. Quercetin also attenuates atherosclerosis in ApoE(−/−) gene-knockout mice by alleviating inflammation, improving NO bioavailability, and inducing heme oxygenase-1 (Loke et al., 2010). Adhesion molecules and matrix metalloproteinases are key proteins for several processes involved in atherosclerotic plaque formation such as infiltration of inflammatory cells. Quercetin was able to reduce

TNFα-induced upregulation of the adhesion molecules of vascular cell adhesion molecule-1 (VCAM-1), intercellular adhesion molecule-1 (ICAM-1), and monocyte chemoattractant protein-1 (MCP-1) in human endothelial and vascular smooth muscle cells. However, the quercetin metabolites, quercetin 3′-sulfate, quercetin 3-glucuronide, and 3′-methyl-quercetin 3-glucuronide, had no effect on TNFα-induced upregulation of adhesion molecule or chemokine expression (Winterbone et al., 2009). Quercetin downregulates both PMA- and TNFα-induced ICAM-1 expression via inhibiting both AP-1 activation and the JNK pathway. The molecular mechanisms by which quercetin may counteract inflammatory gene expression have not yet been fully elucidated. Quercetin inhibits TNFα production as well as inducible nitric oxide synthase (iNOS) expression and NO production in LPS-activated macrophages, an effect that has been associated with the inhibition of the NF-κB pathway. In addition, quercetin is able to stimulate the expression of the anti-inflammatory cytokine IL-10 (Comalada et al., 2006).

In a recent study by Boesch-Saadatmandi et al. (2010), the effect of on inflammatory gene expression quercetin and its major metabolites quercetin-3-glucuronide (Q3G) and isorhamnetin was investigated in murine RAW264.7 macrophages. Quercetin and isorhamnetin but not Q3G significantly decreased TNFα mRNA and protein levels. Antiinflammatory properties of quercetin and isorhamnetin were accompanied by an increase in heme oxygenase 1 protein levels, a downstream target of the transcription factor Nrf 2, known to antagonize chronic inflammation. Furthermore, proinflammatory microRNA-155 was downregulated by quercetin and isorhamnetin but not by Q3G.

2.1.1 LDL oxidation

Low-density lipoprotein (LDL) oxidation is proinflammatory and proatherogenic and is strictly involved in the initiation, progression, and potentially, in the destabilization of atherosclerotic lesions. Minimally oxidized LDL stimulates endothelial cells to produce chemokines and other factors that are responsible for the recruitment and penetration of monocytes into the arterial wall and the proliferation and differentiation of monocytes/macrophages. When LDL particles become further oxidized, highly oxidized LDL are preferentially taken up by macrophage cells via scavenger receptors, resulting in the formation of foam cells. Studies in human populations have shown that circulating oxidized LDLs are associated with preclinical atherosclerosis, coronary arterial atherosclerosis, acute coronary syndrome, and vulnerable plaques. Therefore, it has been suggested that a promising strategy to reduce the risk of atherosclerosis could be the dietary supplementation with antioxidants such as quercetin. Quercetin and quercetin-3-O-glucuronide protect LDL from neutrophil-mediated modification, mainly through the inhibition of myeloperoxidase, potentially reducing the risk of atherosclerosis.

A study carried out on LDL receptor gene-knockout (LDLR$^{-/-}$) mice demonstrated that quercetin significantly upregulates the hepatic expression of the antiatherogenic gene, paraoxonase1, with concomitantly increased serum paraoxonase1 activity (Leckey et al., 2010), an additional mechanism by which quercetin can protect LDL from oxidation and play a protective role in atherosclerosis.

2.2 Vascular Relaxation

The endothelium plays a fundamental role in maintaining vascular homeostasis. In particular, endothelial cells produce many biologically active compounds involved in local regulation of blood flow, blood pressure, and vascular tone. Among these substances, the most important is nitric oxide (NO). Cardiovascular risk factors such as diabetes and smoking alter the redox state in the vessel, a condition that can lead to endothelial dysfunction and atherosclerosis. Endothelial dysfunction and the reduction of NO production are early biomarkers of vascular disorders. Oxidative stress, caused by endothelial dysfunction and loss of NO, alters several physiological functions such as platelet aggregation, leukocyte adhesion, and blood flow in the endothelium.

In a study carried out in aortic rings isolated from streptozotocin (STZ)-induced diabetic rat, quercetin induced a dose–dependent vasorelaxation at early stages of diabetes development, and this response follows a NO- and prostaglandin-dependent process. In a study, the effects of quercetin were compared with those of the antioxidant ascorbic acid (vitamin C) on the reactivity of aortic rings from spontaneously hypertensive rats (SHR). The results showed that acute exposure to quercetin improves endothelium-dependent vascular relaxation and reduces α_1–adrenergic-receptor-mediated contractions of isolated hypertensive aortae, with greater potency than ascorbic acid. This suggests a better vascular protective effect with this flavonoid than with ascorbic acid in SHR model of hypertension and possibly, in human cardiovascular diseases. In a study by Xu et al. (2007), structure–activity relationships (SAR) for vascular relaxation effects were examined for 17 different flavonoids using porcine coronary arteries. Among the 17 flavonoids examined in this study, quercetin was one of the most effective relaxation agents, and interestingly, the comparison of rutin with quercetin demonstrated that the presence of a glycosylation group greatly reduced the relaxation effect.

2.3 Antiplatelet Activity

Platelet activation and aggregation play a critical role in the pathogenesis of acute coronary syndromes, and it has been shown that antiplatelet therapy reduces cardiovascular disease risk. Platelets play a fundamental role in hemostasis by facilitating the repair of minor vascular injuries through the formation of aggregates over tears within artery walls. Dysfunction in platelet activation leads to thrombosis that causes the blocking of cardiac arteries by thrombi resulting in myocardial infarction. Although a specific mechanism for quercetin antiplatelet activity has not been established, a number of investigations of possible mechanisms have been reported. You et al. (1999) showed that quercetin inhibits lipoxygenase, reducing the generation of arachidonic acid metabolites. Gryglewski et al. (1987) concluded that quercetin is antithrombotic because it is selectively bound to mural platelet thrombi and owing to its free radical scavenging properties, resuscitate biosynthesis and action of endothelial prostacyclin and endothelium-derived relaxing factor. Quercetin was also found to inhibit two essential processes involved in platelet activation and aggregation: collagen-stimulated Ca^{2+} mobilization from intracellular stores and collagen-stimulated whole-cell protein tyrosine phosphorylation. Navarro-Nunez et al. (2009) analyzed the effects of quercetin on thrombin-induced platelet activation through the assessment of its effects on the specific signaling cascades downstream of protease-activated receptor (PAR)1 and PAR4 and demonstrated that quercetin inhibits the responses of platelets mediated by both PAR1 agonist peptide (AP) and PAR4 AP, via inhibition of calcium mobilization, granule release, and aggregation. Moreover, this study showed that quercetin does not compete for thrombin binding, and thus, receptor antagonism does not seem to account for platelet inhibition with this compound. Recently, Wright et al. (2010) demonstrated that the antiaggregant effects of quercetin and its *in vivo* metabolites are associated with inhibition of Fyn kinase activity and tyrosine phosphorylation of Syk and phospholipase Cγ. They also observed that the principal functional groups attributed to potent inhibition were a planar, C-4 carbonyl substituted, and C-3 hydroxylated C ring, in addition to a B ring catechol moiety.

Rutin, a glycoside of the flavonol quercetin, inhibits the activation of phospholipase C, followed by the inhibition of PKC activity and thromboxane A_2 formation, thereby leading to the inhibition of the phosphorylation of P47 and intracellular calcium mobilization, finally resulting in the inhibition of human platelet aggregation. A study compared the capacity of quercetin and rutin to prevent platelet aggregation, and the results showed that quercetin is about six times more effective than rutin (Gryglewski et al., 1987). The *in vivo* antiaggregant effects of quercetin have not been demonstrated yet.

2.4 Hypertension

Hypertension is the term used to describe high blood pressure, and it has been recognized as one of the major risk factors for developing cardiovascular diseases. Quercetin antihypertensive effects were analyzed only in animal models of hypertension: SHR, a genetic model of multifactorial hypertension; L-NAME-induced hypertension (LIH), in which hypertension is caused by the inhibition of NO synthase with N-nitro-L-arginine methyl ester (L-NAME); deoxycorticosterone acetate (DOCA)-salt, a model of volume-dependent hypertension, which is triggered by administration of NaCl and characterized by a suppressed plasma renin level due to sodium retention; the Dahl salt-sensitive rats that are genetically predisposed to develop hypertension when they receive NaCl; two-kidney, one-clip (2K1C) Goldblatt hypertensive rat, which is a model of renovascular hypertension with reduced blood flow to one kidney; and obese Zucker rat, a genetic model of metabolic syndrome, demonstrating elevated blood pressure.

Quercetin's antihypertensive effect was observed for the first time by Duarte et al. (2001) in a study carried out in SHRs that received a single oral daily dose of 10 mg kg^{-1} of quercetin for 5 weeks. Interestingly, they measured a significant reduction in systolic, diastolic, and mean arterial blood pressure and heart rate in hypertensive rats, but they did not observe any effect in normotensive rats. Emura et al. (2007) investigated the antihypertensive effect of orally administered isoquercitrin (EMIQ), a water-soluble glycoside of quercetin produced from rutin by enzymatic treatment, in SHRs. The systolic blood pressure in SHR-administered EMIQ was significantly lower than that in the control group, and the effect of EMIQ was higher than equimolar administration of quercetin, possibly due to a higher bioavailability. In L-NAME-induced hypertensive rat, quercetin markedly inhibited the development of L-NAME-induced hypertension, and this effect was accompanied by a partial or full prevention of most of the effects induced by L-NAME. In most cases, these effects were dose dependent, but none of them were observed in normotensive animals. In DOCA-salt hypertensive rats, quercetin (10 mg kg^{-1}) was able to inhibit the development of DOCA-salt-induced hypertension with the same efficacy as the Ca^{2+} channel blocker verapamil (Galisteo et al., 2004). Two studies have observed that quercetin reduces elevated systolic blood pressure in Dahl salt-sensitive rats (Mackraj et al., 2008). In obese Zucker rats, a daily dose of quercetin (2 or 10 mg kg^{-1}) for 10 weeks induced a progressive reduction in blood pressure without an effect on the control lean Zucker rats (Rivera et al., 2008). The effects of oral quercetin treatment (10 mg kg^{-1}) quercetin were analyzed in 2K1C rats, and results demonstrated that quercetin reduced systolic blood pressure in this animal model.

2.5 Myocardial Ischemia/Reperfusion

Myocardial infarction is the acute condition of necrosis of the myocardium that occurs as a result of critical imbalance between coronary blood supply and myocardial demand. Myocardial ischemia followed by reperfusion results in tissue injury termed ischemia/reperfusion injury, which is characterized by decreased myocardial contractile function, occurrence of arrhythmias, and development of tissue necrosis. Reperfusion may be considered as a double-faced Janus event: although it is essential for the survival of the heart, it paradoxically induces new cellular damage that reduces the positive effects of reperfusion itself. Of the numerous mechanisms implicated in the pathobiology of reperfusion injury, oxidative stress has been suggested as a key mechanism of cellular damage in ischemia/reperfusion (I/R) injury.

In an *in vitro* model of I/R, we showed that quercetin elicits two different antioxidant mechanisms: direct and indirect. The first one refers to its classical ability to react with free radicals, while the indirect mechanism highlights the enhancement of the endogenous antioxidant defense system. In particular, using DNA microarrays, we demonstrated that quercetin induces glutathione-S-transferase, NADPH-quinone oxidoreductase, thioredoxin reductase, heme oxygenase, and increased reduced glutathione content in primary cardiomyocytes (Angeloni et al., 2008). Using the same I/R model, we also demonstrated that quercetin is able to protect cardiac cells acting as both an antioxidant and a modulator of the signal transduction pathway related to apoptosis (Angeloni et al., 2007). Bartekova et al. (2010) demonstrated that quercetin is able to protect Langendorff perfused rat hearts during 25 min global ischemia at 37 °C. In particular, they observed that quercetin administered before ischemia had a weaker effect on infarct size limitation than quercetin applied during reperfusion, probably due to the vasodilatatory effect of quercetin applied during reperfusion, which has been demonstrated by several authors. Kolchin Iu et al. (1991) observed, in experimental myocardial infarction in dogs, that the administration of quercetin solution (50 mg kg^{-1}) improved the contractile function of the left ventricular myocardium, decreased the incidence of heart rate and conductivity disorders, contributed to limitation of the ischemic damage area, exerted the protective effect on the ultrastructure of the coronary arteries, improved the coronary circulation, and prevented the intravascular thrombus formation. In addition, Ikizler et al. (2007) reported that quercetin has the capacity to protect the myocardial tissue against global ischemia and reperfusion injury with a higher efficacy if the molecule is administered as a chronic treatment protocol for 7 days rather than an acute therapy. The cardioprotective action of quercetin was also supported by Annapurna et al. (2009) who observed the cardioprotective effects of quercetin and rutin in I/R injury in both normal and diabetic rats and ascribed the protection in part to the attenuation of oxidative stress and moderate increment in antioxidant reserves. Interestingly, in this study, the authors observed a strong cardioprotection of quercetin on acute treatment just before reperfusion. A possible rationale for the discrepancies between these two studies is the route of administration of drug, which affects its availability in the circulatory system. In the study by Annapurna et al., quercetin was administered through the intraperitoneal route, which ensures better absorption of the drug than the oral route used by Ikizler.

I/R can also lead to an acute inflammatory process with the release of multiple cytokines and reactive oxygen species. Reperfusion is generally associated with a reduction of endogenous NO production resulting from endothelial dysfunction and tissue damage linked to neutrophil infiltration. Experimental studies in animals have shown that quercetin reduces the contractile dysfunction of the heart, the infarct size, and the pattern of protein expression changes (including iNOS and NADPH oxidase isoforms NOX2) induced by cardiac ischemia.

Another mechanism by which quercetin protects against I/R injury is its ability to reduce the expression of matrix metalloproteinases (MMP-2 and MMP-9) and to stabilize the atherosclerotic plaque. In fact, most acute coronary events result from a rupture in the atherosclerotic plaque, thrombus formation, and the subsequent myocardial ischemia.

2.6 Cardiac Hypertrophy

Cardiac hypertrophy is a homeostatic response to diverse pathophysiological stimuli characterized by thickening of the heart muscle. Although cardiac hypertrophy is a compensatory response in the early phase, it is followed by decompensation and can lead to heart failure. Inhibition of cardiac hypertrophy leads to a significant reduction in cardiovascular mortality and morbidity.

It has been reported that quercetin counteracts cardiomyocyte hypertrophy induced by angiotensin II, inhibiting both protein kinase C and tyrosine protein kinase. Yoshizumi et al. (2001) demonstrated that quercetin is able to prevent angiotensin-II-induced vascular smooth muscle cell hypertrophy, thanks to its inhibitory effect on Src homology and collagen (Shc)-dependent and phosphatidylinositol 3-kinase-dependent JNK activation. A study carried out on rats consuming a standard or quercetin supplemented chow before abdominal aortic constriction showed that quercetin supplementation prevented cardiac hypertrophy compared with untreated rats (Jalili et al., 2006).

In a recent study, Han et al. (2009) demonstrated that quercetin appears to block the development of cardiac hypertrophy induced by pressure overload in rats and that these effects may be mediated through reduced oxidant status and inhibition of ERK1/2, p38 MAP kinase, Akt, and GSK-3-beta activities. Yoshizumi et al. (2002) reported that quercetin 3-O-β-glucuronide prevents angiotensin-II-induced vascular smooth muscle cell hypertrophy through the inhibition of JNK and the AP-1 signaling pathways. Another quercetin *in vivo* metabolite, 3,3′,4′,5,7-pentamethylquercetin, a methylated form of quercetin, reduces angiotensin-II-induced cardiac hypertrophy in rats (Mao et al., 2009).

3. SAFETY OF QUERCETIN

Quercetin becomes oxidized into various oxidation products during its antioxidative activities. It has been shown that oxidation products such as semiquinone radicals and quinones display various toxic effects due to their ability of arylating protein thiols. Moreover, quercetin quinone is very reactive toward thiols and can instantaneously form an adduct with GSH, giving GSQ. GSQ is not stable and dissociates continuously into GSH and QQ with a half-life of 2 min, but as long as the GSH concentration is high, it will offer protection against quercetin quinone by trapping it as GSQ. However, when the GSH concentration is low, the dissociated quercetin quinone will react with other thiol groups, leading to toxic effects such as increased membrane permeability or loss of activity of enzymes that contain a critical SH-group. The toxicity induced by quercetin quinone has been defined as the quercetin paradox, that is, the conversion of quercetin into a potential toxic product while offering protection by scavenging ROS. However, to our knowledge, no studies have observed the *in vivo* formation and possible toxicity of quercetin quinone. Quercetin has also been reported to display genotoxic effects *in vitro*.

Interestingly, these mutagenic effects of quercetin are predominantly shown in bacteria and are suggested to require quinone formation as mediators as well. However, more recent *in vitro* studies indicated that quercetin is protective against genotoxicants and therefore regarded as antimutagenic. In 1999, the International Agency for Research on Cancer concluded that quercetin is not classified as carcinogenic to humans. It has also been demonstrated that quercetin, administered orally to rats at dose levels of up to 2000 mg kg^{-1} body weight, did not show evidences of carcinogenicity or genotoxic potential, and a recent comprehensive overview and critical examination of the scientific literature supported the safety of quercetin (Harwood et al., 2007). In conclusion, with particular respect to humans, quercetin is well tolerated as an addition to food.

GLOSSARY

Bioavailability Describes the amount of a substance that reaches the blood stream or becomes available at the targeted place in the body after administration.

Matrix metalloproteinases (MMPs) are zinc-dependent endopeptidases that are capable of degrading all kinds of extracellular matrix proteins. These enzymes play a key role in many biological processes such as embryogenesis, wound healing, and angiogenesis; normal tissue remodeling; and in diseases such as atheroma, cancer, arthritis, and tissue ulceration.

NF-κB is a transcription factor found in almost all animal cell types and is involved in cellular responses to stimuli such as stress, cytokines, free radicals, ultraviolet irradiation, and oxidized LDL. NF-κB plays a fundamental role in regulating the immune response to infection.

Nuclear factor (erythroid-derived 2)-like 2 (Nrf2) is the master transcription factor that regulates the antioxidant response because it is able to induce fundamental antioxidant genes.

Oxidative stress condition in which the presence of excessive levels of reactive oxygen/nitrogen species in the cell is not balanced by antioxidants.

Tumor necrosis factor α (TNFα) is a multifunctional cytokine that possesses a wide range of proinflammatory actions with effects on lipid metabolism, coagulation, insulin resistance, and the function of endothelial cells lining blood vessels. TNF is described as a regulatory cytokine because it controls the release of other cytokines necessary to counteract disease or infection.

REFERENCES

Angeloni, C., Spencer, J.P., Leoncini, E., Biagi, P.L., Hrelia, S., 2007. Role of quercetin and its in vivo metabolites in protecting H9c2 cells against oxidative stress. Biochimie 89, 73–82.

Angeloni, C., Leoncini, E., Malaguti, M., et al., 2008. Role of quercetin in modulating rat cardiomyocyte gene expression profile. American Journal of Physiology. Heart and Circulatory Physiology 294, H1233–H1243.

Annapurna, A., Reddy, C.S., Akondi, R.B., Rao, S.R., 2009. Cardioprotective actions of two bioflavonoids, quercetin and rutin, in experimental myocardial infarction in both normal and streptozotocin-induced type I diabetic rats. Journal of Pharmacy and Pharmacology 61, 1365–1374.

Bartekova, M., Carnicka, S., Pancza, D., et al., 2010. Acute treatment with polyphenol quercetin improves postischemic recovery of isolated perfused rat hearts after global ischemia. Canadian Journal of Physiology and Pharmacology 88, 465–471.

Boesch-Saadatmandi, C., Loboda, A., Wagner, A.E., et al., 2010. Effect of quercetin and its metabolites isorhamnetin and quercetin-3-glucuronide on inflammatory gene expression: role of miR-155. The Journal of Nutritional Biochemistry 22, 293–299.

Comalada, M., Ballester, I., Bailon, E., et al., 2006. Inhibition of pro-inflammatory markers in primary bone marrow-derived mouse macrophages by naturally occurring flavonoids: analysis of the structure–activity relationship. Biochemical Pharmacology 72, 1010–1021.

Duarte, J., Perez-Palencia, R., Vargas, F., et al., 2001. Antihypertensive effects of the flavonoid quercetin in spontaneously hypertensive rats. British Journal of Pharmacology 133, 117–124.

Egert, S., Wolffram, S., Bosy-Westphal, A., et al., 2008. Daily quercetin supplementation dose-dependently increases plasma quercetin concentrations in healthy humans. Journal of Nutrition 138, 1615–1621.

Emura, K., Yokomizo, A., Toyoshi, T., Moriwaki, M., 2007. Effect of enzymatically modified isoquercitrin in spontaneously hypertensive rats. Journal of Nutritional Science and Vitaminology (Tokyo) 53, 68–74.

Galisteo, M., Garcia-Saura, M.F., Jimenez, R., et al., 2004. Effects of chronic quercetin treatment on antioxidant defence system and oxidative status of deoxycorticosterone acetate-salt-hypertensive rats. Molecular and Cellular Biochemistry 259, 91–99.

Gryglewski, R.J., Korbut, R., Robak, J., Swies, J., 1987. On the mechanism of antithrombotic action of flavonoids. Biochemical Pharmacology 36, 317–322.

Han, J.J., Hao, J., Kim, C.H., et al., 2009. Quercetin prevents cardiac hypertrophy induced by pressure overload in rats. Journal of Veterinary Medical Science 71, 737–743.

Harwood, M., Danielewska-Nikiel, B., Borzelleca, J.F., et al., 2007. A critical review of the data related to the safety of quercetin and lack of evidence of in vivo toxicity, including lack of genotoxic/carcinogenic properties. Food and Chemical Toxicology 45, 2179–2205.

Ikizler, M., Erkasap, N., Dernek, S., Kural, T., Kaygisiz, Z., 2007. Dietary polyphenol quercetin protects rat hearts during reperfusion: enhanced antioxidant capacity with chronic treatment. Anadolu Kardiyoloji Dergisi 7, 404–410.

Jalili, T., Carlstrom, J., Kim, S., et al., 2006. Quercetin-supplemented diets lower blood pressure and attenuate cardiac hypertrophy in rats with aortic constriction. Journal of Cardiovascular Pharmacology 47, 531–541.

Kolchin Iu, N., Maksiutina, N.P., Balanda, P.P., et al., 1991. The cardioprotective action of quercetin in experimental occlusion and reperfusion of the coronary artery in dogs. Farmakologiia i Toksikologiia 54, 20–23.

Kottra, G., Daniel, H., 2007. Flavonoid glycosides are not transported by the human Na+/glucose transporter when expressed in Xenopus laevis oocytes, but effectively inhibit electrogenic glucose uptake. Journal of Pharmacology and Experimental Therapeutics 322, 829–835.

Leckey, L.C., Garige, M., Varatharajalu, R., et al., 2010. Quercetin and ethanol attenuate the progression of atherosclerotic plaques with concomitant up regulation of paraoxonase1 (PON1) gene expression and PON1 activity in LDLR-/- mice. Alcoholism, Clinical and Experimental Research 34, 1535–1542.

Loke, W.M., Proudfoot, J.M., Hodgson, J.M., et al., 2010. Specific dietary polyphenols attenuate atherosclerosis in apolipoprotein E-knockout mice by alleviating inflammation and endothelial dysfunction. Arteriosclerosis, Thrombosis, and Vascular Biology 30, 749–757.

Mackraj, I., Govender, T., Ramesar, S., 2008. The antihypertensive effects of quercetin in a salt-sensitive model of hypertension. Journal of Cardiovascular Pharmacology 51, 239–245.

Maffei, F., Tarozzi, A., Carbone, F., et al., 2007. Relevance of apple consumption for protection against oxidative damage induced by hydrogen peroxide in human lymphocytes. British Journal of Nutrition 97, 921–927.

Mao, Z., Liang, Y., Du, X., Sun, Z., 2009. 3,3′,4′,5,7-Pentamethylquercetin reduces angiotensin II-induced cardiac hypertrophy and apoptosis in rats. Canadian Journal of Physiology and Pharmacology 87, 720–728.

Navarro-Nunez, L., Rivera, J., Guerrero, J.A., et al., 2009. Differential effects of quercetin, apigenin and genistein on signalling pathways of protease-activated receptors PAR(1) and PAR(4) in platelets. British Journal of Pharmacology 158, 1548–1556.

Rivera, L., Moron, R., Sanchez, M., Zarzuelo, A., Galisteo, M., 2008. Quercetin ameliorates metabolic syndrome and improves the inflammatory status in obese Zucker rats. Obesity (Silver Spring) 16, 2081–2087.

Winterbone, M.S., Tribolo, S., Needs, P.W., Kroon, P.A., Hughes, D.A., 2009. Physiologically relevant metabolites of quercetin have no effect on adhesion molecule or chemokine expression in human vascular smooth muscle cells. Atherosclerosis 202, 431–438.

Wright, B., Moraes, L.A., Kemp, C.F., et al., 2010. A structural basis for the inhibition of collagen-stimulated platelet function by quercetin and structurally related flavonoids. British Journal of Pharmacology 159, 1312–1325.

Xu, Y.C., Leung, S.W., Yeung, D.K., et al., 2007. Structure–activity relationships of flavonoids for vascular relaxation in porcine coronary artery. Phytochemistry 68, 1179–1188.

Yoshizumi, M., Tsuchiya, K., Kirima, K., et al., 2001. Quercetin inhibits Shc- and phosphatidylinositol 3-kinase-mediated c-Jun N-terminal kinase activation by angiotensin II in cultured rat aortic smooth muscle cells. Molecular Pharmacology 60, 656–665.

Yoshizumi, M., Tsuchiya, K., Suzaki, Y., et al., 2002. Quercetin glucuronide prevents VSMC hypertrophy by angiotensin II via the inhibition of JNK and AP-1 signaling pathway. Biochemical and Biophysical Research Communications 293, 1458–1465.

You, K.M., Jong, H.G., Kim, H.P., 1999. Inhibition of cyclooxygenase/lipoxygenase from human platelets by polyhydroxylated/methoxylated flavonoids isolated from medicinal plants. Archives of Pharmacal Research 22, 18–24.

FURTHER READING

Bischoff, S.C., 2008. Quercetin: potentials in the prevention and therapy of disease. Current Opinion in Clinical Nutrition and Metabolic Care 11, 733–740.

Boots, A.W., Li, H., Schins, R.P., et al., 2007. The quercetin paradox. Toxicology and Applied Pharmacology 222, 89–96.

Boots, A.W., Haenen, G.R., Bast, A., 2008. Health effects of quercetin: from antioxidant to nutraceutical. European Journal of Pharmacology 585, 325–337.

Crozier, A., Jaganath, I.B., Clifford, M.N., 2009. Dietary phenolics: chemistry, bioavailability and effects on health. Natural Product Reports 26, 1001–1043.

Moon, Y.J., Wang, L., DiCenzo, R., Morris, M.E., 2008. Quercetin pharmacokinetics in humans. Biopharmaceutics and Drug Disposition 29, 205–217.

Murota, K., Terao, J., 2003. Antioxidative flavonoid quercetin: implication of its intestinal absorption and metabolism. Archives of Biochemistry and Biophysics 417, 12–17.

Nikolic, M., Nikic, D., Petrovic, B., 2008. Fruit and vegetable intake and the risk for developing coronary heart disease. Central European Journal of Public Health 16, 17–20.

Perez-Vizcaino, F., Duarte, J., 2010. Flavonols and cardiovascular disease. Molecular Aspects of Medicine 31, 478–494.

Perez-Vizcaino, F., Duarte, J., Jimenez, R., Santos-Buelga, C., Osuna, A., 2009. Antihypertensive effects of the flavonoid quercetin. Pharmacological Reports 61, 67–75.

Williams, R.J., Spencer, J.P., Rice-Evans, C., 2004. Flavonoids: antioxidants or signalling molecules? Free Radical Biology and Medicine 36, 838–849.

CHAPTER 14

Vitamin K, Coronary Calcification and Risk of Cardiovascular Disease

G.W. Dalmeijer, Y.T. van der Schouw, J.W.J. Beulens
University Medical Center Utrecht, Utrecht, The Netherlands

1. VITAMIN K

Vitamin K was discovered in the early 1930s by the nutritional biochemist Hendrik Dam as an antihemorrhagic factor in chickens (Dam and Schonheyder, 1934). Vitamin K is a fat-soluble vitamin that occurs in two biologically active forms; phylloquinone (vitamin K_1) and menaquinones (vitamin K_2) with side chains based on a number of repeating prenyl units; this number being given as a suffix, that is, menaquinone-n, (MK-n). Vitamin K is a group name for a number of related compounds, which have a 2-methylated-1,4-naphthoquinone ring structure in common, and vary in the aliphatic side chain attached at the 3-position (Figure 14.1). It is generally accepted that the naphthoquinone ring is the functional group, and therefore the mechanism of action is similar for all K-vitamins. However, side-chain-related differences may be expected with respect to intestinal absorption, transport, tissue distribution, and bio-availability. These differences are caused by the different hydrophobicity of the various side chains and by the different food matrices in which they occur (Cranenburg et al., 2007).

The major dietary source of vitamin K is the plant form, phylloquinone, which is widely distributed in foods. Leafy green vegetables and vegetable oils (soybean, cottonseed, canola, and olives) are the largest contributors to dietary intakes (Booth et al., 1996). Dietary relevant menaquinones range from MK-4 through MK-10. The richest dietary sources of menaquinones are fermented foods. For that reason, there is a geographic distribution in menaquinone intake. In the Western diet, the richest dietary sources of menaquinones are cheese and curd (MK-8 and MK-9), whereas in Japan, natto, fermented soy beans, (MK-7) is the richest dietary source of menaquinones (Shearer and Newman, 2008). Many of the longer-chain menaquinones are also produced by intestinal bacteria, and historically these forms were believed to be an important source of vitamin K. However, their contribution to vitamin K status is now considered insignificant; their low bioactivity may be due to their location in bacterial membranes and consequent poor absorption from the gut (Cranenburg et al., 2007).

It has been demonstrated that the bioavailability of vitamin K is dependent on the nature of the food matrix (Cranenburg et al., 2007). It was found that phylloquinone

Bioactive Food as Dietary Interventions for Cardiovascular Disease
http://dx.doi.org/10.1016/B978-0-12-396485-4.00012-8

© 2013 Elsevier Inc.
All rights reserved.

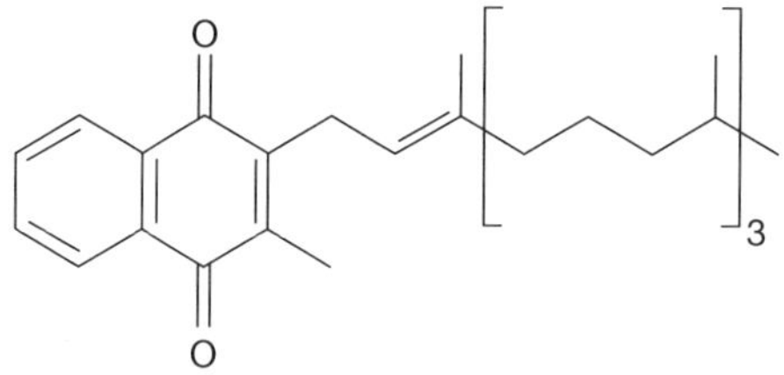

Figure 14.1 Phylloquinone and menaquinone.

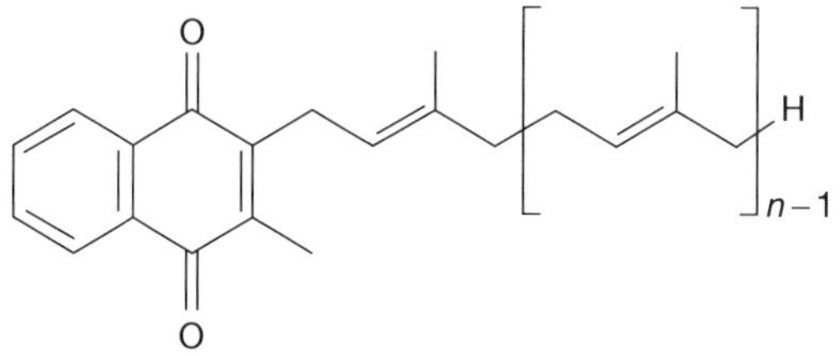

absorption from vegetables is very poor, namely 5–10% without concomitant fat intake and 10–15% if taken together with fat, whereas menaquinone absorption from dairy products and natto was much better, probably almost complete. Another difference between phylloquinone and the long-chain menaquinones (not MK-4) is the half-life time. Phylloquinone has a disappearance curve with an apparent half-life time of 1.5 h, whereas menaquinones have more complex disappearance curves with a very long half-life time (Schurgers et al., 2007b).

The adequate intake for vitamin K is established at 90 µg per day for women and 120 µg per day for men, based on median intakes from food as estimated from NHANES III (1998–1994) (National Research Council, 2000). These recommendations are set to meet requirements for hemostasis. The liver as main site for clotting factor synthesis, however, efficiently extracts vitamin K from the circulation, which could lead to insufficient amount to cover requirements of extra-hepatic tissues, including the vascular wall (Cranenburg et al., 2007). However, this distribution could differ for phylloquinone and menaquinones.

Phylloquinone is predominantly transported with the triacylglycerol-rich fraction, which is mainly cleared by the liver. Phylloquinone is therefore cleared very effectively from circulation by the liver to function as a cofactor for proteins in blood coagulation (Cranenburg et al., 2007). Accumulation and utilization of phylloquinone in extra-hepatic tissues such as the vessel wall is therefore lower than that in hepatic tissues. Menaquinones, on the other hand, are found in both triacylglycerol-rich lipoprotein and low-density lipoprotein, mainly though these low-density lipoprotein menaquinones are

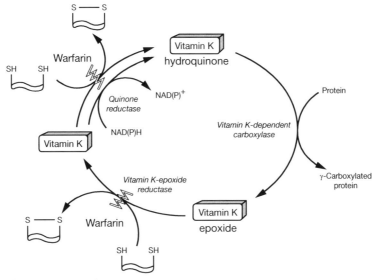

Figure 14.2 The vitamin K cycle.

transported to extra-hepatic tissues. This is confirmed by higher accumulation and utilization of menaquinone-4 than phylloquinone in extra-hepatic tissues such as the vessel wall (Spronk et al., 2003).

As a cofactor to the carboxylase that generates gamma–carboxyglutamic acid, vitamin K undergoes a cycle of oxidation and reduction that allows reuse (see Figure 14.2). Vitamin K-epoxide reductase (VKOR) ensures the reutilization of vitamin K after it has been oxidized in the carboxylase reaction. On a molecular level, VKOR reduces vitamin K epoxide (KO) in two steps: first to vitamin K quinine (K), and subsequently to vitamin K hydroquinone (KH$_2$), the latter being the active cofactor of gamma–glutamyl carboxylase (GGCX); this process is shown in Figure 14.2. Anticoagulants such as warfarin block the reduction of vitamin K oxide to vitamin K, explaining their antagonistic effects on this cycle. Polymorphisms of VKORC1 and GGCX affect the necessary warfarin dose in coagulation (Mushiroda et al., 2006). Such single nucleotide polymorphisms (SNPs) could therefore also influence coronary calcification.

Vitamin K functions as a cofactor for the enzyme GGCX, catalyzing the gamma–glutamyl carboxylation of certain glutamic acid residues (Gla) in proteins (Cranenburg et al., 2007). These vitamin K–dependent proteins include the hepatic–coagulation factors prothrombin, factors VII, IX, and X (Cranenburg et al., 2007). Vitamin K also functions as a cofactor for extra-hepatic Gla-proteins in bone, such as osteocalcin, and the vessel wall, such as matrix Gla-protein (MGP). MGP is a powerful inhibitor of vascular calcification (Shanahan et al., 1998). Coronary calcification is a strong, independent predictor of coronary events. MGP knock-out mice develop severe vascular calcification

(Luo et al., 1997). In humans, MGP loss-of-function mutations also increase coronary calcification, and impaired carboxylation of MGP is associated with vascular calcification (Cranenburg et al., 2007). The anticoagulant warfarin, a vitamin K antagonist, indeed inhibits carboxylation not only of coagulation factors but also of MGP and increases vascular calcification in humans and rats (Koos et al., 2005; Price et al., 1998). These effects are prevented in warfarin-treated rats by vitamin K-rich diets (Schurgers et al., 2007a). Vitamin K could therefore reduce coronary calcification and eventually cardiovascular disease (CVD) through carboxylation of MGP (see Figure 14.2).

To further support this hypothesis, a few studies investigated whether VKORC1 SNPs associated with reduced formation of the active vitamin K form increased CVD risk. Two of these studies conclude that VKORC1 may serve as a novel genetic marker for the risk of CVD (Teichert et al., 2008; Wang et al., 2006), while Watzka et al. (2007) did not find an association between VKORC1 genotype and CVD risk. Similarly, the first human studies investigating the association between plasma MGP and CVD also showed inconsistent results (O'Donnell et al., 2006; Schurgers et al., 2005). However, this is probably due to the measurement of total plasma MGP instead of caroboxylated or uncarboxylated MGP.

In the next part, the evidence on the relations between vitamin K intake and arterial calcification, cardiovascular disease (CHD), and stroke risk is reviewed.

2. VITAMIN K AND ARTERIAL CALCIFICATION

While the genetic and biochemical studies establish that inadequate carboxylation of MGP results in abnormal calcification, there are limited observational data linking an inadequate intake of vitamin K with vascular calcification (Table 14.1).

One study investigated the association between vitamin K intake and aortic atherosclerosis. In this nested case-control study, postmenopausal women ($n = 113$) with aortic atherosclerosis reported 42.9 μg per day (95% confidence interval (CI): −6.6; 92.5) lower vitamin K intake than women without atherosclerosis, after adjustment for age. In the age group 60–69 years, the vitamin K intake was 74.8 μg per day (95% CI: 135.1; 14.6) lower in the women with calcification, while there was no significant difference in the 70–79 age group (Jie et al., 1995).

2.1 Phylloquinone

Four cross-sectional studies investigated the association between phylloquinone intake and calcification, but none of these found an association. In the Rotterdam cohort study (Geleijnse et al., 2004), the mean intake of phylloquinone was similar across categories of aortic calcification (249.2, 249.0, and 245.0 μg per day for mild, moderate, and severe stages, respectively). Cross-sectional analyses from this study showed that the intake of phylloquinone was not significantly associated with moderate or severe aortic

Table 14.1 Vitamin K and Arterial Calcification

Study	Study design	Participants	Measurement	Exposure/intervention	Endpoint	Result
Jie et al. (1995)	Nested case–control study	34 women with aortic calcification and 79 without aortic calcification	FFQ	Vitamin K intake: Cases: 189.9 ± 15.5 µg per day Controls: 243.6 ± 15.32 µg per day	Aortic atherosclerosis	Phylloquinone ↓
Villines et al. (2005)	Cross-sectional study	807 participants, aged 39–45 years	The Block Dietary Questionnaire	Phylloquinone intake: 115.2 ± 79.0 µg per day	CAC	Phylloquinone ↔
Maas et al. (2007b)	Cross-sectional study	1689 women, aged 49–70 years	FFQ	Phylloquinone intake: 216.6 µg per day (BAC+) and 210.7 µg per day (BAC−) Menaquinone intake: 26.9 µg per day (BAC+) and 29.4 µg per day (BAC−)	BAC	Phylloquinone ↔ Menaquinone ↔
Beulens et al. (2009)	Cross-sectional study	564 postmenopausal women, aged 49–70 years	FFQ	Phylloquinone intake: 217.0 ± 92.3 µg per day Menaquinone intake: 31.6 ± 12.3 µg per day	CAC	Phylloquinone ↔ Menaquinone ↓
Geleijnse et al. (2004)	Cross-sectional study	4473 men and women, aged 55 years and over	FFQ	Phylloquinone intake: men; 257.1 ± 116.1 µg per day, women; 244.3 ± 131.9 µg per day Menaquinone intake: men; 30.8 ± 18.0 µg per day, women; 27.0 ± 15.1 µg per day	CAC	Phylloquinone ↔ Menaquinone ↓

Continued

Table 14.1 Vitamin K and Arterial Calcification—cont'd

Study	Study design	Participants	Measurement	Exposure/intervention	Endpoint	Result
Braam et al. (2004)	RCT	181 women, aged 50–60 years	Group 1: placebo Group 2: supplement; minerals, vitamin D Group 3: Supplement: minerals vitamin D, phylloquinone	1 mg per day phylloquinone for 3 years	Elastic properties	Phylloquinone ↓
Shea et al. (2009)	RCT	388 adults, aged 60–80 years	Group 1: Multivitamin Group 2: Multivitamin with phylloquinone	Intervention: 500 µg per day phylloquinone for 3 years	CAC	Phylloquinone ↓

↑ High phylloquinone/menaquinone intake was associated with increased calcification.
↓ High phylloquinone/menaquinone intake was associated with reduced calcification.
↔ There was no association between phylloquinone/menaquinone intake and calcification.

calcification (Geleijnse et al., 2004). Villines et al. (2005) studied 807 consecutive active-duty US Army personnel, 39–45 years old, without known CHD and showed that the mean intake of phylloquinone was similar in subjects with (114.2 ± 78.7 µg per day) and without (119.2 ± 80.3 µg per day) coronary artery calcification (CAC). After full adjustment, there was no association between phylloquinone intake and the presence of CAC. Maas et al. (2007b) carried out a study among 1689 women, aged 49–70 years. The prevalence of breast arterial calcification (BAC) was similar (11%) across quartiles of phylloquinone intake. However, the clinical significance of breast artery calcification for future coronary disease is controversial, because its association with prevalent coronary heart disease is weak. In a study among 564 postmenopausal women, Beulens et al. (2009) found that phylloquinone intake was not associated with CAC with a relative risk (RR) of 1.17 (95% CI: 0.96; 1.42; $p_{trend} = 0.11$) of the highest versus the lowest quartile.

Two randomized trials investigated the association between phylloquinone intake and calcification. Braam et al. (2004) assessed the effect of 3 years of daily phylloquinone (1 mg per day), minerals, and vitamin D supplementation on vascular health in 181 post-menopausal women. They measure the vessel wall characteristics of the common carotid artery with ultrasound. The investigators concluded that a supplement containing phylloquinone, minerals, and vitamin D had a beneficial effect on the elastic properties of the arterial vessel wall. However, owing to the design of the study, it was not possible to distinguish whether these effects are due to phylloquinone alone or due to the combination of phylloquinone, minerals, and vitamin D. Shea et al. (2009) performed a randomized trial in 388 healthy older adults; 200 adults received a multivitamin with an additional 500 µg per day of phylloquinone, and 188 adults received a multivitamin alone. There was no difference in CAC progression between the two groups. However, in a subgroup analysis of subjects who were $\geq 85\%$ adherent to supplementation, there was less CAC progression in the phylloquinone group than in the control group ($p = 0.03$). Furthermore, when restricting to subjects with pre-existing CAC, those who received phylloquinone supplements had 6% less progression than did those who received the multivitamin alone ($p = 0.04$).

Overall, the two intervention studies with phylloquinone supplementation found small beneficial effects of phylloquinone intake on the arterial vessel wall, while none of the observational studies observed an association between phylloquinone intake and calcification. This discrepancy could be explained by the relative high doses of phylloquinone in the intervention studies compared with phylloquinone intake in the observational studies. Doses of 1 mg per day and 0.5 mg per day were used in the trials, while the mean intake of phylloquinone in the observational studies varied between 0.1 and 0.25 mg per day. It could also be explained by the better absorption of phylloquinone from supplements compared with phylloquinone from food products (Schurgers and Vermeer, 2000). The randomized trials, however, do provide evidence that high doses of phylloquinone can indeed reduce coronary calcification.

2.2 Menaquinones

Three of the four previously mentioned cross-sectional studies also investigated associ-ations of menaquinones intake and coronary calcification (Beulens et al., 2009; Geleijnse et al., 2004; Maas et al., 2007a). In the Rotterdam study, Geleijnse et al. (2004) found that menaquinones intake was lower in subjects with severe aortic calcification (25.6 µg per day) than in subjects with moderate or mild calcification (28.6 and 28.8 µg per day, respectively; $p = 0.001$). For severe calcification, a strong inverse relationship with mena-quinone intake was found with odds ratios (ORs) for severe calcification of 0.71 (95% CI: 0.50, 1.00) and 0.48 (95% CI; 0.32, 0.71) in the mid- and upper tertiles of menaquinones intake respectively, compared with the lower tertile. Maas et al. (2007a) showed that the prevalence of BAC was less common in the highest (9%) quartile of menaquinones in-take, compared with the lowest quartile (13%). This study by Geleijnse et al. (2004) showed a similar association with an OR of 0.7 (95% CI: 0.5; 1.1), although it did not reach significance. Finally, Beulens et al. (2009) showed that high menaquinones intake was associated with reduced CAC with an RR of 0.80 (95% CI: 0.65; 0.98; $p_{trend} = 0.03$) of the highest versus the lowest quartile. In conclusion, high menaquinone intake was associated with a modestly reduced risk of arterial calcification in two of the three cross-sectional studies (Table 14.1) (Beulens et al., 2009; Geleijnse et al., 2004). We are not aware of any randomized trials that investigated the association of menaquinones intake and the risk of arterial calcification.

3. VITAMIN K INTAKE AND RISK OF CORONARY HEART DISEASE

3.1 Phylloquinone

To date, four prospective cohort studies investigated the relation between phylloquinone intake and the risk of coronary heart disease. Erkkila et al. (2005, 2007) investigated the association between phylloquinone intake and CVD risk in two cohorts. In the Nurses' Health Study (Erkkila et al., 2005), over 72 000 female nurses, aged 38–65 years, were followed for 16 years. After adjustment for CHD risk factors, diet, and lifestyle, high phylloquinone intake was associated with a decreased risk of CHD with an RR of 0.84 (95% CI: 0.71; 1.00) for the highest versus lowest quartile. In a subsequent study among 40 087 men who participated in the Health Professionals' Follow-up Study, though, a significantly reduced risk was only observed in the age-adjusted model (RR: 0.79; 95% CI: 0.69; 0.91) (Erkkila et al., 2007). After adjustment for CHD risk factors, diet, and lifestyle, the association attenuated to a nonsignificant model (RR: 0.91; 95% CI: 0.77; 1.06). The authors therefore concluded that phylloquinone intake may just be a marker for a heart-healthy diet instead of biologically linked to CHD.

Similarly, in the Rotterdam cohort, Geleijnse et al. (2004) showed that after adjust-ment for CHD risk factors, diet, and lifestyle, high phylloquinone intake was not associated with a decreased risk of CHD with an RR of 0.89 (95% CI: 0.63; 1.25) for the highest versus the lowest tertile. Finally, in the Prospect-EPIC cohort, phylloquinone intake was not associated with the risk of CHD (HR: 1.00; 95% CI: 1.00; 1.02) after adjustment for CHD risk factors, diet, and lifestyle (Gast et al., 2009).

In conclusion, high phylloquinone intake has not been associated with a reduced risk of CHD in four cohort studies once the statistical analysis is adjusted for CHD risk factors, diet, and lifestyle factors associated with coronary heart disease (Table 14.2).

3.2 Menaquinones

Two of the previously mentioned cohort studies also investigated the relation of mena-quinones intake with the risk of CHD. In the Rotterdam cohort (Geleijnse et al., 2004), the RR of incident CHD was reduced in the upper tertile of menaquinones intake compared with the lower tertile (0.59) (95% CI: 0.40; 0.86). Similarly, the risk of CHD mortality was reduced in the upper tertile of menaquinone intake compared with the lowest tertile (0.43) (95% CI: 0.24; 0.77). In the prospect-EPIC cohort (Gast et al., 2009), the investigators also observed an inverse association between menaquinone intake and the risk of CHD with a hazard ratio (HR) of 0.91 (95% CI: 0.85; 1.00, p-value 0.08) per 10 µg per day of menaquinones intake. This association was mainly due to menaquinone subtypes MK-7, MK-8, and MK-9.

The two cohort studies (Gast et al., 2009; Geleijnse et al., 2004), which examined the effects of menaquinones intake on the incidence of CHD, reported a significantly reduced risk of CHD with higher menaquinone intake (Table 14.2). These findings suggest that an adequate intake of menaquinone could be important for CHD prevention.

4. VITAMIN K INTAKE AND RISK OF STROKE

Two cohort studies, Nurses' Health Study (Erkkila et al., 2005) and the Health Professionals Study (Erkkila et al., 2007), investigated the association between phylloquinone intake and the incidence of stroke (Table 14.3). Neither study found significant association between phylloquinone and the incidence of stroke. The association between menaquinones intake and the incidence of stroke has not been investigated to date.

5. CONCLUSION

Although animal experiments and other basic studies show compelling evidence linking vitamin K intake to a reduced coronary calcification and risk of CVD, the evidence from human observational and intervention studies is scarce and inconsistent. Observational studies have shown no associations between the intake of phylloquinone and arterial calcification, incidence of CHD, or stroke. Nevertheless, the results of intervention studies look promising as they showed improved vascular elasticity and reduced progression

Table 14.2 Vitamin K Intake and Risk of Coronary Heart Disease

Study	Study design	Participants	Measurement	Exposure/intervention	Endpoint	Result
Erkkila et al. (2005)	Cohort study	72 874 females, aged 38–65 years	Semiquantitative FFQ	Phylloquinone intake: 184 ± 106 μg per day	CHD	Phylloquinone ↔ Menaquinone
Erkkila et al. (2007)	Cohort study	40 087 males, aged 40–75 years	Semiquantitative FFQ	Phylloquinone intake: 165 μg per day	CHD	phylloquinone ↔ Menaquinone ↓
Geleijnse et al. (2004)	Cohort study	4807 adults, aged 55 years and over	FFQ	Phylloquinone intake: men; 257.1 ± 116.1 μg per day, women; 244.3 ± 131.9 μg per day Menaquinone intake: men; 30.8 ± 18.0 μg per day, women; 27.0 ± 15.1 μg per day	CHD	Phylloquinone ↔ Menaquinone ↓
Gast et al. (2009)	Cohort study	16 057 women, aged 49–70 years	FFQ	Phylloquinone intake: 211.7 ± 100.3 μg per day Menaquinone intake: 29.1 ± 12.8 μg per day	CHD	Phylloquinone ↔ Menaquinone ↓

↑ High phylloquinone/menaquinone intake was associated with increased CHD risk.
↓ High phylloquinone/menaquinone intake was associated with reduced CHD risk.
↔ There was no association between phylloquinone/menaquinone intake and CHD risk.

Table 14.3 Vitamin K Intake and Risk of Stroke

Study	Study design	Participants	Measurement	Exposure/ intervention	Endpoint	Result
Erkkila et al. (2005)	Cohort study	72 874 women, aged 38– 65 years	Semiquantitative FFQ	Phylloquinone intake: 184 ± 106 µg per day	Stroke	Phylloquinone $\leftrightarrow$
Erkkila et al. (2007)	Cohort study	40 087 men, aged 40–75 years	Semiquantitative FFQ	Phylloquinone intake: 165 µg per day	Stroke	Phylloquinone $\leftrightarrow$

↑ High phylloquinone intake was associated with increased stroke risk.
↓ High phylloquinone intake was associated with reduced stroke risk.
↔ There was no association between phylloquinone/menaquinone intake and stroke risk.

of coronary calcification after phylloquinone supplementation. The relatively high doses of phylloquinone in the intervention studies or better absorption of phylloquinone supplements could explain these differences (Schurgers and Vermeer, 2000). For menaquinones intake, observational studies consistently show inverse associations of menaquinones intake with arterial calcification and CHD risk. These findings suggest that an adequate intake of menaquinones could be important for arterial calcification reduction and CHD prevention. However, these results should be confirmed by randomized controlled trials of menaquinone supplementation and coronary calcification.

Although the data from animal experiments and certain human observational and intervention studies are promising, the exact role of phylloquinone and menaquinones in the etiology of coronary calcification and cardiovascular disease in human remains to be established. Studies using biomarkers of vitamin K intake and status in relation to cardiovascular diseases and randomized controlled trials on vitamin K intake and coronary calcification are needed to further establish these relations.

REFERENCES

Beulens, J.W., Bots, M.L., Atsma, F., et al., 2009. High dietary menaquinone intake is associated with reduced coronary calcification. Atherosclerosis 203 (2), 489–493.

Booth, S.L., Pennington, J.A., Sadowski, J.A., 1996. Food sources and dietary intakes of vitamin K-1 (phylloquinone) in the American diet: data from the FDA Total Diet Study. Journal of the American Dietetic Association 96 (2), 149–154.

Braam, L.A., Hoeks, A.P., Brouns, F., Hamulyak, K., Gerichhausen, M.J., Vermeer, C., 2004. Beneficial effects of vitamins D and K on the elastic properties of the vessel wall in postmenopausal women: a follow-up study. Thrombosis and Haemostasis 91 (2), 373–380.

Cranenburg, E.C., Schurgers, L.J., Vermeer, C., 2007. Vitamin K: the coagulation vitamin that became omnipotent. Thrombosis and Haemostasis 98 (1), 120–125.

Dam, H., Schonheyder, F., 1934. A deficiency disease in chicks resembling scurvy. Biochemistry Journal 28 (4), 1355–1359.

Erkkila, A.T., Booth, S.L., Hu, F.B., et al., 2005. Phylloquinone intake as a marker for coronary heart disease risk but not stroke in women. European Journal of Clinical Nutrition 59 (2), 196–204.

Erkkila, A.T., Booth, S.L., Hu, F.B., Jacques, P.F., Lichtenstein, A.H., 2007. Phylloquinone intake and risk of cardiovascular diseases in men. Nutrition, Metabolism, and Cardiovascular Diseases 17 (1), 58–62.

Gast, G.C., de Roos, N.M., Sluijs, I., et al., 2009. A high menaquinone intake reduces the incidence of coronary heart disease. Nutrition, Metabolism, and Cardiovascular Diseases 19 (7), 504–510.

Geleijnse, J.M., Vermeer, C., Grobbee, D.E., et al., 2004. Dietary intake of menaquinone is associated with a reduced risk of coronary heart disease: the Rotterdam Study. Journal of Nutrition 134 (11), 3100–3105.

Jie, K.S., Bots, M.L., Vermeer, C., Witteman, J.C., Grobbee, D.E., 1995. Vitamin K intake and osteocalcin levels in women with and without aortic atherosclerosis: a population-based study. Atherosclerosis 116 (1), 117–123.

Koos, R., Mahnken, A.H., Muhlenbruch, G., et al., 2005. Relation of oral anticoagulation to cardiac valvular and coronary calcium assessed by multislice spiral computed tomography. The American Journal of Cardiology 96 (6), 747–749.

Luo, G., Ducy, P., McKee, M.D., et al., 1997. Spontaneous calcification of arteries and cartilage in mice lacking matrix GLA protein. Nature 386 (6620), 78–81.

Maas, A.H., van der Schouw, Y.T., Atsma, F., et al., 2007a. Breast arterial calcifications are correlated with subsequent development of coronary artery calcifications, but their aetiology is predominantly different. European Journal of Radiology 63 (3), 396–400.

Maas, A.H., van der Schouw, Y.T., Beijerinck, D., et al., 2007b. Vitamin K intake and calcifications in breast arteries. Maturitas 56 (3), 273–279.

Mushiroda, T., Ohnishi, Y., Saito, S., et al., 2006. Association of VKORC1 and CYP2C9 polymorphisms with warfarin dose requirements in Japanese patients. Journal of Human Genetics 51 (3), 249–253.

National Research Council, 2000. Dietary Reference Intakes for Vitamin A, Vitamin K, Arsenic, Boron, Chromium, Copper, Iodine, Iron, Manganese, Molybdenum, Nickel, Silicon, Vanadium, and Zinc. National Academy Press, Washington.

O'Donnell, C.J., Shea, M.K., Price, P.A., et al., 2006. Matrix Gla protein is associated with risk factors for atherosclerosis but not with coronary artery calcification. Arteriosclerosis, Thrombosis, and Vascular Biology 26 (12), 2769–2774.

Price, P.A., Faus, S.A., Williamson, M.K., 1998. Warfarin causes rapid calcification of the elastic lamellae in rat arteries and heart valves. Arteriosclerosis, Thrombosis, and Vascular Biology 18 (9), 1400–1407.

Schurgers, L.J., Vermeer, C., 2000. Determination of phylloquinone and menaquinones in food. Effect of food matrix on circulating vitamin K concentrations. Haemostasis 30 (6), 298–307.

Schurgers, L.J., Teunissen, K.J., Knapen, M.H., et al., 2005. Novel conformation-specific antibodies against matrix gamma-carboxyglutamic acid (Gla) protein: undercarboxylated matrix Gla protein as marker for vascular calcification. Arteriosclerosis, Thrombosis, and Vascular Biology 25 (8), 1629–1633.

Schurgers, L.J., Spronk, H.M., Soute, B.A., Schiffers, P.M., DeMey, J.G., Vermeer, C., 2007a. Regression of warfarin-induced medial elastocalcinosis by high intake of vitamin K in rats. Blood 109 (7), 2823–2831.

Schurgers, L.J., Teunissen, K.J., Hamulyak, K., Knapen, M.H., Vik, H., Vermeer, C., 2007b. Vitamin K-containing dietary supplements: comparison of synthetic vitamin K1 and natto-derived menaquinone-7. Blood 109 (8), 3279–3283.

Shanahan, C.M., Proudfoot, D., Farzaneh-Far, A., Weissberg, P.L., 1998. The role of Gla proteins in vascular calcification. Critical Reviews in Eukaryotic Gene Expression 8 (3–4), 357–375.

Shea, M.K., O'Donnell, C.J., Hoffmann, U., et al., 2009. Vitamin K supplementation and progression of coronary artery calcium in older men and women. American Journal of Clinical Nutrition 89 (6), 1799–1807.

Shearer, M.J., Newman, P., 2008. Metabolism and cell biology of vitamin K. Thrombosis and Haemostasis 100 (4), 530–547.

Spronk, H.M., Soute, B.A., Schurgers, L.J., Thijssen, H.H., De Mey, J.G., Vermeer, C., 2003. Tissue-specific utilization of menaquinone-4 results in the prevention of arterial calcification in warfarin-treated rats. Journal of Vascular Research 40 (6), 531–537.

Teichert, M., Visser, L.E., van Schaik, R.H., et al., 2008. Vitamin K epoxide reductase complex subunit 1 (VKORC1) polymorphism and aortic calcification: the Rotterdam Study. Arteriosclerosis, Thrombosis, and Vascular Biology 28 (4), 771–776.

Villines, T.C., Hatzigeorgiou, C., Feuerstein, I.M., O'Malley, P.G., Taylor, A.J., 2005. Vitamin K1 intake and coronary calcification. Coronary Artery Disease 16 (3), 199–203.

Wang, Y., Zhang, W., Zhang, Y., et al., 2006. VKORC1 haplotypes are associated with arterial vascular diseases (stroke, coronary heart disease, and aortic dissection). Circulation 113 (12), 1615–1621.

Watzka, M., Nebel, A., El Mokhtari, N.E., et al., 2007. Functional promoter polymorphism in the VKORC1 gene is no major genetic determinant for coronary heart disease in Northern Germans. Thrombosis and Haemostasis 97 (6), 998–1002.

CHAPTER 15

A Review of the Antioxidant Actions of Three Herbal Medicines (*Crataegus monogyna, Ginkgo biloba,* and *Aesculus hippocastanum*) on the Treatment of Cardiovascular Diseases

L.M. McCune

BotanyDoc Education and Consulting Services, Tucson, AZ, USA

1. INTRODUCTION

According to the Centers for Disease Control and Prevention (CDC) and the American Heart Association, heart disease is the leading cause of death in the United States with a mortality rate of more than a quarter of total deaths in 2004. Risk factors associated with heart disease include inactivity, obesity, diabetes, cigarette smoking, high blood pressure, and high cholesterol (CDC, 2010). Metabolic syndrome, defined as having at least three of the five risk factors (high blood pressure, high cholesterol, high waist circumference, high fasting blood glucose, and high serum triglycerides) had a prevalence of 34% in the United States between the years 2003 and 2006. High blood pressure and cardiovascular damage are also key factors in the development of many of the complications of heart disease and diabetes such as kidney disease and peripheral neuropathies (Lloyd-Jones et al., 2010). Angina (pain from decreased blood flow to the heart), coronary syndrome, heart failure, pulmonary embolism, arrhythmias, aortic valve disorders, or bacterial endocarditis are some of the cardiovascular diseases that account for the most deaths worldwide, with heart disease responsible for 7.2 million deaths in 2004 (WHO, 2010).

Low levels of endogenous (human produced) antioxidants are common to those diagnosed with cardiovascular disease, diabetes, or metabolic syndrome. Antioxidants, whether endogenous or exogenous/dietary, have the ability to decrease many of the components and complications of cardiovascular diseases including the damage caused by oxidants in the aftermath of ischemic heart failure. The ability of exogenous antioxidants to influence health parameters may be through indirect action on endogenous antioxidants and their effects on enzyme systems. Atherosclerosis, the buildup of inflammation, foam cells, platelets, fatty deposits, and scar tissue in arteries, is one of the leading

© 2013 Elsevier Inc.
All rights reserved.

components of cardiovascular diseases. The levels of endogenous antioxidants are important to stem the damage caused by atherosclerosis, ischemia events, hypercholesterolemia, hypertriglyceridemia, and hyperglycemia. Flavonoids and other antioxidants from plant products have the ability to influence cholesterol, triglyceride metabolism, and the induction of inflammatory cytokines (Zern and Fernandez, 2005). Experiments on cardiovascular parameters frequently focus on the ability of exogenous antioxidant compounds to scavenge oxidants, reduce inflammation, affect LDL levels, reduce platelet aggregation, and affect endothelium relaxation and coronary contractions.

Many research articles have ascribed the benefits of various fruit and vegetable consumption in reducing the risk of cardiovascular diseases to their antioxidant flavonoids, carotenoids, vitamin C/ascorbic acid, and vitamin E/tocopherol content. The American Heart Association promotes the consumption of fruits and vegetables in part because, as shown in the Zutphen Elderly Study, the consumption of flavonoids was inversely related to coronary heart disease incidence (Howard and Kritchevsky, 1997). In addition, the protective health benefits of the so-called 'French Paradox' and 'Mediterranean diet' has been attributed to the flavonoids and other antioxidants in the grapes, fruits, vegetables, and nuts that are abundant in these diets (Zern and Fernandez, 2005). Over 5000 flavonoids have been characterized including the well-represented myricetin, kaempferol, and quercetin. Their strong antioxidant activity is often associated with available hydroxyl groups and double bond structures.

Some of the specific food plants that have had extensive research related to their antioxidant and cardioprotective abilities include tea, cocoa, wine/grapes, cranberry, soy, garlic and onion, turmeric, fenugreek, ginger, and capsaicin species. Another source of plant antioxidants and cardiovascular protectant compounds is herbal medicines. The German Commission E Monographs (Blumenthal, 1998), the standard reference for prescription herbal products in some of the countries of Europe, lists the following plants for treatment of cardiovascular indications: Ginkgo biloba leaf extract (*Ginkgo biloba* L.), onion (*Allium cepa* L.), motherwork herb (*Leonuri cardiacae* L.), hawthorn leaf with flower (*Crataegus monogyna* Jaquin emend. Lindmand or *C. laevigata* (Poiret) de Candolle*)*, lily of the valley herb (*Convallariae majalis* L.), pheasants eye herb (*Adonidis vernalis* L.), squill (*Urginea maritime* (L.) Baker), butcher's bloom (*Ruscus aculeatus* L.), camphor (*Cinnamomum camphora* (L.) Siebold), lavender flower (*Lavandulae angustifolia* Miller), rosemary leaf (*Rosmarinus officinalis* L.), scotch broom herb (*Cytisus scoparius* (L.) Link), garlic (*Allium sativum* L.), soy lecithin and phospholipid (*Glycine max* (L.) Merrill), Indian snakeroot (*Rauwolfia serpentine* (L.) Bentham ex Kurz), arnica flower (*Arnica montana* L. or *A. chamissonis* Less. subsp. *foliosa* (Nutt.) Maguiere), sweet clover (*Melilotus officinalis* (L.) Pallas and/or *M. altissimus* Thuillier), and horse chestnut seed (*Aesculus hippocastanum* L.). This chapter focuses on a literature review of three of these herbal medicines long associated with the treatment of cardiovascular disease symptoms: hawthorn, ginkgo, and horse chestnut seed.

2. HAWTHORN

Hawthorn (*Crataegus monogyna* or *laevigata* frequently referred to as *C. oxyacantha*) has other common names such as may bush and white thorn and is found in Europe, North America, and Asia as a deciduous tree in the Rosaceae family (Anon, 2010). It has been used traditionally for menstrual flow, kidney stones, as a diuretic, astringent and, most commonly, a cardiac tonic. The Commission E Monographs lists the leaf with flower as an approved herb because of the scientific data available prior to 1993, whereas there was limited scientific support and therefore unapproved status, for the berry, flower, or leaves alone (Blumenthal, 1998). Hawthorn was one of the top five prescribed phytomedicines in Germany in 1996 with retail sales in millions of US$. Dosage rates have been given as 250–500 mg per day of standardized extracts containing 18% oligomeric proanthocyanidins (Anon, 2010) or 30–169 mg procyanidins/epicatechin (Blumenthal, 1998) for a minimum of 6 weeks.

Hawthorn contains polycyclic flavonoids including epicatechin, chlorogenic acid, rutin, isoquercitin, and hyperoside (Dasqupta et al., 2010). The oligomeric procyanidins present contain multiple groups of catechins and epicatechin (Blumenthal, 1998). Vitexin-4″-O-glucoside and vitexin-2″-O-rhamnoside have been described as the major flavonoids present in hawthorn leaves that are readily absorbed when the products are fed to rats (Ma et al., 2010). In one study, it was the chlorogenic acid found in leaves and flowers that had the most antioxidant activity of the compounds identified and tested in a DPPH–HPLC system (Raudonis et al., 2009), while the oliogomeric procyanidins have been shown to have the greatest free radical scavenging activity and inhibition of elastase (important in damage after ischemia) in an ischemia-reperfusion model in rats (Chatterjee et al., 1997). Many of the flavonoids of hawthorn have induced increased coronary blood flow and relaxation in guinea pig hearts (Schüssler et al., 1995). Results in animal studies have indicated that hawthorn's compounds have the ability to increase heart contractions and blood flow, protect endothelium relaxation, reduce heart damage after ischemic events, and reduce the incidence of cholesterol following high-fat diets (Miller, 1998). It is thought that the antiarrhythmic action of hawthorn is via repolarizing of potassium channels, while its other actions make it appear similar to either phosphodiesterase inhibitors or cardiac glycosides (Guo et al., 2008).

In a meta-analysis of eight human clinical trials (studies that were randomized, placebo controlled, and double-blind), it was shown that exercise tolerance, pressure-heart rate product, fatigue, and maximal workload of those with chronic heart failure were improved with daily doses of hawthorn (Pittler et al., 2003). It was also shown that hawthorn has antiarrhythmic properties. In these clinical trials, the dosage rates were between 160 and 1800 mg per day of standardized extracts containing leaf and flower for 3–16 weeks. The adverse effects were mild and less than the placebo. These results were consistent with a review of 14 trials in 2009 (Guo et al., 2008).

Hawthorn has been well tolerated historically and in clinical trials (Hedley, 2001). In some animal studies, there is suggested interference with digoxin, a common medication for heart patients. One study (Dasqupta et al., 2010) used two different brands of extracts of hawthorn berries added directly to isolated drug-free serum and serum of patients on digoxin followed by testing in two different immunoassays and isolated rat cardiomyocytes. One of the immunoassays for digoxin recorded interference with the hawthorn extracts, whereas the other brand of immunoassay did not. In the rat cardiomyocytes, the combined use of digoxin and hawthorn did not show an additive effect, causing the authors to conclude that they may bind to the same binding sites (Na^+/K^+ adenosine triphophatase). Further studies are needed in humans to determine the bioavailability, absorption, distribution, transport, and metabolism of hawthorn extracts to support these results. At least in rats the absorption of orally administered extract causes hawthorn's active flavonoids to be preferentially represented by epicatechin (Chang et al., 2005). The difference between results of extract added directly to serum and orally administered extract could be determined with more human pharmacokinetic research.

3. GINKGO

Ginkgo (*Ginkgo biloba* L.) is an ancient tree species that has been used as a heart medicine in Chinese phytomedicine since at least 1509 (Chan et al., 2007) (Figure 15.1). It has also been used traditionally for lung ailments, brain function, and inner ear disorders. The German Commission E Monographs (Blumenthal, 1998) listed the leaf extract as an approved herb due to established results in experimental research. In the United States, it is one of the top-selling herbal supplements with over 16 million US$ in sales in the mass market in 2009 and $4 276 489 in the US natural and heath food retailers alone (Cavalier et al., 2010).

Ginkgo leaves have diterpene terpenoids (chiefly the ginkgolides and bilobalide) and flavonoids (including quercetin, kaempferol, and isorhamnetin). Extracts are usually standardized to about 25% flavone glycosides and 5% terpene lactones (Chan et al., 2007) and below 5 ppm ginkgolic acids. Suggested dosages are between 120 and 240 mg daily in multiple increments (Blumenthal, 1998).

A review of the scientific literature specifically related to ginkgo's use for cardiovascular disease (Mahady, 2002) identified clinical data supporting antioxidant activity (protection of endogenous ascorbic levels and free-radical–induced lipid peroxidation) and inhibition of platelet aggregation. *In vivo* and *in vitro* data have also identified numerous actions of Ginkgo's antioxidants in limiting the lipid peroxidation, destruction of endothelium relaxing factor, and postischemic production of free radicals associated with many of the aspects of cardiovascular disease. Its free radical scavenging action has been responsible for protecting nitric oxide and prostaglandin I_2 activity, thereby ensuring continued blood flow via smooth muscle relaxation (Chan et al., 2007). In isolated guinea

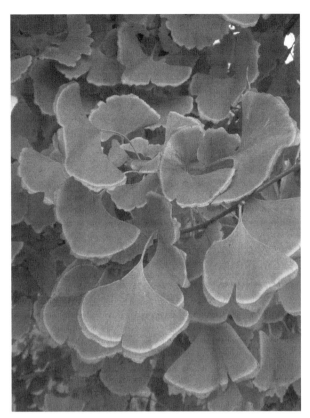

Figure 15.1 *Ginkgo biloba* leaves.

pig and rat hearts, ginkgo's flavonoids improved coronary blood flow via enhanced vasor-elaxation and aorta contractions that were likely mediated by nitric oxide and cyclic GMP phosphodiesterase. Decreased incidence of arrhythmias and increased hypoxia tolerance have also been observed in studies on rat myocardium (Mahady, 2002).

Although much of the current research focuses on the use of ginkgo for memory and cerebral issues, clinical trials have reported antioxidant activity, improved blood flow, and anti-inflammatory properties against cardiovascular disease development. In a human clinical trial of 60 healthy elderly adults, it was found that an injectable ginkgo extract preparation improved brachial artery endothelial vasomotor function (flow-mediated dilation) and coronary artery blood flow (Wu et al., 2008a). It was also determined in 80 coronary artery disease patients that a dose of the same injectable gingko extract resulted in similarly improved coronary artery blood flow partially through mediation of nitric oxide and endothelin-1 balance (Wu et al., 2008b). In a pilot study of eight high-risk cardiovascular patients consuming ginkgo at 240 mg per day for 2 months, atherosclerotic nanoplaque formation was seen to decrease concurrently with an increase in superoxide dismutase generation and a decrease in oxidized low-density lipoprotein (oxLDL) levels (Rodriguez et al., 2007).

Although ginkgo has been well tolerated in clinical trials (Kleijnen and Knipschild, 1992; Mahady, 2002), there have been reports of excess bleeding (Chan et al., 2007) and concerns over the potential for poisoning related to 4-O-methylpyridoxine (ginkgotoxin) found in the seeds of ginkgo. Potential side effects include dizziness, headache, palpitations, allergic skin conditions, and gastrointestinal complaints (Chan et al., 2007). Colalto (2010) reviewed numerous research articles investigating potential drug interactions of ginkgo with no conclusive evidence to indicate interactions or excess bleeding. However, some of the studies were contradictory and the between-subject variability large enough to warrant some caution when taking warfarin or digoxin until further studies are conducted. A recent report by Kuller et al. (2010) on the large Ginkgo Evaluation of Memory (GEM) trial indicated no evidence for a reduction in cardiovascular events over a period of 6 years of ginkgo administration. Although those on ginkgo had a significantly less number of events than those on placebo, the total number of events was very small.

4. HORSE CHESTNUT SEED

Horse chestnut seed (*Aesculus hippocastanum* L.), of the family Hippocastanceae, is a medicinal tree species cultivated widely for ornamental and shade purposes. It has been used traditionally to alleviate rheumatism, diarrhea, sports injuries, stomach ache, hemorrhoids, varicose veins, and as an analgesic for chest pain. Horse chestnut is related to the buckeye trees found in North America but not the edible sweet chestnut, *Castanea sativa* of the family Fagaceae. Horse chestnut is one of the top 20 herbal supplements sold in the United States with sales of $558 946 in 2009 in the mass market alone (Cavalier et al., 2010).

Extracts of horse chestnut are commonly standardized to about 20% of triterpene saponin glycosides (the natural mix of these is commonly referred to as aescin). Aescin is found in *A. hippocastanum* seeds at the rate of 9.5% dry matter as well as the flavonoids quercetin, kaempherol, epicatechin, and anthocyanins; and the fatty acids lauric acid, palmitic acid, myristic acid, stearic acid, arachidic acid, and oleic acid (Srijayanta et al., 1999). The concentration of flavonoids can increase to 11% dry matter in a purified extract, which may explain the potent bioactivity of horse chestnut (Kapusta et al., 2007).

Experiments in animal and cell culture systems have demonstrated the effectiveness of horse chestnut in decreasing inflammation and platelet aggregation, increasing venous contractions and protecting venous endothelium relaxation. In bovine mesenteric veins and arteries, an extract of up to 2 mg ml^{-1} aescin caused contractions thought to be partially mediated through the 5-HT$_{2A}$ receptors (Felixsson et al., 2010). In ADP-induced human platelet aggregation studies, it was determined that horse chestnut extract reduced platelet aggregation. Speculation of the components responsible for the reduction includes coumarin and quercetin (Felixson et al., 2010). Aescin, a mixture of saponins, has been shown to have synergistic anti-inflammatory effects with glucocorticoids (corticosterone) in mouse paw edema and rat pleuritis models. Besides, inhibition of the inflammatory agents, tumor necrosis factor α, nitric oxide, and interleukin 1β was observed in an LPS-stimulated murine macrophage RAW264.7 cell system (Xin et al., 2010). The antioxidant effects of a horse chestnut extract have been examined in mice given a high-fat diet (Kücükkurt et al., 2010). The level of fat in this diet caused significant increases in malondialdehyde (a marker of lipid peroxidation), a decrease in reduced glutathione (important in endogenous antioxidant systems), and an increase in the antioxidant enzymes Cu–Zn superoxide dismutase and catalase. Administration of the extract caused a significant decrease in malondialdehyde, an increase in reduced glutathione, and a return to normal levels of superoxide dismutase and catalase. The extract also improved symptoms of liver dysfunction (fat vacuoles, inflammatory patches, necrosis, and fibrosis) in both the high-fat diet and control diet groups.

Endothelial dysfunction is a precursor to hypertension, atherosclerotic disease, hypercholesterolemia, and chronic venous insufficiency (CVI). There are many studies on the effects of horse chestnut extracts on the traits and symptoms of CVI (these can include varicose veins, venous ulcers, leg-tiredness, swelling, and the hardening of the skin caused by lipidermatosclerosis). In human varicose vein segments, aescin caused a significant improvement in endothelium-dependent relaxation upon the administration of acetylcholine (Carrasco et al., 2009). Similar protection of the endothelium has been seen in rat aorta segments as well as an ability to promote contractions in arterial smooth muscle (Carrasco and Vidrio, 2007). Speculation on mechanisms involved includes the increased permeability to calcium and the subsequent enhancement of endothelial nitric oxide synthase 3 as well as the protection and enhancement of proteoglycan synthesis (an important component of the endothelium) (Pettler and Ernst, 2006).

In a pilot trial, a topically applied phospholipid gel preparation of aescin caused a return to near-normal concentrations of plasma-free radicals in venous hypertensive microangiopathy patients (Ricci et al., 2004). Seventeen randomized controlled trials using orally administered horse chestnut extract (standardized to aescin) in patients suffering from CVI have been reviewed (Pettler and Ernst, 2006). It was concluded that the extract improves leg pain, leg volume, leg circumference, swelling, and itching. Dosages in these trials ranged from 100 to 150 mg aescin daily. The adverse events were mild, with six studies listing gastrointestinal complaints, dizziness, itching, nausea, and headache in 1–36% of the patients.

5. CONCLUDING STATEMENTS

The three herbal treatments reviewed above are all well tolerated in clinical trials with indications of benefits to heart disease patients. Since concerns have been raised on bleeding with ginkgo, it should not be taken with warafin or, because of the chance of interference, with digoxin. As none of the studies have been carried out on children or pregnant women, they cannot be recommended for them at this time.

This chapter has focused on only three of the many herbs, foods, and spices that possess antioxidant activity and the potential to treat cardiovascular diseases in humans. The search for cardiovascular medicines should encompass the many different cultural traditional medical systems of the world and their use of plant products to maintain health as well as to treat the symptoms of cardiovascular disease. Medicinal plants included in the German Commission E Monographs include those with a history of experimental support in Europe with a bias toward English-speaking academia. Certainly in Traditional Chinese Medicine there are many herbs and spices, often used in combination, that are prescribed for the treatment of cardiovascular diseases (Ceylan-Isik, 2008). In India, the Ayurvedic health system encompasses the use of many plant products including the much-researched ginger, turmeric, and fenugreek. Indigenous People's traditional food systems and medicinal plants should likewise be examined as culturally appropriate strategies to counteract the increasing prevalence of cardiovascular diseases and type 2 diabetes associated with a move away from traditional lifestyles.

Herbal medicine, almost by definition, is the application of a group of compounds rather than single pure entities. These compounds can have synergistic or antagonistic properties that affect how the compounds interact and the potential to affect multiple aspects of a disease. The multiple actions of each of the three herbal medicines above illustrate this point. Further research is needed in human pharmacokinetics of bioactive components from herbal medicines, foods, and spices. Only then can the *in vitro* experiments, injections into animals and human ingestion trials be brought together to determine the mechanisms of action of plant products on cardiovascular health.

6. SUMMARY

- Plant products, whether food, herb, or spice, can contribute antioxidants to ameliorate symptoms of cardiovascular diseases.
- Hawthorn can improve exercise tolerance, pressure-heart rate product, fatigue, maximal workload, and has antiarrhythmic properties.
- Gingko's antioxidant and anti-inflammatory properties improve brachial artery endothelial vasomotor function (flow-mediated dilation) and coronary artery blood flow.
- Horse chestnut seed decreases inflammation and platelet aggregation, increases venous contractions, and protects venous endothelium relaxation in animal and cell studies, while in humans it has been shown to improve conditions of CVI.
- The search for plant medicines should encompass the food, herb, and spice use of cultures around the world. Human pharmacokinetic studies are needed on plants used for food, herbs, and spice.

GLOSSARY

Arrhythmia Abnormal heart rhythm.

Atherosclerosis The buildup of fatty material that leads to hardening and narrowing of the arteries.

Cardiomyocytes Specialized muscle cells that make up the walls of the heart.

Endothelium The layer of cells that line the inside of blood vessels.

Ischemia Inadequate blood supply, and therefore oxygen, to a part of the body.

LDL Low-density lipoprotein that carries cholesterol in the blood stream, often referred to as the 'bad cholesterol' in blood measurements.

Lipid peroxidation The damage caused (often to cell membranes) by the deterioration of cell lipids from electron removal by free radicals.

Microangiopathy Disease of the small blood vessels.

Peripheral neuropathies Nerve damage to the extremities (such as fingers, toes, penis) often leading to the lack of function and damage to these tissues.

Pharmacokinetics How a chemical is changed by the body via its absorption, bioavailability, metabolism, and excretion.

REFERENCES

Anon, 2010. Crataegus oxycantha (Hawthorn) monograph. Alternative Medicine Review 15, 164–167.

Blumenthal, M. (Ed.), 1998. The Complete German Commission E Monographs: Therapeutic Guide to Herbal Medicines. Integrative Medicine Communications, Boston, MA.

Carrasco, O.F., Vidrio, H., 2007. Endothelium protectant and contractile effects of the antivaricose principle escin in rat aorta. Vascular Pharmacology 47, 68–73.

Carrasco, O.F., Ranero, A., Hong, E., Vidrio, H., 2009. Endothelial function impairment in chronic venous insufficiency: effect of some cardiovascular protectant agents. Angiology 60, 763–771.

Cavalier, C., Rea, P., Lynch, M.E., Blumenthal, M., 2010. Herbal supplement sales rise in all channels in 2009. Herbalgram 86, 62–65.

CDC, 2010. Heart Disease Facts. http://www.cdc.gov/heartdisease/facts.htm.

Chan, P.C., Xia, Q., Fu, P.P., 2007. *Ginkgo biloba* leave extract: biological, medicinal, and toxicological effects. Journal of Environmental Science and Health Part C 25, 211–244.

Chang, Q., Zuo, Z., Ho, W.K., Chow, M.S., 2005. Comparison of the pharmacokinetics of hawthorn phenolics in extract versus individual pure compound. Journal of Clinical Pharmacology 45, 106–112.

Chatterjee, S.S., Koch, E., Jaggy, H., Krzeminski, T., 1997. In vitro and in vivo studies on the cardioprotective action of oligomeric procyanidins in a *Crataegus* extract of leaves and blooms. Arzneimittelforschung 47, 821–825.

Colalto, C., 2010. Herbal interactions on absorption of drugs: mechanisms of action and clinical risk assessment. Pharmacological Research 62, 207–227.

Ceylan-Isik, A.F., Fliethman, R.M., Wold, L.E., Ren, J., 2008. Herbal and traditional Chinese medicine for the treatment of cardiovascular complications in diabetes mellitus. Current Diabetes Reviews 4, 320–328.

Dasqupta, A., Kidd, L., Poindexter, B.J., Bick, R.J., 2010. Interference of hawthorn on serum digoxin measurements by immunoassays and pharmacodynamic interaction with digoxin. Archives of Pathology and Laboratory Medicine 134, 1188–1192.

Felixsson, E., Persson, I.A.-L., Eriksson, A.C., Persson, K., 2010. Horse chestnut extract contracts bovine vessels and affects human platelet aggregation through 5-HT2A receptors: An in vitro study. Phytotherapy Research 24, 1297–1301.

Guo, R., Pittler, M.H., Ernst, E., 2008. Hawthorn extract for treating chronic heart failure (review). Cochrane Database of Systematic Reviews 1, CD005312.

Hedley, C., 2001. Humours, hearts and hawthorn. European Journal of Herbal Medicine 5, 27–31.

Howard, B., Kritchevsky, D., 1997. Phytochemicals and cardiovascular disease: a statement for Healthcare Professionals from the American Heart Association. Circulation 95, 2591–2593.

Kapusta, I., Janda, B., Szajwaj, B., et al., 2007. Flavonoids in horse chestnut (Aesculus hippocastanum) seeds and powdered waste water byproducts. Journal of Agricultural Food Chemistry 55, 8485–8490.

Kleijnen, J., Knipschild, P., 1992. Ginkgo biloba for cerebral insufficiency. British Journal of Clinical Pharmacology 34, 352–358.

Kücükkurt, I., Ince, S., Keles, H., et al., 2010. Beneficial effects of Aesculus hippocastanum L. seed extract on the body's own antioxidant defense system on subacute administration. Journal of Ethnopharmacology 129, 18–22.

Kuller, L.H., Ives, D.G., Fitzpatrick, A.L., et al., 2010. Does Ginkgo biloba reduce the risk of cardiovascular events? Circulation: Cardiovascular Quality Outcomes 3, 41–47.

Lloyd-Jones, D., Adams, R.J., Brown, T.M., et al., 2010. Heart disease and stroke statistics 2010 update: a report from the American Heart Association. Circulation 121, e46–e215.

Ma, L.Y., Liu, R.H., Xu, X.D., Yu, M.Q., Zhang, Q., Liu, H.L., 2010. The pharmacokinetics of C-glycosyl flavones of Hawthorn leaf flavonoids in rat after single dose oral administration. Phytomedicine 17, 640–645.

Mahady, G.B., 2002. Ginkgo biloba for the prevention and treatment of cardiovascular disease: a review of the literature. Journal of Cardiovascular Nursing 16, 21–32.

Miller, A.L., 1998. Botanical influences on cardiovascular disease. Alternative Medical Review 3, 422–431.

Pittler, M.H., Schmidt, K., Ernst, E., 2003. Hawthorn extract for treating chronic heart failure: meta-analysis of randomized trials. American Journal of Medicine 114, 665–674.

Pittler, M.H., Ernst, E., 2010. Horse chestnut seed extract for chronic venous insufficiency. Cochrane Database of Systematic Reviews 9, CD003230.

Raudonis, R., Jakstas, V., Burdulis, D., Benetis, R., Janulis, V., 2009. Investigation of contribution of individual constituents to antioxidant activity in herbal drugs using postcolumn HPLC method. Medicina (Kaunas) 45, 382–394.

Ricci, A., Ruffini, I., Cesarone, M.R., et al., 2004. Variations in plasma free radicals with topical aescin + essential phospholipids gel in venous hypertension: new clinical data. Angiology 55, S11–S14.

Rodrıguez, M., Ringstad, L., Schafer, P., et al., 2007. Reduction of atherosclerotic nanoplaque formation and size by Ginkgo biloba (EGb 761) in cardiovascular high-risk patients. Atherosclerosis 192, 438–444.

Schüssler, M., Hölzl, J., Fricke, U., 1995. Myocardial effects of flavonoids from Crataegus species. Arzneimittelforschung 45, 842–845.

Srijayanta, S., Raman, A., Goodwin, B.L., 1999. A comparative study of the constituents of Aesculus hippocastanum and Aesculus indica. Journal of Medicinal Food 2, 45–50.

WHO, 2010. Cardiovascular diseases (CVDs). http://www.who.int/mediacentre/factsheets/fs317/en/index.html.

Wu, Y.Z., Li, S.Q., Cui, W., Zu, X.G., Du, J., Wang, F.F., 2008a. Ginkgo biloba extract improves coronary blood flow in healthy elderly adults: role of endothelium-dependent vasodilation. Phytomedicine 15, 164–169.

Wu, Y.Z., Li, S.Q., Zu, X.G., Du, J., Wang, F.F., 2008b. Ginkgo biloba extract improves coronary artery circulation in patients with coronary artery disease: contribution of plasma nitric oxide and endothelin-1. Phytotherapy Research 22, 734–739.

Xin, W., Zhang, L., Sun, F., et al., 2010. Escin exerts synergistic anti inflammatory effects with low doses of glucocorticoids in vivo and in vitro. Phytomedicine 10.1016/j.phymed.2010.08.013.

Zern, T.L., Fernandez, M.L., 2005. Cardioprotective effects of dietary polyphenols. Journal of Nutrition 135, 2291–2294.

FURTHER READING

Etkin, N.L. (Ed.), 1994. Eating on the Wild Side: The Pharmacologic, Ecologic, and Social Implications of Using Noncultigens. The University of Arizona Press, Tucson, AZ.

Lewis, W.H., Elvin-Lewis, M.P.F., 2003. Medical Botany: Plants Affecting Human Health, 2nd edn. John Wiley & Sons, Hoboken, NJ.

Schultes, R.E., Von Reis, S. (Eds.), 1995. Ethnobotany: Evolution of a Discipline. Dioscorides Press, Portland, OR.

Tyler, V.E., 1993. The Honest Herbal: A Sensible Guide to the Use of Herbs and Related Remedies, 3rd edn. Pharmaceutical Products Press, Binghamton, NY.

RELEVANT WEBSITES

http://abc.herbalgram.org/site/PageServer?pagename=Homepage – American Botanical Council.

http://www.ars-grin.gov/duke/ – Dr. Duke's Phytochemical and Ethnobotanical Databases.

http://www.napralert.org/ – NAPRALERT: Natural products alert database.

CHAPTER 16

Grape Polyphenols in Heart Health Promotion

E.M. Seymour, S.L. Hummel, M.G. Kondoleon, A. Kirakosyan, P.B. Kaufmanz, S.F. Bolling

University of Michigan Health System, Ann Arbor, MI, USA

1. INTRODUCTION

Observational studies indicate that cardiac mortality is inversely associated with higher wine consumption. However, some populations with higher wine intake also consume more fats, exercise less, and smoke more cigarettes than neighboring populations. This seemingly illogical finding has been coined the 'French paradox.' Wine consumption, particularly red wine, may play a role in the protective association of the French paradox. The cardioprotective constituents in wine are unknown, but numerous studies suggest that the phytochemical compounds from grapes may play a causative role.

Grape products appear to exert numerous effects of interest to healthy cardiovascular function. As discussed here, clinical trials and animal studies with purple grape juice suggest cardioprotective effects through enhanced vasodilation, reduced platelet aggregation, reduced oxidation of macromolecules, and enhanced plasma antioxidant capacity. The fact that both wine and grape juice confer cardiovascular benefits suggests some shared critical compounds and/or mechanism of effect. However, the grape constituents responsible for the health benefits remain unclear.

2. GRAPE CHEMISTRY AND BIOAVAILABILITY

2.1 Chemistry

Phenolic compounds in grapes can arbitrarily be divided into four groups: simple phenols, flavonoids, anthocyanins, and stilbenes. Grape phytochemicals are often called polyphenols because of their common phenolic acid group. Differences in the degree of oxidation and hydroxylation of the phenolic rings lead to a large family structure with essential differences in biological behavior, bioavailability, and efficacy. Grape polyphenols of potential medical interest are found within the skins, seeds, vine stems, and leaves. Furthermore, differences in polyphenol content exist between grape components (juice, pomace, and seed), different varietals of grape, and different agricultural regions (Fuleki and Ricardo-Da-Silva, 2003). Grape phenols and polyphenols exist as free compounds, as

Bioactive Food as Dietary Interventions for Cardiovascular Disease
http://dx.doi.org/10.1016/B978-0-12-396485-4.00014-1

© 2013 Elsevier Inc.
All rights reserved.

255

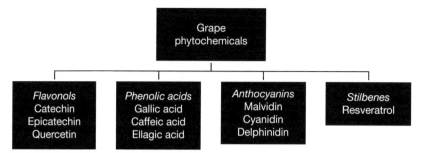

Figure 16.1 Subclasses of grape phytochemicals and some representative compounds. Anthocyanins in foods are most commonly conjugated to one or more sugars.

glycoside polymers or as part of larger-molecular-weight oligomeric chains or structures. Figure 16.1 illustrates these groups and some of their representative compounds.

The most common polyphenols in grape skin and pomace include phenolic acids, anthocyanidins, flavonols, and large-molecular-weight poly-galloyl polyflavan-3-ols. These components are found in fresh grapes, grape juice, wine, and grape skin extract. Grape seed extract contains mainly larger-molecular-weight compounds of repeating flavan-3-ol units esterified to gallic acid, with larger chains than those found in grape skin. Relative to grape skin, grape seed extract contains high-molecular-weight flavonols called proanthocyanidins (Shi et al., 2003). The chemical constituents of grape seeds and stems are often found in wine due to prolonged exposure to macerated grapes during vinification. It remains unknown which grape constituents offer greatest biologic and health effect or if these components act synergistically.

2.2 Bioavailability

Bioavailability is assessed by examining the absorption, distribution, metabolism, and excretion of a given compound. Research on phytochemical bioavailability is critical to the advancement of research in bioactive components from foods. Such studies could allow identification of the effective constituents for positive health effects and the comparison of grape product efficacy. For many years, little was known about the bioavailability of polyphenols due to difficulties in reliable quantification in tissues. Recent advances in instrumentation now permit detailed metabolomic profiling of compound bioavailability.

Polyphenols are altered extensively during metabolism; the molecular forms reaching the peripheral circulation and tissues are different from those present in foods. As used here, the term 'metabolism' describes the typical modifications that occur during or after absorption of compounds from ingested food. Most polyphenol glucosides are deglycosylated by β-glucosidases in the small intestine. Next, many compounds are glucuronidated in the small intestine. Glucuronides enter the hepatic portal vein and travel to the liver where they may be further methylated, glucuronidated, or sulfated. In the liver, polyphenols and their conjugates are metabolized by the phase II drug-metabolizing enzymes. The resulting molecules are glucuronate and sulfate conjugates, with or without methylation across the catechol functional group, and many molecules are conjugated multiple times. Compounds not absorbed in the small intestine can be further metabolized in the large intestine. Catabolism of polyphenols generally occurs as a result of microbial activity in the colon (Gonthier et al., 2003). The end products of this catabolism can then be utilized by the local microflora or absorbed into circulation. In summary, the plasma metabolites of phytochemicals are commonly conjugates (e.g., sulfates and glucuronates) of the parent aglycone or conjugates of methylated parent aglycones.

The half-life of plasma polyphenolic constituents and their metabolites is within hours, but recent studies now that constituents can be incorporated into body tissues which could extend their biologic effects including genetic modification. In fact, many experimental studies with phytochemical-rich products have demonstrated a biologic effect while not showing significant plasma presence of the parent constituents. As a result, there is increasing speculation that enterohepatic conjugates or colonic metabolites of the parent compounds are actually responsible for the observed biologic effects (Silberberg et al., 2006). The predominance of polyphenol metabolites and conjugates over parent compounds has important consequences for biomedical research in this area. Polyphenol metabolites are chemically distinct from their parent compounds, differing in size, polarity, and ionic form. Consequently, their physiologic behavior is likely to be different from that of the parent compounds. Therefore, *in vitro* studies (like cell culture studies) or *ex vivo* studies (as with isolated platelets or monocytes) with the parent constituents will not likely yield useful information regarding possible disease-modifying effects afforded by grape product ingestion. This limitation is critical to consider when interpreting the clinical significance of such studies using grape polyphenols.

Concerning efficacy of bioavailable compounds, the effective constituents in grape products are unknown. Published studies concerning grape polyphenol bioavailability have been focused on the plasma and urine kinetics of low-molecular-weight flavonoid constituents like epicatechin (Vinson et al., 2001), on anthocyanins like malvidin-3-glucoside (Bub et al., 2001), and on stilbenes like trans-resveratrol (Meng et al., 2004). Among grape products, perhaps the greatest controversy concerns the possible efficacy of proanthocyanidin-rich products like grape seed extract. *In vitro*, in an aqueous milieu, grape seed proanthocyanidins have extraordinary antioxidant capacity. However, proanthocyanidins are condensed tannins of high molecular weight and are not likely bioavailable in their native form (Rasmussen et al., 2005). The controversy arises from the assertion and commercial promotion of proanthocyanidin-rich supplements as having superior antioxidant capability. In fact, it is uncertain if their promising antioxidant capacity from *in vitro* studies is sustained *in vivo*. For grape seed extract, it is likely that only the few, lowest-molecular-weight constituents can be absorbed directly and then conjugated.

An alternative hypothesis is that the proanthocyanidin polymers are metabolized by colonic microflora to alternate, absorbable phenolic acid compounds (Ward et al., 2004).

3. HUMAN STUDIES – CARDIOVASCULAR EFFECTS

3.1 Reduced Platelet Aggregation

Anti-platelet therapy is an important target in the treatment of cardiovascular disorders. Platelets that are beneficial and essential for blot clotting can also serve a deleterious role in atherosclerosis. Increased platelet aggregation, as a result of increased platelet sensitivity and activation, contributes to the initiation and progression of atherosclerosis and to the occurrence of thrombotic events. Platelet aggregation is associated with an increased release of reactive oxidative species that can oxidize LDL. In addition, aggregated platelets increased platelet–vessel wall interactions. These effects of platelets result in damage to the vascular endothelium and in the potentiation of atherosclerosis. In addition to their role in the initiation of atherosclerosis, platelets also contribute to atherosclerosis progression by releasing various growth and chemotactic factors that accelerate the proliferation and migration of smooth muscle cells. Therefore, reducing the activity of platelets would potentially reduce development and progression of heart disease.

The human trials summarized in Table 16.1 reveal that diverse grape products have demonstrated anti-platelet activity. In these supplementation trials, the *in vivo* potential of platelets to adhere and aggregate is simulated *ex vivo* by agonists like thrombin, collagen, and ADP. The studies show that diverse grape products lowered platelet aggregation and increased the resistance of platelets to agonist-mediated activation. However, it appears that this benefit may be attenuated in subjects with risk factors for heart disease.

3.2 Enhanced Vasodilation

Nitric oxide (NO) plays a crucial role in the homeostasis of the vascular tone by acting as a vasodilator. As a dynamic mediator of vascular compliance, NO is a freely diffusible gas that acts as an intracellular and intercellular messenger. The half-life of NO under physiological conditions is measured in seconds, as NO is avidly scavenged by superoxide anions and heme-containing molecules, especially hemoglobin. NO is formed from the guanidine-nitrogen terminal of L-arginine by nitric oxide synthases. Most of the cellular actions of NO are explained by the activation of the cytosolic enzyme-soluble guanylate cyclase that catalyzes the formation of cyclic guanosine monophosphate (cGMP). Increased cGMP activates protein kinase G that phosphorylates a number of proteins involved in vasodilation. In addition to the depressor effect of vasodilation, NO inhibits platelet adherence to the endothelium. Enhanced NO production or availability would thereby enhance vasodilation, lower blood pressure, and reduce platelet aggregation.

Table 16.1 Human Studies of Reduced Platelet Aggregation Effects from Grape Products

Product (reference)	Dose/day	Days	Sample	Relevant biomarkers affected ($p < 0.05$)	Relevant biomarkers not affected ($p > 0.05$)
Grape juice (Freedman et al., 2001)	7 ml/kg	14	20 healthy subjects	Increased platelet nitric oxide release, Lower-platelet aggregation, platelet superoxide	
Wine vs. wine extract (Hansen, 2005)	375 ml or wine extract	28	69 healthy men and women	Wine decreased fibrinogen, grape extract had no effect	Clotting factor VIIc
Red wine, white wine, grape juice, grape juice + resveratrol (Pace 1996)	500 ml grape juice 375 ml red + white wine	28	24 healthy men	Both wines decreased platelet reactivity to thrombin. Resveratrol-supplemented juice decreased platelet reactivity to thrombin	
Purple grape juice (Keevil et al., 2000)	7.5 ml/kg	10	10 healthy subjects	Decreased platelet aggregation	
Wine vs. grape juice (Coimbra et al., 2005)	250 ml 500 ml	14	16 (8 men, 8 women, all with elevated cholesterol)		Platelet aggregation
Grape seed extract (Clifton, 2004)	2 g/day	5	28 healthy subjects		Tissue-type plasminogen activator, plasminogen activator inhibitor-1
Grape juice (Albers et al., 2004)	7 ml/kg	14	20 subjects with coronary heart disease		Platelet aggregation, P selectin, thromboxane B2
Grape juice (Dohadwala et al., 2011)	7 ml/kg	56	64 subjects with stage I hypertension		Soluble CD40

The effect of grape product ingestion on *in vivo* NO dynamics is of great clinical interest. *In vitro* studies with grape polyphenols have indicated delayed NO degradation by phosphodiesterase 5 (Dell'Agli et al., 2005), which would prolong NO availability. In addition, incubating arterial rings in a tissue bath with grape juice increased endothelial-dependent vasorelaxation by a nitric oxide-dependent mechanism (Fitzpatrick et al., 1993). Also, NO bioavailability is negatively impacted by oxidative stress, from which NO is oxidized to non-dilatory peroxynitrite. In humans, the impact of grape products on vasodilation is measured by blood pressure, by flow-mediated vasodilation of the brachial artery by ultrasound, and by indexes of improved NO availability. Studies summarized in Table 16.2 show that diverse grape products can improve vasodilation and/or reduce blood pressure. It remains unknown if these changes in blood pressure confer greater resistance to eventual hypertensive pathologies like heart failure or stroke.

4. POTENTIAL MECHANISMS OF EFFECT

4.1 Antioxidant Effects

Grape products limit tissue and systemic oxidative stress in several animal models. Proposed mechanisms of this effect include direct scavenging of free radicals and/or improved endogenous antioxidant defense. If able to provide an *in vivo* antioxidant effect in humans, grape polyphenol intake may modify diverse contributors to cardiovascular morbidity and mortality. Several grape products are capable of providing antioxidant effects, which can be measured directly by enhanced plasma antioxidant capacity or indirectly by reduced plasma oxidative stress and/or reduced oxidative damage of biomolecules. As summarized in Table 16.3, grape products can enhance plasma antioxidant capacity, decrease oxidation of LDL, and lower 8-isoprostane, a lipid oxidation product that serves as a systemic marker of oxidative stress. In addition, these effects were demonstrated in both healthy subjects and at-risk subjects. The impact on antioxidant capacity seems to vary, which may be an effect of altered time of sampling. Antioxidant capacity varies relative to food intake and meal content.

4.2 Anti-inflammatory Effects

Inflammation is a key contributor to the progression of many forms of heart disease. Inflammation directly damages target tissue and promotes the formation of reactive oxygen species that can damage neighboring tissue. *In vitro* and animal studies suggest that grape polyphenols have the potential to modulate eicosanoid metabolism (Li et al., 2001). The 5-lipoxygenase pathway, in particular, is an important target because it is involved in the synthesis of leukotrienes. These powerful mediators of inflammation play a role in cellular processes that contribute to atherosclerosis. *In vivo* studies examining anti-inflammatory effects of grape products are more limited and are summarized in Table 16.4. Measurements include

Table 16.2 Human Studies of Enhanced Vasodilation Effects from Grape Products

Product (reference)	Dose/day	Days	Sample	Relevant biomarkers affected ($p < 0.05$)	Relevant biomarkers not affected ($p > 0.05$)
Wine versus wine extract (Hansen, 2005)	375 ml or wine extract	28	69 healthy men and women		Blood pressure
Red wine versus de-alcoholized red wine (Agewall)	250 ml of either	1 (2×)	12 healthy subjects	Increased resting blood flow and heart rate, enhanced flow-mediated vasodilation by de-alcoholized red wine	Heart rate
Grape seed extract (Ward et al., 2005)	1 g	42	69 hypertensive men		Blood pressure, brachial artery vasodilation
Grape juice (Freedman et al., 2001)	7 ml/kg	14	20 healthy subjects	Increased platelet nitric oxide release	
Grape juice (Stein et al., 1999)	7.7 ml/kg	14	15 adults with coronary artery disease	Increased flow-mediated vasodilation	
Grape juice (Park et al., 2009)	5.5 ml/kg	56	40	Blood pressure	
Wine vs. grape juice (Coimbra et al., 2005)	250 ml 500 ml	14	16 (8 men, 8 women, all with high cholesterol)	Increased flow-mediated vasodilation, wine additionally decreased nitroglycerine-mediated vasodilation	Blood pressure
Grape seed extract (Clifton, 2004)	2 g/day	5	28 healthy subjects	Increased flow-mediated vasodilation	Plasma nitrate
Grape juice (Dohadwala et al., 2011)	7 ml/kg	56	64 subjects with stage I hypertension	Decreased nocturnal blood pressure (24 h ambulatory)	Arterial stiffness, office blood pressure

Continued

Table 16.2 Human Studies of Enhanced Vasodilation Effects from Grape Products—cont'd

Product (reference)	Dose/day	Days	Sample	Relevant biomarkers affected (p < 0.05)	Relevant biomarkers not affected (p > 0.05)
Grape seed extract (Sivaprakasapillai et al., 2009)	150 or 300 mg	28	27 subjects with metabolic syndrome	Blood pressure	
Grape seed extract (Kar et al., 2009)	600 mg	28	32 subjects		Endothelium-dependent vasodilation
Whole grape powder (Chaves et al., 2009)	36 g, 36 g 2 ×	1, 21	Healthy subjects	Flow-mediated dilation	Blood pressure
Grape juice (Park et al., 2009)	5.5 ml/ kg	56	21 healthy subjects	Blood pressure	

Table 16.3 Human Studies of Antioxidant Effects of Grape Products

Product (reference)	Dose/day	Days	Total subjects	Relevant biomarkers affected ($p < 0.05$)	Relevant biomarkers not affected ($p > 0.05$)
Red wine (Nigdikar et al., 1998)	375 ml	14	9 healthy men	Decreased plasma Lipid peroxides	
Grape polyphenol extract (Vigna et al., 2003)	300 mg	28	24 male smokers	Decreased plasma lipid oxidation, increased lag time for LDL oxidation	
Grape seed extract (Preuss et al., 2000)	100 mg	60	40 subjects with high cholesterol	Decreased autoantibodies to oxidized LDL	
Grape juice (Stein et al., 1999)	7.7 ml/kg	14	15 adults with coronary artery disease	Increased lag time to LDL oxidation	
Whole grape powder (Zern et al., 2005)	36 g	28	24 pre- and 20 post menopausal women	Decreased urine 8-isoprostane	LDL oxidative stress
Grape seed extract (Ward et al., 2005)	1 g	42	69 hypertensive men		Oxidized LDL, plasma and urine 8-isoprostane
Grape polyphenol extract (Nutall, 1998)	300 mg	5	20 healthy subjects	Increased serum antioxidant capacity	
Purple grape juice (Day et al., 1997)	125 ml	7	7 healthy subjects	Increased serum antioxidant capacity	LDL oxidation
Grape seed extract (Vinson et al., 2001)	600 mg	9	9 healthy subjects 8 subjects with high cholesterol	Increased serum antioxidant capacity in subjects with high cholesterol	
Grape juice (Freedman et al., 2001)	7 ml/kg	14	20 healthy subjects	Increased plasma antioxidant capacity, decreased platelet superoxide release	
Grape juice (Albers et al., 2004)	7 ml/kg	14	20 healthy subjects	Decreased platelet superoxide release	
Grape juice (O'Bryne, 2002)	10 ml/kg	14	15 healthy subjects	Increased serum antioxidant capacity, increased lag time to LDL oxidation	

Continued

Table 16.3 Human Studies of Antioxidant Effects of Grape Products—cont'd

Product (reference)	Dose/day	Days	Total subjects	Relevant biomarkers affected ($p < 0.05$)	Relevant biomarkers not affected ($p > 0.05$)
Grape seed extract (Clifton, 2004)	2 g	5	28 healthy subjects		Oxidized LDL, urinary 8-isoprostane
Grape juice (Rowe et al., 2011)	360 ml	63	85 healthy subjects		Plasma antioxidant capacity
Grape seed extract (Sivaprakasapillai et al., 2009)	150 or 300 mg	28	27 subjects with metabolic syndrome		Oxidized LDL
Grape seed extract (Kar et al., 2009)	600 mg	28	32 subjects	Whole blood glutathione	Serum antioxidant capacity
Whole grape powder (Chaves et al., 2009)	36 g, 36 g 2×	1, 21	Healthy subjects	Serum antioxidant capacity after 21 days	Serum antioxidant capacity after one acute dose
Grape juice (Hollis et al., 2009)	480 ml	84	27 healthy subjects		Serum antioxidant capacity

Table 16.4 Human Studies of Reduced Inflammation Effects of Grape Products

Product (reference)	Dose/day	Days	Sample	Relevant biomarkers affected ($p < 0.05$)	Relevant biomarkers not affected ($p > 0.05$)
Whole grape powder (Zern et al., 2005)	36 g	28	24 pre-menopausal and 20 post-menopausal women	Decreased plasma tumor necrosis factor alpha	
Red wine, white wine, grape juice, grape juice + resveratrol (Pace 1996)	500 ml grape juice 375 ml red + white wine	28	24 healthy men	Both wines decreased plasma thromboxane B2	Neither juice affected thromboxane B2
Grape seed extract (Ward et al., 2005)	1 g	42	69 hypertensive men		Plasma C-reactive protein, white blood cell count
Grape juice (Polagruto et al., 2003)	6–9 ml/kg	5	28 healthy subjects	Increased plasma PGI_2,	Plasma leukotriene LTA_4
Grape seed extract (Clifton, 2004)	2 g/day	5	28 healthy subjects		Plasma C-reactive protein, vascular cellular adhesion molecule–1, intercellular adhesion molecule–1
Grape juice (Albers et al., 2004)	7 ml/kg	14	20 subjects with coronary heart disease	Decreased soluble CD40, platelet superoxide release	Interleukin 8, C-reactive protein
Grape juice (Dohadwala et al., 2011)	7 ml/kg	56	64 subjects with stage I hypertension		C-reactive protein
Grape seed extract (Kar et al., 2009)	600 mg	28	32 subjects	Plasma C-reactive protein	
Grape juice (Rowe et al., 2011)	360 ml	63	85 healthy subjects	T-cell ($\gamma\delta$) proliferation	C-reactive protein, serum amyloid α

thromboxanes and leukotrienes, interleukins, tumor necrosis factor, C-reactive protein, and cell adhesion molecules. Collectively, these studies show that diverse grape products can lower systemic and local markers of inflammation.

5. TRANSLATIONAL FRONTIERS

5.1 Preclinical Promise

Recent animal studies suggest that chronic intake of grape products reduces the development of cardiovascular diseases rather than just surrogate markers as presently studied in humans. For example, in atherosclerosis-prone mice, intake of whole grape powder (for 10 weeks) reduced atherosclerotic lesion area, serum oxidative stress, macrophage-mediated oxidation of LDL, and macrophage uptake of oxidized LDL, but increased serum antioxidant capacity (Fuhrman et al., 2005). In hypertensive rats, intake of whole grape powder (for 18 weeks) reduced the degree of hypertension, cardiac remodeling, cardiac fibrosis, and diastolic dysfunction. In addition, these phenotypic effects correlated with altered cardiac genes relevant to inflammation and antioxidant defense (Seymour et al., 2008, 2010), suggesting direct nutrigenomic effects from regular grape intake. In obese hamsters, intake of grape seed extract (for 12 weeks) reduced abdominal fat, plasma insulin, and leptin but increased adiponectin. Grape seed extract also reduced fasting glucose and insulin resistance (Decorde et al., 2008). Finally, insulin-resistant rats fed different grape extracts (for 6 weeks) showed reduced hypertension and cardiac hypertrophy (from the anthocyanin-rich grape fraction) and reduced insulin resistance and hypertriglyceridemia (from the proanthocyanin-rich fraction) (Al-Awwadi et al., 2005). Further comparative studies are needed to elucidate nutrigenomic and phenotypic effects of grape product intake in relevant models of heart disease.

5.2 Clinical and Translational Challenges

Oxidative stress and inflammation are now implicated in a diverse array of human cardiovascular pathology including coronary artery disease and heart failure. As shown in Tables 16.1–16.4, the initial clinical experience with grape-based products shows significant promise in reducing surrogate markers of cardiovascular risk. However, translating these potential benefits into clearly defined outcome benefits in humans presents several challenges. As previously discussed, the effects of grape-based dietary supplementation may vary by the product used. Habitual dietary patterns could enhance or blunt the cardiovascular effects of grape products. However, current methods to measure micronutrient intake are imperfect and until recently were not well-suited to estimate phytochemical intake. Assessment of adherence to grape-based supplements may be complex, since information is still emerging about which grape components are absorbed and how they are metabolized.

As clinical/translational studies progress from enrolling fairly healthy patients to those with more severe cardiovascular pathology and associated comorbidities, assessing the safety and potential benefit of grape-based products will become more complex. As an example, frequently indicated medications such as renin–angiotensin–aldosterone system blocking agents and HMG-CoA reductase inhibitors (statins) may also reduce oxidative stress and inflammation, which could blunt the effects of grape products. Drug–supplement interactions are possible as well, as grape seed extract variably inhibits CYP3A4 (a liver cytochrome that metabolizes many common medications).

As evidenced by the variability in Tables 16.3 and 16.4, assessment of changes in systemic oxidative stress and inflammation may not be sufficient to assess the physiologic response to grape products. The effects may be primarily nutrigenomic and mediated by very small quantities of polyphenolic compounds. Accordingly, obtaining relevant cells to assess gene expression profiles will be a critical step in understanding the potential cardiovascular benefits of grape products in humans. Myocardial tissue may be obtained during cardiac surgery or via endomyocardial biopsy, but these invasive approaches are not indicated in most patients and are particularly poorly suited to investigating differences pre-and posttreatment. Investigating gene profiles in easily harvested circulating immune cells or endothelial cells obtained via recently developed, low-risk biopsy techniques may provide an appropriate avenue to assess the effects of grape products on oxidative stress, inflammation, and vascular dysfunction.

REFERENCES

Agewall, S., Wright, S., Doughty, R.N., et al., 2000. Does a glass of red wine improve endothelial function? European Heart Journal 21 (1), 74–78.

Al-Awwadi, N.A., Araiz, C., Bornet, A., et al., 2005. Extracts enriched in different polyphenolic families normalize increased cardiac NADPH oxidase expression while having differential effects on insulin resistance, hypertension, and cardiac hypertrophy in high-fructose-fed rats. Journal of Agricultural and Food Chemistry 53 (1), 151–157.

Albers, A.R., Varghese, S., Vitseva, O., et al., 2004. The antiinflammatory effects of purple grape juice consumption in subjects with stable coronary artery disease. Arteriosclerosis, Thrombosis, and Vascular Biology 24 (11), e179–e180.

Bub, A., Watzl, B., Heeb, D., et al., 2001. Malvidin-3-glucoside bioavailability in humans after ingestion of red wine, dealcoholized red wine and red grape juice. European Journal of Nutrition 40 (3), 113–120.

Chaves, A.A., Joshi, M.S., Coyle, C.M., et al., 2009. Vasoprotective endothelial effects of a standardized grape product in humans. Vascular Pharmacology 50 (1–2), 20–26.

Clifton, P.M., 2004. Effect of grape seed extract and quercetin on cardiovascular and endothelial parameters in high-risk subjects. Journal of Biomedicine and Biotechnology 2004 (5), 272–278.

Coimbra, S.R., Lage, S.H., Brandizzi, L., et al., 2005. The action of red wine and purple grape juice on vascular reactivity is independent of plasma lipids in hypercholesterolemic patients. Brazilian Journal of Medical and Biological Research 38 (9), 1339–1347.

Day, A.P., Kemp, H.J., Bolton, C., et al., 1997. Effect of concentrated red grape juice consumption on serum antioxidant capacity and low-density lipoprotein oxidation. Annals of Nutrition and Metabolism 41 (6), 353–357.

Decorde, K., Teissedre, P.L., Auger, C., et al., 2008. Phenolics from purple grape, apple, purple grape juice and apple juice prevent early atherosclerosis induced by an atherogenic diet in hamsters. Molecular Nutrition and Food Research 52 (4), 400–407.

Dell'Agli, M., Galli, G.V., Vrhovsek, U., et al., 2005. In vitro inhibition of human cgmp-specific phospho-diesterase-5 by polyphenols from red grapes. Journal of Agricultural and Food Chemistry 53 (6), 1960–1965.

Dohadwala, M.M., Hamburg, N.M., Holbrook, M., et al., 2011. Effects of concord grape juice on ambulatory blood pressure in prehypertension and stage 1 hypertension. American Journal of Clinical Nutrition 92 (5), 1052–1059.

Fitzpatrick, D.F., Hirschfield, S.L., Coffey, R.G., 1993. Endothelium-dependent vasorelaxing activity of wine and other grape products. The American Journal of Physiology 265 (2 Pt 2), H774–H778.

Freedman, J.E., Parker 3rd, C., Li, L., et al., 2001. Select flavonoids and whole juice from purple grapes inhibit platelet function and enhance nitric oxide release. Circulation 103 (23), 2792–2798.

Fuhrman, B., Volkova, N., Coleman, R., Aviram, M., 2005. Grape powder polyphenols attenuate athero-sclerosis development in apolipoprotein e deficient (e0) mice and reduce macrophage atherogenicity. The Journal of Nutrition 135 (4), 722–728.

Fuleki, T., Ricardo-Da-Silva, J.M., 2003. Effects of cultivar and processing method on the contents of cat-echins and procyanidins in grape juice. Journal of Agricultural and Food Chemistry 51 (3), 640–646.

Gonthier, M.P., Cheynier, V., Donovan, J.L., et al., 2003. Microbial aromatic acid metabolites formed in the gut account for a major fraction of the polyphenols excreted in urine of rats fed red wine polyphenols. The Journal of Nutrition 133 (2), 461–467.

Hollis, J.H., Houchins, J.A., Blumberg, J.B., Mattes, R.D., 2009. Effects of concord grape juice on appetite, diet, body weight, lipid profile, and antioxidant status of adults. Journal of the American College of Nutrition 28 (5), 574–582.

Kar, P., Laight, D., Rooprai, H.K., et al., 2009. Effects of grape seed extract in type 2 diabetic subjects at high cardiovascular risk: a double blind randomized placebo controlled trial examining metabolic markers, vascular tone, inflammation, oxidative stress and insulin sensitivity. Diabetic Medicine 26 (5), 526–531.

Keevil, J.G., Osman, H.E., Reed, J.D., Folts, J.D., 2000. Grape juice, but not orange juice or grapefruit juice, inhibits human platelet aggregation. The Journal of Nutrition 130 (1), 53–56.

Li, W.G., Zhang, X.Y., Wu, Y.J., Tian, X., 2001. Anti-inflammatory effect and mechanism of proantho-cyanidins from grape seeds. Acta Pharmacologica Sinica 22 (12), 1117–1120.

Meng, X., Maliakal, P., Lu, H., et al., 2004. Urinary and plasma levels of resveratrol and quercetin in humans, mice, and rats after ingestion of pure compounds and grape juice. Journal of Agricultural and Food Chemistry 52 (4), 935–942.

Nigdikar, S.V., Williams, N.R., Griffin, B.A., Howard, A.N., 1998. Consumption of red wine polyphenols reduces the susceptibility of low-density lipoproteins to oxidation in vivo. American Journal of Clinical Nutrition 68 (2), 258–265.

Park, Y.K., Lee, S.H., Park, E., et al., 2009. Changes in antioxidant status, blood pressure, and lymphocyte DNA damage from grape juice supplementation. Annals of the New York Academy of Sciences 1171, 385–390.

Polagruto, J.A., Schramm, D.D., Wang-Polagruto, J.F., et al., 2003. Effects of flavonoid-rich beverages on prostacyclin synthesis in humans and human aortic endothelial cells: association with ex vivo platelet function. Journal of Medicinal Food 6 (4), 301–308.

Preuss, H.G., Wallerstedt, D., Talpur, N., et al., 2000. Effects of niacin-bound chromium and grape seed proanthocyanidin extract on the lipid profile of hypercholesterolemic subjects: a pilot study. Journal of Medicine 31 (5–6), 227–246.

Rasmussen, S.E., Frederiksen, H., Struntze Krogholm, K., Poulsen, L., 2005. Dietary proanthocyanidins: occurrence, dietary intake, bioavailability, and protection against cardiovascular disease. Molecular Nutrition and Food Research 49 (2), 159–174.

Rowe, C.A., Nantz, M.P., Nieves, C., et al., 2011. Regular consumption of concord grape juice benefits human immunity. Journal of Medicinal Food.

Seymour, E.M., Singer, A.A., Bennink, M.R., et al., 2008. Chronic intake of a phytochemical-enriched diet reduces cardiac fibrosis and diastolic dysfunction caused by prolonged salt-sensitive hypertension. The Journals of Gerontology. Series A, Biological Sciences and Medical Sciences 63 (10), 1034–1042.

Seymour, E.M., Bennink, M.R., Watts, S.W., Bolling, S.F., 2010. Whole grape intake impacts cardiac peroxisome proliferator-activated receptor and nuclear factor kappab activity and cytokine expression in rats with diastolic dysfunction. Hypertension 55 (5), 1179–1185.

Shi, J., Yu, J., Pohorly, J.E., Kakuda, Y., 2003. Polyphenolics in grape seeds-biochemistry and functionality. Journal of Medicinal Food 6 (4), 291–299.

Silberberg, M., Morand, C., Mathevon, T., et al., 2006. The bioavailability of polyphenols is highly governed by the capacity of the intestine and of the liver to secrete conjugated metabolites. European Journal of Nutrition 45 (2), 88–96.

Sivaprakasapillai, B., Edirisinghe, I., Randolph, J., et al., 2009. Effect of grape seed extract on blood pressure in subjects with the metabolic syndrome. Metabolism 58 (12), 1743–1746.

Stein, J.H., Keevil, J.G., Wiebe, D.A., et al., 1999. Purple grape juice improves endothelial function and reduces the susceptibility of ldl cholesterol to oxidation in patients with coronary artery disease. Circulation 100 (10), 1050–1055.

Vigna, G.B., Costantini, F., Aldini, G., et al., 2003. Effect of a standardized grape seed extract on low-density lipoprotein susceptibility to oxidation in heavy smokers. Metabolism 52 (10), 1250–1257.

Vinson, J.A., Proch, J., Bose, P., 2001. Meganatural((r)) gold grapeseed extract: in vitro antioxidant and in vivo human supplementation studies. Journal of Medicinal Food 4 (1), 17–26.

Ward, N.C., Croft, K.D., Puddey, I.B., Hodgson, J.M., 2004. Supplementation with grape seed polyphenols results in increased urinary excretion of 3-hydroxyphenylpropionic acid, an important metabolite of proanthocyanidins in humans. Journal of Agricultural and Food Chemistry 52 (17), 5545–5549.

Ward, N.C., Hodgson, J.M., Croft, K.D., et al., 2005. The combination of vitamin c and grape-seed polyphenols increases blood pressure: a randomized, double-blind, placebo-controlled trial. Journal of Hypertension 23 (2), 427–434.

Zern, T.L., Wood, R.J., Greene, C., et al., 2005. Grape polyphenols exert a cardioprotective effect in pre- and postmenopausal women by lowering plasma lipids and reducing oxidative stress. The Journal of Nutrition 135 (8), 1911–1917.

CHAPTER 17

Cacao for the Prevention of Cardiovascular Diseases

M. Jenny, S. Schroecksnadel, J.M. Gostner, F. Ueberall, D. Fuchs

Innsbruck Medical University, Innsbruck, Austria

ABBREVIATIONS

5-HIAA 5-Hydroxyindoleacetic acid
ACS Acute coronary syndrome
AMI Acute myocardial infarction
CAD Coronary artery disease
CRP C-reactive protein
GTP Guanosine triphosphate
H_2O_2 Hydrogen peroxide
IDO Indoleamine 2,3-dioxygenase
IFN-γ Interferon-γ
IL Interleukin
LDL Low-density lipoprotein
NAD^+ Nicotinamide adenine dinucleotide
NF-κB Nuclear factor-κB
NOS Nitric oxide synthase
O_2^- Superoxide
ORAC Oxygen radical absorbance capacity
PBMC Peripheral blood mononuclear cells
PHA Phytohemagglutinin
ROS Reactive oxygen species
T5H Tryptophan-5-hydroxylase
TDO Tryptophan 2,3-dioxygenase
Th T-helper (cells)

1. INTRODUCTION

Cacao, sometimes also called cocoa, refers to the dry powder derived from the beans of the evergreen cocoa tree *Theobroma cacao* L. (Sterculiaceae or alternatively Malvaceae) by grinding the seeds and removing the cocoa butter from the dark and bitter cocoa solids. For more than 4000 years, from the ancient people of Olmec, Maya, and Aztec cultures up to the present, the fruits of *T. cacao* have been used as food and as a medicinal remedy, and consumption of cacao has always been associated with regalement and a sense of

Bioactive Food as Dietary Interventions for Cardiovascular Disease
http://dx.doi.org/10.1016/B978-0-12-396485-4.00015-3

© 2013 Elsevier Inc.
All rights reserved.

delight. Especially, the indigenous people of Central and South America still use the fruits of *T. cacao* as a traditional medicine. Historically, the most consistent applications of cacao for medicinal purposes are appetite-stimulating, relaxing, and mood-enhancing effects. Today, about 100 therapeutic applications of cacao are described involving the gastro-intestinal, nervous, cardiovascular, and immune systems. Several *in vitro* and *in vivo* studies suggest that the active constituents of cacao exhibit protective effects against diseases associated with inflammation and impaired immune function such as cardiovascular disease and cancer (Corti et al., 2009; Galleano et al., 2009).

The term cardiovascular disease comprises several classes of disturbances, which involve primarily the heart and the vascular system and usually refer to diseases associated with atherosclerosis. Atherosclerosis is a multifactorial disease, which progresses through several stages and requires the cooperative action of many cell types in different organ systems (Ramsey et al., 2010). The major pathophysiological consequences arise from chronic inflammatory processes and increased levels of oxidative stress in the arteries and veins, which cause oxidation of lipids and proteins (Chisolm and Steinberg, 2000). The *oxidative modification hypothesis of atherogenesis*, which states that oxidation of low-density lipoprotein (LDL) is an early event in the development of atherosclerosis, suggests that consumption of antioxidants should prevent oxidation of LDL and thereby reduce the risk or progression of atherosclerosis. However, this assumption is controversially discussed in the literature and has not been conclusively proven in clinical trials. In this regard, it was suggested that in addition to a direct radical absorbance capacity, an antioxidant for the treatment of oxidative stress-related diseases should provide further properties such as the interference with enzymes involved in cytoprotective mechanisms. Owing to the crucial role of inflammation in the pathogenesis of atherosclerosis, the desired pharmacological action of a beneficial antioxidant for the treatment of cardiovascular diseases should also include a potential to counteract inflammatory mechanisms (Brigelius-Flohé et al., 2005).

2. DIETARY ANTIOXIDANTS

In general, most herbs and fruits are believed to exhibit antioxidant activities, which are proposed to positively influence oxidative stress-related diseases. Antioxidants are reducing agents, inhibiting oxidation of other molecules by being oxidized themselves. They terminate radical-driven chain reactions and thus protect cells from the damaging effects of oxidation. Most of the proposed mechanisms for the potentially beneficial effects of cacao on health have been attributed to the high amount of polyphenolic compounds in cacao beans, such as the flavan-3-ol monomers epicatechin, catechin, gallocatechin, or epigallocatechin and their oligomeric derivatives known as procyanidins. Accordingly, several *in vitro* and *in vivo* studies could demonstrate that cacao flavonoids have the capacity to act as potent antioxidants due to their ability to reduce free radical formation and to scavenge free radicals (Corti et al., 2009; Galleano et al., 2009). In humans, for example, cacao has been shown to counteract lipid peroxidation and to lower plasma levels of oxidized LDL in hypercholesterolemic patients (Tokede et al., 2011). Measurements of the antioxidant capacity of cacao and chocolate products from major brands in the United States revealed that natural cacao powder contained the highest levels of antioxidant capacity with an oxygen radical absorbance capacity (ORAC) value between 720 and 875 µmol Trolox equivalents g^{-1} (Miller et al., 2006). Due to their content of polyphenolic compounds, black tea, green tea, and red wine also have gained attention as being potentially healthy for the cardiovascular system. However, cacao contains remarkable higher amounts of total phenolics and flavonoids and exhibits also higher total antioxidant capacities than teas and red wine, which suggests that cacao should be even more beneficial to cardiovascular health.

Although flavonol-rich cacao has the potential to augment an individual's antioxidant defense system, there is emerging evidence that antioxidants in general can also influence cellular mechanisms such as signaling pathways and gene expression. Accordingly, the reported effects of cacao on human health cannot be attributed exclusively to its radical scavenging capacity. In this regard, cacao compounds were shown to interfere with several inflammatory pathways, for example, by improving or normalizing eicosanoid production, platelet activation, nitric oxide-dependent activities, and cytokine production. For all these effects, the extent of cacao present in chocolate is considered to be of utmost importance. Recently, dark chocolate was demonstrated to induce coronary vasodilation, to improve coronary vascular function, and to decrease platelet adhesion within short time after consumption. These beneficial effects seem to go along with a significant reduction of serum oxidative stress and were positively correlated with changes in serum epicatechin concentrations. Thus, cacao and cacao-derived products with a high content of pure cacao have the potential to positively modulate oxidative stress and the inflammatory status, both of which are hallmarks of cardiovascular diseases.

Flavonols from cacao have been shown to mediate various anti-inflammatory effects, such as the modulation of cytokine production, for example, inhibition of interleukin (IL)-2 and IL-4 or stimulation of IL-1β and IL-5 in mitogen-stimulated peripheral blood mononuclear cells (PBMC) (Corti et al., 2009; Galleano et al., 2009). Suppression of the IL-2- or interferon (IFN)-γ-induced Th-1 type immune response and its downstream biochemical pathways by extracts of cacao was shown in several studies and agrees well with findings of us and others that antioxidants such as vitamin C and E, resveratrol but also green and black tea or wine, generally exhibit suppressive properties on activated immune cells. Recently, we could show significant suppressive effects of cacao extracts on secretion of pro-inflammatory IFN-γ by T-cells and related biochemical pathways in human macrophages, such as degradation of tryptophan by indoleamine 2,3-dioxygenase (IDO) and formation of the pteridine neopterin, which is derived from guanosine triphosphate (GTP) via GTP-cyclohydrolase I (Figure 17.1; Werner et al., 1989). In the *in vitro* model of freshly isolated PBMC (Jenny et al., 2011), cacao extracted in water

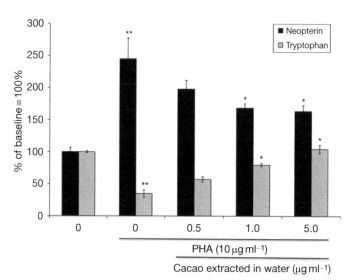

Figure 17.1 Concentrations of neopterin and tryptophan expressed as % of baseline in the supernatants of unstimulated and phytohemagglutinin (PHA)-stimulated PBMC pretreated or not with increasing concentrations of cacao extracted in water. Results shown are the mean values ± S.E.M. of four independent experiments run in duplicates ($^{**}p < 0.005$, compared with unstimulated cells; $^{*}p < 0.05$, compared with PHA-stimulated cells). *Adapted from Jenny, M., Santer, E., Klein, A., et al., 2009. Cacao extracts suppress tryptophan degradation of mitogen-stimulated peripheral blood mononuclear cells. Journal of Ethnopharmacology 122, 261–267.*

significantly and dose-dependently suppressed degradation of tryptophan and formation of neopterin, which was induced by the mitogen phytohemagglutinin (PHA) (Jenny et al., 2009). At concentrations of 1–5 µg ml^{-1}, the water extract of cacao was able to completely inhibit tryptophan degradation, so that baseline levels of tryptophan in the culture medium remained unchanged. In this chapter, the implications of these suppressive capacities of cacao for the prevention of cardiovascular diseases are discussed.

3. THE ROLE OF TRYPTOPHAN METABOLISM AND NEOPTERIN FORMATION IN CARDIOVASCULAR DISEASE

3.1 Tryptophan and Indoleamine 2,3-Dioxygenase

The essential amino acid tryptophan is required for protein synthesis and serves as a precursor of a large number of metabolites in human nutrition and metabolism. About 95% of dietary tryptophan is metabolized by the kynurenine pathway, the primary route of tryptophan degradation in mammalian cells, leading to the formation of metabolites such as nicotinamide adenine dinucleotide (NAD^+), kynuramines, kynurenic acid, quinolinic acid, and picolinic acid. The main biological function of the kynurenine pathway involves the regulation of plasma levels of tryptophan by the clearance of excess circulating

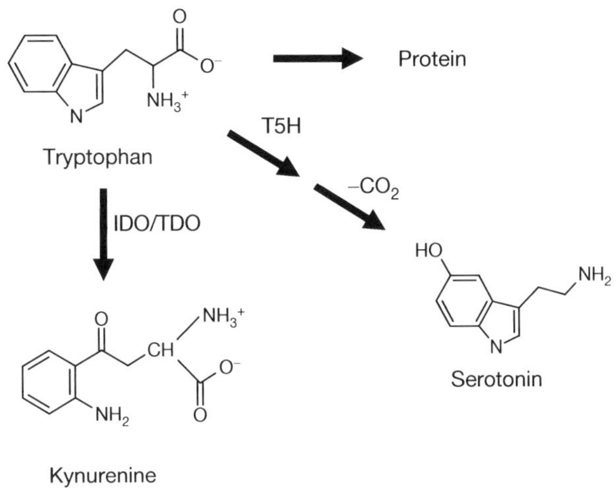

Figure 17.2 The essential amino acid tryptophan is required for protein biosynthesis and is converted by tryptophan 2,3-dioxygenase (TDO) in the liver and by indoleamine 2,3-dioxygenase (IDO) in various tissues and cells to kynurenine. Tryptophan also serves as a precursor of serotonin (5-hydroxytryptamine) biosynthesis, which is initiated by tryptophan-5-hydroxylase (T5H).

tryptophan. The biosynthesis of kynurenines and NAD^+ is initialized by the predominantly hepatic tryptophan 2,3-dioxygenase (TDO) and IDO, which is expressed in various peripheral cells such as macrophages and cells of the central nervous system (Werner et al., 1989). While TDO accepts only tryptophan as a substrate and is activated primarily by glucocorticoids, IDO metabolizes also 5-hydroxytryptophan, serotonin (5-hydroxytryptamine), and tryptamine and is preferentially induced by Th1-type cytokine IFN-γ and some other pro-inflammatory stimuli. Consequently, the second important pathway of tryptophan metabolism is the serotonin pathway, in which hydroxylation of tryptophan is initiated by the rate-limiting enzyme tryptophan-5-hydroxylase (T5H) yielding the neurotransmitter serotonin, which appears to be strongly involved in the pathogenesis of mood disorders and depression (Figure 17.2; Widner et al., 2002).

During inflammatory responses, IDO-triggered tryptophan degradation is an important mechanism of the antimicrobial and antiproliferative response of the human immune defense system. In the course of the Th1-type immune response against intracellular pathogens such as viruses, parasites, and bacteria, T-cells are activated and release large amounts of cytokines, such as IL-2 and IFN-γ. Pro-inflammatory cytokine IFN-γ is probably the most important multiplier of antimicrobial and antitumoral host defense mediating a variety of physiological and cellular responses, for example, induction of high amounts of reactive oxygen species (ROS), such as H_2O_2 and O_2^-, by macrophages and other cells, which are directed to suppress the growth and proliferation of cells and pathogens (Schroecksnadel et al., 2010). ROS are capable to interfere with various redox-sensitive intracellular signal-transduction cascades involving, for example,

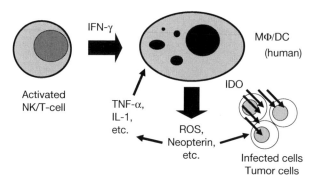

Figure 17.3 The immune response includes several cells and the production of various mediators. One of the most important components of the T-helper (Th)1-type immune response is the pro-inflammatory cytokine interferon-γ (IFN-γ), which is secreted mainly from activated T-cells and natural killer (NK) cells. Apart from the immunomodulatory properties of IFN-γ, the main goal of this cytokine is to limit the growth of pathogens and malignant cells. To achieve this purpose, various pathways are initiated by IFN-γ, of which many are directed to deprive essential nutrients. Within this strategy, degradation of tryptophan by indoleamine 2,3-dioxygenase (IDO) and formation of reactive oxygen species (ROS) and neopterin in human macrophages (MΦ) and dendritic cells (DC) are involved, which also contribute to accelerate the production of other important pro-inflammatory mediators such as tumor necrosis factor-α (TNF-α) and intetleurkin-1 (IL-1).

activation of nuclear factor-κB (NF-κB), which in turn potentiates the production of pro-inflammatory cytokines such as TNF-α and IL-1. Consequently, accumulation of ROS further amplifies the Th1-type immune response and thereby acts as positive modulators in addition to pro-inflammatory Th1-type cytokines (Figure 17.3).

T-cell-derived IFN-γ involves also stimulation of IDO enzyme activity in human macrophages and dendritic cells, which converts tryptophan into N-formylkynurenine that is subsequently deformylated to kynurenine (Figure 17.2; Werner et al., 1989). The resulting depletion of tryptophan in the circulation inhibits protein synthesis and limits the growth of intracellular microorganisms such as bacteria, parasites, and viruses, but also of highly proliferating tumor cells. The growth of the intracellular bacteria *Chlamydia pneumonia,* for example, can effectively be suppressed by the activity of IDO, not only upon IFN-γ-induced macrophage activation but also upon activated aortic smooth muscle cells. However, tryptophan depletion via activation of IDO in IFN-γ-stimulated macrophages and dendritic cells was also found to decelerate the T-cell response and thereby may represent an auto-regulatory mechanism, which attenuates the cellular immune response, for example, in atheroma formation. Additionally, tryptophan availability and IDO activity also seem to inhibit the oxidation of LDL, most likely because IDO requires the superoxide anion for cleavage of the indole ring structure, and metabolites of kynurenine appear to suppress oxidation of lipoproteins. Thus, activation of IDO may also contribute to downregulate foam cell formation.

3.2 Neopterin and GTP-Cyclohydrolase I

In parallel with tryptophan degradation, IFN-γ stimulates GTP-cyclohydrolase I in human monocyte-derived macrophages and dendritic cells to produce neopterin (D-erythro-1,2,3-trihydroxypropyl-pterin), representing another marker for the activation of the T-cell/macrophage axis (Figure 17.3; Murr et al., 2002). Based on a constitutive enzyme deficiency in the biosynthesis of tetrahydrobiopterin, neopterin is produced at the expense of biopterin derivatives. 5,6,7,8-Tetrahydrobiopterin serves as a cofactor of several amino acid monooxygenases involved in the oxidation of tryptophan, phenylalanine, and tyrosine and also of nitric oxide synthase (NOS). Under certain environmental conditions, neopterin may act in a pro-oxidant manner (Hoffmann et al., 2003). In this regard, neopterin was found, for example, to support LDL oxidation *in vitro* or to amplify oxidation of the vasodilatory molecule NO to form peroxynitrite. Thus, increased production of neopterin may counteract the formation of NO and thereby give rise to vasoconstriction and raised blood pressure.

Significant associations between plasma levels of IFN-γ, neopterin, and accelerated tryptophan degradation have been found in various diseases associated with an activated cell-mediated immune response, such as virus infections, heart diseases, autoimmune diseases, malignant disorders, and allograft rejection episodes (Table 17.1; Schroecksnadel et al., 2006).

Neopterin represents a marker of increased risk and progression of cardiovascular diseases and may play an important role in the pathogenesis of atherosclerosis (De Rosa et al., 2011; Fuchs et al., 2009). The relationship between neopterin levels and atherosclerosis has been assessed in several studies. Increased levels of inflammatory markers such as fibrinogen, ferritin, C-reactive protein (CRP), and also neopterin correlate strongly with the extent of vascular diseases and allow the prediction of disease progression (Avanzas et al., 2005; Grammer et al., 2009; Pedersen et al., 2011). Circulating neopterin concentrations were shown to be higher in patients with ischemic heart disease, hypertension, and acute coronary syndrome (ACS). Furthermore, neopterin concentrations have been reported to be significantly elevated in patients with cerebrovascular and peripheral artery atherosclerosis, chronic limb ischemia, and carotid artery disease. In patients with carotid artery disease, neopterin has been associated with an increased rate of transient ischemic attacks and stroke. The relation between elevated neopterin levels and atheromatous coronary artery disease (CAD) and an even more pronounced elevation in patients with acute myocardial infarction (AMI) is also established. Some studies have reported only a weak albeit significant correlation between circulating neopterin and the extent of coronary atheromatous disease. However, several studies have shown a correlation between circulating neopterin and the presence of multiple complex (vulnerable) plaques in patients with unstable and stable CAD. Multiple complex coronary plaques are known to be associated with rapid progression of CAD and

Table 17.1 List of Clinical Conditions, Which Are Associated with Accelerated Tryptophan Degradation and Enhanced Neopterin Formation and Their Association with Clinical Findings

Clinical diagnosis	Additional specific findings
Infectious diseases	
HIV-1 infection	Correlation with stage, improvement during antiretroviral therapy, prediction of outcome, association with neuropsychiatric symptoms
Septicemia	Prediction of outcome
Heart diseases	
Congestive heart failure	Correlation with disease activity
Coronary artery disease	Prediction of outcome
Autoimmunity	
Rheumatoid arthritis	Correlation with disease activity
Systemic lupus erythematosus	Correlation with disease activity
Cancer	
Colorectal cancer	Prediction of outcome, association with neuropsychiatric symptoms
Malignant melanoma	Prediction of outcome
Gynecological cancer	Prediction of outcome
Bronchus carcinoma	Prediction of outcome
Transplant rejection	
Kidney allograft recipients	Prediction of rejection
Liver allograft recipients	Prediction of rejection
Cytokine treatment	
Interferon-α, Interleukin-2	Association with neuropsychiatric symptoms

adverse prognosis in patients with CAD. Thus, measurement of neopterin concentrations in the plasma of patients provides comprehensive information regarding the risk of cardiovascular events, when macrophage activation is implicated, for example, upon rapid progression of CAD and atheromatous plaque disruption. In comparison with CRP (Grammer et al., 2009), neopterin has been shown to be an even more sensitive marker of inflammation, which is involved in the pathogenesis of several inflammation-associated diseases and can be used not only to predict the outcome of a disease but also to monitor the effectiveness of a medication.

Regarding tryptophan degradation in connection with cardiovascular diseases, lower serum tryptophan concentrations and higher kynurenine concentrations were shown in patients with atheromatous plaques and in patients suffering from myocardial infarction or angina pectoris, when compared with healthy controls (Niinisalo et al., 2008; Pedersen et al., 2011; Wirleitner et al., 2003). Significant correlations between markers of immune activation such as neopterin and IDO activity could also be shown in patients with coronary heart disease, indicating that enhanced tryptophan degradation is immune-mediated and not due to reduced dietary intake of tryptophan. However, the down regulatory effect of IDO seems to exhibit only a capacity to delay and not to entirely suppress inflammatory cascades, but IDO may be responsible for certain adverse effects of chronic diseases that involve depressive mood disorders (Widner et al., 2002). In fact, patients with major depression frequently show decreased plasma tryptophan concentrations due to enhanced degradation, which also corresponds with increased concentrations of immune activation markers. Accumulation of neurological active kynurenine metabolites, such as quinolinic acid, may further contribute to the development of neurological/psychiatric disorders. Thus, IDO seems to represent a link between the immunological network and neuroendocrine functions with far-reaching implications to the psychological status of patients.

4. CACAO TO ENHANCE MOOD

Apart from the strong anti-inflammatory effect of cacao, its influence on IDO could relate to the mood-enhancing effects attributed to cacao. If our *in vitro* findings hold true for the situation *in vivo*, cacao should be able to slow down inflammation-associated tryptophan degradation and thus improve the availability of tryptophan for biosynthesis of serotonin. There are a number of reports implicating a role of cytokine-induced IDO in psychiatric diseases, and several studies showed that the mood is negatively influenced by the depletion of tryptophan (Widner et al., 2002). Such a scenario agrees well with the known capacity of cacao to improve mood, lift spirits, and make people feel good. In atypical depression and in seasonal affective disorder, chocolate craving was reported to be a form of self-medication in having an impact on brain neurotransmitters. Likewise, chocolate has been characterized to have antidepressant benefits. Accordingly, several psychoactive constituents including anandamines, caffeine, or phenylethylamine have been identified in cacao. However, the achievable plasma levels of these compounds after ingestion of a typical serving of cacao are assumed to be too low to take effect. Nevertheless, inhibition of IDO activity by cacao may mimic a kind of oral tryptophan supplementation, which has been shown to result in enhanced concentrations of the serotonin metabolite 5-hydroxyindoleacetic acid (5-HIAA) in the cerebrospinal fluid and conversely diets devoid of tryptophan resulted in impaired cerebral serotonin formation. At least in the gastrointestinal tract one can assume the presence of all cacao compounds at effectual concentrations, at which they could also increase the availability of tryptophan and production of serotonin. A great proportion of serotonin (about 95%) in the human body is synthesized and stored in the gastrointestinal tract acting as a paracrine messenger to modulate sensation, secretion, and motility. According to this, ingestion of cacao products or administration of polyphenols present in cacao could play an important role in the modulation of tryptophan availability and consequently the disposability of serotonin.

5. CONCLUSION

The beneficial and protective effects of cacao in diseases associated with oxidative stress and inflammation have been shown in a number of *in vitro* and *in vivo* studies. Evidence of the suppressive capacity of cacao on IFN-γ stimulated downstream pathways, such as degradation of tryptophan and formation of neopterin in human macrophages, which have been shown to be disturbed in several atherosclerosis-related disease, suggests that ingestion of pure cacao (preferentially dissolved in water) may be recommended for the prevention of cardiovascular disease. Additionally, we propose another mechanism for the mood-elevating effect of cacao due to its capacity to enhance the availability of tryptophan for serotonin synthesis. Increased serotonin levels may improve quality of life, especially in patients suffering from oxidative stress and inflammatory conditions.

REFERENCES

Avanzas, P., Arroyo-Espliguero, R., Quiles, J., Roy, D., Kaski, J.C., 2005. Elevated serum neopterin predicts future adverse cardiac events in patients with chronic stable angina pectoris. European Heart Journal 26, 457–463.

Brigelius-Flohé, R., Kluth, D., Banning, A., 2005. Is there a future for antioxidants in atherogenesis? Molecular Nutrition & Food Research 49, 1083–1089.

Chisolm, G.M., Steinberg, D., 2000. The oxidative modification hypothesis of atherogenesis: an overview. Free Radical Biology & Medicine 28, 1815–1826.

Corti, R., Flammer, A.J., Hollenberg, N.K., Lüscher, T.F., 2009. Cocoa and cardiovascular health. Circulation 119, 1433–1441.

De Rosa, S., Cirillo, P., Pacileo, M., et al., 2011. Neopterin: from forgotten biomarker to leading actor in cardiovascular pathophysiology. Current Vascular Pharmacology 9, 188–199.

Fuchs, D., Avanzas, P., Arroyo-Espliguero, R., et al., 2009. The role of neopterin in atherogenesis and cardiovascular risk assessment. Current Medicinal Chemistry 16, 4644–4653.

Galleano, M., Oteiza, P.I., Fraga, C.G., 2009. Cocoa, chocolate, and cardiovascular disease. Journal of Cardiovascular Pharmacology 54, 483–490.

Grammer, T.B., Fuchs, D., Böhm, B.O., Winkelmann, B.R., Maerz, W., 2009. Neopterin as a predictor of total and cardiovascular mortality in individuals undergoing angiography (The Ludwigshafen Risk and Cardiovascular Health Study). Clinical Chemistry 55, 1135–1146.

Hoffmann, G., Wirleitner, B., Fuchs, D., 2003. Potential role of immune system activation associated production of neopterin derivatives in humans. Inflammation Research 52, 313–321.

Jenny, M., Klieber, M., Zaknun, D., et al., 2011. In vitro testing for anti-inflammatory properties of compounds employing peripheral blood mononuclear cells freshly isolated from healthy donors. Inflammation Research 60, 127–135.

Jenny, M., Santer, E., Klein, A., et al., 2009. Cacao extracts suppress tryptophan degradation of mitogen-stimulated peripheral blood mononuclear cells. Journal of Ethnopharmacology 122, 261–267.

Miller, K.B., Stuart, D.A., Smith, N.L., et al., 2006. Antioxidant activity and polyphenol and procyanidin contents of selected commercially available cocoa-containing and chocolate products in the United States. Journal of Agricultural and Food Chemistry 54, 4062–4068.

Murr, C., Widner, B., Wirleitner, B., Fuchs, D., 2002. Neopterin as a marker for immune system activation. Current Drug Metabolism 3, 175–187.

Niinisalo, P., Raitala, A., Pertovaara, M., et al., 2008. Indoleamine 2,3-dioxygenase activity associates with cardiovascular risk factors: the Health 2000 study. Scandinavian Journal of Clinical and Laboratory Investigation 68, 767–770.

Pedersen, E.R., Midttun, Ø., Ueland, P.M., et al., 2011. Systemic markers of interferon-γ-mediated immune activation and long-term prognosis in patients with stable coronary artery disease. Arteriosclerosis, Thrombosis, and Vascular Biology 31, 698–704.

Ramsey, S.A., Gold, E.S., Aderem, A., 2010. A systems biology approach to understanding atherosclerosis. EMBO Molecular Medicine 2, 79–89.

Schroecksnadel, K., Frick, B., Winkler, C., Fuchs, D., 2006. Crucial role of interferon-gamma and stimulated macrophages in cardiovascular disease. Current Vascular Pharmacology 4, 205–213.

Schroecksnadel, S., Jenny, M., Kurz, K., et al., 2010. LPS-induced NF-kappaB expression in THP-1Blue cells correlates with neopterin production and activity of indoleamine 2,3-dioxygenase. Biochemical and Biophysical Research Communications 399, 642–646.

Tokede, O.A., Gaziano, J.M., Djoussé, L., 2011. Effects of cocoa products/dark chocolate on serum lipids: a meta-analysis. European Journal of Clinical Nutrition 65, 879–886.

Werner, E.R., Werner-Felmayer, G., Fuchs, D., et al., 1989. Parallel induction of tetrahydrobiopterin biosynthesis and indoleamine 2,3-dioxygenase activity in human cells and cell lines by interferon-gamma. Biochemical Journal 262, 861–866.

Widner, B., Laich, A., Sperner-Unterweger, B., Ledochowski, M., Fuchs, D., 2002. Neopterin production tryptophan degradation and mental depression: what is the link? Brain, Behavior, and Immunity 16, 590–595.

Wirleitner, B., Rudzite, V., Neurauter, G., et al., 2003. Immune activation and degradation of tryptophan in coronary heart disease. European Journal of Clinical Investigation 33, 550–554.

CHAPTER 18

Phytoestrogens and the Role in Cardiovascular Health: To Consume or Not to Consume?

H. Hwang, J.P. Konhilas
University of Arizona, Tucson, AZ, USA

ABBREVIATIONS

AHA American Heart Association
ER Estrogen receptor
FDA Food and Drug Administration
LDL Low-density lipoprotein
MCP-1 Monocyte chemoattractant protein-1
NO Nitric oxide
eNOS Endothelial NO synthase

1. BACKGROUND AND SIGNIFICANCE

For the past 20–30 years, there has been a dramatic increase in soy consumption worldwide, which is largely attributed to the widely held perception that soy foods and their biologically active compounds, phytoestrogens, confer health benefits. The notion that a soy diet may be beneficial for human health is suggested by lower incidences of cardiovascular and hormone-dependent diseases (such as breast and prostate cancers) in many Asian countries (Keys et al., 1984). In these regions, soy-based products are major dietary components and are regularly consumed (Anderson et al., 1999; Barnes et al., 1995; Setchell and Cassidy, 1999). Early experimental studies and clinical trials investigating the potential impact of soy have generally supported the role of soy protein in promoting cardiovascular health, as well as ameliorating common symptoms that afflict women, such as osteoporosis, breast cancer, and postmenopausal hot flashes (Anderson et al., 1995).

A landmark, meta-analysis of 38 clinical trials published in 1995 (Anderson et al., 1995) has largely supported these cardiovascular health claims for soy protein such that in 1999, the US Food and Drug Administration (FDA) approved soy protein as an effective dietary component for reducing coronary heart disease (Food labeling: health claims: soy protein and coronary artery disease, 1999). This was followed up in 2000 by the American Heart Association affirming the FDA's soy health claim (AHA) stating

Bioactive Food as Dietary Interventions for Cardiovascular Disease
http://dx.doi.org/10.1016/B978-0-12-396485-4.00016-5

© 2013 Elsevier Inc.
All rights reserved.

that the intake of soy protein with a diet low in saturated fat and cholesterol is recommended and may reduce the risk of coronary heart disease (Erdman, 2000). Since then, numerous studies on soy protein and its biologically active components, particularly soy isoflavones, have been intensively carried out.

Unlike the results of these early studies, the latest data have been mixed. The benefits have often been negligible or, at best, modest. Negative impacts of soy intake have also been reported (Konhilas and Leinwand, 2007). Recently, after re-evaluating the soy protein/phytoestrogen data, the AHA eventually removed its endorsement from 2000, stating that the ostensible cardiovascular health benefits afforded by soy protein are unfounded. Specifically, the AHA stated that there is no clear evidence that soy isoflavones, the most abundant bioactive phytoestrogens in soy products, benefit cardiovascular health (Sacks et al., 2006). Furthermore, there has been a growing concern over the long-term dietary use of these plant-derived compounds, because phytoestrogens can bind endogenous estrogen receptors (ERs) and potentially behave as endocrine disruptors, adversely affecting human health (Rozman et al., 2006).

There is a search for effective dietary alternatives to the typical "Western" diet that is high in saturated fats and carbohydrates. Despite the potential adverse effects and conflicting results over the use of soy phytoestrogens for cardiovascular health, the attitude of the general public toward soy intake and phytoestrogens remains quite positive. Given that cardiovascular disease is the leading cause of death in developed countries and that soy phytoestrogens are found in many of today's prepared and processed foods on the market, it is vital to critically assess the impact of soy and its bioactive compounds on cardiovascular health and understand the potential risks and benefits.

2. PHYTOESTROGENS AND BIOLOGY, CHEMISTRY, AND PHARMACOKINETICS

Phytoestrogens are plant-derived estrogens that are structurally similar to 17-β estradiol (Figure 18.1), the major endogenous estrogen present in females (also present in males), with the capability of exerting various biological effects comparable to those of estrogens. Isoflavones, coumestans, and lignans are three major categories of phytoestrogens. Isoflavones are a class of isoflavonoids and are perhaps the most studied soy phytoestrogens with estrogenic properties (Setchell, 1998). The common sources of isoflavones are soy protein isolate; textured soy flour; miso, soy-based bacon bits and burgers; and soybeans (Patisaul and Jefferson, 2010). It is important to note that the concentrations of isoflavones contained in these soy products can be variable depending on the types of soybeans used, timing of harvest, processing techniques, and environmental factors (Patisaul and Jefferson, 2010). For example, ethanol extraction, a commonly used method to isolate soy protein, produces soy protein isolate devoid of isoflavones.

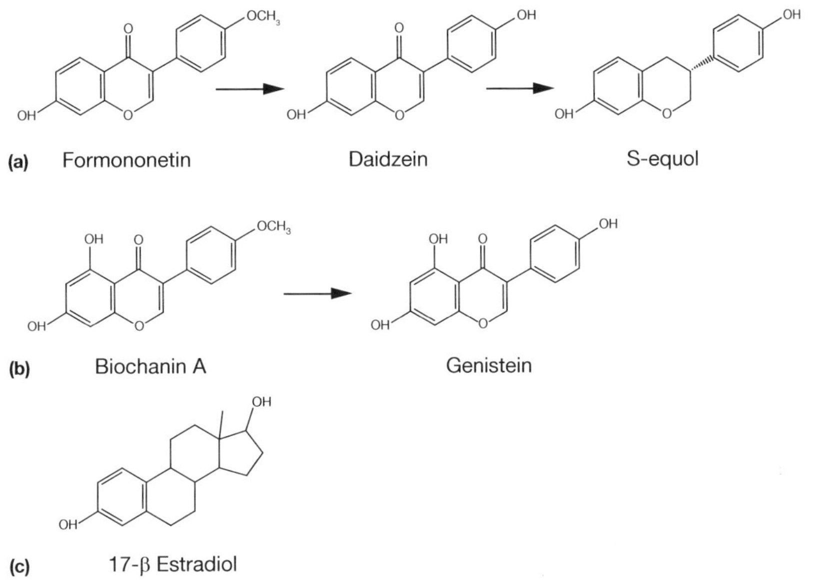

Figure 18.1 Chemical structures and the bioformations of daidzein (a), equol (a), and genistein (b). The structure of 17β-estradiol (c) is provided for comparison.

Conversely, because isoflavones function as plant phytoalexins (plant antibiotics), isoflavone content in harvested soy crop can drastically increase upon exposure to environmental stresses such as low humidity or destructive bacteria (Eldridge and Kwolek, 1983). Thus, isoflavone content varies considerably in soy products, even within the same type or brand. This may underlie individual variation in the postprandial plasma level of isoflavones and subsequently exert differential biological effects (Verkasalo et al., 2001b).

2.1 Daidzein and Genistein

Daidzein and genistein are ruminal demethylation products of the isoflavones, biochanin A and formononetin, respectively (Setchell et al., 2001, 2002), and are the most abundant forms of soy phytoestrogens (Figure 18.1). These isoflavones are present in soy protein and foods as either unconjugated aglycones (daidzein and genistein) or conjugated glycosides (daidzin and genistin). Glycosidic isoflavones are not readily bioavailable because of the sugar-binding moiety that prohibits enterocyte crossing. Thus, hydrolysis, usually mediated by intestinal bacteria, is required for gut absorption and bioavailability. On hydrolysis, unconjugated aglycones are produced, which can be further metabolized into p-ethylphenol (genistein) and equol (daidzein). In the body, these compounds can go through reconjugation to glucuronides and are excreted in the urine (Setchell et al., 2001). Although the half-life of genistein and daidzein is relatively short (8 h), it is important to note that the excretion of genistein is much slower than that of daidzein, suggesting that genistein may impart greater biological actions than daidzein (Busby et al., 2002).

2.2 Equol

Equol was first identified from the urine of pregnant mares from which the name equol was originated (Figure 18.1a). It is exclusively a daidzein metabolite produced by intestinal bacterial metabolism in humans (Setchell et al., 2003b). Equol exists as diastereoisomers, S- or R-isomer, distinguished by the presence or absence of a double bond in the heterocyclic ring structure. Humans exclusively produce the S-equol isomer from daidzein metabolism. S-Equol exerts most of the biological effects that are attributed to equol. The plasma concentration of equol after consumption of soy products is relatively higher than any other isoflavone (Gu et al., 2006; Zubik and Meydani, 2003). Equol is also known to have greater estrogenic potency compared to its parent compound daidzein evidenced by a stronger induction of target gene expressions, probably resulting in a greater biological impact (Morito et al., 2001; Shutt and Cox, 1972). Moreover, a greater fraction (~50%) of circulating equol is present in the plasma as an unbound form, a form that is readily available for the ER binding, than any other isoflavones (~5% for genistein and ~18% for daidzein) (Nagel et al., 1998).

For these reasons, some suggest that the ability to produce equol is a critical factor that potentially determines whether the biological impact of isoflavones (Setchell et al., 2002) is beneficial or detrimental and that the equol producers more likely benefit from the intake of isoflavones than those who are not equol producers (Setchell et al., 2002). In line with this contention, in a randomized, placebo-controlled crossover study, favorable effects on blood–lipid profiles were observed only in individuals with equol-producing capability (Meyer et al., 2004). In contrast, another study reported that regular consumption of soy protein containing isoflavones by individuals with mild levels of plasma cholesterol did not reduce levels of plasma cholesterol, independent of whether the subjects were equol producers or not (Thorp et al., 2008). Thus, the notion that equol producers could be advantageous over nonequol producers in reducing risks of especially cardiovascular disease remains unclear.

2.3 Resveratrol

Although human exposure to phytoestrogens occurs primarily through consumption of soy foods, resveratrol is also a phytoestrogen that has recently gained considerable attention. Functionally, it is better known as a compound linked to the "French paradox," the phenomenon that, despite a higher intake of saturated fat, the Italian and French populations tend to have a lower incidence of cardiovascular disease compared with European and US counterparts. Resveratrol is found mainly in grape seeds and grape skins, and like most phytoestrogens, has a polyphenolic ring structure that enables it to act as an estrogen mimetic and bind ERs. Resveratrol exists as cis- and trans-isoforms, but the trans form is known to exert most of the biological action. Much of the biological action is known to be mediated through interaction with ERs. In addition, it has also been shown that resveratrol has a biological activity that is independent of ER activation, such as antioxidant, anti-inflammatory, and vasodilatory actions (Basly et al., 2000; Fremont, 2000; Robb et al., 2008; Wallerath et al., 2002). Among other suggested biological roles, resveratrol has been shown to extend life span in animal models. In one particular study, mice fed with a high-calorie diet along with resveratrol demonstrated improved survival and a reduction in adverse health effects compared to mice fed with a high-calorie diet only (Baur et al., 2006). The mechanism of resveratrol's anti-aging effects is mediated through Sir2 (Sirt1 in mammalian cells), a conserved deacetylase, similar to a mouse model of calorie restriction (Baur et al., 2006; Lee et al., 2008).

3. BIOLOGICAL MODES OF ACTION: ESTROGENIC, ANTIESTROGENIC, AND ER INDEPENDENT MODES OF ACTION

The presence of a phenolic ring structure enables phytoestrogens to act as estrogen agonists and/or antagonists. Although factors other than chemical structure can also affect their biological modes of action (e.g., phytoestrogen concentrations, receptor status, and estrogen levels), the traditional estrogenic effects of phytoestrogens essentially depend on binding affinity to ERs. On binding to ERs, phytoestrogens can initiate transcription much like estrogen by recruiting coactivators, activating estrogen-response elements, and/or binding early immediate genes (Konhilas and Leinwand, 2007; Kushner et al., 2000). The antiestrogenic activities of phytoestrogens are likely related to their ability to compete with endogenous estrogen for ER occupancy (Picherit et al., 2000). Given that the degree by which estrogen exerts its biological activity is determined by the ER occupancy, competitive inhibition for ER binding may underlie the basis of biological efficacy (Nagel et al., 1998).

Two isoforms of ER, α and β, are known to be present, which differ in their C-terminal ligand binding and N-terminal transactivation domains. Estrogen has equal binding affinity for both ER α and β, whereas daidzein and genistein have preferential binding affinity for ER β (Kuiper et al., 1997). ER α and β are differentially expressed throughout the body and are uniquely involved in gene regulation. Differential gene regulation is achieved by recruiting distinct sets of coactivators and corepressors, the differential binding affinity of phytoestrogens may implicate their distinct aspects of biological impact (Moggs and Orphanides, 2001). In a recent study of ER subtype expression, ER β expression was found to be enhanced in the vascular wall of women with coronary artery disease, while ER α predominated in the control group of women without disease. Thus, isoflavone phytoestrogens that selectively target ER β

subtype may provide cardiovascular benefit for women with coronary heart disease, presumably through improved vascular function (Cruz et al., 2008).

Phytoestrogens are capable of disrupting normal endocrine function and can cause breeding abnormalities in animals. The most well-documented incidence pertaining to estrogenic mode of action is an outbreak of infertility in sheep in Australia. These sheep were grazing red clover that had a high percentage of isoflavone formononetin, which was being biotransformed into equol by intestinal bacteria (Figure 18.2) (Bennetts et al., 1946; Bradbury and White, 1954). Switching sheep to a genetically modified clover lacking isoflavones ameliorated the infertility. Similarly, an episode involving animals living in North American zoos, which experienced decreasing fertility and liver disease because of their soy isoflavone-rich diet, is also such an example (Setchell et al., 1987).

Unlike detrimental effects to animal fertility, the effects of isoflavones on human reproductive function have not been adequately identified. This may be partly due to differences in isoflavone exposure between humans and animals. Notably, the isoflavone content that caused the clover disease in Australian sheep was estimated to be around 20–100 g per day. These amounts are 1333- to 2000-folds higher than the amount of isoflavones that can be achieved by humans ($15–50 \text{ mg day}^{-1}$) fed an isoflavone–rich diet (Nagata et al., 1998; Wakai et al., 1999). Thus, despite the ability of phytoestrogens to act as endocrine disruptors and impact animal fertility, it is unlikely that humans with a typical soy diet will achieve comparable levels of biologically active isoflavones to impact human fertility.

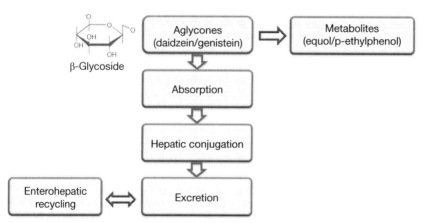

Figure 18.2 Absorption and metabolism of daidzein and genistein in the body. Glycosidic isoflavones are not readily bioavailable because of the sugar-binding moiety that prohibits enterocyte crossing. Hydrolysis is required for gut absorption and bioavailability. On hydrolysis, unconjugated aglycones are produced, which can be further metabolized into *p*-ethylphenol (genistein) and equol (daidzein). In the body, these compounds can go through reconjugation to glucuronides and are excreted in the urine.

Two possible exceptions are the use of soy-based infant formula and the intake of high-supplementary isoflavones. In the United States, 25% of infants are reportedly fed a soy protein-based infant formula (Badger et al., 2002). Although infant formula contains a relatively low content of isoflavones, which likely depends on batches and sources of isoflavones (Patisaul and Jefferson, 2010), the volume intake (6–9 mg kg^{-1} day^{-1}) could be enough to substantially increase plasma levels of isoflavones. Specifically, infants fed soy-based formulas can be exposed to an isoflavone dose that is five- to tenfold higher than that of adults consuming modest amounts of soy protein foods, posing a potential developmental health risk (Setchell et al., 1998). Still, little is known about intake of soy infant formula and the long-term health impacts. Concerning the potential detrimental effects associated with the use of high-supplementary isoflavones, there was a clinical case study reporting that intake of high-supplementary isoflavones could affect female reproductive health (Chandrareddy et al., 2008). In this report, symptoms of abnormal uterine bleeding, endometrial pathology, and dysmenorrhea in females were eliminated after removing the isoflavone supplement from the diet, suggesting that high-supplementary intake of isoflavones, at least in humans may do more harm than good. Interestingly, laboratory animals with soy protein being their major dietary component, readily consume 60–80 mg kg^{-1} day^{-1} of isoflavones on a daily basis throughout their life span without adverse effects on breeding capability (Brown and Setchell, 2001).

Isoflavones and resveratrol bind to ERs but with a much weaker binding affinity than endogenous estrogen (100, 1000, and 7000 times weaker for daidzein, genistein, and resveratrol) (Adlercreutz et al., 1995; Bowers et al., 2000). Despite the weak binding properties of these phytoestrogens, it is possible to achieve biologically effective levels following intake of soy foods to compete with endogenous estrogen for ERs. Specifically, most estrogen that circulates in the blood is bound to albumin and/or sex-hormone-binding globulin (Nagel et al., 1998). Only a small fraction ($<5\%$) of the circulating estrogen is a free, unbound form that is available for the ER occupancy. Although the levels of estrogen are variable during menstrual cycle, total plasma estrogen ranges from less than 50 (at menstruation) to 200 pg ml^{-1} (at the peak of follicular development). Considering the bound and unbound forms of circulating estrogen, the amount of free, unbound estrogen available for ER occupancy is approximately 2.5–10 pg ml^{-1}. In a typical Japanese diet, the plasma level of genistein can reach as high as 4 μM (Adlercreutz et al., 1993; Setchell, 1998) of which, approximately 5% is present as the unbound form, an amount that is well beyond the biologically effective levels of estrogen (Verkasalo et al., 2001a). Moreover, the binding affinity of daidzein and equol for plasma protein is so low that 18% of plasma daidzein and 50% of plasma equol are present as unbound forms, effectively increasing their bioavailability for ER occupancy (Garreau et al., 1991; Nagel et al., 1998). From these data, it is likely that after intake of soy products, the plasma levels of isoflavones can easily exceed the levels that are achieved by endogenous estrogen and are biologically active and potentially impact a wide range of cellular and molecular targets.

In addition to functional effects similar to estrogen, phytoestrogens have biological properties that are not related to estrogen. Specifically, genistein is a potent inhibitor of protein tyrosine kinases and has the ability to regulate cell growth and proliferation and inhibit activation of growth factors (Akiyama et al., 1987; Kim et al., 1998). Such actions of genistein can potentially slow the rate of tumorigenesis, which is in fact the rationale for the use of isoflavones in patients with or at risk of developing breast cancer (Wright et al., 1995). There is also evidence that genistein has antioxidant and anti-inflammatory properties implicating a role as a cardioprotective agent (Ruiz-Larrea et al., 1997). Among isoflavones with known antioxidant properties, equol is shown to have much more potent antioxidant capabilities than genistein or daidzein presumably because of its ability to readily donate an electron/hydrogen to free radicals (Mitchell et al., 1998). The suggestion is that individuals with equol-producing ability may perhaps be better protected against exposure to oxidative stress, which could result in reduced risks of cardiovascular disease (see below). Overall, phytoestrogens are unique compounds with multiple biological effects, whose modes of action involve both ER-dependent and ER-independent mechanisms. Although they bind to ERs weakly, the bioavailability and preferential binding to ER β confer phytoestrogens as significant biologically relevant compounds.

4. PHYTOESTROGENS AND CARDIOVASCULAR HEALTH

Risks for coronary artery disease substantially increase in postmenopausal women, purportedly because of a loss of estrogen production. Estrogen replacement therapy (hormone replacement therapy) is a conventional approach to treating postmenopausal symptoms. However, some evidence suggests that the risks that accrue from hormone replacement therapy could exceed the potential benefits. In a recent study from the Women's Health Initiative, increased risks for developing breast cancer, heart attacks, and strokes in association with hormone replacement therapy were reported (Rossouw et al., 2002).

Because phytoestrogens are nonsteroidal, dietary estrogens, they have been considered as an alternative to hormone replacement therapy (Paech et al., 1997). Moreover, phytoestrogens are suggested to play a role in reducing risks for coronary heart disease and promoting cardiovascular health. Here, evidence for and against the purported benefits of soy protein/phytoestrogens in promoting cardiovascular health is presented (Figure 18.3). Interestingly, we have reported a negative effect of soy rodent chow on a genetic model of heart disease suggesting alternative pathways targeted by isoflavones (Stauffer et al., 2006). Here, the focus is on isoflavone phytoestrogens and their effects on cholesterol lowering, vascular function, and regulation of blood pressure and the ability to enhance antioxidant and anti-inflammatory capacities.

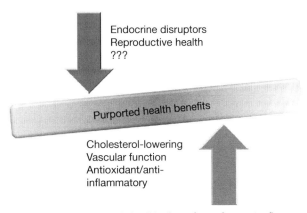

Figure 18.3 Summary of the purported health benefits of soy isoflavones. Consumption of phytoestrogen in the form of a soy-based diet is an attractive dietary alternative and may reduce the risks of developing coronary heart disease. Possible mechanisms could involve cholesterol-lowering effects, improved vascular function, and antioxidant activity. Since soy phytoestrogens can also play a role as endocrine disruptors that may adversely affect human health, it is important to make dietary choices accordingly.

4.1 Cholesterol-Lowering Effects

The incidence of cardiovascular disease in Asian adult populations is typically lower than that in Western countries. It is possible that the lower incidence of cardiovascular disease is related to higher amount of soy foods in their diet, exerting favorable effects on blood–lipid profile, a well–established risk factor for coronary heart disease. In fact, the FDA's health claims that daily intake of soy protein reduces risk factors, albeit marginally (less than 3%), for cardiovascular disease was largely based on the cholesterol-lowering (total and low-density lipoprotein; LDL) effects of soy protein. Yet, the validity of these data suggesting the potential benefit of soy isoflavones on cholesterol is being questioned. For example, the AHA recently reversed its endorsement of soy products after a retrospective meta–analysis found no effect of soy proteins or plant estrogens on lipids and/or lipid profiles (Sacks et al., 2006).

An important question in these studies is whether the soy isoflavones themselves are even responsible for the presumed benefits. Support for the biological role of soy isoflavones was demonstrated in studies where the cholesterol-lowering effects were absent when soy protein depleted of isoflavones was administered (Crouse et al., 1999; Wangen et al., 2001). Specifically, textured soy protein, which contained half soy flour and half soy protein concentrate, was effective in reducing blood cholesterol, whereas soy protein isolate whose isoflavones had been removed during the process of ethanol extraction, failed to show the efficacy. These results suggest that isoflavones are likely the responsible compounds for the hypocholesterolemic effects. However, conflicting results have also been reported (Hodgson et al., 1998; Nestel et al., 1997;

Simons et al., 2000). In these studies, there was a favorable impact of soy protein on blood–lipid profile, regardless of whether the soy protein contained isoflavones or not (Demonty et al., 2003). Taken together, it is likely that soy protein plays a role in lowering blood cholesterol. However, it is not clear whether soy isoflavones are responsible for the impact of soy protein on lipid profiles.

4.2 Vascular Function

Vascular function is often studied by measuring endothelial function and arterial compliance, a measure of distensibility in major arterial vasculature. Abnormalities in vascular function are associated with increased risks for future cardiovascular events. Thus, improvements in arterial compliance and endothelial function can be viewed as protective against future cardiovascular events.

Most studies investigating the effects of phytoestrogens on vascular function have been carried out in postmenopausal women whom often exhibit a rapid decline in endothelial function compared to age-matched men (Taddei et al., 1996). Notably, one study examined the dose-dependent impact of isoflavones on vascular function (Walker et al., 2001). To investigate whether genistein influences endothelium-dependent vasodilation, multiple doses of genistein ($10–300$ nmol min^{-1}, each dose for 6 min) were infused into the forearm brachial artery of healthy human subjects (Walker et al., 2001). Brachial infusion of genistein potentiated endothelium-dependent vasodilation in response to acetylcholine and induced dose-dependent increases in blood flow. Intriguingly, this effect was blocked by an inhibitor of nitric oxide (NO), suggesting that genistein caused NO-dependent vasodilation (Walker et al., 2001).

This was also confirmed in other studies by demonstrating that the vasodilatory effects of isoflavones were mediated through increased production of NO (Karamsetty et al., 2001; Squadrito et al., 2002; van der Schouw et al., 2002). Likewise, in an experimental model of diet-induced atherosclerosis, postmenopausal monkeys receiving an isoflavone-rich soy diet showed an endothelium-mediated vasodilatory response to acetylcholine, whereas control animals receiving a low dose of isoflavones had a constrictive response. Furthermore, intravenous administration of genistein caused dilation in these animals with previously constricted coronary vasculature (Honore et al., 1997). However, the findings that report the efficacy of isoflavones on improved vascular function are contradicted by a study in which purified soy isoflavones (80 mg day^{-1}) failed to show increased flow-mediated arterial dilation in postmenopausal women (Simons et al., 2000).

Systemic arterial compliance, an important cardiovascular risk factor, was also tested. In double-blinded, placebo-controlled, randomized trials of postmenopausal women, both purified soy and red clover phytoestrogens significantly increased arterial compliance (Nestel et al., 1997, 1999). Intriguingly, these effects occurred in the absence of changes in plasma lipid profile. Collectively, this evidence, albeit limited, indicates that isoflavones may act as a potent vasodilator and improve arterial compliance, including NO-dependent vascular endothelial function. This may underlie the basis of cardiovascular health-promoting effects of phytoestrogens and improved blood pressure regulation discussed below.

4.3 Blood Pressure

Studies investigating the effect of soy protein with or without isoflavones on blood pressure are less conclusive (Hodgson et al., 1999; Teede et al., 2001, 2006). In a randomized, double-blinded study of normotensive men and postmenopausal women, intake of soy protein resulted in a small but a significant reduction (5 mmHg) in mean blood pressure (Teede et al., 2001). However, these data contradicted the results of a clinical trial using supplementary isoflavones (30 mg of genistein, 16 mg of biochanin A, 1 mg of daidzein, and 8 mg of formononetin) that failed to show any blood pressure-lowering effect (Teede et al., 2001). Interestingly, this study also reported a decline in endothelial function in male subjects receiving the isoflavone supplement, posing a potential cardiovascular health risk (Teede et al., 2001). Likewise, a single dose of purified unconjugated isoflavones at amounts ($2–16$ mg kg^{-1}) that exceed normal dietary intake ($0.5–1$ mg kg^{-1}) in healthy postmenopausal women had minimal impact on blood pressure (Bloedon et al., 2002). Overall, the impact of isoflavones on blood pressure is not convincing. The available studies demonstrate a marginal or no effect of isoflavones on blood pressure. Additional study is required to fully resolve whether isoflavones have impact on the regulation of blood pressure.

4.4 Antioxidant and Anti-Inflammatory Effects

Activation of oxidative and inflammatory pathways contributes to the progression of atherosclerosis and increases the incidence of coronary events. Since phytoestrogens have antioxidant and anti-inflammatory capacity, administration of these compounds may reduce the incidence of coronary heart disease.

Phytoestrogens show antioxidant effects on cholesterol oxidation, and this prevention of cholesterol oxidation may partially underlie the cardiovascular health benefits demonstrated in human (Jenkins et al., 2002; Tikkanen et al., 1998; Wiseman et al., 2000) and animal studies (Register et al., 2005). Healthy volunteers who received soy isoflavone (12 mg genistein and 7 mg daidzein) bars for 2 weeks showed protection against LDL oxidation, resistance to copper-mediated oxidation *ex vivo*, and marked prolongation of lag time to LDL oxidation (Tikkanen et al., 1998). Likewise, consumption of soy containing naturally occurring amounts of isoflavones reduced lipid peroxidation in humans and increased the resistance of LDL to oxidation compared with a soy diet without iso-flavones (Wiseman et al., 2000). These clinical findings are in line with an animal study reporting that a soy diet increased the expression of antioxidant genes, including endo-thelial NO synthase (eNOS), manganese superoxide dismutase, and cytochrome c oxi-dase (Mahn et al., 2005). Conversely, a soy-deficient diet decreased eNOS and antioxidant gene expression, accompanied by impaired endothelial function and elevated blood pressure. These phenotypes were reversed following refeeding with a soy-containing diet.

Isoflavones may also impart antiatherosclerotic actions through cholesterol-independent mechanisms. In a mouse model of apolipoprotein E knockout, a soy-containing diet reduced atherosclerotic lesions without affecting blood cholesterol levels (Register et al., 2005). Likewise, the inhibitory effect of a soy protein diet on atherosclerosis in mice required neither alterations in plasma cholesterol contents nor the presence of LDL receptors that are suggested to be involved in cholesterol-lowering effects of isoflavones (Adams et al., 2002a).

These data may indicate that the antioxidant properties of isoflavones may play a larger role in the antiatherosclerotic impact. Monocyte binding to endothelium and the subsequent migration into the intimal layer is an initial step for atherosclerosis. This process is promoted by increased transcription, and thus, activation, of these adhesion molecules. It has been suggested that phytoestrogens can attenuate atheroscle-rosis by reducing gene transcription of adhesion molecules and their subsequent migration to the atherosclerotic lesion. Indeed, in a nonhuman primate model of atherosclerosis consuming a moderately atherogenic diet, an isoflavone dose equivalent to $129 \, \text{mg day}^{-1}$ exerted an anti-inflammatory effect specific for serum soluble vascular cell adhesion molecule-1 (Adams et al., 2002b). In a study of human endothe-lial cells cocultured with monocytes, genistein was shown to reduce the expression of intracellular and vascular adhesion molecules (Takahashi et al., 1996). Similar findings have also been reported in rodents-fed soy-based diets (Adams et al., 2002a). In a model of apolipoprotein E-deficient mice, intake of a dietary soy protein isolate supplemented with isoflavones ameliorated atherosclerotic lesions, which was in turn accompanied by reduced expression of monocyte chemoattractant protein-1 (MCP-1). This suggests that the reduction in atherosclerotic lesions observed in these mice is mediated by the inhibition of MCP-1, leading to reduced monocyte migration (Nagarajan et al., 2008).

Although these studies indicate the antioxidant capacity of phytoestrogens (primarily prevention of LDL oxidation), they only implicate a potential role for phytoestrogens in reducing the risk for coronary heart disease. This potential benefit of phytoestrogens on cardiovascular health can be mediated through enhanced antioxidant capacity, improved endothelial function, diminished LDL oxidation, and consequently, reduced stress-induced inflammation.

5. CONFOUNDING FACTORS TO CONSIDER

Results from the clinical, nutritional, and biological studies of soy protein show both positive and negative results regarding the efficacy of soy phytoestrogens/isoflavones in the prevention of cardiovascular disease. It is possible that confounding factors that were unknown and/or neglected at the time of study might have contributed to the incongruous findings. Heterogeneity of participants (e.g., variations in baseline LDL cholesterol levels and equol producer vs. nonequol producer), variability of phytoestrogen doses and dietary compositions, and presence of preexisting disease may all affect the study outcomes. Recognition that the nutritional study outcomes are confounded by various factors is an initial step to better understand the roles of phytoestrogens in cardiovascular health.

Intake of phytoestrogens in the human nutritional studies can be variable because of timing of harvest, use of a particular soy crop, and types of soybeans used among other reasons. Studies often fail to measure blood isoflavones, and individual isoflavone intake is frequently derived from a food-frequency questionnaire (Verkasalo et al., 2001b; van der Schouw et al., 2002). This is an important issue because the biological modes of action of phytoestrogens and the effects are shown to be dose dependent (Kuiper et al., 1998; Patel et al., 2001; Walker et al., 2001). Specifically, ER binding of isoflavones occurs in the nanomolar range, whereas antioxidant activity of isoflavones requires a much higher dose (Kuiper et al., 1998; Patel et al., 2001). Consistent with the dose-dependency of isoflavones, in a study of human fetal endothelial cells, genistein rapidly activated eNOS at a nanomolar (100 nM) range (Joy et al., 2006), whereas it inhibits protein tyrosine kinase at micromolar (10–50 μM) concentrations (Chu et al., 2005).

In addition to variation in dietary phytoestrogen content and the differential biological impact, there is interindividual variation in isoflavone metabolism that can contribute to inconsistent study outcomes. By and large, not all humans are able to produce equol (Lampe et al., 1998; Setchell et al., 2003a). The equol-producing ability, which was originally coined when limited numbers of individuals (only 4 in 6) fed a soy diet excreted equol in their urine (Setchell et al., 1984), is considerably variable among different adult populations. Approximately 60% Asian adult populations fed a soy-rich diet are readily capable of producing equol from daidzein metabolism, presumably because of the presence of intestinal equol-producing bacteria (Fujimoto et al., 2008; Song et al., 2006; Watanabe et al., 1998), while the incidence (approximately 30%) is much lower in Western populations (Lampe et al., 1998; Rowland et al., 2000). Thus, it is clear that there is marked interindividual and interregional variation in the ability to produce equol from isoflavone metabolism. This may contribute largely and underlie the basis to the inconsistent findings of soy phytoestrogens on human cardiovascular health.

Furthermore, a previous meta-analysis demonstrated that the impact of a soy diet on serum lipids depended on the initial serum cholesterol concentration (Anderson et al., 1995). When a substantial portion of an animal protein diet was replaced with soy, normo-cholesterolemic individuals often tended to be unresponsive to isoflavone exposure (Hodgson et al., 1998), whereas individuals with higher initial cholesterol level showed a more robust response (Anderson et al., 1995; Potter et al., 1998). The implication from these studies is that variations in baseline cholesterol levels could affect the study outcomes. Besides individual differences in isoflavone metabolism and initial serum cholesterol, existing disease may also confound study outcomes. In a recent meta-analysis of double-blind, randomized, placebo-controlled trials of postmenopausal women, isoflavone supplementation showed improved flow-mediated endothelial function only in women with a low (<5.2%) baseline flow-mediated dilation, suggesting that preexisting disease alters the effectiveness of isoflavones (Li et al., 2010).

Finally, nutritional studies are often carried out using animal models. The strength of animal studies is that the experimental conditions are readily controlled. Thus, potential confounding variables such as doses of phytoestrogens and dietary compositions can be minimized. The weakness of animal studies is that the biological effects often differ from those in humans. For example, phytoestrogen metabolism in animals differs from that of humans. Most animals are capable of producing the daidzein metabolite equol, whereas not all humans have this ability (Lampe et al., 1998; Setchell et al., 2003a). The concentration of circulating equol is also typically higher in rodents and nonhuman primates than in humans, partially because of a slower urinary clearance (Brown and Setchell, 2001; Gu et al., 2006). Thus, it is clear that not all species are created equal in terms of how they metabolize phytoestrogens. For this reason, species-specific differences in phytoestrogen metabolism must be considered when results of animal studies are extrapolated to humans. Overall, it is conceivable that the variation of phytoestrogen intake, interindividual variability, and interregional variability in phytoestrogen metabolism may partially underlie the incongruous findings.

6. SUMMARY AND CONCLUDING REMARKS

Soy is a rich source of highly bioactive compounds that have distinct biological properties implicating an important role as a dietary component. Phytoestrogens can exert a wide range of cellular and molecular effects at levels that can be achieved through food intake. However, the role of soy phytoestrogens on cardiovascular health is largely inconsistent. Consumption of soy protein may have a favorable impact, albeit marginal, on blood lipid profiles, which presumably lowers the risk of cardiovascular incidences. However, neither beneficial nor detrimental effects of phytoestrogens on serum cholesterol and blood pressure are often reported. The beneficial effects on vascular function appear to be more consistent. Nevertheless, there is emerging evidence that phytoestrogens may affect cardiovascular health through mechanisms involving enhanced antioxidant and anti-inflammatory capacities. Inconsistency in some of the findings may stem from variations in isoflavone content, individual difference in isoflavone metabolism and baseline cholesterol levels, variations in doses, and possibly dietary composition.

What can we say about soy phytoestrogens as heart-healthy dietary alternative? Soy products contain various nutrients, including high-polyunsaturated and low-saturated fats, fiber, and vitamins, that are all potentially beneficial for long-term cardiovascular health. For this reason, moderate consumption of phytoestrogen in the form of a soy-based diet is an attractive dietary alternative and may confer meaningful long-term cardiovascular benefits. On the other hand, given the existing evidence that soy phytoestrogens play a role as endocrine disruptors that may adversely affect human health, use of phytoestrogen supplement should be approached with caution until the safety and efficacy are proven.

ACKNOWLEDGMENTS

This work was supported by NIH grant (HL 098256) and by a National and Mentored Research Science Development Award (K01 AR052840) from the NIH awarded to J.P. Konhilas.

REFERENCES

Adams, M.R., Golden, D.L., Anthony, M.S., Register, T.C., Williams, J.K., 2002a. The inhibitory effect of soy protein isolate on atherosclerosis in mice does not require the presence of ldl receptors or alteration of plasma lipoproteins. Journal of Nutrition 132, 43–49.

Adams, M.R., Golden, D.L., Register, T.C., et al., 2002b. The atheroprotective effect of dietary soy iso-flavones in apolipoprotein e-/- mice requires the presence of estrogen receptor-alpha. Arteriosclerosis, Thrombosis, and Vascular Biology 22, 1859–1864.

Adlercreutz, H., Markkanen, H., Watanabe, S., 1993. Plasma concentrations of phyto-oestrogens in Japanese men. The Lancet 342, 1209–1210.

Adlercreutz, C.H., Goldin, B.R., Gorbach, S.L., et al., 1995. Soybean phytoestrogen intake and cancer risk. Journal of Nutrition 125, 757s–770s.

Akiyama, T., Ishida, J., Nakagawa, S., et al., 1987. Genistein, a specific inhibitor of tyrosine-specific protein kinases. Journal of Biological Chemistry 262, 5592–5595.

Anderson, J.W., Johnstone, B.M., Cook-Newell, M.E., 1995. Meta-analysis of the effects of soy protein intake on serum lipids. The New England Journal of Medicine 333, 276–282.

Anderson, J.J., Anthony, M.S., Cline, J.M., Washburn, S.A., Garner, S.C., 1999. Health potential of soy isoflavones for menopausal women. Public Health Nutrition 2, 489–504.

Badger, T.M., Ronis, M.J., Hakkak, R., Rowlands, J.C., Korourian, S., 2002. The health consequences of early soy consumption. Journal of Nutrition 132, 559s–565s.

Barnes, S., Peterson, T.G., Coward, L., 1995. Rationale for the use of genistein-containing soy matrices in chemoprevention trials for breast and prostate cancer. Journal of Cellular Biochemistry. Supplement 22, 181–187.

Basly, J.P., Marre-Fournier, F., Le Bail, J.C., Habrioux, G., Chulia, A.J., 2000. Estrogenic/antiestrogenic and scavenging properties of (E)- and (Z)-resveratrol. Life Sciences 66, 769–777.

Baur, J.A., Pearson, K.J., Price, N.L., et al., 2006. Resveratrol improves health and survival of mice on a high-calorie diet. Nature 444, 337–342.

Bennetts, H.W., Underwood, E.J., Shier, F.L., 1946. A specific breeding problem of sheep on subterranean clover pastures in Western Australia. Australian Veterinary Journal 22, 2–12.

Bloedon, L.T., Jeffcoat, A.R., Lopaczynski, W., et al., 2002. Safety and pharmacokinetics of purified soy isoflavones: single-dose administration to postmenopausal women. American Journal of Clinical Nutrition 76, 1126–1137.

Bowers, J.L., Tyulmenkov, V.V., Jernigan, S.C., Klinge, C.M., 2000. Resveratrol acts as a mixed agonist/antagonist for estrogen receptors alpha and beta. Endocrinology 141, 3657–3667.

Bradbury, R.B., White, D.E., 1954. Estrogens and related substances in plants. Vitamins and Hormones 12, 207–233.

Brown, N.M., Setchell, K.D., 2001. Animal models impacted by phytoestrogens in commercial chow: implications for pathways influenced by hormones. Laboratory Investigation 81, 735–747.

Busby, M.G., Jeffcoat, A.R., Bloedon, L.T., et al., 2002. Clinical characteristics and pharmacokinetics of purified soy isoflavones: single-dose administration to healthy men. American Journal of Clinical Nutrition 75, 126–136.

Chandrareddy, A., Muneyyirci-Delale, O., Mcfarlane, S.I., Murad, O.M., 2008. Adverse effects of phytoestrogens on reproductive health: a report of three cases. Complementary Therapies in Clinical Practice 14, 132–135.

Chu, L., Zhang, J.X., Norota, I., Endoh, M., 2005. Differential action of a protein tyrosine kinase inhibitor, genistein, on the positive inotropic effect of endothelin-1 and norepinephrine in canine ventricular myocardium. British Journal of Pharmacology 144, 430–442.

Crouse 3rd, J.R., Morgan, T., Terry, J.G., Ellis, J., Vitolins, M., Burke, G.L., 1999. A randomized trial comparing the effect of casein with that of soy protein containing varying amounts of isoflavones on plasma concentrations of lipids and lipoproteins. Archives of Internal Medicine 159, 2070–2076.

Cruz, M.N., Agewall, S., Schenck-Gustafsson, K., Kublickiene, K., 2008. Acute dilatation to phytoestrogens and estrogen receptor subtypes expression in small arteries from women with coronary heart disease. Atherosclerosis 196, 49–58.

Demonty, I., Lamarche, B., Jones, P.J., 2003. Role of isoflavones in the hypocholesterolemic effect of soy. Nutrition Reviews 61, 189–203.

Eldridge, A.C., Kwolek, W.F., 1983. Soybean isoflavones: effect of environment and variety on composition. Journal of Agricultural and Food Chemistry 31, 394–396.

Erdman Jr., J.W., 2000. Soy protein and cardiovascular disease: a statement for healthcare professionals from the nutrition committee of the AHA. Circulation 102, 2555–2559.

Food Labeling: Health Claims: Soy Protein And Coronary Artery Disease, 1999. Food and Drug Administration, HHS: final rule: soy protein and coronary heart disease. Federal Register 64, 57700–57733.

Fremont, L., 2000. Biological effects of resveratrol. Life Sciences 66, 663–673.

Fujimoto, K., Tanaka, M., Hirao, Y., et al., 2008. Age-stratified serum levels of isoflavones and proportion of equol producers in Japanese and Korean healthy men. Prostate Cancer and Prostatic Diseases 11, 252–257.

Garreau, B., Vallette, G., Adlercreutz, H., et al., 1991. Phytoestrogens: new ligands for rat and human alpha-fetoprotein. Biochimica et Biophysica Acta 1094, 339–345.

Gu, L., House, S.E., Prior, R.L., et al., 2006. Metabolic phenotype of isoflavones differ among female rats, pigs, monkeys, and women. Journal of Nutrition 136, 1215–1221.

Hodgson, J.M., Puddey, I.B., Beilin, L.J., Mori, T.A., Croft, K.D., 1998. Supplementation with isoflavonoid phytoestrogens does not alter serum lipid concentrations: a randomized controlled trial in humans. Journal of Nutrition 128, 728–732.

Hodgson, J.M., Puddey, I.B., Beilin, L.J., et al., 1999. Effects of isoflavonoids on blood pressure in subjects with high-normal ambulatory blood pressure levels: a randomized controlled trial. American Journal of Hypertension 12, 47–53.

Honore, E.K., Williams, J.K., Anthony, M.S., Clarkson, T.B., 1997. Soy isoflavones enhance coronary vascular reactivity in atherosclerotic female macaques. Fertility and Sterility 67, 148–154.

Jenkins, D.J., Kendall, C.W., Jackson, C.J., et al., 2002. Effects of high- and low-isoflavone soyfoods on blood lipids, oxidized LDL, homocysteine, and blood pressure in hyperlipidemic men and women. American Journal of Clinical Nutrition 76, 365–372.

Joy, S., Siow, R.C., Rowlands, D.J., et al., 2006. The isoflavone Equol mediates rapid vascular relaxation: Ca^{2+}-independent activation of endothelial nitric-oxide synthase/Hsp90 involving ERK1/2 and Akt phosphorylation in human endothelial cells. Journal of Biological Chemistry 281, 27335–27345.

Karamsetty, M.R., Klinger, J.R., Hill, N.S., 2001. Phytoestrogens restore nitric oxide-mediated relaxation in isolated pulmonary arteries from chronically hypoxic rats. Journal of Pharmacology and Experimental Therapeutics 297, 968–974.

Keys, A., Menotti, A., Aravanis, C., et al., 1984. The seven countries study: 2,289 deaths in 15 years. Preventive Medicine 13, 141–154.

Kim, H., Peterson, T.G., Barnes, S., 1998. Mechanisms of action of the soy isoflavone genistein: emerging role for its effects via transforming growth factor beta signaling pathways. American Journal of Clinical Nutrition 68, 1418s–1425s.

Konhilas, J.P., Leinwand, L.A., 2007. The effects of biological sex and diet on the development of heart failure. Circulation 116, 2747–2759.

Kuiper, G.G., Carlsson, B., Grandien, K., et al., 1997. Comparison of the ligand binding specificity and transcript tissue distribution of estrogen receptors alpha and beta. Endocrinology 138, 863–870.

Kuiper, G.G., Lemmen, J.G., Carlsson, B., et al., 1998. Interaction of estrogenic chemicals and phytoestrogens with estrogen receptor beta. Endocrinology 139, 4252–4263.

Kushner, P.J., Agard, D.A., Greene, G.L., et al., 2000. Estrogen receptor pathways to AP-1. The Journal of Steroid Biochemistry and Molecular Biology 74, 311–317.

Lampe, J.W., Karr, S.C., Hutchins, A.M., Slavin, J.L., 1998. Urinary equol excretion with a soy challenge: influence of habitual diet. Proceedings of the Society for Experimental Biology and Medicine 217, 335–339.

Lee, I.H., Cao, L., Mostoslavsky, R., et al., 2008. A role for the NAD-dependent deacetylase Sirt1 in the regulation of autophagy. Proceedings of the National Academy of Sciences of the United States of America 105, 3374–3379.

Li, S.H., Liu, X.X., Bai, Y.Y., et al., 2010. Effect of oral isoflavone supplementation on vascular endothelial function in postmenopausal women: a meta-analysis of randomized placebo-controlled trials. American Journal of Clinical Nutrition 91, 480–486.

Mahn, K., Borras, C., Knock, G.A., et al., 2005. Dietary soy isoflavone induced increases in antioxidant and eNOS gene expression lead to improved endothelial function and reduced blood pressure in vivo. The FASEB Journal 19, 1755–1757.

Meyer, B.J., Larkin, T.A., Owen, A.J., Astheimer, L.B., Tapsell, L.C., Howe, P.R., 2004. Limited lipid-lowering effects of regular consumption of whole soybean foods. Annals of Nutrition and Metabolism 48, 67–78.

Mitchell, J.H., Gardner, P.T., Mcphail, D.B., Morrice, P.C., Collins, A.R., Duthie, G.G., 1998. Antioxidant efficacy of phytoestrogens in chemical and biological model systems. Archives of Biochemistry and Biophysics 360, 142–148.

Moggs, J.G., Orphanides, G., 2001. Estrogen receptors: orchestrators of pleiotropic cellular responses. EMBO Reports 2, 775–781.

Morito, K., Hirose, T., Kinjo, J., et al., 2001. Interaction of phytoestrogens with estrogen receptors alpha and beta. Biological and Pharmaceutical Bulletin 24, 351–356.

Nagarajan, S., Burris, R.L., Stewart, B.W., Wilkerson, J.E., Badger, T.M., 2008. Dietary soy protein isolate ameliorates atherosclerotic lesions in apolipoprotein E-deficient mice potentially by inhibiting monocyte chemoattractant protein-1 expression. Journal of Nutrition 138, 332–337.

Nagata, C., Takatsuka, N., Kurisu, Y., Shimizu, H., 1998. Decreased serum total cholesterol concentration is associated with high intake of soy products in Japanese men and women. Journal of Nutrition 128, 209–213.

Nagel, S.C., Vom Saal, F.S., Welshons, W.V., 1998. The effective free fraction of estradiol and xenoestrogens in human serum measured by whole cell uptake assays: physiology of delivery modifies estrogenic activity. Proceedings of the Society for Experimental Biology and Medicine 217, 300–309.

Nestel, P.J., Yamashita, T., Sasahara, T., et al., 1997. Soy isoflavones improve systemic arterial compliance but not plasma lipids in menopausal and perimenopausal women. Arteriosclerosis, Thrombosis, and Vascular Biology 17, 3392–3398.

Nestel, P.J., Pomeroy, S., Kay, S., et al., 1999. Isoflavones from red clover improve systemic arterial compliance but not plasma lipids in menopausal women. Journal of Clinical Endocrinology and Metabolism 84, 895–898.

Paech, K., Webb, P., Kuiper, G.G., et al., 1997. Differential ligand activation of estrogen receptors ERalpha and ERbeta at AP1 sites. Science 277, 1508–1510.

Patel, R.P., Boersma, B.J., Crawford, J.H., et al., 2001. Antioxidant mechanisms of isoflavones in lipid systems: paradoxical effects of peroxyl radical scavenging. Free Radical Biology & Medicine 31, 1570–1581.

Patisaul, H.B., Jefferson, W., 2010. The pros and cons of phytoestrogens. Frontiers in Neuroendocrinology 31, 400–419.

Picherit, C., Dalle, M., Neliat, G., et al., 2000. Genistein and daidzein modulate in vitro rat uterine contractile activity. The Journal of Steroid Biochemistry and Molecular Biology 75, 201–208.

Potter, S.M., Baum, J.A., Teng, H., Stillman, R.J., Shay, N.F., Erdman Jr., J.W., 1998. Soy protein and isoflavones: their effects on blood lipids and bone density in postmenopausal women. American Journal of Clinical Nutrition 68, 1375s–1379s.

Register, T.C., Cann, J.A., Kaplan, J.R., et al., 2005. Effects of soy isoflavones and conjugated equine estrogens on inflammatory markers in atherosclerotic, ovariectomized monkeys. Journal of Clinical Endocrinology and Metabolism 90, 1734–1740.

Robb, E.L., Page, M.M., Wiens, B.E., Stuart, J.A., 2008. Molecular mechanisms of oxidative stress resistance induced by resveratrol: specific and progressive induction of MnSod. Biochemical and Biophysical Research Communications 367, 406–412.

Rossouw, J.E., Anderson, G.L., Prentice, R.L., et al., 2002. Risks and benefits of estrogen plus progestin in healthy postmenopausal women: principal results from the Women's Health Initiative randomized controlled trial. Journal of the American Medical Association 288, 321–333.

Rowland, I.R., Wiseman, H., Sanders, T.A., Adlercreutz, H., Bowey, E.A., 2000. Interindividual variation in metabolism of soy isoflavones and lignans: influence of habitual diet on equol production by the gut microflora. Nutrition and Cancer 36, 27–32.

Rozman, K.K., Bhatia, J., Calafat, A.M., et al., 2006. NTP-CERHR expert panel report on the reproductive and developmental toxicity of genistein. Birth Defects Research. Part B, Developmental and Reproductive Toxicology 77, 485–638.

Ruiz-Larrea, M.B., Mohan, A.R., Paganga, G., Miller, N.J., Bolwell, G.P., Rice-Evans, C.A., 1997. Antioxidant activity of phytoestrogenic isoflavones. Free Radical Research 26, 63–70.

Sacks, F.M., Lichtenstein, A., Van Horn, L., Harris, W., Kris-Etherton, P., Winston, M., 2006. Soy protein, isoflavones, and cardiovascular health: an American Heart Association Science Advisory for professionals from the Nutrition Committee. Circulation 113, 1034–1044.

Setchell, K.D., 1998. Phytoestrogens: the biochemistry, physiology, and implications for human health of soy isoflavones. American Journal of Clinical Nutrition 68, 1333s–1346s.

Setchell, K.D., Cassidy, A., 1999. Dietary isoflavones: biological effects and relevance to human health. Journal of Nutrition 129, 758s–767s.

Setchell, K.D., Borriello, S.P., Hulme, P., Kirk, D.N., Axelson, M., 1984. Nonsteroidal estrogens of dietary origin: possible roles in hormone-dependent disease. American Journal of Clinical Nutrition 40, 569–578.

Setchell, K.D., Gosselin, S.J., Welsh, M.B., et al., 1987. Dietary estrogens – a probable cause of infertility and liver disease in captive cheetahs. Gastroenterology 93, 225–233.

Setchell, K.D., Zimmer-Nechemias, L., Cai, J., Heubi, J.E., 1998. Isoflavone content of infant formulas and the metabolic fate of these phytoestrogens in early life. American Journal of Clinical Nutrition 68, 1453s–1461s.

Setchell, K.D., Brown, N.M., Desai, P., et al., 2001. Bioavailability of pure isoflavones in healthy humans and analysis of commercial soy isoflavone supplements. Journal of Nutrition 131, 1362s–1375s.

Setchell, K.D., Brown, N.M., Lydeking-Olsen, E., 2002. The clinical importance of the metabolite equol – a clue to the effectiveness of soy and its isoflavones. Journal of Nutrition 132, 3577–3584.

Setchell, K.D., Brown, N.M., Desai, P.B., et al., 2003a. Bioavailability, disposition, and dose-response effects of soy isoflavones when consumed by healthy women at physiologically typical dietary intakes. Journal of Nutrition 133, 1027–1035.

Setchell, K.D., Faughnan, M.S., Avades, T., et al., 2003b. Comparing the pharmacokinetics of daidzein and genistein with the use of 13C-labeled tracers in premenopausal women. American Journal of Clinical Nutrition 77, 411–419.

Shutt, D.A., Cox, R.I., 1972. Steroid and phyto-oestrogen binding to sheep uterine receptors in vitro. Journal of Endocrinology 52, 299–310.

Simons, L.A., Von Konigsmark, M., Simons, J., Celermajer, D.S., 2000. Phytoestrogens do not influence lipoprotein levels or endothelial function in healthy, postmenopausal women. The American Journal of Cardiology 85, 1297–1301.

Song, K.B., Atkinson, C., Frankenfeld, C.L., et al., 2006. Prevalence of daidzein-metabolizing phenotypes differs between Caucasian and Korean American women and girls. Journal of Nutrition 136, 1347–1351.

Squadrito, F., Altavilla, D., Morabito, N., et al., 2002. The effect of the phytoestrogen genistein on plasma nitric oxide concentrations, endothelin-1 levels and endothelium dependent vasodilation in postmenopausal women. Atherosclerosis 163, 339–347.

Stauffer, B.L., Konhilas, J.P., Luczak, E.D., Leinwand, L.A., 2006. Soy diet worsens heart disease in mice. The Journal of Clinical Investigation 116, 209–216.

Taddei, S., Virdis, A., Ghiadoni, L., et al., 1996. Menopause is associated with endothelial dysfunction in women. Hypertension 28, 576–582.

Takahashi, M., Kitagawa, S., Masuyama, J.I., et al., 1996. Human monocyte-endothelial cell interaction induces synthesis of granulocyte-macrophage colony-stimulating factor. Circulation 93, 1185–1193.

Teede, H.J., Dalais, F.S., Kotsopoulos, D., Liang, Y.L., Davis, S., Mcgrath, B.P., 2001. Dietary soy has both beneficial and potentially adverse cardiovascular effects: a placebo-controlled study in men and postmenopausal women. Journal of Clinical Endocrinology and Metabolism 86, 3053–3060.

Teede, H.J., Giannopoulos, D., Dalais, F.S., Hodgson, J., Mcgrath, B.P., 2006. Randomised, controlled, cross-over trial of soy protein with isoflavones on blood pressure and arterial function in hypertensive subjects. Journal of the American College of Nutrition 25, 533–540.

Thorp, A.A., Howe, P.R., Mori, T.A., et al., 2008. Soy food consumption does not lower LDL cholesterol in either equol or nonequol producers. American Journal of Clinical Nutrition 88, 298–304.

Tikkanen, M.J., Wahala, K., Ojala, S., Vihma, V., Adlercreutz, H., 1998. Effect of soybean phytoestrogen intake on low density lipoprotein oxidation resistance. Proceedings of the National Academy of Sciences of the United States of America 95, 3106–3110.

Van Der Schouw, Y.T., Pijpe, A., et al., 2002. Higher usual dietary intake of phytoestrogens is associated with lower aortic stiffness in postmenopausal women. Arteriosclerosis, Thrombosis, and Vascular Biology 22, 1316–1322.

Verkasalo, P.K., Appleby, P.N., Allen, N.E., Davey, G., Adlercreutz, H., Key, T.J., 2001a. Soya intake and plasma concentrations of daidzein and genistein: validity of dietary assessment among eighty British women (Oxford arm of the European Prospective Investigation into Cancer and Nutrition). British Journal of Nutrition 86, 415–421.

Verkasalo, P.K., Appleby, P.N., Davey, G.K., Key, T.J., 2001b. Soy milk intake and plasma sex hormones: a cross-sectional study in pre- and postmenopausal women (EPIC-Oxford). Nutrition and Cancer 40, 79–86.

Wakai, K., Egami, I., Kato, K., Kawamura, T., et al., 1999. Dietary intake and sources of isoflavones among Japanese. Nutrition and Cancer 33, 139–145.

Walker, H.A., Dean, T.S., Sanders, T.A., Jackson, G., Ritter, J.M., Chowienczyk, P.J., 2001. The phytoestrogen genistein produces acute nitric oxide-dependent dilation of human forearm vasculature with similar potency to 17beta-estradiol. Circulation 103, 258–262.

Wallerath, T., Deckert, G., Ternes, T., et al., 2002. Resveratrol, a polyphenolic phytoalexin present in red wine, enhances expression and activity of endothelial nitric oxide synthase. Circulation 106, 1652–1658.

Wangen, K.E., Duncan, A.M., Xu, X., Kurzer, M.S., 2001. Soy isoflavones improve plasma lipids in normocholesterolemic and mildly hypercholesterolemic postmenopausal women. American Journal of Clinical Nutrition 73, 225–231.

Watanabe, S., Yamaguchi, M., Sobue, T., et al., 1998. Pharmacokinetics of soybean isoflavones in plasma, urine and feces of men after ingestion of 60 g baked soybean powder (kinako). Journal of Nutrition 128, 1710–1715.

Wiseman, H., O'reilly, J.D., Adlercreutz, H., et al., 2000. Isoflavone phytoestrogens consumed in soy decrease F(2)-isoprostane concentrations and increase resistance of low-density lipoprotein to oxidation in humans. American Journal of Clinical Nutrition 72, 395–400.

Wright, J.D., Reuter, C.W., Weber, M.J., 1995. An incomplete program of cellular tyrosine phosphory-lations induced by kinase-defective epidermal growth factor receptors. Journal of Biological Chemistry 270, 12085–12093.

Zubik, L., Meydani, M., 2003. Bioavailability of soybean isoflavones from aglycone and glucoside forms in American women. American Journal of Clinical Nutrition 77, 1459–1465.

CHAPTER 19

Probiotic Species on Cardiovascular Disease: The Use of Probiotics to Reduce Cardiovascular Disease Risk Factors

H. Chen, J.P. Konhilas
University of Arizona, Tucson, AZ, USA

ABBREVIATIONS

ACE Angiotensin I converting enzyme
BSH Bile salt hydrolase
CVD Cardiovascular disease
DBP Diastolic blood pressure
GDCA Glycodeoxycholic acid
HCAEC Human coronary artery endothelial cells
HDL High-density lipoprotein
LDL Low-density lipoprotein
LPS Lipopolysaccharide
SBP Systolic blood pressure
SFA Saturated fatty acids
SHR Spontaneous hypertensive rats
SOD Superoxide dismutase
TAG Triglyceride
TAS Total antioxidant status
TBARS Thiobarbituric acid reactive substances
TDCA Taurodeoxycholic acid
TLRs Toll-like receptors
TNF-α Tumor necrosis factor-α

1. INTRODUCTION

Cardiovascular disease (CVD), which is usually used to refer to disease conditions related to atherosclerosis, is the leading cause of illness and death in industrialized countries. In 2006, CVD alone accounted for 34.3% of all deaths or 1 out of every 2.9 deaths in the United States (Lloyd-Jones et al., 2009). Many risk factors have been associated with the development of atherosclerosis, such as hypertension, dyslipoproteinemia, and diabetes or impaired glucose tolerance (insulin resistance) (Guttmacher et al., 2003). Recently, it has been revealed that inflammation plays a role in the pathogenesis of CVD. In regards to

Bioactive Food as Dietary Interventions for Cardiovascular Disease
http://dx.doi.org/10.1016/B978-0-12-396485-4.00017-7

© 2013 Elsevier Inc.
All rights reserved.

the prevention of CVD, epidemiologic studies and randomized clinical trials have provided compelling evidence that coronary heart disease is largely preventable (Cooper et al., 2000). Currently, prevention and initial treatment of CVD are primarily focused on diet and lifestyle interventions (Artinian et al., 2010). Studies suggest that proper management of CVD risk factors may result in improved morbidity and mortality. In addition, the high cost of medical therapy and patient compliance to this therapy are major limitations to risk management. Therefore, alternative strategies for CVD prevention and treatment, such as probiotic dietary therapy, have received considerable attention by scientific community.

By FAO/WHO definition, probiotics are viable microorganisms that confer health benefits to the host once consumed in adequate amounts. Microbes such as *Lactobacillus* and *Bifidobacterium* are the most common organisms used as probiotics. These probiotics are commonly consumed as adjuvant of fermented foods such as yogurt, soy yogurt, or as dietary supplements. Several studies in animals and humans have shown that probiotics and probiotic dairy products may protect against CVD by lowering CVD risk factors. This chapter will focus on the effects of probiotics and probiotic dairy products on CVD risk factors in both animal models and humans with particular attention given to the mechanisms by which these effects might be exerted.

2. HYPOCHOLESTEROLEMIC EFFECT OF PROBIOTICS

Hypercholesterolemia has been identified as a major risk factor of CVD, increasing the risk of a heart attack threefold over individuals with normal blood lipid profiles. The possible cholesterol-lowering effect of probiotic bacteria was first suggested by the early observations of Mann & Spoerry (Mann and Spoerry, 1974). They discovered that high consumption of fermented milk reduced serum cholesterol levels despite the weight gain in African men of the Maasai tribe. Since then, research has been done on the hypocholesterolemic potential of probiotics, in both animal models and human clinical trials. Although far from being conclusive, results from animal and human studies suggest that probiotics have cholesterol-lowering capacity, especially probiotics from fermented dairy products.

2.1 Animal Studies

In a cholesterol-fed rabbit model, 30-day oral administration of a soy product fermented by *Enterococcus faecium* CRL 183 and *Lactobacillus jugurti* 416 caused an 18.4% reduction in total cholesterol and a 17.8% increase in the high-density lipoprotein (HDL) fraction (Rossi et al., 2000). In another study, *Lactobacillus plantarum* PH04, isolated from infant feces, was fed to hypercholesterolemic mice. Compared with the control group, serum cholesterol and triglycerides (TAGs) were, respectively, 7 and 10% lower in the experimental group (Nguyen et al., 2007). Similarly, feeding rats a cholesterol-enriched diet along with milk yogurt or soy yogurt supplemented with the probiotics, *Bifidobacterium lactis* (Bb-12) or *Bifidobacterium longum* (Bb-46) for 5 weeks resulted in lower levels of total plasma cholesterol, very low-density lipoprotein (VLDL), and low-density lipoprotein (LDL) cholesterol. Interestingly, the hypocholesterolemic effect was strain specific. Yogurt or soy yogurt containing Bb-46 was more effective in the low-ering of plasma and liver cholesterol levels than yogurt or soy yogurt containing Bb-12 (Abd El-Gawad et al., 2005). Another study using rats on a cholesterol-rich diet showed daily *Lactobacillus acidophilus* 4356 supplementation at a daily dose of 109 colony forming units (CFU) significantly lowered total serum cholesterol, LDL cholesterol, and TAG concentrations without a change in serum HDL cholesterol concentrations (Huang et al., 2010).

Models, other than rats and mice, demonstrated similar results. In cholesterol-fed rabbits, oral administration of *E. faecium* CRL 183 suspension by gavage resulted in improved lipid profiles by increasing the HDL level by 43% and lowing TAG level by 50% (Cavallini et al., 2009). Research conducted on male hamsters fed a high-cholesterol diet showed that after an 8 week intake of milk fermented by *Lactobacillus* strains (NTU 101 and 102) demonstrated about a 20% decrease in total serum (and liver) cholesterol levels. Although there was a decrease in LDL, HDL decreased as well (Chiu et al., 2006). Similarly, hyperlipidemic hamsters administered (8 weeks) a fermented milk–soy milk supplemented with *Monordia charantia* fermented by *Lactobacillus paracasei subsp. paracasei* NTU 101 showed lowered serum cholesterol and TAG, reduced athero-sclerotic plaque in aorta, increased superoxide dismutase (SOD) and total antioxidant status (TAS) activity, and reduced thiobarbituric acid reactive substances (TBARS). All of the above suggested that this fermented soy milk product was effective in prevent-ing and retarding the hyperlipidemia-induced oxidative stress and atherosclerosis in hyperlipidemic hamsters model (Tsai et al., 2009).

2.2 Human Studies

Compared to the study results from animal models, the cholesterol-lowering effect of probiotics in human trials is more controversial. While some studies showed significant lipid-lowering effects of probiotics, others did not. It must be noted that most human trials are randomized, double-blind, and placebo-controlled studies. In one study that included 48 normocholesterolemic healthy, male human subjects, 6 weeks oral intake of soy product fermented with *E. faecium* and *L. jugurti* demonstrated a 10% increase in HDL-cholesterol (Rossi et al., 2003). In another study, 70 overweight subjects ingested yogurt fermented with one strain of *E. faecium* and two strains of *Streptococcus thermophilus* on a daily basis for 8 weeks. These study subjects showed reduced LDL-cholesterol by 8.4% (Agerholm-Larsen et al., 2000). In a trial including 90 young healthy women, daily consumption of probiotic yogurt fermented by *L. acidophilus* La5 and

B. lactis Bb12 for 6 weeks increased plasma HDL and lowered LDL levels. While both probiotic and conventional yogurt decreased the total/HDL cholesterol ratio, only probiotic yogurt showed elevated HDL levels (Sadrzadeh-Yeganeh et al., 2010). In two independent studies involving a total of 69 hypercholesterolemic human subjects, effects of consumption of one daily serving of fermented milk by *L. acidophilus* L1 on serum lipids for 3–4 months were examined. The daily intake of fermented milk resulted in a moderate decrease of total serum cholesterol (2.4–3.2%) (Anderson and Gilliland, 1999).

However, the hypocholesterolemic effects of probiotic products have not always been observed in human trials. Several studies have demonstrated minimal, if any, impact of probiotics on lipid profiles. In a study involving 80 volunteers with elevated cholesterol levels, daily intake of a capsule containing *L. acidophilus* for 6 months did not cause any change in serum lipids throughout the study (Lewis and Burmeister, 2005). Similarly, daily intake of a capsule containing *Lactobacillus fermentum* 10 weeks failed to lower serum cholesterol levels in human subjects with elevated cholesterol to start (Simons et al., 2006).

Interestingly, all studies that failed to show cholesterol-lowering activity used bacteria-containing capsules instead of fermented milk or soy products as the method of probiotic delivery. This indicates that the hypocholesterolemic effect may be from the fermented milk product and not directly from the probiotics. Moreover, these data also suggest that the hypocholesterolemic effect of probiotics may be strain specific.

3. MECHANISM OF HYPOCHOLESTEROLEMIC EFFECT OF PROBIOTICS

Several mechanisms have been proposed for mediating the cholesterol-lowering effects of probiotics. However, these studies addressing the mechanism of probiotic efficacy have been tested both *in vitro* and *in vivo*. Most of the *in vivo* studies conducted so far have focused on simply verifying the lipid-lowering effects of probiotics, rather than the mechanisms of this effect.

3.1 Enzymatic Deconjugation of Bile Salt by Bile Salt Hydrolase from Probiotics

Bile is synthesized in the liver from cholesterol. It is then stored and concentrated in the gall bladder, and released into the duodenum upon ingestion of food. Bile consists of cholesterol, phospholipids, conjugated bile acids, bile pigments, and electrolytes. Recycling of conjugated bile salts occurs along the proximal and distal ileum, where they are reabsorbed actively into the hepatic portal circulation, a process called enterohepatic circulation. However, once deconjugated by bile salt hydrolase (BSH) from probiotics, bile acids are less soluble and absorbable by the intestines, leading to their elimination in feces. As a result, more cholesterol needs to be utilized to synthesize new bile acids, which in turn causes the lowering of serum cholesterol (Begley et al., 2006). In an *in vitro* study using microencapsulated *L. plantarum* 80 (pCBH1), BSH was able to effectively break down conjugated bile acids, glycodeoxycholic acid (GDCA), and taurodeoxycholic acid (TDCA) (Jones et al., 2004). Furthermore, BSH activity has been identified in many other probiotic species (Lambert et al., 2008; Patel et al., 2010). Therefore, bile salt deconjugation by BSH of probiotics may be a common mechanism for mediating the hypocholesterolemic effect. In addition, an inverse relationship between fecal excretions of bile acids and levels of total cholesterol in blood plasma was observed from rats fed a cholesterol-enriched diet with probiotic supplementation (Abd El-Gawad et al., 2005).

3.2 Assimilation of Cholesterol by Probiotics

Several human gut-derived lactic acid bacteria and bifidobacteria strains have shown the capacity to consume cholesterol *in vitro* (Pereira and Gibson, 2002). It has been previously reported that media cholesterol can be removed by binding to cellular surfaces of strains of *Lactobacillus gasseri*. Interestingly, the cholesterol-binding ability was strain specific (Usman and Hosono, 1999). Another study showed that lipids absorbed by probiotics were predominantly found in the membrane, suggesting that cholesterol was incorporated into the cellular membrane of the cells. Although growing cells removed more cholesterol than dead cells, the heat-killed cells could still remove cholesterol from media, suggesting that some cholesterol was bound to the cellular surface (Usman and Hosono, 1999). In a recent study, a fluorescent probe was used to label the phospholipid bilayer of probiotic cells to determine the possible locations of the incorporated cholesterol within the membrane. Enrichment of cholesterol was found in the regions of the phospholipid tails, upper phospholipids, and polar heads of the cellular membrane phospholipid bilayer in cells that were grown in the presence of cholesterol, indicating incorporation of cholesterol in those regions (Lye et al., 2010).

3.3 Conversion of Cholesterol into Coprostanol

Conversion of cholesterol into coprostanol decreases the amount of cholesterol being absorbed, leading to a reduced concentration in the physiological cholesterol pool, which in turn results in lowered serum cholesterol levels. It has been reported that cholesterol dehydrogenase (isomerase) produced by strains of *Sterolibacterium denitrificans* was responsible for catalyzing the transformation of cholesterol to cholest-4-en-3-one, an intermediate cofactor in the conversion of cholesterol to coprostanol (Chiang et al., 2008). In a recent study, the conversion of cholesterol to coprostanol by strains of lactobacilli was evaluated using fluorometric assays. Both intracellular and extracellular cholesterol reductases were detected in all strains of probiotics examined. The decrease of cholesterol concentration in the medium upon fermentation by probiotics was accompanied by increased concentrations of coprostanol in the media (Lye et al., 2010).

4. HYPOTENSIVE EFFECT OF FERMENTED MILK PRODUCT

Hypertension is a major risk factor in CVD and its related complications. The disease affects approximately 1 billion individuals worldwide, and approximately 7.1 million deaths per year can be attributed to hypertension (Chobanian et al., 2003). Because of its high prevalence, severe consequences, and especially its association with CVD, hypertension has become a worldwide health challenge. Reduction in blood pressure, as small as 10–12 mmHg in systolic blood pressure (SBP) or 5 mmHg in diastolic blood pressure (DBP), may reduce the risk of stroke by 40%, coronary heart disease by 16%, and all-cause mortality by 13% (Collins and MacMahon, 1994). Over the last two decades, the blood pressure-lowering potential of fermented milk products has been tested in both animal models and human trials.

4.1 Animal Studies

The blood pressure-lowering effects of milk products fermented by different probiotics species have been intensively studied using spontaneous hypertensive rats (SHRs). Interestingly, both transient and long-term hypotensive benefits have been observed. In two separate studies, feeding SHRs sour milk fermented by *Lactobacillus helveticus* and *Saccharomyces cerevisiae* (Ameal S product) or a yogurt product supplemented with *L. helveticus* CPN4 strain led to a significant decrease in SBP 6 h after feeding (Nakamura et al., 1995; Yamamoto et al., 1999). Similar results following with fermented, caseinate-enriched milk supplemented with *L. helveticus* R211 and R389 or skim milk fermented by *Enterococcus faecalis* (CECT 5727, 5728, 5826, and 5827) 5 and 4 h postfeeding, respectively (Leclerc et al., 2002). With regards to long-term hypotensive effects, it was reported that 12–23 weeks of oral administration resulted in significant drops in SBP using several strains of probiotics (Nakamura et al., 1996; Sipola et al., 2001, 2002).

4.2 Human Studies

The results from human (randomized, double-blind, placebo-controlled) studies are less consistent. Studies involving mildly hypertensives demonstrated that 8 weeks of oral intake (Ameal S or Evolus products) reduced SBP by ~14 and 10 mmHg, respectively (Hata et al., 1996; Seppo et al., 2003). Similar results were obtained in healthy (Kawase et al., 2000) or hypertensive volunteers (Seppo et al., 2003). On the other hand, no significant blood pressure change was observed in hypertensive human subjects (89 human subjects included) after 24 weeks (12 weeks of low dosage, followed by 12 weeks of high dosage) of oral administration of probiotic-containing milk (Jauhiainen and Korpela, 2007) or milk fermented with *L. helveticus* (Usinger et al., 2010). In a trial involving 135 Dutch subjects with elevated SBP, consumption of fermented milk for 8 weeks did not culminate in decreased blood pressure when compared with control group (Engberink et al., 2008).

5. MECHANISMS OF BLOOD PRESSURE LOWERING

The exact blood pressure-lowering mechanism of fermented milk products is still unknown. It is generally accepted that bioactive peptides generated during the fermentation process of milk play an important role in the blood pressure-lowering effect. Thus, the impact of these probiotic-generated peptides on pressure control mechanisms has been studied, with a particular focus on the renin–angiotensin system (RAS). RAS is a hormone system that regulates blood pressure and water (fluid) balance. In RAS, renin acts on angiotensinogen, the inactive precursor, thus releasing the decapeptide angiotensin I. Then, angiotensin I is converted to angiotensin II by angiotensin I converting enzyme (ACE). Angiotensin II is a strong vasoconstrictor that induces release of aldosterone and, therefore, increases sodium concentration and further increases blood pressure. Also, ACE inactivates bradykinin, which is another potent vasodilator (Roland et al., 2007). So far, many peptides that inhibit ACE have been identified from fermented milk products.

It was first reported that αs1- and β-casein hydrolysates by the *L. helveticus* CP790 proteinase inhibit ACE activity. Accordingly, oral administration of these hydrolysates showed antihypertensive activity in SHRs (Yamamoto et al., 1994). Two peptides (Val–Pro–Pro [VPP] and Ile–Pro–Pro [IPP]) in Calpis sour milk were identified as inhibitors of ACE (Nakamura et al., 1995) and long-term (>9 weeks) intake of *L. helveticus* fermented milk containing IPP, VPP peptides attenuated hypertension in SHRs (Jauhiainen et al., 2005; Sipola et al., 2001, 2002). In addition, single oral administration of the sour milk or corresponding inhibitory units of these peptides significantly decreased SBP in SHRs (Nakamura et al., 1995). Subsequently, it was reported that fermented milk containing these peptides reduces blood pressure in SHR better than fermented milk lacking these peptides (Fuglsang et al., 2002).

With respect to humans, a clinical study conducted on 30 hospital outpatient subjects suggested that these two peptides and sour milk did significantly lower both the SBP and DBP in the treatment group, but not in a placebo-controlled group (Hata et al., 1996). The observed hypotensive effect of the milk appears to be associated with the amount of peptides involved. Thus, fermented milk, which contains more peptides, has a greater hypotensive effect than milk containing less peptides (Sipola et al., 2002). On the contrary, in some studies, fermented milk alone has shown better effect than peptides alone, suggesting that other components in the fermented milk also contribute to the antihypertensive effect (Jauhiainen et al., 2005; Sipola et al., 2002). Recently, these two peptides have been shown able to prevent the development of malignant hypertension in a rat transgenic malignant hypertension model, which overexpresses human renin and human angiotensinogen genes (Jauhiainen et al., 2010).

Besides VPP and IPP, there are many other peptides from fermented milk products have been identified as ACE inhibitory peptides in different *in vitro* studies (Minervini et al., 2003; Yamamoto et al., 1999). Also, ACE inhibitory peptides have been identified and tested from milk products fermented by bacterial species other than *Lactobacillus* species. Milk fermented with *E. faecalis* CECT 5727, revealed two peptides, LHLPLP and LVYPFPGPIPNSLPQNIPP, which showed angiotensin converting enzyme–inhibitory (ACEI) activity; this hypotensive activity was observed in SHR after oral administration. In addition, the presence of these antihypertensive peptides was confirmed in fermented milk prepared with other selected strains of *E. faecalis* (CECT 5728, 5826, and 5827) as well (Quirûs et al., 2007). Finally, the bioactive peptides from cell wall fragments of *Lactobacillus casei* YIT9018 also showed antihypertensive activity (Sawada et al., 1990).

6. ALTERNATIVE TARGETS OF BIOACTIVE PEPTIDES

Although ACE inhibition seems to be the primary target, the peptide Lys–Val–Leu–Pro–Val–Pro–Gln was identified as having strong antihypertensive effects, despite low anti-ACE activity (Maeno et al., 1996). Another peptide alpha–lactorphin, which is derived from α-lactalbumin, has been shown to lower blood pressure in SHRs via opioid receptors (Nurminen et al., 2000). This suggestion is that the antihypertensive effect of probiotics may result from alternative targets other than ACE.

7. EFFECTS OF PEPTIDES OTHER THAN BLOOD PRESSURE-LOWERING EFFECT

Peptides from fermented milk products have demonstrated multiple targets. In this regard, VPP and IPP peptides were associated with improved endothelium–dependent relaxation in SHRs (Jauhiainen et al., 2005). In an *in vitro* study using SHR mesenteric arteries, these peptides had a protective effect on the endothelial function. In addition, administration of VPP and IPP peptides improved vascular endothelial function in 24 human subjects with mild hypertension, which appears to be independent of their blood pressure-lowering effects (Hirota et al., 2007). In a recent double-blind parallel group intervention study, long-term intervention (24 weeks) with peptide milk reduced arterial stiffness in hypertensive human subjects as compared to controls (Jauhiainen and Korpela, 2007). Therefore, it is likely that the overall antihypertensive effect from consumption of fermented milk products may result from the combinatorial action of probiotic-derived peptides on multiple targets including ACE, vascular, and endothelial cells.

8. LIPOPOLYSACCHARIDE (LPS), INFLAMMATION, CVD, AND PROBIOTICS

The traditional view of atherosclerosis as a lipid storage disorder has been replaced by the new concept that atherosclerosis is mostly an inflammatory disorder and thus the inflammatory response plays a central role in every step of atherosclerosis development (Ross, 1999, Hansson, 2005). For example, the fatty streak, generally taken as the earliest type of lesion of atherosclerosis, is an inflammatory lesion, including macrophages and T lymphocytes (Stary et al., 1994) and is present in every phase of atherosclerosis development (Hansson et al., 1989). Currently, the role of Toll-like receptors (TLRs) and macrophages in atherosclerosis is emerging as important for the pathogenesis of atherosclerosis. TLRs bind molecules with pathogen-like molecular patterns, and initiate a signal cascade, which leads to cell activation (Janeway and Medzhitov, 2002). Cells in human atherosclerotic lesions display a spectrum of TLRs (Edfeldt et al., 2002). Recently, TLR4 has been shown to play an essential role in the development of atherosclerosis. Knockout of TLR4 inhibited the development of atherosclerosis in apoE-knockout mice (Hayashi et al., 2010). Similarly, TLR4 knockout has been associated with reductions in lesion size, lipid content, and macrophage infiltration in apoE−/− mice fed a high-cholesterol diet for 6 months (Michelsen et al., 2004). On the other hand, stimulation of TLR2, led to a significant increase in atherosclerotic plaque development in ApoE knockout mice (Schoneveld et al., 2005).

Activation of TLR4 is triggered by the agonist LPS, also called endotoxin, which is an outer membrane component of gram-negative bacteria and is composed of oligosaccharides and acylated saturated fatty acids (SFA). Free SFA have been reported to bind and activate TLR4 (Lee et al., 2001; 2003) suggesting a potential role of LPS as the proinflammatory mediator in atherosclerosis (Stoll et al., 2004). The prospective results from the Bruneck study suggest that endotoxemia constitutes a strong risk factor for the development of atherosclerosis, especially for smokers (Wiedermann et al., 1999). Moreover, results from a large population study implicated a strong association between chronic infections and atherosclerosis development, even in low-risk subjects. Interestingly, a wide range of infections usually caused by gram negative bacteria, such as respiratory and urinary tract infections, were associated with an increased risk for atherosclerosis, while infections from viruses were not (Kiechl et al., 2001).

On the same note, animal studies revealed that weekly injections of LPS accelerated the development of atherosclerotic lesions in rabbits on hypercholesterolemic diets and in apoE-deficient mice (Lehr et al., 2001). All the above evidence suggests that chronic exposure to endotoxin may be an important pathogenic and trigger factor for the development of atherosclerosis. Further evidence of LPS activity was shown in an *in vitro* study, where LPS activated human coronary artery endothelial cells (HCAEC) resulting in increased proinflammatory cytokine secretion as well as elevated levels of cell adhesion molecules. The observed HCAEC activation was shown to be mediated by LPS through TLR4 (Zeuke et al., 2002). Similarly, LPS-dependent activation of arterial smooth muscle through TLR4 signaling lead to a proinflammatory phenotype in vascular smooth muscle cells, including increased proinflammatory cytokine secretion.

Although nutritional SFA can trigger an inflammatory response by acting directly on TLR4 (Shi et al., 2006), a high-fat diet may also, indirectly, contribute to a proinflammatory environment and subsequent activation of TLR4. It has been demonstrated in diet-induced obesity models that dietary fat may increase LPS absorption through (1) a change of gut microbial composition and gut permeability, (2) an increase in LPS absorption by facilitating its incorporation into chylomicrons (Ghoshal et al., 2009), and (3) TLR4-mediated enterocyte phagocytosis and translocation of gram-negative bacteria across the intestinal barrier resulting in an increase of plasma LPS (Neal et al., 2006). In support of these data, gut microbiota control through antibiotic treatment resulted in decreased metabolic endotoxemia, reduced inflammatory tone, and increased glucose tolerance (Cani et al., 2008; Membrez et al., 2008). Similarly, genetically obese mice treated with an LPS inhibitor led to decreased inflammation and metabolic abnormalities. Finally, reduced plasma LPS level by antibiotic treatment reduced the occurrence of visceral adipose tissue inflammation, oxidative stress, and macrophage infiltration markers in high-fat fed mice, implicating LPS as an important trigger for inflammation (Cani et al., 2008). All of the above suggest that LPS–TLR4 signaling may be responsible for the inflammatory response in diet-induced obesity.

9. IMPROVING INSULIN RESISTANCE ASSOCIATED WITH INFLAMMATION

It is now clear that a low-grade inflammatory response is associated with obesity, insulin resistance, and diabetes, all of which are important risk factors for CVDs (Wellen and Hotamisligil, 2005). It was first reported that tumor necrosis factor-α (TNF-α), an important inflammatory factor, was overexpressed in adipose tissue from rodent models of obesity and diabetes. Neutralization of TNF-α in obese rat model caused a significant increase in the peripheral uptake of glucose in response to insulin. Therefore, it is possible that inflammation, specifically TNF-α, may play an important role in obesity, insulin resistance, and diabetes (Hotamisligil et al., 1993). A similar increase of TNF-α expression was also observed in the adipose and muscle tissues of obese humans (Hotamisligil et al., 1995; Kern et al., 1995; Saghizadeh et al., 1996).

TNF-α has been demonstrated to regulate adipocyte metabolism at multiple levels, from transcriptional regulation to hormone receptor signaling, which eventually leads to changes in the overall metabolism of adipocytes (Sethi and Hotamisligil, 1999). In addition, it has been shown that overproduction of TNF-α is closely associated with obese-induced insulin resistance. On the other hand, TNF-α-deficient obese mice were protected from obese-induced insulin resistance (Uysal et al., 1997). Besides TNF-α, other inflammatory mediators also exhibit similar expression and impact insulin action in a manner similar to that of TNF-α during obesity (Dandona et al., 2004; Pickup, 2004). Therefore, by reducing LPS level and LPS-induced inflammation, probiotics may be able to improve the insulin resistance associated with inflammation, which in turn will benefit the long-term outcome of CVD.

10. CONCLUSIONS AND FUTURE DIRECTIONS

The body of evidence regarding the potential benefit of probiotics for CVD is continually growing. Although the animal studies appear to be clearer regarding this potential benefit, the human studies are not. The lack of consistency with the human studies is not surprising given the multiple confounders associated with these types of study designs. The challenge for future investigators is to address these confounding issues in a controlled manner. More importantly, it is critical to delineate the impact of probiotics in a strain-dependent manner. That is, the impact of specific strains of probiotics on independent risk factors has not been addressed. Nevertheless, the foundation for the use of probiotics as a central *preventative* component for CVD has been established.

ACKNOWLEDGMENTS

This work was supported by NIH grant (HL 098256) and by a National and Mentored Research Science Development Award (K01 AR052840) from the NIH awarded to J.P. Konhilas.

REFERENCES

Abd El-Gawad, I.A., El-Sayed, E.M., Hafez, S.A., El-Zeini, H.M., Saleh, F.A., 2005. The hypocholesterolaemic effect of milk yoghurt and soy-yoghurt containing bifidobacteria in rats fed on a cholesterol-enriched diet. International Dairy Journal 15, 37–44.

Agerholm-Larsen, L., Raben, A., Haulrik, N., Hansen, A.S., Manders, M., Astrup, A., 2000. Effect of 8 week intake of probiotic milk products on risk factors for cardiovascular diseases. European Journal of Clinical Nutrition 54, 288–297.

Anderson, J.W., Gilliland, S.E., 1999. Effect of fermented milk (yogurt) containing Lactobacillus acidophilus L1 on serum cholesterol in hypercholesterolemic humans. Journal of the American College of Nutrition 18, 43–50.

Artinian, N.T., Fletcher, G.F., Mozaffarian, D., et al., 2010. On behalf of the American Heart Association Prevention Committee of the Council on Cardiovascular Nursing, Interventions to promote physical activity and dietary lifestyle changes for cardiovascular risk factor reduction in adults: A scientific statement from the American Heart Association. Circulation 122, 406–441.

Begley, M., Hill, C., Gahan, C.G., 2006. Bile salt hydrolase activity in probiotics. Applied and Environmental Microbiology 72, 1729–1738.

Cani, P.D., Bibiloni, R., Knauf, C., et al., 2008. Changes in gut microbiota control metabolic endotoxemia-induced inflammation in high-fat diet-induced obesity and diabetes in mice. Diabetes 57, 1470–1481.

Cavallini, D.C., Bedani, R., Bomdespacho, L.Q., Vendramini, R.C., Rossi, E.A., 2009. Effects of probiotic bacteria, isoflavones and simvastatin on lipid profile and atherosclerosis in cholesterol-fed rabbits: A randomized double-blind study. Lipids in Health and Disease 8, 1.

Chiang, Y.-R., Ismail, W., Heintz, D., Schaeffer, C., van Dorsselaer, A., Fuchs, G., 2008. Study of anoxic and oxic cholesterol metabolism by Sterolibacterium denitrificans. Journal of Bacteriology 190, 905–914.

Chiu, C.-H., Lu, T.-Y., Tseng, Y.-Y., Pan, T.-M., 2006. The effects of *Lactobacillus*-fermented milk on lipid metabolism in hamsters fed on high-cholesterol diet. Applied Microbiology and Biotechnology 71, 238–245.

Chobanian, A.V., Bakris, G.L., Black, H.R., et al., 2013. The National High Blood Pressure Education Program Coordinating Committee, Seventh Report of the Joint National Committee on prevention, detection, evaluation, and treatment of high blood pressure. Hypertension 42, 1206–1252.

Collins, R., Macmahon, S., 1994. Blood pressure, antihypertensive drug treatment and the risks of stroke and of coronary heart disease. British Medical Bulletin 50, 272–298.

Cooper, R., Cutler, J., Desvigne-Nickens, P., et al., 2000. Trends and disparities in coronary heart disease, stroke, and other cardiovascular diseases in the United States: Findings of the national conference on cardiovascular disease prevention. Circulation 102, 3137–3147.

Dandona, P., Aljada, A., Bandyopadhyay, A., 2004. Inflammation: The link between insulin resistance, obesity and diabetes. Trends in Immunology 25, 4–7.

Edfeldt, K., Swedenborg, J., Hansson, G.K., Yan, Z.-Q., 2002. Expression of toll-like receptors in human atherosclerotic lesions: A possible pathway for plaque activation. Circulation 105, 1158–1161.

Engberink, M.F., Schouten, E.G., Kok, F.J., van Mierlo, L.A.J., Brouwer, I.A., Geleijnse, J.M., 2008. Lactotripeptides show no effect on human blood pressure: Results from a double-blind randomized controlled trial. Hypertension 51, 399–405.

Fuglsang, A., Nilsson, D., Nyborg, N.C., 2002. Cardiovascular effects of fermented milk containing angiotensin-converting enzyme inhibitors evaluated in permanently catheterized, spontaneously hypertensive rats. Applied and Environmental Microbiology 68, 3566–3569.

Ghoshal, S., Witta, J., Zhong, J., de Villiers, W., Eckhardt, E., 2009. Chylomicrons promote intestinal absorption of lipopolysaccharides. Journal of Lipid Research 50, 90–97.

Guttmacher, A.E., Collins, F.S., Nabel, E.G., 2003. Cardiovascular disease. The New England Journal of Medicine 349, 60–72.

Hansson, G.R.K., 2005. Inflammation, atherosclerosis, and coronary artery disease. The New England Journal of Medicine 352, 1685–1695.

Hansson, G., Jonasson, L., Seifert, P., Stemme, S., 1989. Immune mechanisms in atherosclerosis. Arteriosclerosis, Thrombosis, and Vascular Biology 9, 567–578.

Hata, Y., Yamamoto, M., Ohni, M., Nakajima, K., Nakamura, Y., Takano, T., 1996. A placebo-controlled study of the effect of sour milk on blood pressure in hypertensive subjects. The American Journal of Clinical Nutrition 64, 767–771.

Hayashi, C., Madrigal, A.G., Liu, X., et al., 2010. Pathogen-mediated inflammatory atherosclerosis is mediated in part via toll-like receptor 2-induced inflammatory responses. Journal of Innate Immunity 2, 334–343.

Hirota, T., Ohki, K., Kawagishi, R., et al., 2007. Casein hydrolysate containing the antihypertensive tripeptides Val-Pro-Pro and Ile-Pro-Pro improves vascular endothelial function independent of blood pressure-lowering effects: Contribution of the inhibitory action of angiotensin-converting enzyme. Hypertension Research 30, 489–496.

Hotamisligil, G.S., Shargill, N.S., Spiegelman, B.M., 1993. Adipose expression of tumor necrosis factor-alpha: Direct role in obesity-linked insulin resistance. Science 259, 87–91.

Hotamisligil, G.S., Arner, P., Caro, J.F., Atkinson, R.L., Spiegelman, B.M., 1995. Increased adipose tissue expression of tumor necrosis factor-alpha in human obesity and insulin resistance. The Journal of Clinical Investigation 95, 2409–2415.

Huang, Y., Wang, J., Cheng, Y., Zheng, Y., 2010. The hypocholesterolaemic effects of Lactobacillus acidophilus American Type Culture Collection 4356 in rats are mediated by the down-regulation of Niemann-Pick C1-Like 1. British Journal of Nutrition 104, 807–812.

Janeway, C.A., Medzhitov, R., 2002. Innate Immune Recognition. Annual Review of Immunology 20, 197–216.

Jauhiainen, T., Korpela, R., 2007. Milk peptides and blood pressure. The Journal of Nutrition 137, 825S–829S.

Jauhiainen, T., Vapaatalo, H., Poussa, T., Kyronpalo, S., Rasmussen, M., Korpela, R., 2005. Lactobacillus helveticus fermented milk lowers blood pressure in hypertensive subjects in 24-h ambulatory blood pressure measurement. American Journal of Hypertension 18, 1600–1605.

Jauhiainen, T., Pilvi, T., Cheng, Z.J., et al., 2010. Milk products containing bioactive tripeptides have an antihypertensive effect in double transgenic rats (dTGR) harbouring human renin and human angiotensinogen genes. Journal of Nutrition and Metabolism 2010, 287030–287035.

Jones, M.L., Chen, H., Ouyang, W., Metz, T., Prakash, S., 2004. Microencapsulated genetically engineered Lactobacillus plantarum 80 (pCBH1) for bile acid deconjugation and its implication in lowering cholesterol. Journal of Biomedicine and Biotechnology 2004, 61–69.

Kawase, M., Hashimoto, H., Hosoda, M., Morita, H., Hosono, A., 2000. Effect of administration of fermented milk containing whey protein concentrate to rats and healthy men on serum lipids and blood pressure. Journal of Dairy Science 83, 255–263.

Kern, P.A., Saghizadeh, M., Ong, J.M., Bosch, R.J., Deem, R., Simsolo, R.B., 1995. The expression of tumor necrosis factor in human adipose tissue. Regulation by obesity, weight loss, and relationship to lipoprotein lipase. The Journal of Clinical Investigation 95, 2111–2119.

Kiechl, S., Egger, G., Mayr, M., et al., 2001. Chronic Infections and the risk of carotid atherosclerosis: Prospective results from a large population study. Circulation 103, 1064–1070.

Lambert, J.M., Bongers, R.S., de Vos, W.M., Kleerebezem, M., 2008. Functional analysis of four bile salt hydrolase and penicillin acylase family members in Lactobacillus plantarum WCFS1. Applied and Environmental Microbiology 74, 4719–4726.

Leclerc, P.-L., Gauthier, S.F., Bachelard, H., Santure, M., Roy, D., 2002. Antihypertensive activity of casein-enriched milk fermented by Lactobacillus helveticus. International Dairy Journal 12, 995–1004.

Lee, J.Y., Sohn, K.H., Rhee, S.H., Hwang, D., 2001. Saturated fatty acids, but not unsaturated fatty acids, induce the expression of cyclooxygenase-2 mediated through toll-like receptor 4. The Journal of Biological Chemistry 276, 16683–16689.

Lee, J.Y., Ye, J., Gao, Z., et al., 2003. Reciprocal modulation of toll-like receptor-4 signaling pathways involving MyD88 and phosphatidylinositol 3-kinase/AKT by saturated and polyunsaturated fatty acids. The Journal of Biological Chemistry 278, 37041–37051.

Lehr, H.-A., Sagban, T.A., Ihling, C., et al., 2001. Immunopathogenesis of atherosclerosis: Endotoxin accelerates atherosclerosis in rabbits on hypercholesterolemic diet. Circulation 104, 914–920.

Lewis, S.J., Burmeister, S., 2005. A double-blind placebo-controlled study of the effects of Lactobacillus acidophilus on plasma lipids. European Journal of Clinical Nutrition 59, 776–780.

Lloyd-Jones, D., Adams, R., Carnethon, M., et al., 2009. Heart disease and stroke statistics – 2009 update: A report from the American Heart Association Statistics Committee and Stroke Statistics Subcommittee. Circulation 119, e21–e181.

Lye, H.S., Rusul, G., Liong, M.T., 2010. Removal of cholesterol by lactobacilli via incorporation and conversion to coprostanol. Journal of Dairy Science 93, 1383–1392.

Maeno, M., Yamamoto, N., Takano, T., 1996. Identification of an antihypertensive peptide from casein hydrolysate produced by a proteinase from Lactobacillus helveticus CP790. Journal of Dairy Science 79, 1316–1321.

Mann, G.V., Spoerry, A., 1974. Studies of a surfactant and cholesteremia in the Maasai. The American Journal of Clinical Nutrition 27, 464–469.

Membrez, M., Blancher, F., Jaquet, M., et al., 2008. Gut microbiota modulation with norfloxacin and ampicillin enhances glucose tolerance in mice. The FASEB Journal 22, 2416–2426.

Michelsen, K.S., Wong, M.H., Shah, P.K., et al., 2004. Lack of Toll-like receptor 4 or myeloid differentiation factor 88 reduces atherosclerosis and alters plaque phenotype in mice deficient in apolipoprotein E. Proceedings of the National Academy of Sciences of the United States of America 101, 10679–10684.

Minervini, F., Algaron, F., Rizzello, C.G., Fox, P.F., Monnet, V., Gobbetti, M., 2003. Angiotensin I-converting-enzyme-inhibitory and antibacterial peptides from Lactobacillus helveticus PR4 proteinase-hydrolyzed caseins of milk from six species. Applied and Environmental Microbiology 69, 5297–5305.

Nakamura, Y., Yamamoto, N., Sakai, K., Takano, T., 1995. Antihypertensive effect of sour milk and peptides isolated from it that are inhibitors to angiotensin I-converting enzyme. Journal of Dairy Science 78, 1253–1257.

Nakamura, Y., Masuda, O., Takano, T., 1996. Decrease of tissue angiotensin I-converting enzyme activity upon feeding sour milk in spontaneously hypertensive rats. Bioscience, Biotechnology, and Biochemistry 60, 488–489.

Neal, M.D., Leaphart, C., Levy, R., et al., 2006. Enterocyte TLR4 mediates phagocytosis and translocation of bacteria across the intestinal barrier. Journal of Immunology 176, 3070–3079.

Nguyen, T.D., Kang, J.H., Lee, M.S., 2007. Characterization of Lactobacillus plantarum PH04, a potential probiotic bacterium with cholesterol-lowering effects. International Journal of Food Microbiology 113, 358–361.

Nurminen, M.-L., Sipola, M., Kaarto, H., et al., 2000. [alpha]-Lactorphin lowers blood pressure measured by radiotelemetry in normotensive and spontaneously hypertensive rats. Life Sciences 66, 1535–1543.

Patel, A., Singhania, R., Pandey, A., Chincholkar, S., 2010. Probiotic bile salt hydrolase: Current developments and perspectives. Applied Biochemistry and Biotechnology 162, 166–180.

Pereira, D.I., Gibson, G.R., 2002. Cholesterol assimilation by lactic acid bacteria and bifidobacteria isolated from the human gut. Applied and Environmental Microbiology 68, 4689–4693.

Pickup, J.C., 2004. Inflammation and activated innate immunity in the pathogenesis of type 2 diabetes. Diabetes Care 27, 813–823.

Quirûs, A., Ramos, M., Muguerza, B., et al., 2007. Identification of novel antihypertensive peptides in milk fermented with Enterococcus faecalis. International Dairy Journal 17, 33–41.

Roland, E.S., Karl, F.H., Markus, P.S., Bernhard, M.W.S., 2007. Renin-angiotensin system and cardiovascular risk. The Lancet 369, 1208–1219.

Ross, R., 1999. Atherosclerosis – an inflammatory disease. The New England Journal of Medicine 340, 115–126.

Rossi, E.A., Vendramini, R.C., Carlos, I.Z., et al., 2000. Effects of a novel fermented soy product on the serum lipids of hypercholesterolemic rabbits. Arquivos Brasileiros de Cardiologia 74, 213–216.

Rossi, E.A., Vendramini, R.C., Carlos, I.Z., de Oliveira, M.G., de Valdez, G.F., 2003. Effect of a new fermented soy milk product on serum lipid levels in normocholesterolemic adult men. Archivos Latinoamericanos de Nutrición 53, 47–51.

Sadrzadeh-Yeganeh, H., Elmadfa, I., Djazayery, A., Jalali, M., Heshmat, R., Chamary, M., 2010. The effects of probiotic and conventional yoghurt on lipid profile in women. British Journal of Nutrition 103, 1778–1783.

Saghizadeh, M., Ong, J.M., Garvey, W.T., Henry, R.R., Kern, P.A., 1996. The expression of TNF alpha by human muscle. Relationship to insulin resistance. The Journal of Clinical Investigation 97, 1111–1116.

Sawada, H., Furushiro, M., Hirai, K., Motoike, M., Watanabe, T., Yokokura, T., 1990. Purification and characterization of an antihypertensive compound from Lactobacillus casei. Agricultural and Biological Chemistry 54, 3211–3219.

Schoneveld, A.H., Oude Nijhuis, M.M., Van Middelaar, B., Laman, J.D., De Kleijn, D.P.V., Pasterkamp, G., 2005. Toll-like receptor 2 stimulation induces intimal hyperplasia and atherosclerotic lesion development. Cardiovascular Research 66, 162–169.

Seppo, L., Jauhiainen, T., Poussa, T., Korpela, R., 2003. A fermented milk high in bioactive peptides has a blood pressure-lowering effect in hypertensive subjects. The American Journal of Clinical Nutrition 77, 326–330.

Sethi, J.K., Hotamisligil, G.S., 1999. The role of TNF[alpha] in adipocyte metabolism. Seminars in Cell & Developmental Biology 10, 19–29.

Shi, H., Kokoeva, M.V., Inouye, K., Tzameli, I., Yin, H., Flier, J.S., 2006. TLR4 links innate immunity and fatty acid-induced insulin resistance. The Journal of Clinical Investigation 116, 3015–3025.

Simons, L.A., Amansec, S.G., Conway, P., 2006. Effect of Lactobacillus fermentum on serum lipids in subjects with elevated serum cholesterol. Nutrition, Metabolism, and Cardiovascular Diseases 16, 531–535.

Sipola, M., Finckenberg, P., Santisteban, J., Korpela, R., Vapaatalo, H., Nurminen, M.L., 2001. Long-term intake of milk peptides attenuates development of hypertension in spontaneously hypertensive rats. Journal of Physiology and Pharmacology 52, 745–754.

Sipola, M., Finckenberg, P., Korpela, R., Vapaatalo, H., Nurminen, M.L., 2002. Effect of long-term intake of milk products on blood pressure in hypertensive rats. The Journal of Dairy Research 69, 103–111.

Stary, H., Chandler, A., Glagov, S., et al., 1994. A definition of initial, fatty streak, and intermediate lesions of atherosclerosis. A report from the Committee on Vascular Lesions of the Council on Arteriosclerosis, American Heart Association. Circulation 89, 2462–2478.

Stoll, L.L., Denning, G.M., Weintraub, N.L., 2004. Potential role of endotoxin as a proinflammatory mediator of atherosclerosis. Arteriosclerosis, Thrombosis, and Vascular Biology 24, 2227–2236.

Tsai, T.Y., Chu, L.H., Lee, C.L., Pan, T.M., 2009. Atherosclerosis-preventing activity of lactic acid bacteria-fermented milk-soymilk supplemented with Momordica charantia. Journal of Agricultural and Food Chemistry 57, 2065–2071.

Usinger, L., Jensen, L.T., Flambard, B., Linneberg, A., Ibsen, H., 2010. The antihypertensive effect of fermented milk in individuals with prehypertension or borderline hypertension. Journal of Human Hypertension 24, 678–683.

Usman, Hosono, A., 1999. Bile tolerance, taurocholate deconjugation, and binding of cholesterol by Lactobacillus gasseri strains. Journal of Dairy Science 82, 243–248.

Uysal, K.T., Wiesbrock, S.M., Marino, M.W., Hotamisligil, G.S., 1997. Protection from obesity-induced insulin resistance in mice lacking TNF-alpha function. Nature 389, 610–614.

Wellen, K.E., Hotamisligil, G.K.S., 2005. Inflammation, stress, and diabetes. The Journal of Clinical Investigation 115, 1111–1119.

Wiedermann, C.J., Kiechl, S., Dunzendorfer, S., et al., 1999. Association of endotoxemia with carotid atherosclerosis and cardiovascular disease: Prospective results from the Bruneck study. Journal of the American College of Cardiology 34, 1975–1981.

Yamamoto, N., Akino, A., Takano, T., 1994. Antihypertensive effect of the peptides derived from casein by an extracellular proteinase from Lactobacillus helveticus CP790. Journal of Dairy Science 77, 917–922.

Yamamoto, N., Maeno, M., Takano, T., 1999. Purification and characterization of an antihypertensive peptide from a yogurt-like product fermented by Lactobacillus helveticus CPN4. Journal of Dairy Science 82, 1388–1393.

Zeuke, S., Ulmer, A.J., Kusumoto, S., Katus, H.A., Heine, H., 2002. TLR4-mediated inflammatory activation of human coronary artery endothelial cells by LPS. Cardiovascular Research 56, 126–134.

CHAPTER 20

Dairy Foods and Cardiovascular Diseases

N.J. Correa-Matos*, S.B. Vaghefi[†]
*Brooks College of Health, University of North Florida, Jacksonville, FL, USA
[†]University of North Florida, St. Johns, FL, USA

ABBREVIATIONS

CLA Conjugated linoleic acid
CRP C-reactive protein
CVD Cardiovascular diseases
ICAM-1 Intracellular adhesion molecule 1
IL Interleukin
LDL Low-density lipoprotein
NF-κB Nuclear factor kappa B
VLDL Very low density lipoprotein

1. PREVALENCE OF CARDIOVASCULAR DISEASES IN THE UNITED STATES

Cardiovascular disease (CVD) is the leading cause of morbidity and mortality in the United States. According to the Center for Disease Control and Prevention (Heron, 2007), one in four Americans die from the consequences of heart disease regardless of gender and ethnicity. Coronary artery disease is the most prevalent type of CVD among Americans. The cost for the treatment of CVDs exceeds 300 billion dollars per year (CDC, 2005). In the United States, the most common risks factors for CVDs are sedentary life, obesity, high blood pressure, cigarette smoking, and unhealthy dietary habits such as diets high in saturated fat and high cholesterol, low or no intake of fruits and vegetables, and comorbidities such as diabetes. Four major risks factors contributing to atherosclerosis are smoking, high blood pressure, atherogenic lipoproteins, and hyperglycemia (Ross, 1999). These factors can predispose individuals to a series of local and systemic inflammatory responses that can affect the blood vessels, either by narrowing or blocking them, causing myocardial infarction or heart attacks, chest pain, strokes, or death.

Bioactive Food as Dietary Interventions for Cardiovascular Disease
http://dx.doi.org/10.1016/B978-0-12-396485-4.00018-9

© 2013 Elsevier Inc.
All rights reserved.

319

2. MECHANISM OF INFLAMMATION

The vascular circulation of lipid–rich lipoproteins can lead to deposition of fatty streaks in the blood vessels. The presence of the fatty streaks will start a cascade of immune reactions secondary to the presence of these unwanted particles attached to the blood vessels, interfering with the normal movement of blood through the circulatory system. Immune cells (macrophages and leukocytes) will migrate to the injured site, causing the narrowing of the blood vessels. The passage of large atherogenic lipoproteins – very low–density lipoprotein (VLDL) and low–density lipoprotein (LDL) – through the narrowed blood vessel can cause the accumulation of the cholesterol in the already formed fatty streak producing an atherosclerotic lesion. This injurious event will eventually elicit the following responses: (Pearson et al., 2003):

1. Oxidation of the LDL–fraction by nitric oxide eliciting the formation of "foam" cells, leading to an additional damage to the smooth vascular endothelium causing further injurious stimuli to the already damaged tissue. These activities cause more inflammation and subsequent vessel narrowing, and blot clots can complete the process of blockages.
2. The secretion of adhesion molecules will facilitate the migration of monocytes to the subendothelial tissue, causing subsequent damage to the smooth muscle cells, promoting the rupture of the plaque in the inflamed tissue leading to blood clot or thrombosis.

Immune responses occurring during the development of CVD lead to local and systemic inflammations. Inflammatory processes in CVDs are ongoing processes that occur in all stages of atherosclerosis. A local as well as a systemic response will occur from the time the plaque is growing to the overall body response to inflammation (Libby and Ridker, 1999; Figure 20.1).

Examination of the inflammatory cascade leads to production of several biomarkers that can be seen in CVDs. The oxidation of LDL–cholesterol can elicit an inflammatory response from the innate immune system, with an increase in macrophages and dendritic cells that can promote the transcription of proinflammatory cytokines such as interleukin–1 (IL–1), which causes low grade fever, as well as IL–2, IL–6, and IL–8 among others. Adhesion molecules such as intracellular cell adhesion molecule (ICAM–1) will bring more immune cells to the lesion. Consequent production of leukocytes and acute phase molecules such as C–reactive protein (CRP) can turn this localized inflammation to a systemic one. The most common biomarkers used in clinical settings because of the essays availability are the white blood cells, CRP, and fibrinogen (Libby and Ridker, 1999). Other markers of inflammation, such as ICAM–1, NF–κB (which is a nuclear factor that increases cellular transcription and synthesis of TNF–α), interleukins IL–1, IL–2, IL–6, and IL–8 that require more specific treatment of the samples, become difficult because of unavailability of assays in the clinical setting. Owing to the limitations in the analyses of some of the biomarkers, clinicians are using the analysis of total cholesterol, oxidized LDL–cholesterol lipoproteins, and overall lipid profile in conjunction with available biomarkers to assess inflammation in CVD.

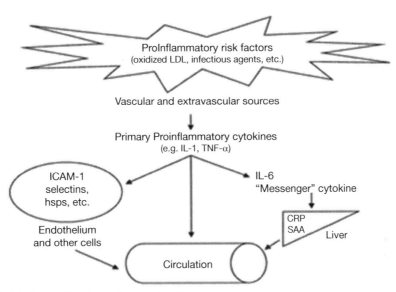

Figure 20.1 Inflammation in cardiovascular disease.

2.1 Role of Obesity as a Cause of Inflammation

New research is focusing on the proinflammatory markers produced by the enlarged adipocytes in obese patients with hypertension and CVD. A reduction in serum adiponectin, an anti–inflammatory and cholesterol-lowering cytokine produced by adipocytes (Mantzoros et al., 2006), and an increase in *resistin* is associated with insulin resistance, obesity, and increased risks of inflammation such as elevated total cholesterol. Adiponectin release is lower in the evening compared to the mornings, in both obese and postmenopausal women, increasing the risk for insulin resistance and elevated levels of inflammatory markers – CRP, IL-6, and TNF-α – therefore, increasing the risk for inflammation (Engeli et al., 2003) and vascular endothelial damage. Because the protective effect of adiponectin is lower in the evening, women consuming large meals at night can increase the risk of obesity and the process of inflammation (Ouchi et al., 2003).

3. ROLE OF SELECTED FOODS IN THE PREVENTION OF INFLAMMATION IN CVD

Many food bioactive components and nutrients have been associated with beneficial effects in preventing inflammation thus risk of heart disease. Some of them include the following.

3.1 Dairy Products

Consumption of milk has been associated with an increase in morbidity and mortality due to the fat content in milk. Studies linked the saturated fatty acids in milk with increase in

LDL-cholesterol and atherogenic plaque and inflammation due to its LDL oxidation. Conversely, other studies have shown that milk consumption has been associated with a reduction in mortality, especially in men. A protective benefit of milk was observed in men who drank more than one-third of a pint a day (Ness et al., 2001) compared to nondrinkers. Similar results were observed in men participating in The Seven Day Adventist Study (Snowdon et al., 1984) when consuming about 2–8 oz glasses a day. Studies in women showed a slightly greater benefit in low- and nonfat milk drinkers compared to the ones that consume whole milk. Moreover, students with lactovegetarians found reduced mortality risks in the ones consuming more than 8 oz/day compared to the ones consuming less. These studies were unable to demonstrate higher risks in whole milk drinkers compared to low- or nonfat milk drinkers. This may be due to other components in milk that are protective or the fact that lactovegetarians follow a diet high in fruit and vegetables and fiber, which is protective against CVD. These points are discussed later in this chapter.

Consumption of dairy products has been shown to be beneficial for patients with hypertension, CVD (Alonso et al., 2005), and weight maintenance. Factors contributing to this benefit are magnesium, fatty acids, calcium, casein, and vitamin D. The effect of magnesium reducing CRP and ICAM inflammatory factors has been discussed earlier.

Although milk is high in saturated fatty acids and can increase LDL cholesterol, not all the LDL particles are atherogenic and less likely to be oxidized. LDL atherogenic particles from lauric (12:0) and myristic (14:0) acids are the ones that are smaller (with less fat content) than the large less-dense LDL particles contained in milk and most likely to be oxidized (Siri-Tarino et al., 2010). Studies have shown that nonfat milk consumption has an effect in lowering cholesterol levels; however, the results are inconclusive (St-Onge et al., 2000). In a study with 35 healthy adults consuming nonfat, low-fat dairy products, or carbohydrate loaded foods daily for 2 months, plasma concentrations of proinflammatory TNF-α was reduced; however, values for ICAM were unaffected (Van Meijl and Mensink, 2010).

A lipid component in milk, known as conjugated linoleic acid (CLA), which is a polyunsaturated fatty acid occurring naturally in milk (Reynolds and Roche, 2010), has been studied in cell culture reducing the activation of the proinflammatory nuclear factor NF-κB. The reduced activity of this nuclear factor is responsible for inhibition of the synthesis of proinflammatory cytokines (Losche et al., 2005).

In a study with obese rodents receiving a diet supplemented with linoleic acid or CLA for 6 weeks, it was found that markers of inflammation, triglycerides, and VLDL-cholesterol were reduced (Moloney et al., 2007). Studies of trans fats in humans are lacking, however, data from *in-vitro* studies found a positive association between CVD and milk consumption (Woodside et al., 2008).

Casein, a protein component in milk, has shown to have effects in reducing inflammatory markers in cultured cells (Vordenbäumen et al., 2011). Same effects have been seen in other mammals' milk, such as goat's and donkey's, where both milks reduce inflammation via the release of the vasodilator nitric oxide, a potent antagonist for inflammatory markers against atherosclerosis (Jirillo et al., 2010). Another protein component in milk, whey, has been shown to have similar functions as calcium in reducing adipogenesis, increasing lipolysis, and maintaining healthy weight (Zemel, 2001).

Vitamin D, an important component in milk, has shown to reduce platelet aggregation and clot formation via the plasminogen activator's inhibitor-1 (PAI-1). Studies with low levels of activated vitamin D showed to increase clot formation, TNF-α, and IL-1. Although data with human cells showed that 1,25 OH (D3) reduced inflammation and clot formation by NF-κB inactivation. More research is needed to look at the exact mechanism of this benefit of vitamin D in CVDs, considering that elevated levels have opposite effects, by increasing renin–angiotensin system and eventually increasing vascular resistance and blood pressure (Chen et al., 2010).

Calcium components in milk impacts CVDs by two mechanisms: control of blood pressure and reduction in inflammation by inhibiting adipogenesis. Milk calcium lowers the levels of 1,25 dihydroxyvitamin D [1,25 OH (D3)]. The low level of 1,25 OH (D3) prevents calcium influx to cell, which results in less vascular resistance and reduction in blood pressure. The calcium influx inactivates adipocytes' hormone-sensitive lipase via dephosphorylation, reducing lipolysis and promoting adipogenesis by increasing triglycerides stores. This effect has shown to be abolished in high-calcium diets, which caused increased fat loss and a reduction in adipocyte-related inflammation. This mechanism is the one that confers calcium the "antiobesity effect" explained in the studies presented by Zemel (2001).

Although milk contains some sodium, the amounts are not sufficient to induce urinary calcium losses, which is the most common issue with high-salt diets and hypertension. A case–control study with hypertensive adults consuming diets supplemented with dairy products found a significant reduction in blood pressure and intracellular calcium compared to controls (Hilpert et al., 2009).

Milk contains the disaccharide lactose that has shown to have little effect in increasing LDL-cholesterol and risk of insulin resistance. If milk consumption is substituted with carbohydrate, the excess of carbohydrate will result in lipogenesis and production of the fatty acid palmitate (16:0), which have been shown to increase triglycerides, reduce HDL, inhibit the action of LDL receptor, and increase the concentration of small, oxidized LDL-cholesterol particles.

A meta-analysis that included more than ten human subjects in cohort studies was not able to support negative effects of dairy consumption on CVDs (Elwood et al., 2010), suggesting a protective effect in heart disease due to the multiple bioactive components acting together and sometimes synergistically (Zemel, 2001) in preventing further heart damage. Goldbohm et al. (2011) in a prospective cohort study in Netherlands found that consumption of dairy products over 10 years had no effect in the mortality rates among men but in women, intake of dairy fat slightly increased mortality in all causes including ischemic heart disease. They, however, suggest that more research may elucidate a protective effect of fermented dairy products on mortality from stroke.

3.2 Nuts

The role of tree nuts (almonds, hazelnuts, walnuts, pistachios, macadamias, and cashews) in CVD is diverse. Although nuts contain high amounts of lipids, these are composed mostly of omega-3 and omega-6 polyunsaturated fatty acids, sterols, and vitamin E, which have been known to have heart-healthy benefit as shown in Table 20.1 (Ros et al., 2010).

Recent studies have shown that consumption of nuts has a lowering effect on total blood cholesterol (Sabaté et al., 2006). Epidemiological studies demonstrated a reduced relative risk for CVD in individual consuming nuts twice a day compared to ones who did not consume nuts (Li et al., 2009; Sabaté et al., 2006). Similarly, data from 25 clinical studies found that the daily consumption of 2.5 oz of nuts reduced total blood cholesterol about 5% and LDL-cholesterol about 8% (Lefevre et al., 2005). This level of reduction in both total and LDL-cholesterol decreases the formation of the atherogenic plaque and eventually, inflammation in these individuals.

Table 20.1 Energy and Fat Content and Average Fatty Acid and Sterol Composition of Nuts per 28-g Serving

Nuts[a]	Energy (kcal)	Fat (g (% En))	SFA (g)	MUFA (g)	PUFA (g)	LA (g)	ALA (g)	PS (mg)
Almonds	162	14.2 (78.9)	1.1	9.0	3.4	3.4	0.0	33.6
Brazil nuts (dried)	183	18.6 (91.5)	4.2	6.9	5.8	5.7	0.0	NR
Cashews	154	13.0 (76.0)	2.6	7.6	2.2	2.2	0.0	44.2
Hazelnuts	176	17.0 (86.9)	1.3	12.8	2.2	2.2	0.0	26.9
Macadamia nuts	201	21.2 (94.9)	3.4	16.5	0.4	0.4	0.1	32.5
Peanuts	149	13.8 (83.4)	1.9	6.8	4.4	4.4	0.0	61.6
Pecans	193	20.2 (94.2)	1.7	11.4	6.0	5.8	0.3	28.6
Pine nuts (dried)	188	19.2 (91.9)	1.4	5.3	9.5	9.3	0.0	39.5
Pistachios	156	12.4 (71.5)	1.5	6.5	3.8	3.7	0.1	59.9
Walnuts	183	18.3 (90.0)	1.7	2.5	13.2	10.7	2.5	20.2

ALA, α-linolenic acid; En, energy; LA, linoleic acid; MUFA, monounsaturated fatty acids; PS, plant sterols; PUFA, polyunsaturated fatty acids; SFA, saturated fatty acids.
[a] Data are for raw nuts, except when specified.
Data from U.S. Department of Agriculture available from: http://www.nal.usda.gov/fnic/cgi-bin/nut_search.pl. Reprinted with permission from Ros et al. (2010).

Nuts have also shown to reduce the levels of serum inflammatory biomarkers: CRP, IL6, ICAM-1, and fibrinogen (Jiang et al., 2006), ICAM-1 and to increase the anti-inflammatory marker of adiponectin (Mantzoros et al., 2006).

It seems that the type of nuts and their components influence the reduction in different inflammatory markers, suggesting that they act in different steps of the metabolic pathway. In a study of subjects with high levels of cholesterol, the consumption of more than 1 oz of almonds twice a day showed reduction in the inflammatory marker CRP, whereas the consumption of walnuts 1–3 servings a day increased the levels of CRP, even though it is high in the anti-inflammatory marker α-linoleic acid. It seems that the cardioprotective effect of walnuts is observed by the amount of MUFA through the antioxidant mechanism.

The high concentration of monounsaturated fatty acids in almonds also has shown a higher resistance to oxidation, which can favorably aid in reducing inflammation (Blomhoff et al., 2006). The high levels of magnesium observed in almonds and cashews to be about 80 mg and 75 mg/1 oz, respectively (NIH, accessed: January 2011), showed an inverse relationship with inflammatory markers CRP and ICAM-1 (Song et al., 2007).

Cashews are also high in MUFA, but in studies so far have not shown improvements in CRP (Mukuddem-Petersen et al., 2007). Furthermore, consumption of cashews did not lower total cholesterol. However, Brazil nuts (2 nuts/day) have shown to improve the activity of glutathione peroxidase, which is a potent endogenous antioxidant and because of its components, selenium, β-sitoesetrol, and α-tocopherol, help to reduce inflammation (Thomson et al., 2008).

Walnuts contain high amounts of PUFA (linoleic and α-linoleic acids) and have been widely studied on its cardioprotective effects (24). Diets containing 30–108 g/day (1–4 oz) showed reductions in total ($\sim$10 mg/dl) and LDL ($\sim$9 mg/dl) cholesterol after 2–4 months consumption (Sabaté et al., 2010) and maintained over 6 months (Torabian et al., 2010). Another study with obese and control patients for a period over a year showed significant HDL increments with walnut consumption (Tapsell et al., 2009). This is important since increasing HDL is possible usually by increasing physical activity or loosing significant amount of body fat. Another benefit of walnuts is that they contain natural vasodilators (L-arginine which leads to the production of nitric oxide) and antioxidants (vitamin E and phenolic compounds) to prevent oxidation-induced inflammation (López-Uriarte et al., 2009).

3.3 Fish and Fish Oils

Salmon, tuna, trout, sardines, herring, and fish oil contain high amounts of omega-3-fatty acids eicopentaenoic and docosahexaenoic acid. Consumption of 2 oz of these varieties of fish twice a week has shown to reduce risk factors for inflammation such as triglycerides and cholesterol. Also, it has been shown to reduce inflammation, reduce platelet aggregation, and prevent damage to endothelial vascular function. Owing to the inflammatory properties of omega-6-fatty acids (corn, soy, and safflower oil), it is recommended to have a balance between omega-3 and omega-6-fatty acids. The best way to accomplish this objective is to reduce the function of the inflammatory marker prostaglandin E-2 and leukotrienes that are produced by the arachidonic acid (AA) in omega-6-fatty acids. It is recommended to keep a specific ratio of omega-6 to omega-3 (e.g., 4:2) to prevent inflammation in CVD (Park and Mozaffarian, 2010). It is important to note that some fish have high amounts of mercury and this can also cause an increase in oxidation and damage to the heart (Mozaffarian, 2009).

Fish is a good source of the mineral selenium (which can also be found in yeast, grains, seafood, liver, meat chicken, and eggs), that have been shown to act as an antioxidant that can prevent LDL oxidation and further cause damage to the endothelium.

3.4 Coffee

Several bioactive components in coffee can reduce inflammation by their actions as antioxidants, free radical scavengers, vasodilators, endothelial functions promoters, and reducing homocysteine levels. The release of these components is dependent on the type of coffee and its preparation. Roasting, boiling, and filtering the coffee can affect the release of caffeine, dipertene oils (cafestol and kahweol), and polyphenols (chlorogenic acid – CGA, caffeic acid, and quinic acid).

Boiled coffee has a higher concentration of compounds called dipertenes (cafestol and kahweol) when compared to the filtered coffee. In a 10-week study with men, levels of LDL-cholesterol increased in subjects consuming boiled coffee compared to those consuming filtered coffee (Forde et al., 1985). *In vitro* studies, found a direct relationship between dipertenes concentration and LDL receptor inhibition, allowing more small LDL particles to form the plaque and be subjected to oxidation (Bonita et al., 2007). This relationship, however, is not evidenced in human studies to date. However, it is believed to be due to apoptotic function of dipertenes on LDL receptors. The overall effect is the increase of LDL-cholesterol and increased risk of atherosclerosis.

In average, caffeine content ranges between 30 and 175 mg/2 oz of coffee equal to ¼ of a cup (Gilbert et al., 1976) and its benefit as free radical scavenger *in vitro* is observed in quantities as high as four cups. Markers of inflammation in humans have been shown to be reduced by the consumption of moderate coffee drinking of 10 oz or 1 and 1/4 of a cup (300 ml/day) (Bonita et al., 2007). According to the U.S. Nurses' Health Study, levels of CRP were reduced in Type 2 diabetic women consuming caffeinated coffee, with similar effects in healthy women consuming decaffeinated coffee (Lopez-Garcia et al., 2006).

Caffeine-containing soda beverages had no benefits when consumed by hypertensive persons indicating that other components of coffee such as polyphenols can reduce inflammation. Filtered coffee seems to modulate inflammatory markers and improve endothelial function. However, these effects were negated in heavy drinkers. It was observed that drinking doses of less than 6.5 oz or ¾ of a cup (200 ml/day) modulated the inflammatory response while this response increased with larger doses of six cups/day (48 oz/day) in both men and women (Zampelas et al., 2004).

Polyphenols play an important role as antioxidants. One of the two major polyphenols, caffeic acid, has shown an antioxidant potential that can last as long as 2 h after the consumption of doses of 6.5 oz or ¾ of a cup (200 ml) of coffee (Bonita et al., 2007). A weekly consumption of 24 oz (3 cups)/day showed a reduction in LDL-oxidation in Japanese participants. The other polyphenol, CGA, has a beneficial effect of improving endothelial function, promoting vasodilation (by increasing nitric oxide) and reducing homocysteine levels in humans after a 12-week intake of 140 mg caffeine per day (around 1/5 of a teaspoon) (Umemura et al., 2006). The magnesium component of coffee can also increase vasodilatation (Higdon and Frei, 2006) and have a synergistic effect with polyphenols.

3.5 Tea

The flavonoid compounds found in tea modulate inflammatory responses and confer several benefits in CVDs. Black and green tea flavonoids have shown to produce health benefits in CVD in amounts as low as 2–3 cups/day (2 gm of tea in hot water can produce up to 200 mg of flavonoids (Hodgson and Croft, 2010). The major flavonoids in green tea are flavanols catechins (epicatechins, epicatechingallate (ECG), epigallocatechin (EGC), and epigallocatechingallate (EGCG)), whereas the flavonoids in black tea are teaflavins and tearubigins. All of them have shown to improve endothelial function through production of nitric oxide, reduction of LDL-cholesterol, reduction of oxidation, and reduction of CRP (Hodgson, 2006); however, the effects in humans have been inconsistent and thus more research is needed.

3.6 Red Wine and Red Grape

The antioxidant benefit of the polyphenol anthocyanin has shown to prevent CVDs by reducing inflammation, preventing LDL-cholesterol oxidation, and reducing fibrin, which is responsible for blood clots. A study conducted in adults consuming 200–300 ml of red wine per day supplemented with red grape extracts for 4 weeks found reduction of cardiovascular risks factors; however, studies related to the actual effect of the phenolic compounds or the alcohol are still inconclusive (Hansen et al., 2005).

3.7 Chocolate

Flavanol compounds in cocoa – epicatechin, catechin, and procyanidin – play a role in reducing inflammation by different mechanisms. One of the mechanism in which particularly (−) epicatechin reduces inflammation is by the modulation of NF-κB, which is the nuclear factor that triggers the transcription of proinflammatory cytokines such as IL-2, IL-1β, and TNF-α among others (Selmi et al., 2008). The modulation of IL-2 results in a reduction in aggregation molecules. The modulation of IL-1β preserved endothelial function and prevented adhesion molecules aggregation fibrin and the reduced the nitric oxide cascade, preventing thrombosis. The effects of flavanol inhibiting the inflammatory pathway of leukotrienes via reduction in cyclooxygenases have been observed as early as 2 h after consumption (Schewe et al., 2002). The reduction in platelets activation has been observed 6 h after cocoa consumption (Rein et al., 2000). The antioxidant effect of flavanol in the release of nitric oxide was observed in humans consuming cocoa supplemented drinks for a period of 5 days (Fisher et al., 2003). Most of the antioxidant effects have been observed in dark chocolate (Selmi et al., 2008) in addition to improvements in arterial wall function. Evidence suggests that cocoa consumption provide long-term benefits in modulation of oxidative stress.

3.8 Vitamins: Folic Acid, Vitamin B12 and B6

These water-soluble vitamins play an important role in prevention of CVDs. Sources of folate are found in deep green leafy vegetables, whereas vitamins B12 and B6 are mostly found in meat products. Folate and B12 are the vitamins involved in methyl transfer metabolism. In order for folic acid to be active and involved in cell synthesis and repair, the 5-methyl THF form must be demethylated by vitamin B12, which transfers this methyl to homocysteine to form methionine, another activator of cell synthesis. Elevated levels of serum homocysteine have been shown to increase vascular damage and inflammation cascade, increasing risks for CVD (Blom and Smulders, 2011). Furthermore, Vitamin B6 has been shown to reduce homocysteine levels by producing cysteine and eliminating it in the urine. Adequate levels of these three vitamins play a role in the reduction of risks factors associated with inflammatory response in cardiovascular system. It is important to keep the levels within the Dietary Reference Intakes (DRI) of 400 µg/day of folate for adult male and female; 2.4 µg/day of vitamin B12 for adult male and female; and 1.3–1.7 and 1.3–1.5 µg of vitamin B6 for an adult male and female, respectively.

4. SUMMARY

Food and nutrients play an important role in the prevention and reduction of inflammation in CVD as presented in this chapter. Dairy products confer many nutrients and biochemical components that reduce inflammation, endothelial damage, and induce vasodilation. These food components include casein, magnesium, vitamin D, and calcium. Fatty fish and fish oil contain a higher concentration of omega-3 polyunsaturated fatty acids that has anti-inflammatory properties. Consumption of about 2 oz of nuts per day has shown to reduce the risk factors for inflammation such as total cholesterol and proinflammatory cytokines. Dietary fiber can help to reduce risk factors by aiding in healthy weight maintenance, nutrient absorption, and through the end product of fiber fermentation butyrate. Butyrate can reduce inflammation via reduction of NF-κB and PGE_2. Additionally, the increased amounts of vitamins and minerals such as magnesium found in dietary fiber sources, such as fruits and vegetables, can reduce the risk factors and add to benefits. The role of vitamin B6, vitamin B12, and selenium in reducing oxidative stress has been widely investigated. The role of antioxidants in preventing the oxidation of LDL-cholesterol and further inflammation via the action of vitamins E and C, selenium and polyphenols – resveratrol (in red grapes and red wine), and reducer of inflammation as anthocyanins, flavonoids, and flavanols (as in chocolates) are discussed. Adiposity also increases inflammation and atherosclerosis, so healthy weight maintenance provides benefits in the prevention and treatment of CVD as well as reducing the risks factor for CVD including sedentary living, high consumption of saturated fats and sodium, high cholesterol and blood pressure, alcohol, and smoking. A balanced diet that provides adequate calories for age, height, weight, gender, rich in fruits, vegetables, nuts, dairy products and controlled in fats and a physically active lifestyle will help to reduce inflammation in CVD.

REFERENCES

Alonso, A., Buena, J.J., Delgado-Rodriguez, M., Martinez, J.A., Martinez-Gonzalez, M.A., 2005. Low-fat dairy consumption and reduced risk of hypertension: the Seguimiento Universidad de Navarra (SUN) cohort. The American Journal of Clinical Nutrition 82, 972–979.

Blom, H.J., Smulders, Y., 2011. Overview of homocysteine and folate metabolism. With special references to cardiovascular disease and neural tube defects. Journal of Inherited Metabolic Disease 34(1), 75–81 Epub 2010 Sep 4.

Blomhoff, R., Carlsen, M.H., Frost Andersen, L., Jacobs Jr., D.R., 2006. Health benefits of nuts: potential role of antioxidants. The British Journal of Nutrition 96 (Suppl. 2), S52–S60.

Bonita, J.S., Mandarano, M., Shuta, D., Vinson, J., 2007. Coffee and cardiovascular disease: in vitro, cellular, animal, and human studies. Pharmacological Research 55(3), 187–198 Epub 2007 Jan 26.

Centers for Disease Control and Prevention, 2005. Racial/ethnic and socioeconomic disparities in multiple risk factors for heart disease and stroke – United States, 2003. Morbidity and Mortality Weekly Report 54(5), 113–117.

Chen, Y., Kong, J., Sun, T., et al., 2010. 1, 25-Dihydroxyvitamin D (3) suppresses inflammation-induced expression of plasminogen activator inhibitor-1 by blocking nuclear factor-κB activation. Archives of Biochemistry and Biophysics 507(2), 241–247.

Elwood, P.C., Pickering, J.E., Givens, D.I., Gallacher, J.E., 2010. The consumption of milk and dairy foods and the incidence of vascular disease and diabetes: an overview of the evidence. Lipids 45(10), 925–939.

Engeli, S., Feldpausch, M., Gorzelniak, K., et al., 2003. Association between adiponectin and mediators of inflammation in obese women. Diabetes 52, 942–947.

Fisher, N.D., Hughes, M., Gerhard-Herman, M., Hollenberg, N.K., 2003. Flavanol-rich cocoa induces nitric-oxide-dependent vasodilation in healthy humans. Journal of Hypertension 21, 2281–2286.

Forde, O.H., Knutsen, S.F., Arnesen, E., Thelle, D.S., 1985. The Tromso heart study: coffee consumption and serum lipid concentrations in men with hypercholesterolaemia: a randomised intervention study. British Medical Journal 290, 893–895.

Gilbert, R.M., Marshman, J.A., Schwieder, M., Berg, R., 1976. Caffeine content of beverages as consumed. Canadian Medical Association Journal 7, 114(3), 205–208.

Goldbohm, R.A., Chorus, A.M., Garre, F.G., Schouten, L.J., Van den Brandt, P.A., 2011. Dairy consumption and 10-y total and cardiovascular mortality: a prospective cohort study in the Netherlands. The American Journal of Clinical Nutrition 93(3), 615–627.

Hansen, A.S., Marckmann, P., Dragsted, L.O., Finné Nielsen, IL., Nielsen, SE., Grønbaek, M., 2005. Effect of red wine and red grape extract on blood lipids, haemostatic factors, and other risk factors for cardiovascular disease. European Journal of Clinical Nutrition 59 (3), 449–455.

Heron, M.P., 2007. Deaths: leading causes for cardiovascular diseases 2004 [PDF–3.2M]. National Vital Statistics Reports. 2007; 56(5) National Center for Health Statistics, Hyattsville, MD.

Higdon, J.V., Frei, B., 2006. Coffee and health: a review of recent human research. Critical Reviews in Food Science and Nutrition 46(2), 101–102.

Hilpert, K.F., West, S.G., Bagshaw, D.M., et al., 2009. Effects of dairy products on intracellular calcium and blood pressure in adults with essential hypertension. Journal of the American College of Nutrition 28(2), 142–149.

Hodgson, J.M., 2006. Effects of tea and tea flavonoids on endothelial function and blood pressure: a brief review. Clinical and Experimental Pharmacology and Physiology 33 (9), 838–841.

Hodgson, J.M., Croft, K.D., 2010. Tea flavonoids and cardiovascular health. Molecular Aspects of Medicine 31(6), 495–502.

Jiang, R., Jacobs Jr., D.R., Mayer-Davis, E., et al., 2006. Nut and seed consumption and inflammatory markers in the multi-ethnic study of atherosclerosis. American Journal of Epidemiology 163, 222–231.

Jirillo, F., Jirillo, E., Magrone, T., 2010. Donkey's and goat's milk consumption and benefits to human health with special reference to the inflammatory status. Current Pharmaceutical Design 16 (7), 859–863.

Lefevre, M., Champagne, C.M., Tulley, R.T., et al., 2005. Individual variability in cardiovascular disease risk factor responses to low-fat and low-saturated-fat diets in men: body mass index, adiposity, and insulin resistance predict changes in LDL cholesterol. The American Journal of Clinical Nutrition 82, 957–963.

Li, T.Y., Brennan, A.M., Wedick, N.M., et al., 2009. Regular consumption of nuts is associated with a lower risk of cardiovascular disease in women with type 2 diabetes. Journal of Nutrition 139(7), 1333–1338.

Libby, P., Ridker, P.M., 1999. Novel inflammatory markers of coronary risk: theory versus practice. Circulation 100 (11), 1148–1150.

Lopez-Garcia, E., van Dam, R.M., Qi, L., Hu, F.B., 2006. Coffee consumption and markers of inflammation and endothelial dysfunction in healthy and diabetic women. The American Journal of Clinical Nutrition 84, 888–893.

López-Uriarte, P., Bulló, M., Casas-Agustench, P., et al., 2009. Nuts and oxidation: a systematic review. Nutrition Reviews 67, 497–5080.

Losche, C.E., Draper, E., Leavy, O., Kelleher, D., Mills, KH., Roche, HM., 2005. Conjugated linoleic acid suppresses NF-kappa B activation and IL-12 production in dendritic cells through ERK-mediated IL-10 induction. Journal of Immunology 175, 4990–4998.

Mantzoros, C.S., Williams, C.J., Manson, J.A., et al., 2006. Adherence to the Mediterranean dietary pattern is positively associated with plasma adiponectin concentrations in diabetic women. The American Journal of Clinical Nutrition 84, 328–335.

Moloney, F., Toomey, S., Noone, E., et al., 2007. Antidiabetic effects of cis-9, trans–11-conjugated linoleic acid may be mediated via anti-inflammatory effects in white adipose tissue. Diabetes 56, 574–582.

Mozaffarian, D., 2009. Fish, mercury, selenium and cardiovascular risk: current evidence and unanswered questions. International Journal of Environmental Research and Public Health 6, 1894–1916.

Mukuddem-Petersen, J., Stonehouse, W., Jerling, J.C., Hanekom, S.M., White, Z., 2007. Effects of a high walnut and high cashew nut diet on selected markers of the metabolic syndrome: a controlled feeding trial. The British Journal of Nutrition 97, 1144–1153.

National Academy of Sciences. Institute of Medicine. Food and Nutrition Board. Dietary References Intakes, 2010. Available at: http://fnic.nal.usda.gov/nal_display/index.php?info_center=4&tax_level=3&tax_

subject=256&topic_id=1342&level3_id=5140&level4_id=0&level5_id=0&placement_default=0 (accessed 11 January 2011).

Ness, A.R., Smith, G.D., Hart, C., 2001. Milk, coronary heart disease and mortality. Journal of Epidemiology and Community Health 55 (6), 379–382.

Ouchi, N., Ohishi, M., Kihara, S., et al., 2003. Association of hypoadiponectinemia with impaired vasoreactivity. Hypertension 42, 231–234.

Park, K., Mozaffarian, D., 2010. Omega-3 fatty acids, mercury, and selenium in fish and the risk of cardiovascular diseases. Current Atherosclerosis Reports 12 (6), 414–422.

Pearson, T.A., Mensah, G.A., Alexander, R.W., Anderson, J.L., 2003. Markers of inflammation and cardiovascular disease: application to clinical and public health practice: a statement for healthcare professionals from the Centers for Disease Control and Prevention and the American Heart Association. Circulation 107, 499–511.

Rein, D., Paglieroni, T.G., Pearson, D.A., et al., 2000. Cocoa and wine polyphenols modulate platelet activation and function. The Journal of Nutrition 130, 2120S–2126S.

Reynolds, C.M., Roche, H.M., 2010. Conjugated linoleic acid and inflammatory cell signalling. Prostaglandins, Leukotrienes, and Essential Fatty Acids 82 (4–6), 199–204.

Ros, E., Tapsell, L.C., Sabaté, J., 2010. Nuts and berries for heart health. Current Atherosclerosis Reports 12 (6), 397–406.

Ross, R., 1999. Atherosclerosis: an inflammatory disease. The New England Journal of Medicine 340, 115–126.

Sabaté, J., Oda, K., Ros, E., 2010. Nut consumption and blood lipid levels: a pooled analysis of 25 intervention trials. Archives of Internal Medicine 170, 821–827.

Sabaté, J., Salas-Salvadó, J., Ros, E., 2006. Nuts: nutrition and health outcomes. The British Journal of Nutrition 96 (Suppl. 2), S1–S102.

Schewe, T., Kuhn, H., Sies, H., 2002. Flavonoids of cocoa inhibit recombinant human 5-lipoxygenase. The Journal of Nutrition 132, 1825–1829.

Selmi, C., Cocchi, C.A., Lanfredini, M., Keen, C.L., Gershwin, M.E., 2008. Chocolate at heart: the anti-inflammatory impact of cocoa flavanols. Molecular Nutrition & Food Research 52 (11), 1340–1348.

Siri-Tarino, P.W., Sun, Q., Hu, F.B., Krauss, R.M., 2010. Saturated fatty acids and risk of coronary heart disease: modulation by replacement nutrients. Current Atherosclerosis Reports 12 (6), 384–390.

Snowdon, D.A., Phillips, R.L., Fraser, G.E., 1984. Meat consumption and fatal ischemic heart disease. Preventive Medicine 13 (5), 490–500.

Song, Y., Li, T.Y., van Dam, R.M., Manson, J.E., Hu, F.B., 2007. Magnesium intake and plasma concentrations of markers of systemic inflammation and endothelial dysfunction in women. The American Journal of Clinical Nutrition 85, 1068–1074.

St-Onge, M.P., Farnworth, E.R., Jones, P.J., 2000. Consumption of fermented and nonfermented dairy products: effects on cholesterol concentrations and metabolism. The American Journal of Clinical Nutrition 71, 674–681.

Tapsell, L.C., Batterham, M.J., Teuss, G., et al., 2009. Long-term effects of increased dietary polyunsaturated fat from walnuts on metabolic parameters in type II diabetes. European Journal of Clinical Nutrition 63, 1008–1015.

Thomson, C.D., Chisholm, A., McLachlan, S.K., Campbell, J.M., 2008. Brazil nuts: an effective way to improve selenium status. The American Journal of Clinical Nutrition 87, 379–384.

Torabian, S., Haddad, E., Cordero-MacIntyre, Z., et al., 2010. Long-term walnut supplementation without dietary advice induces favorable serum lipid changes in free-living individuals. European Journal of Clinical Nutrition 64, 274–279.

Umemura, T., Ueda, K., Nishioka, K., et al., 2006. Effects of acute administration of caffeine on vascular function. The American Journal of Cardiology 98, 1538–1541.

Van Meijl, L.E., Mensink, R.P., 2010. Effects of low-fat dairy consumption on markers of low-grade systemic inflammation and endothelial function in overweight and obese subjects: an intervention study. The British Journal of Nutrition 104 (10), 1523–1527.

Vordenbäumen, S., Braukmann, A., Petermann, K., et al., 2011. Casein α s1 is expressed by human monocytes and upregulates the production of GM-CSF via p38 MAPK. Journal of Immunology 186 (1), 592–601.

Woodside, J.V., McKinley, M.C., Young, I.S., 2008. Saturated and trans fatty acids and coronary heart disease. Current Atherosclerosis Reports 10 (6), 460–466.

Zampelas, A., Panagiotakos, D.B., Pitsavos, C., Chrysohoou, C., Stefanadis, C., 2004. Associations between coffee consumption and inflammatory markers in healthy persons: the ATTICA study. The American Journal of Clinical Nutrition 80 (4), 862–867.

Zemel, M.B., 2001. Calcium modulation of hypertension and obesity: mechanisms and implications. Journal of the American College of Nutrition 20 (5 Suppl.), 428S–435S.

CHAPTER 21

Red Palm Oil Carotenoids
Potential Role in Disease Prevention

A.J.S. Benadé
Cape Peninsula University of Technology, Cape Town, South Africa

ABBREVIATIONS

BCO β, β-Carotene-15, 15′-mono-oxygenase
CRP C-reactive protein
CVD Cardiovascular disease
IOM Institute of Medicine
LDL Low-density lipoprotein
RAE Retinol activity equivalents
RPO Red palm oil

1. BACKGROUND

Crude oil obtained from the mesocarp of the oil palm, *Elaeis guiniensis*, is one of the richest known sources of biological active carotenoids, which impart the characteristic orange-red color and also offer some oxidative protection to the oil (Goh et al., 1985).

However, during conventional refining processes, all carotenoids present in crude palm oil are destroyed. This has led to the development of a number of modified refining processes to produce edible oil retaining provitamin A activity. One of these modified refining processes developed by the Palm Oil Research Institute of Malaysia produces a refined red palm oil (RPO) of the highest quality while retaining 80% of the carotenoids originally present in the crude palm oil. This product is now available in the market. The carotene content is stable for 9 months when the oil is stored at 30 °C and for over 1 year when stored at 10 °C (Choo et al., 1993).

2. CAROTENOID CONTENT OF RPO

Malaysian crude palm oil normally contains 500–700 ppm carotenoids, of which 35% is α- and 56% is β-carotene. The refined red palm olein, however, contains 513 ppm carotene, of which 44% is α- and 33.3% β-carotene (Bonnie and Choo, 1999). Table 21.1 shows the spectrum of carotenoid content of crude palm oil and refined red palm olein.

Bioactive Food as Dietary Interventions for Cardiovascular Disease
http://dx.doi.org/10.1016/B978-0-12-396485-4.00019-0

© 2013 Elsevier Inc.
All rights reserved.

333

Table 21.1 Carotene Composition (%)

Carotene	Crude palm oil	Red palm olein
α-Carotene	35.1	44.2
β-Carotene	56.0	33.3
cis-α Carotene	2.5	7.5
Phytoene	1.3	3.6
Lycopene	1.3	3.6
δ-Carotene	0.8	3.3
cis-β-Carotene	0.7	0.7
ζ-Carotene	0.7	0.6
β-Zeacarotene	0.7	1.6
γ-Carotene	0.3	0.6
Neurosporene	0.3	—
α-Zeacarotene	0.2	—
Phytofluene	0.1	0.7

Source: Bonnie, T.Y.P., Choo, Y.M., 1999. Valuable minor constituents of commercial red palm olein: carotenoids, vitamin E, ubiquinones and sterols. In: Proceedings of the Porim International Palm Oil Congress (Chemistry and Technology) Kuala Lumpur, Malaysia, Palm Oil Research Institute of Malaysia, pp. 97–108.

3. BIOLOGICAL SIGNIFICANCE OF DIETARY CAROTENOIDS

Carotenoids were shown to influence diverse molecular and cellular processes, which can provide the basis for the effects of carotenoids on human health and disease prevention.

Some carotenoids are called provitamin A compounds because they are precursors of retinol and retinoic acid. Of all the known carotenoids, about 50 display provitamin A activity. The type of carotenoids found in human plasma is determined by the extent to which people consume diets rich in green, yellow/red, or yellow/orange vegetables. Major carotenoid concentrations in the blood are lycopene (20–40%), β-carotene (15–30%), β-cryptoxanthin (13–20%), lutein (10–20%), α-carotene (5–10%), and zeaxanthin (1–5%) (Kritchevsky, 1999).

Carotenoids can also exert their biological activity in disease prevention via several mechanisms. These include antioxidant activity, gap junctional intercellular communication, anti-inflammatory and antitumor promoting property, induction of detoxication enzymes, and inhibition of cholesterol synthesis (Fuhrman et al., 1997; Khachik et al., 1999).

3.1 Carotenoids as Provitamin A

Plant foods such as RPO, dark green leafy vegetables, yellow and orange fruits, and red/orange roots and tubers are rich in provitamin A carotenoids, particularly β-carotene, α-carotene, and β-cryptoxanthin. Considerable research has gone into establishing the nutritional equivalency of retinol and β-carotene when they are ingested as purified compounds and as they are present in the complex matrices of foods. The vitamin A nutritional value of retinol- and carotenoid-containing foods are defined as 'retinol equivalents,' which describes the amount of vitamin A, whether from retinol or from carotenoid precursors with the biological activity of 1 µg of all-*trans*-retinol. The Dietary Reference Intakes published by the Institute of Medicine (IOM) and Health Canada (2002) are expressed in a new unit of bioactivity, the retinol activity equivalent (RAE). One microgram of RAE is equal to 1 µg of all-*trans*-retinol, 2 µg of all-*trans*-β-carotene in oil, 12 µg of β-carotene in foods, and 24 µg of other provitamin A carotenoids in foods.

As the bioactivity of carotenoids differs with the type of foods in which they are present, these factors are considered as average values. Based on the IOM bioactivity values, β-carotene in oil has a bioactivity six times that found in vegetables. If it is assumed that this factor could also be applied to other provitamin carotenoids in oil, then 4 µg of other carotenoids is equal to 1 µg RAE. These factors were used to calculate the RAE content of refined red palm olein, which is given in Table 21.2.

In Table 21.3, the carotenoid content of refined red palm olein is compared with those of tomatoes.

In Table 21.4, the RAE content of refined red palm olein is compared with those of different food items.

The degree of bioconversion of provitamin A sources to vitamin A is determined by the vitamin A status of the host (Ribaya-Mercado et al., 2000). Cleavage of β-carotene to

Table 21.2 Carotenoid Content of Refined Red Palm Olein

Carotenoid	Content (µg/100 g)	RAE
α-Carotene	22675	5669
β-Carotene	17083	8542
cis-α-Carotene	3848	962
γ-Carotene	1692	423
β-Zeacarotene	820	205
Other	5182	—
Total	51300	15801

Modified after Schrimshaw (2000).

Table 21.3 Carotenoid Content of Refined Red Palm Olein and Tomatoes

Carotenoid	Red palm olein[a] (µg g^{-1})	Tomatoes[b] (µg g^{-1})
α-Carotene	226.7	1.01
β-Carotene	170.8	4.49
Lycopene	18.5	25.7
Phytoene	18.5	18.6
Phytofluene	3.6	8.2

[a] Assuming a carotene content of 513 ppm.
[b] From Campbell et al. (2004).

Table 21.4 Carotenoid Content: RAE

Food items	Retinol activity equivalents (RAE) per 100 g (edible portion)	Activity: % of red palm olein
Red palm olein[a]	15 801	100
Carrots	1000	6.33
Leafy vegetables	343	2.17
Apricots	125	0.79
Tomatoes	50	0.32
Bananas	15	0.09
Orange juice	4	0.03

[a] Assuming a carotene content of 513 ppm.
Modified after Schrimshaw (2000).

vitamin A by the enzyme β, β-carotene-15, 15′-mono-oxygenase (BCO) in the small intestine is tightly regulated. Activity of BCO is affected by the vitamin A status of the individual (Parvin and Sivakumar, 2000), which is possibly mediated via a negative feedback regulation mechanism involving retinoic acid and its nuclear receptors (Bachmann et al., 2002).

3.1.1 Value of RPO as a source of provitamin A

Results from several intervention studies using RPO or RPO-based products as part of the daily diet of population groups at risk of subclinical vitamin A deficiencies have invariably confirmed the value of RPO in alleviating subclinical vitamin A deficiency.

3.1.1.1 RPO in the maternal diet

Canfield and Kaminsky (2000) studied the effect of refined RPO supplementation in a population of lactating mothers and their nursing infants in the Honduras. Mothers received 15 mg of β-carotene as refined RPO on six occasions over a period of 2 weeks. Their results showed that refined RPO in the diet of lactating mothers has the potential to enhance vitamin A status of their nursing infants.

A study conducted by the National Institute of Nutrition at Hyderabad, India, fed 8 ml of RPO daily providing 2200 μg of β-carotene to women for 8 weeks starting 26–28 weeks of gestation (Radhika et al., 2003). Postintervention serum retinol levels of women as well as those of their infants were significantly higher compared to controls receiving groundnut oil.

3.1.1.2 Effect of RPO on vitamin A status of school children

Results from three feeding trials on school children receiving sweet snacks, containing locally produced RPO supplying 2400 μg of β-carotene per day for 1–2 months, showed significant increases in serum retinol levels measured after 30 days of daily supplementation with RPO (Manorama et al., 1997).

Van Stuijvenberg and Benadé (2000) evaluated the effect of biscuits baked with either RPO-based baking fat or a biscuit baked with added synthetic β-carotene on the vitamin A status of school children with 5–11 years of age over a period of 3 months. The biscuits provided 1.23 and 1.17 mg of β-carotene, respectively, and were provided 5 days per week. There was a significant improvement in the subclinical vitamin A deficiency as indicated by the serum retinol concentrations of children in both treatment groups. The effects of the two treatments were found to be similar.

Researchers from the Institute of Nutrition and Food Science, University of Dhaka recently reported a decrease in the prevalence of acute respiratory infection from 38% to 17% in school children aged 13–15 years (Shah et al., 2003). Children consumed four biscuits baked with RPO (containing about 1500 μg of β-carotene) daily over a period of 3 months.

Significant improvements in serum retinol concentrations were also reported in preschool children supplemented with RPO (Sivan et al., 2002). Consumption of 5 ml RPO per day for 10 months in preschoolers in Tamil Nadu, India reduced the prevalence of Bitot's spot 15% compared to 10% in the control group.

4. CAROTENOIDS IN HEALTH AND DISEASE

Carotenoids are known to influence diverse molecular and cellular processes, which could be instrumental in their role in reducing the risk for chronic diseases such as cardiovascular disease (CVD) and cancer.

4.1 Carotenoids and Coronary Heart Disease

Epidemiologic and clinical data showed an inverse association between serum levels of β-carotene and other carotenoids and coronary heart disease (Kritchevsky, 1999). Dietary carotenoids may thus protect against CVD.

The relation between CVD risk and fruit and vegetable consumption was demonstrated by Joshipura et al. (2001), who reported a 20% reduction in the incidence of CVD in individuals who consumed the highest quintile of these foods, compared with individuals in the lowest quintile. It is now well established that the level of serum carotenoids can be readily altered by either increasing or decreasing the consumption of fruit and vegetables (Yeum et al., 2004). An increase in serum carotenoids was reported to be accompanied by a significant decrease in serum oxidizability (Bub et al., 2000). Oxidizability in serum can therefore be modified by diet and is related to the carotenoid content of the serum.

In terms of CVD, β-carotene has been the most widely studied because it is one of the most abundant carotenoids. Several studies examined the effects of β-carotene in the context of fruit and vegetable intake and also confirmed an inverse association between β-carotene intake and the risk of CVD. Data from the Rotterdam study on 4802 men and women free of baseline CVD showed that those in the highest tertile of dietary β-carotene intake had a relative CVD risk half of those in the lowest tertile (Klipstein-Growbusch et al., 2000).

The mechanisms of action of carotenoids in reducing CVD risk include inhibition of cholesterol synthesis and an increase in degradation of low-density lipoprotein (LDL) particles through an enhancement of the macrophage LDL receptor activity (Fuhrman et al., 1997). There is also evidence that carotenoids may reduce the risk of atherosclerosis through inhibition of oxidative damage to LDL; oxidative damage to LDL promotes several key steps in atherogenesis. Carotenoids may also reduce the risk of CVD by reducing inflammation as suggested by the inverse association between serum/plasma C-reactive protein (CRP) concentrations and serum/plasma concentrations of α-carotene, β-carotene, and lycopene concentrations (Kritchevsky et al., 2000).

4.1.1 Carotenoids and cancer

As for cancer, several epidemiologic studies also showed that an increased consumption of foods rich in carotenoids is inversely associated with the incidence of major types of cancer in the western world, for example, carcinoma of the lung, stomach, prostate, mouth, esophagus, colon, or rectum (Riboli and Norat, 2003). A similar association was also reported between the concentration of β-carotene in plasma and the risk for cancer. Although the biological mechanism for such protection is unknown, various possibilities exist. Carotenoids are potent antioxidants and oxidative stress is known to be involved in carcinogenesis. In a model *in vitro* system, Bertram and Bortkiewicz (1995) showed that carotenoids, both with and without provitamin A activity, inhibit carcinogen-induced neoplastic transformation. Their results strongly suggest that carotenoids have intrinsic cancer chemopreventive action in humans.

Although red palm olein has a unique carotenoid content, information of its effect on degenerative diseases is largely unknown. Red palm olein is one of the richest sources of carotenoids and its carotenoid content compares favorably with that of tomatoes in terms of lycopene, phytoene, and phytofluene (Table 21.3). If it is assumed that these phytonutrients in tomatoes are major role players in reducing the risk of degenerative diseases, then it could be hypothesized that red palm olein has the same potential as tomatoes for reducing the risk of degenerative diseases. This, however, needs to be established in carefully designed intervention trials.

4.1.1.1 Supplementation with carotenoids

Clinical studies with carotenoid supplementation and some major clinical trials with β-carotene supplementation showed either no or negative effects on CVD and cancer (Lee et al., 1999). Although the reasons for the discrepancy between the results from supplementation and epidemiologic studies are not clear, it has been postulated that supplementation with a single carotenoid at high doses is not sufficient to elicit effects. It has been suggested that a combination of low concentrations of various carotenoids and other micronutrients as found in fruits and vegetables, rather than in individual supplements, appear to be necessary to affect the diverse molecular and cellular processes, which form the basis for human health and disease prevention (Stahl et al., 1998). In addition, various dietary compounds may provide synergistic effects required for protection against disease.

Based on the observed negative association reported between blood carotenoid concentration, CVD, and cancer in epidemiological studies, it could be argued that only those who have low blood levels of carotenoids will benefit from carotenoid supplementation as was observed in supplementation studies in school children. This hypothesis, however, needs to be tested.

5. SAFETY OF CAROTENOIDS FROM NATURAL FOOD SOURCES

There is no documented evidence that consumption of β-carotene containing natural food sources in moderation has negative health implications. Even when very large amounts of carotene-rich foods are consumed, the only observed side effect was the occasional appearance of carotenodermia, which appears to be harmless and which is characterized by a yellow- or orange-tinted skin. The condition disappears spontaneously shortly after the high intake of carotenoid is discontinued.

Vitamin A has the potential for acute and chronic toxicity, whereas provitamin A carotenoids do not share the same toxic potential. As pointed out earlier, the degree of bioconversion of provitamin A in physiological systems is regulated and determined by the vitamin A status of the host. No adverse effects were reported for any one of the studies in which the value of RPO as provitamin A was evaluated. The duration of these studies varied from 2 weeks to 10 months during which time participants in the study received an estimated 2–5 mg of total carotenoids daily.

Data from animal, human, and laboratory research suggested that a chronically elevated intake of vitamin A, in the order of $3000~\mu g~day^{-1}$, about four times recommended daily intake may increase the risk of osteoporotic bone disease and fracture, at least in older men and women (Melhus et al., 1998). As bioconversion of provitamin A to vitamin A is regulated and determined by the vitamin a status of the host, it could be assumed that the intake of provitamin A carotenoids from fruit, vegetables or RPO by older people with an adequate vitamin a status will not pose a risk for the loss of bone mineral density.

β-Carotene is the only carotenoid that has been studied extensively in several large-scale primary and secondary prevention trials. Questions as to the safety of the ingestion of high doses of β-carotene have been raised by the α-tocopherol β-carotene cancer prevention study in Finland. A statistically significant 18% higher incidence of lung cancer was reported in subjects given 20 mg β-carotene daily compared to subjects receiving a placebo.

Based on a review of published studies, the US Preventative Service Task Force does not recommend that people take β-carotene supplements to lower their risk of developing CVD or cancer (Recommendations from the US Services Task Force, 2003).

6. NUTRITIONAL VALUE OF RPO

The value of including moderate amounts of RPO or RPO products into the daily diet with the purpose of preventing or alleviating subclinical vitamin A deficiency is well documented. It is considered to be a healthful, affordable, and sustainable dietary approach to the prevention of subclinical vitamin A deficiency. RPO has an added benefit in so far that the β-carotene present in oil is considered to have a bioavailability six times that of other plant sources. RPO contains a spectrum of natural carotenoids, which are known to exert their biological activity in disease prevention via several mechanisms. Although concern has been expressed about the palmitic acid content of palm olein, the effect of this fatty acid in palm oil is actually close to neutral in terms of its cholesterol raising capacity (Kritchevsky, 2000).

REFERENCES

Bachmann, H., Desbarats, A., Pattison, P., et al., 2002. Feedback regulation of β, β-carotene 15, 15′-monooxygenase by retinoic acid in rats and chickens. Journal of Nutrition 132, 3616–3622.

Bertram, J.S., Bortkiewicz, H., 1995. Dietary carotenoids inhibit neo- plastic transformation and modulate gene expression in mouse and human cells. American Journal of Clinical Nutrition 62 (Suppl.), 1327S–1336S.

Bonnie, T.Y.P., Choo, Y.M., 1999. Valuable minor constituents of commercial red palm olein: carotenoids, vitamin E, ubiquinones and sterols. Proceedings of the Porim International Palm Oil Congress (Chemistry and Technology). Palm Oil Research Institute of Malaysia, Kuala Lumpur, Malaysia, pp. 97–108.

Bub, A., Watzl, B., Abrahamse, L., et al., 2000. Moderate intervention with carotenoid-rich vegetable products reduces lipid peroxidation in men. Journal of Nutrition 130, 2200–2206.

Campbell, J.K., Canene-Adams, K., Lindshield, B.L., et al., 2004. Tomato phytochemicals and prostate cancer risk. Journal of Nutrition 134, 3486S–3492S.

Canfield, L.M., Kaminsky, R.G., 2000. Red palm oil in the maternal diet improves vitamin A status of lactating mothers and their infants. Food and Nutrition Bulletin 21, 144–148.

Choo, Y.M., Ma, A.N., Ooi, C.K., Yap, S.C., Basiron, Y., 1993. Red Palm Oil – A Carotene Rich Nutritious Oil. Porim Information Series No 11. Palm Oil Research Institute of Malaysia, Kuala Lumpur.

Fuhrman, B., Elis, A., Aviram, M., 1997. Hypocholesterolemic effect of lycopene and β-carotene is related to suppression of cholesterol synthesis and augmentation of LDL receptor activity in macrophages. Biochemical and Biophysical Research Communications 233, 658–662.

Goh, S.H., Choo, Y.M., Ong, A.S.H., 1985. Minor constituents of palm oil. Journal of the American Oil Chemists' Society 62, 237–240.

Institute of Medicine, 2002. Dietary Reference Intakes for Vitamin A, Vitamin K, Arsenic, Boron, Chromium, Copper, Iodine, Iron, Manganese, Moloybdenum, Nickel, Silicon, Vanadium and Zinc. National Academy Press, Washington, DC.

Joshipura, K.J., Hu, F.B., Manson, J.E., et al., 2001. The effect of fruit and vegetable intake on risk for coronary heart disease. Annals of Internal Medicine 134, 1106–1114.

Khachik, F., Betram, J.S., Huang, M.T., Fahey, J.W., Talalay, P., 1999. Dietary carotenoids and their metabolites as potentially useful chemopreventive agents against cancer. In: Packer, L., Hiramatsu, M.,
Yoshikawa, T. (Eds.), Antioxidant Food Supplements in Human Health. Academic Press, Tokyo,
pp. 203–229.

Klipstein-Growbusch, K., Launer, L.J., Geleijnse, J.M., et al., 2000. Serum carotenoids and atherosclerosis.
The Rotterdam study. Atherosclerosis 148, 49–56.

Kritchevsky, S.B., 1999. β-Carotene, carotenoids and the prevention of coronary heart disease. Journal of
Nutrition 129, 5–8.

Kritchevsky, D., 2000. Impact of red palm oil on human nutrition and health. Food and Nutrition Bulletin
21, 182–188.

Kritchevsky, S.B., Bush, A.J., Pahor, M., Gross, M.D., 2000. Serum carotenoids and markers of inflammation in nonsmokers. American Journal of Epidemiology 152, 1065–1071.

Lee, I.M., Cook, N.R., Manson, J.E., Buring, J.E., Hennekens, C.H., 1999. Beta-carotene supplementation
and incidence of cancer and cardiovascular disease: the women's health study. Journal of the National
Cancer Institute 91, 2102–2106.

Manorama, R., Sarita, M., Rukmini, C., 1997. Red palm oil for combating vitamin A deficiency. Asia Pacific Journal of Clinical Nutrition 6, 56–59.

Melhus, H., Michaëlsson, K., Kindmark, A., et al., 1998. Excessive dietary intake of vitamin A is associated
with reduced bone, mineral density and increased risk for hip fracture. Annals of Internal Medicine 129,
770–778.

Parvin, S.G., Sivakumar, B., 2000. Nutriotional status affects intestinal carotene cleavage activity and carotene conversion to vitamin A in rats. Journal of Nutrition 130, 573–577.

Radhika, M.S., Bhaskaram, P., Balakrishna, N., Ramalakshmi, B.A., 2003. Red palm oil supplementation: a
feasible diet-based approach to improve the vitamin A status of pregnant women and their infants. Food
and Nutrition Bulletin 24, 208–217.

Ribaya-Mercado, J.D., Solon, F.S., Solon, M.A., et al., 2000. Bioconversion of plant carotenoids in vitamin
A in Filipino school-aged children varies inversely with vitamin A status. American Journal of Clinical
Nutrition 72, 455–465.

Riboli, E., Norat, T., 2003. Epidemiological evidence of the protective effect of fruit and vegetables on
cancer risk. American Journal of Clinical Nutrition 78, 559S–569S.

Schrimshaw, N.S., 2000. Nutritional potential of red palm oil for combating vitamin A deficiency. Food and
Nutrition Bulletin 21, 195–201.

Shah, Md, Keramat, Ali, Khaleda, Adib, et al., 2003. Effects of beta-carotene on acute respiratory infection in
a girls' school of Dhaka City. Chest and Heart Journal 27, 70–76.

Sivan, Y.S., Alwin Jayakumar, Y., Arumughan, C., et al., 2002. Impact of vitamin A supplementation
through different dosages of red palm oil and retinol palmitate on preschool children. Journal of Tropical
Pediatrics 48, 24–28.

Stahl, W., Junghans, A., de Boer, B., et al., 1998. Carotenoid mixtures protect multilamellar
liposomes against oxidative damage; synergestic effects of lycopene and lutein. FEBS Letters 427,
305–308.

U.S. Preventative Services Task Force, 2003. Summaries for patients taking vitamin A supplements to prevent cardiovascular disease and cancer: recommendations from the U.S. Preventative Services Task
Force. Annals of Internal Medicine 139, 1–76.

van Stuijvenberg, M.E., Benadé, A.J.S., 2000. South African experience with the use of red palm oil to improve the vitamin A status of primary schoolchildren. Food and Nutrition Bulletin 21, 212–214.

Yeum, K.-J., Aldini, G., Johnson, E.J., Russel, R.M., Krinsky, N.I., 2004. Molecular aspects and health
issues. In: Packer, L., Obermüller-Jevic, U., Kraemer, K., Sies, H. (Eds.), Carotenoids and Retinoids.
AOCS Press, Champaign Illinois, pp. 218–228.

FURTHER READING

Acheson, R.M., Williams, D.R., 1983. Does consumption of fruit and vegetables protect against stroke? The
Lancet 1, 1191–1193.

Alpha tocopherol beta-carotene cancer prevention study group, 1994. The effect of vitamin E and beta carotene on the incidence of lung cancer and other cancers in male smokers. The New England Journal of Medicine 330, 1029–1035.

Beck, J., Ferrucci, L., Sun, K., et al., 2008. Circulating oxidized low-density lipoproteins are associated with overweight, obesity, and low serum carotenoids in older community-dwelling women. Nutrition 24, 964–968.

Bendich, A., 2004. From 1989 to 2001: what have we learned about the "Biological actions of beta-carotene"? Journal of Nutrition 134, 225S–230S.

Canfield, L.M., Kaminsky, R.G., Taren, D.L., Shaw, E., Sander, J.K., 2001. Red palm oil in the maternal diet increases provitamin A carotenoids in breast milk and serum of the mother–infant dyad. European Journal of Nutrition 40, 30–38.

Feskanich, D., Singh, V., Willett, W.C., Colditz, G.A., 2002. Vitamin A intake and hip fractures among postmenopausal women. Journal of the American Medical Association 287, 47–57.

Fuhrman, B., Volkova, M., Rosenblat, M., Aviram, M., 2000. Lycopene synergistically inhibits LDL oxidation in combination with vitamin E, glabridin, rosmarinic acid, carnosic acid or garlic. Antioxidants & Redox Signaling 2, 491–506.

Gey, K.F., Stahelin, H.B., Eichholzer, M., 1993. Poor plasma status of carotene and vitamin C is associated with higher mortality from ischemic heart disease and stroke: Basel prospective study. Clinical Investigation 71, 3–6.

Greenberg, E.R., Baron, J.A., Karagas, M.R., et al., 1996. Mortality associated with low plasma concentration of Beta-carotene and the effect of oral supplementation. Journal of the American Medical Association 275, 699–703.

Hennekens, C.H., Buring, J.E., Manson, J.E., et al., 1996. Lack of effect of long-term supplementation with Beta-carotene on the incidence of malignant neoplasms and cardiovascular disease. The New England Journal of Medicine 334, 1145–1149.

Lietz, G., Henry, C.J.K., Mulokozi, G., et al., 2001. Comparison of the effects of supplemental red palm oil and sunflower oil on maternal vitamin A status. American Journal of Clinical Nutrition 71, 501–509.

Micozzi, M.S., Brown, E.D., Taylor, P.R., Wolfe, E., 1988. Carotenodermia in men with elevated carotenoid intake from foods and β-carotene supplements. American Journal of Clinical Nutrition 48, 1061–1064.

Nagendran, B., Unnithan, U.R., Choo, Y.M., Sundram, K., 2000. Characteristics of red palm oil, a carotene- and vitamin E- rich refined oil for food uses. Food and Nutrition Bulletin 21, 189–194.

Nguyen, T.L., 2001. Effects of red palm oil supplementation on vitamin A and Iron status of rural under five children in Vietnam. Proceedings of Food Technology and Nutrition Conference, International Palm Oil Congress, Kuala Lumpur, Malaysia.

Olson, J.A., Krinsky, N.I., 1995. The colorful, fascinating world of the carotenoids: important physiologic modulators. The FASEB Journal 9, 1547–1550.

Parker, S., 1996. Absorption, metabolism and transport of carotenoids. The FASEB Journal 10, 542–551.

Pryor, W.A., Stahl, W., Rock, C.L., 2000. Beta carotene: from biochemistry to clinical trials. Nutrition Reviews 58, 39–53.

Rapola, J.M., Virtamo, J., Haukka, J.K., et al., 1996. Effect of vitamin E and Beta-carotene on the incidence of angina pectoris. A randomized double-blind, controlled trial. Journal of the American Medical Association 275, 693–698.

Riboli, E., Norat, T., 2003. Epidemiologic evidence of the protective effect of fruit and vegetables on cancer risk. American Journal of Clinical Nutrition 78, 559S–569S.

Rissanen, T., Voutilainen, S., Nyyssonen, K., et al., 2003. Serum, lycopene concentrations and carotid atherosclerosis: the Kuopio ischaemic heart disease risk factor study. American Journal of Clinical Nutrition 77, 133–138.

Russel, R.M., 2000. The vitamin A spectrum: from deficiency to toxicity. American Journal of Clinical Nutrition 71, 878–884.

Scrimshaw, N.S., 2000. Nutritional potential of red palm oil for combating vitamin A deficiency. Food and Nutrition Bulletin 21, 195–201.

Sivan, Y.S., Jayakumar, Y.A., Arumughan, C., et al., 2001. Impact of beta-carotene supplementation through red palm oil. Journal of Tropical Pediatrics 47, 67–72.

Sluijs, I., Beulens, J.W., Grobbee, D.E., van der Schouw, Y.T., 2009. Dietary carotenoid intake is associated with lower prevalence of metabolic syndrome in middle-aged and elderly men. Journal of Nutrition 139, 987–992.

Solomons, N.W., Orozco, M., 2003. Alleviation of vitamin A deficiency with palm fruit and its products. Asia Pacific Journal of Clinical Nutrition 12, 373–384.

Stahl, W., Ale-Agha, N., Polidori, M.C., 2002. Non-antioxidant properties of carotenoids. Biological Chemistry 383, 553–558.

Steinberg, D., Parthasarathy, S., Carew, T.E., Khoo, J.C., Witztum, J.L., 1989. Beyond cholesterol. Modifications of low density lipoprotein that increases its atherogenicity. The New England Journal of Medicine 320, 915–924.

Vollset, S.E., Bjelke, E., 1983. Does consumption of fruit and vegetables protect against stroke? The Lancet 2, 742.

Yap, S.C., Choo, Y.M., Ooi, C.K., Ong, A.S.H., Goh, S.H., 1991. Quantitative analysis of carotenes in oil from different palm species. Elaeis 3, 309–318.

CHAPTER 22

Bioactive Compounds in Red Palm Oil Can Modulate Mechanisms of Actions in *In Vitro* Anoxic Perfused Rat Hearts

J. van Rooyen
Cape Peninsula University of Technology, Cape Town, South Africa

1. INTRODUCTION

1.1 Bioactive Compounds in Red Palm Oil

Red palm oil is a refined red-orange commercial oil obtained from the mesocarp of the oil palm (*Elaeis guineensis*). It consists mainly of glycerides and nonglycerides, such as free fatty acids, carotenoids, tocotrienols, tocopherols, sterols, phospholipids, squalene, and hydrocarbons. These compounds synergistically and collectively protect the oil against oxidation (Nagendran et al., 2000).

Red palm oil has a very balanced fatty acid composition – 51%, saturated fatty acids; 38%, monounsaturated fatty acids; and 11%, polyunsaturated fatty acids. The major saturated fatty acid is 38–44% of palmitic acid (C16:0) and 4–5% stearic acid (C18:0). Oleic acid (C18:1) represents 39–44% and linoleic acid (C18:2) 10–12% of the unsaturated fatty acids. What is interesting about the structure of the fatty acids on the triglyceride backbone is that the majority (87%) of the unsaturated fatty acids are situated in the sn-2 position, whereas the saturated fatty acids are mostly in the sn-1 and sn-3 positions (Kritchevsky, 1995). Normally, the sn-2 position monoacylglycerols are readily absorbed in the intestine. This unique structure in the palm oil triglyceride backbone therefore ensures that the unsaturated fatty acids in the sn-2 position are mostly absorbed from the intestine and that the saturated fatty acids in the sn-1 and sn-3 positions ensure stability and protection against oxidation (Small, 1991).

Apart from the fatty acids, red palm oil contains concentrated levels of α-, β-, and γ-carotenes; lycopene; and xanthophylls (500–700 ppm). These components are responsible for the red color of the oil. More than 80% of the carotenes are β-carotene (Lehninger et al., 1993). Red palm oil also contains high levels of provitamin E (600–1000 ppm), with 78–82% being tocotrienols and 18–22% tocopherols (Nagendran et al., 2000). Tocotrienols are 40–60 times more potent than tocopherols as antioxidants (Serbinova et al., 1992). Red palm oil also has the highest content of tocotrienols of all edible oils, with rich bran oil as the only other edible oil that comes close, with just less than a third of the levels contained in red palm oil. Other phytonutrients include sterols

(60–620 ppm), squalene (200–500 ppm), coenzyme Q10 (10–80 ppm), glycolipids (1000–3000 ppm), and triterpene alcohol (40–80 ppm).

The unique composition of refined red palm oil makes it valuable in the food and supplement industry. The underlying complementary action of the individual compounds and the synergistic action of the compounds within the red palm oil further substantiate its efficacy. It has also been shown that the bioavailability of the oil is outstanding (Canfield, 2000; You et al., 2002). Red palm oil is commercially available as a salad dressing as well as in a more concentrated form.

1.2 *In Vitro* Anoxic Perfused Rat Heart Model

The anoxic perfused rat heart model has been used to perform drug testing and examine methods of treatment, both before and after episodes of anoxia. These are commonly known as pre- and postconditioning methods to protect the heart against ischemia/reperfusion injury. The author's aim was to investigate the effect of a dietary supplement on the anoxic perfused rat heart.

After a period of ischemia or anoxia, the major challenge is to overcome the accumulation of reactive oxygen species (ROS) during reperfusion. In this period, there is a burst of oxygen due to the provision of oxygen in the reperfusion fluid. The ROS can influence several pathways that may contribute to cardiac protection. However, the aim was to establish whether a natural compound high in antioxidants and given as dietary supplementation before any anoxic event could actually protect the heart against injury after ischemia/reperfusion when there is a high concentration of ROS, or free radicals, as it is commonly called.

The isolated anoxic perfused rat heart is a relatively inexpensive physiological model that is used to perform basic research to elucidate mechanisms of action and establish a foundation for further research in the area of cardiovascular disease.

In their studies, the authors applied the model of dietary red palm oil supplementation to healthy and unhealthy rats. They discovered a few options of protective mechanisms in red palm oil. These protective mechanisms are aimed at the nitric oxide cyclic-GMP pathway, the phosphatidylinositol 3-kinases (PI3-K), protein kinase (PKB/Akt) pathway, and the apoptotic pathway. The authors also showed that dosage and feeding period of red palm oil may influence the efficacy of these protective mechanisms. In the following sections, the importance of these pathways in cardiac protection and the way dietary red palm oil supplementation may influence these pathways are discussed.

2. INVOLVEMENT OF THE PROSURVIVAL AND APOPTOTIC PATHWAYS IN RED PALM OIL PROTECTION

2.1 Background on Pathways

PKB/Akt is a serine/threonine protein kinase that has been implicated in the protection of the myocardium against ischemia/reperfusion injury when it is phosphorylated

(Hausenloy et al., 2004; Jonassen et al., 2001) in the anoxic rat heart model. PKB/Akt is mainly activated by upstream PI3-kinase (Vanhaesebroeck and Waterfield, 1999), an enzyme activated by extracellular stimuli such as growth and insulin (Lawlor and Alessi, 2001). There is also evidence to suggest that PKB/Akt may be activated independently of PI3-kinase through PKA and/or PDK (Fillipa et al., 1999), cellular stresses, and heat shock proteins (Konishi et al., 1997). Downstream PKB/Akt activation has an effect on different signaling targets that are associated with protection, including BAD and Cas-9 (inhibition of apoptosis), JNK (transcriptional inhibition of apoptosis), and GSK-3β (metabolic regulation of apoptosis); it also stimulates NO production (associated with cardiac protection) (Gang et al., 2005). It would thus seem that targeting PKB/Akt phosphorylation could be a good ploy to help protect the heart against injury in anoxic conditions.

On the other hand, apoptosis is a process of programmed cell death that may be triggered by cellular stress, such as anoxia (Gottlieb et al., 1994). Despite the controversy and difference in opinion between necrosis and apoptosis in the heart model, it has been accepted that cardiac cell loss in models of heart attack is associated with apoptosis (Hochhauser et al., 2003; MacLellan and Schneider, 1997). The major indicators of apoptosis in the ischemic/reperfusion rat heart model are the mitogen-activated protein kinases (MAPKs) (Knight and Buxton, 1996). These include the kinases ERK, JNK, and p38. The caspases are cysteine proteases that cleave poly (ADP-ribose) polymerase (PARP) and ultimately cause apoptosis (Salvesen and Dixit, 1997).

2.2 Experimental Results

In several studies since 2005, it has been shown that dietary supplementation with RPO improved cardiac function after a period of anoxia in the isolated rat heart model. Esterhuyse et al. (2006) showed that animals fed with RPO, in both normal and cholesterol-high diets, exhibited significantly improved postischemic function in a working rat heart model. Engelbrecht et al. (2009) and Thamahane-Katengua (2010) confirmed these results in a Langendorff perfused model. All these studies pursued investigations to elucidate possible protective cellular mechanisms underlying the improved function.

Engelbrecht et al. (2006) aimed to show the involvement of the signaling pathways in this red palm oil–induced protection at different stages of the ischemia/reperfusion protocol. They measured the activation of signaling pathways during ischemia and reperfusion. It was shown that PKB/Akt phosphorylation (associated with protection) was significantly increased during reperfusion in RPO-treated hearts, whereas no change was observed during ischemia. p38 phosporylation was also increased only during reperfusion, whereas JNK phosphorylation (associated with pro-apoptosis) in RPO-treated hearts was reduced significantly during reperfusion. In this study, total p38 phosphorylation was measured. The isoform P38-β is normally associated with protection and p38α

with injury. The fact that an increase in total p38 in RPO-treated hearts was associated with improved recovery provides circumstantial evidence that it may have been the p38-β isoform that was phosphorylated; however, this needs to be verified. The same group also found a significant reduction in cleaved PARP and attenuated caspase-3 activation in hearts treated with RPO. Both these proteases are linked to apoptosis. The interesting aspect of these results was that the beneficial effects of RPO were shown in the reperfusion period and not in the ischemic period. In a follow-up study by Kruger et al. (2007), it was shown that dietary treatment with RPO was also able to protect the heart against ischemia/reperfusion when it was added to a cholesterol-rich diet. As in the work of Engelbrecht et al. (2006), the protective mechanisms were activated in the reperfusion period. It is therefore tempting to argue that RPO exerts its protective properties in the reperfusion period, when we consider the signaling pathways as role players in this protection.

Thamahane-Katengua (2010) partly challenged these results by adding a PKB/Akt inhibitor to hearts that were treated with RPO. The results showed a partial abrogation of reperfusion function. This may indicate that PKB/Akt was probably not the only prosurvival mechanism involved. The results in this study also indicated that a downstream proapoptotic Bcl-2-associated death domain (BAD) may be involved. Although Thamahane-Katengua (2010) showed results obtained from only the reperfusion period, it demonstrated again that RPO played a major protective role in the reperfusion period of the protocol.

The fact that all these studies have shown a protective effect of RPO in reperfusion may suggest that the antioxidant compounds in RPO may play an important role in activating the protective signaling pathways in reperfusion when there is an increase in ROS. At present, it is uncertain which of the bioactives of RPO is responsible for this protection. However, it is inviting to speculate that the combination of fatty acids and antioxidants is responsible for this protection because of a synergistic action among all the bioactives.

3. INVOLVEMENT OF THE NO-cGMP PATHWAY AND MMP IN RED PALM OIL PROTECTION

Several studies over a long period of time have shown that nitric oxide (NO) can protect against ischemia/reperfusion injury (Araki et al., 2000; Bolli, 2001; Maulik et al., 1995). Without spending too much time on the details of this mechanism, we attribute the protection to the increase of cGMP levels in the myocardium. Du Toit et al. (2001) showed that a reduction in the cAMP-to-cGMP ratio may be an underlying mechanism to consider in the protection offered by cGMP. cAMP has, since early in the 1970s, been known to be deleterious to the ischemic myocardium (Podzuweit et al., 1976). Esterhuyse et al. (2006) clearly showed that dietary RPO supplementation improved aortic output recovery after ischemia/reperfusion in models fed both cholesterol-rich and normal diets. The results clearly showed that nitric oxide synthase (NOS) activity was increased and that superoxide dismutase activity, the enzyme responsible for producing peroxynitrate from NO, was unchanged. Intracellular levels of NO subsequently increased, which led to an increase in cGMP levels. A significant increase in cGMP levels was observed during the ischemic period. Newaz et al. (2003) also provided evidence of improved NOS activity and cardiac protection in hypertensive rats in a study in which γ-tocotrienols were credited for the protective effect. These findings suggest that RPO can also protect the heart in the ischemic period, but rather through a different mechanism involving NO–cGMP.

The matrix metalloproteinase 2 (MMP-2) are a group of endopeptidases that may be activated by ROS, which are normally produced during oxidative stress conditions (Rajagopalan et al., 1996). Activated MMP2 is associated with poor recovery and increased infarct size in the heart (Fert-Bober et al., 2008) through mechanisms related to apoptosis and necrosis. Evidence shows that inhibition of MMP2 can improve functional recovery after exposure to ischemia/reperfusion (Bendeck et al., 2003; Krishnamurthy et al., 2009). Bester et al. (2010) have shown that a dietary intake of $7 \, mg \, kg^{-1}$ RPO could reduce infarct size. They argue that MMP2 may be involved in this protection, but further studies are needed to conclusively show that MMP2 are part of the mechanism. However, in the same study, levels of lactate dehydrogenase, a marker for cardiac tissue damage, were significantly reduced in RPO-supplemented hearts. These results and conclusions strengthened the observation of Van Rooyen et al. (2008) who argued that the protective effect of red palm oil is not restricted to only one mechanism and that several mechanisms synergistically aid in this protection. In a follow-up study by Szucs et al. (2011), it was shown, for the first time, that RPO could reduce MMP2 levels before ischemia, and not in reperfusion, in a model where RPO was supplemented with a cholesterol-rich diet. This may argue that the benefit of RPO is achieved before exposure to ischemia/reperfusion injury, almost similar to a preconditioning effect.

4. OPTIMAL FEEDING PERIOD AND DOSAGE OF RED PALM OIL TO OFFER PROTECTION AGAINST ANOXIA

The beneficial effect of red palm oil, and for that matter, any supplement, is always associated with the daily dose and duration of supplementation. Initially, all studies by the Van Rooyen group (Bester et al., 2006, 2010; Engelbrecht et al., 2006; Esterhuyse et al., 2006; Kruger et al., 2007) on red palm oil supplementation in the ischemia/reperfusion anoxic model were performed using a daily dose of $7 \, mg \, kg^{-1}$ diet in the rat model. When this was extrapolated to human consumption, the indication was that a human being should consume $0.58 \, mg \, kg^{-1}$ of red palm oil (Engelbrecht et al., 2006).

This is approximately 40 mg of red palm oil a day for a person weighing 70 kg, which is just more than 2 tablespoons of oil per day. This dose was used in reference to the study of Serbinova et al. (1992) who used a tocotrienol-rich palm oil at a daily dose of 7 mg kg^{-1} diet in rats. At the time of Serbinova's study, no work had been performed with any form of palm oil on the ischemic/reperfusion model. However, during the course of the Van Rooyen investigations, another less concentrated red palm salad oil was also used to investigate the mechanisms and duration of supplementation. This less concentrated red palm salad oil was used at a dosage 10 times the dosage of the concentrated red palm oil. This means that a daily dose of 2000 µl of less concentrated red palm oil was used. Both Engelbrecht et al. (2009) and Thamahane-Katengua (2010) used the less concentrated red palm oil but at higher dosages and still showed RPO's protective effects against ischemia/reperfusion injury. Thamahane-Katengua (2010) also showed that a feeding period of 6 weeks is the optimal supplementation time, with better results being obtained now by continuing the supplementation for 2 more weeks. Diet supplementation for 4 weeks with the RPO salad oil did not achieve the same results that had been published earlier on red palm oil concentrate and ischemia/reperfusion. These results provided circumstantial evidence that concluded and confirmed that there is an optimal supplementation time for red palm oil benefit in this model of anoxic stress. A feeding time of 5 weeks with concentrated red palm oil was effective.

5. RED PALM OIL PROTECTION IN OTHER DISEASE MODELS

The beneficial effect of red palm oil has recently been studied in other models of oxidative stress. Wergeland et al. (2011) hypothesized a possible role for red palm oil treatment in chemotherapy, and Bačová et al. (2011) showed that red palm oil dietary supplementation may also prove beneficial to spontaneously hypertensive rats.

Wergeland et al. (2011) supplemented the diet with 7 mg kg^{-1} (200 µl per day per rat) of red palm oil for 4 weeks. In the last 12 days, rats were treated with daunorubicin as the chemotherapeutic agent. Daunorubicin is known to be toxic to healthy tissue and to cause cardiomyopathy and congestive heart failure (Van Hoff et al., 1977). In these studies, it was shown that while it was being treated with daunorubicin, the heart could be protected against failure of function with an RPO-supplemented diet. It was shown that the MAP kinase pathway was involved in this protection and that the antioxidants in red palm oil were to be credited with this action. Bačová et al. (2011) also used a daily dose of 7 mg kg^{-1} diet (200 µl per day per rat) red palm oil as supplementation.

Preliminary results showed that red palm oil could decrease the blood pressure and blood glucose in a model of spontaneously hypertensive rats. They also showed that red palm oil reduced reperfusion arrhythmias in both control and spontaneously hypertensive rats (Table 22.1).

Table 22.1 The Protective Effect of Red Palm Oil and the Mechanisms Involved in Different Models of Oxidative Stress

Red palm oil: physiological effect	Mechanism	Period of protection	Reference
Increased left ventricular developed pressure (LVDP)	PKB/Akt	Reperfusion	Engelbrecht et al. (2009)
Increased aortic output	PKB/Akt	Reperfusion	Engelbrecht et al. (2006)
	Antiapoptosis	Reperfusion	Engelbrecht et al. (2006)
	NO-cGMP	Ischemia	Esterhuyse et al. (2006)
Decreased infarct size	LDH	Reperfusion	Bester et al. (2010)
	MMP-2	Reperfusion	Bester et al. (2010)
	MMP-2	Preischemic	Szucs et al. (2011)
	PKB/Akt	Reperfusion	Bester et al. (2010)

6. SUMMARY

Results of research on dietary supplementation with RPO in a model of anoxia have clearly shown protective action against ischemia/reperfusion injury. This protection may occur during ischemia via the NO-cGMP pathway, or via the prosurvival signaling pathway, or antiapoptosis during reperfusion. It would also seem that the beneficial effect of RPO cannot be attributed to any one of the bioactives in the oil, and that all the bioactives are collectively responsible for this protection. However, more investigations should be performed to clearly indicate the optimal dosage and supplementation period in the human model.

REFERENCES

Araki, M., Tanaka, M., Hasegawa, K., et al., 2000. Nitric oxide inhibition improved myocardial metabolism independent of tissue perfusion during ischaemia, but not during reperfusion. Molecular and Cellular Cardiology 32 (3), 375–384.

Bačová, V.C., Radošinská, J., Knezl, V., et al., 2011. Tribulová, Beneficial effects of red palm oil demonstrated in spontaneously hypertensive rats. In: Abstract, 21st Annual European Meeting on Hypertension and Cardiovascular prevention, Milan Convention Centre, Milan, Italy, 17–20 June 2011.

Bendeck, M.P., Conde, M., Zhang, M., Nili, M., Strauss, B.H., Farwell, S.M., 2003. Doxycycline modulates smooth muscle cell growth, migration and matrix remodeling after arterial injury. The American Journal of Pathology 160, 1089–1095.

Bester, D.J., Kupai, K., Csont, T., et al., 2010. Dietary red palm oil supplementation reduces myocardial infarct size in an isolated perfused rat heart model. Lipids in Health and Disease 9 (64), 1–9.

Bester, D.J., van Rooyen, J., du Toit, E.F., Esterhuyse, A.J., 2006. Red palm oil protects against the consequences of oxidative stress when supplemented with dislipidaemic diets. Medical Technology SA 20 (1), 3–10.

Bolli, R., 2001. Cardioprotective function of inducible nitric oxide synthase and role of nitric oxide in myocardial ischaemia and preconditioning: An overview of a decade of research. Journal of Molecular and Cellular Cardiology 33, 1897–1918.

Canfield, L.M., 2000. Red palm oil in the maternal diet improves vitamin A status of lactating mothers and infants. Food and Nutrition Bulletin 21 (2), 144–148.

Du Toit, E.F., Meiring, J., Opie, L.H., 2001. Relation of cyclic nucleotide ratios to ischaemic and reperfusion injury in nitric oxide-donor treated hearts. Journal of Cardiovascular Pharmacology 38, 529–538.

Engelbrecht, A.M., Esterhuyse, J., du Toit, E.F., Lochner, A., van Rooyen, J., 2006. p38-MAPK and PKB/Akt, possible role players in red palm oil-induced protection of the isolated perfused rat heart. The Journal of Nutritional Biochemistry 17, 265–271.

Engelbrecht, A.M., Odendaal, L., Du Toit, E.F., et al., 2009. The effect of dietary red palm oil on the functional recovery of the ischaemia/reperfused isolade rat heart: The involvement of the PI3-kinase signaling pathway. Lipids in Health and Disease 8 (18), 1–8.

Esterhuyse, J.S., van Rooyen, J., Strijdom, H., Bester, D., du Toit, E.F., 2006. Proposed mechanism for red palm oil induced cardioprotection in a model of hyperlipidaemia in the rat. Prostaglandins, Leukotrienes, and Essential Fatty Acids 75, 375–384.

Fert-Bober, J., Leon, H., Sawicka, J., et al., 2008. Inhibiting matrix metalloproteinase-2 reduces protein release into coronary effluent from isolated rat hearts during ischaemia-reperfusion. Basic Research in Cardiology 103 (5), 431–443.

Fillipa, N., Sable, C.L., Filloux, C., Hemmings, B., van Obbregheni, E., 1999. Mechanism of protein kinase B activation by cyclic AMP-dependent protein kinase. Molecular and Cellular Biology 19 (7), 4989–5000.

Gang, S., Gaoliang, O., Shideng, B., 2005. The activation of Akt/PKB signaling pathway and cell survival. Journal of Molecular Medicine 9 (1), 59–71.

Gottlieb, R.A., Burleson, K.O., Kloner, R.A., Babior, B.M., Engler, R.L., 1994. Reperfusion injury induces apoptosis in rabbit cardiomyocytes. The Journal of Clinical Investigation 94, 1621.

Hausenloy, D.J., Mocanu, M.M., Yellon, D.M., 2004. Cross-talk between the survival kinases during early reperfusion: Its contribution to ischemic preconditioning. Cardiovascular Research 63, 305–312.

Hochhauser, E., Kivity, S., Offen, D., 2003. Bax ablation protects against myocardial ischemia reperfusion injury in transgenic mice. American Journal of Physiology. Heart and Circulatory Physiology 284, H2351–H2359.

Jonassen, A.K., Sack, M.N., Mjøs, O.D., Yellon, D.M., 2001. Myocardial protection by insulin at reperfusion requires early administration and is mediated via Akt and p70s6 kinase cell-survival signaling. Circulation Research 89, 1–9.

Knight, R.J., Buxton, D.B., 1996. Stimulation of c-Jun kinase and mitogen activated protein kinase by ischaemia and reperfusion in the perfused rat heart. Biochemical and Biophysical Research Communications 218, 83–88.

Konishi, H., Matsuzaki, H., Tanaka, M., et al., 1997. Activation of protein kinase B (Akt/RAC-protein kinase) by cellular stress and its association with heat shock protein Hsp27. FEBS Letters 410, 493–498.

Krishnamurthy, P., Peterson, J.T., Subramanian, V., Singh, M., Singh, K., 2009. Inhibition of matrix metalloproteinases improves left ventricular function in mice lacking osteopontin after myocardial infarction. Molecular and Cellular Biochemistry 322, 53–62.

Kritchevsky, D., 1995. Influence of triglyceride structure on lipid metabolism. Malaysian Oil Technology 4 (1), 23–27.

Kruger, M.J., Engelbrecht, A.M., Esterhuyse, J., du Toit, E.F., van Rooyen, J., 2007. Dietary red palm oil reduces ischaemia-reperfusion injury in rats fed a hypercholesterolaemic diet British. The Journal of Nutrition 97 (4), 653–660.

Lawlor, M.A., Alessi, D.R., 2001. PKB/Akt: A key mediator of cell proliferation, survival and insulin responses?. Journal of Cell Science 114, 2903–2910.

Lehninger, A.L., Nelson, D.L., Cox, M.M., 1993. Principles of Biochemistry, 2nd edn. Worth Publishers, New York 259–262.

MacLellan, W.R., Schneider, M.D., 1997. Death by design: Programmed cell death in cardiovascular biology and disease. Circulation Research 81, 137–144.

Maulik, N., Engelman, D.T., Watanabe, M., et al., 1995. Nitric oxide signaling in ischaemic heart. Cardio-vascular Research 30, 593–601.

Nagendran, B., Unnithan, U.R., Choo, Y.M., Sundram, K., 2000. Characteristics of red palm oil, α-carotene- and vitamin E-rich oil for food uses. Food and Nutrition Bulletin 21 (2), 189–194.

Newaz, M.A., Yousefipour, Z., Nawal, N., Adeed, N., 2003. Nitric oxide synthase activity in blood vessels of spontaneously hypertensive rats: Antioxidant protection by gamma-tocotrienol. Journal of Physiology and Pharmacology 54 (3), 319–327.

Podzuweit, T., Lubbe, W.F., Opie, L.H., 1976. Cyclic adenosine monophosphate, ventricular fibrillation and anti-arrhythmic drugs. The Lancet 14 (1), 341–342 7955.

Rajagopalan, S., Meng, X.P., Ramasamy, S., Harrison, D.G., Galis, Z.S., 1996. Reactive oxygen species produced by macrophage-derived foam cells regulate the activity of vascular matrix metalloproteinases in vitro: Implications for atherosclerotic plague stability. The Journal of Clinical Investigation 98, 2572–2579.

Salvesen, G.S., Dixit, V.M., 1997. Caspases: Intracellular signaling by proteolysis. Cell 91, 443–446.

Serbinova, E., Khavaja, S., Catudioc, J., et al., 1992. Palm oil vitamin E protects against ischemia/reperfusion in the isolated perfused Langendorff heart. Nutrition Research 12 (suppl 1), S203–S215.

Small, D.M., 1991. The effects of glyceride structure on absorption and metabolism. Annual Review of Nutrition 11, 413–434.

Szucs, G., Bester, D.J., Kupai, K., et al., 2011. Dietary red palm oil supplementation decreases infarct size in cholesterol fed rats. Lipids in Health and Disease 10, 103.

Thamahane-Katengua, E.T.M., 2010. The effect of dietary red palm oil supplementation on the PI3K-PKB/Akt signaling in the isolated perfused rat heart. M. Tech Thesis, Cape peninsula University of Technology, South Africa.

Van Hoff, D.D., Rozencweig, M., Layard, M., Slavik, M., Muggia, F.M., 1977. Daunomycin-induced cardiotoxicity in children and adults, A review of 100 cases. The American Journal of Medicine 62, 200–208.

Van Rooyen, J., Esterhuyse, A.J., Engelbrecht, A.M., du Toit, E.F., 2008. Health benefits of a natural carotonoid rich oil: A proposed mechanisms of protection against ischemia/reperfusion injury. Asia Pacific Journal of Clinical Nutrition 17 (Suppl 1), 316–319.

Vanhaesebroeck, B., Waterfield, M.D., 1999. Signaling by distinct classes of phophoinositide 3-kinases. Experimental Cell Research 253, 239–254.

Wergeland, A., Bester, D.J., Sishi, B.J.N., Engelbrecht, A.M., Jonassen, A.K., van Rooyen, J., 2011. Dietary red palm oil protects the heart against the cytotoxic effects of anthracycline. Cell Biochemistry and Function 29 (5), 356–364.

You, C.S., Parker, R.S., Swanson, J.E., 2002. Bioavailability and vitamin A value of carotenes from red palm oil assessed by an extrinsic isotope reference method. Asia Pacific Journal of Clinical Nutrition 11 (7), S438–S442.

CHAPTER 23

The Effect of ʟ-Carnitine Supplement and Its Derivatives on Cardiovascular Disease

M.R. Movahed
University of Arizona Sarver Heart Center, Tucson, AZ, USA

ABBREVIATIONS

ALC Acetyl-ʟ-carnitine
CACT Carnitine-acylcarnitine translocase
CoA Coenzyme A
CPT Carnitine palmitoyl transferase
CRAT Acylcarnitine transferase
DM Diabetes mellitus
eNOS Endothelial nitric oxide synthase
LC ʟ-Carnitine
LDL Low-density lipoprotein
NO Nitric oxide
PDH Pyruvate dehydrogenase
PGI2 Prostacyclin
PLC Propionyl-ʟ-carnitine
PLC Phospholipase C
PVD Peripheral vascular disease
SOD Superoxide dismutase
TCA Tricarboxylic acid
TG Triglyceride
VCAM-1 Vascular cell adhesion molecule-1
VSMCs Vascular smooth muscle cells

1. INTRODUCTION

Cardiovascular disease is the leading cause of death in the United States. Substantial advancement in our knowledge in the recent years has led to the development of numerous active drugs and advancement in technology for the prevention and treatment of various cardiovascular conditions. However, the effect on the reduction in the cardiovascular-related morbidity and mortality has been limited and modest. Furthermore, current treatment modalities are associated with its inherited risk and adverse events. Natural

Bioactive Food as Dietary Interventions for Cardiovascular Disease
http://dx.doi.org/10.1016/B978-0-12-396485-4.00021-9

© 2013 Elsevier Inc.
All rights reserved.

products have gained substantial interest in recent years in the prevention and treatment of various conditions including cardiovascular disease as they are rarely associated with significant adverse events. L-carnitine (LC) is a nonprotein amino acid that is synthesized from the essential amino acids lysine and methionine or (Zammit, 1999) it can be obtained from dietary intake. It is important for the transport of fatty acids into the mitochondria. Myocardial tissue produces more than 60% of its energy through fatty acid oxidation as the main source of energy (Neely and Morgan, 1974). For this reason, the effect of LC on various cardiovascular conditions has found particular interest. Acetyl-L-carnitine (ALC) and propionyl-L-carnitine (PLC) are endogenous derivatives from LC, with PLC having higher affinity for skeletal and cardiac muscles (Siliprandi et al., 1991; Zammit, 1999). LC is an essential cofactor for fatty acid transport into the mitochondria for the metabolism of long-chain fatty acids into the β-oxidation cycle to produce acetyl-CoA for energy production in the form of ATP. Furthermore, through modulation in the acetyl-CoA/CoA ratio and the pyruvate dehydrogenase complex in the mitochondria, LC plays an important role in glucose metabolism (Broderick et al., 1992; Lysiak et al., 1988). Another well-known physiological effect of LC is the role of LC in the efflux of acylcarnitines and other acetyl groups from the cells, reducing accumulation of these intermediates produced by β-oxidation (Chapela et al., 2009). These intermediates have been thought to be important in the pathogenesis of insulin resistance. Accordingly, LC and its analogs have been evaluated in patients with diabetes, congestive heart failure, angina pectoris, acute myocardial infarction, peripheral vascular disease, and diastolic heart failure. The aim of this chapter is to summarize our current knowledge about the effect of LC and its derivate supplement in the treatment of various cardiovascular conditions.

2. THE EFFECT OF LC AND ITS DERIVATES ON THE CARDIOVASCULAR RISK FACTORS

2.1 Diabetes Mellitus and LC Analogs

Patients with diabetes mellitus (DM) are at substantial risk for coronary artery disease, congestive heart failure, stroke, cardiomyopathy, peripheral vascular disease, renal failure, and endothelial dysfunction. This fact has made cardiovascular disease the leading cause of death in this population (Anon, 1999a). Any effort in reducing the risk of DM or better DM treatment can lead to reduction in cardiovascular-related morbidity and mortality. As mentioned earlier, increasing the concentration of fatty acids and lipid metabolites can lead to reduction in insulin sensitivity, one of the important mechanisms for insulin resistance in the heart or muscle (Adams et al., 2009; Zhang et al., 2010) LC plays an important role in the reduction of excess acyl groups from mitochondria by increasing the transport of these products out of the cell or by inhibiting the transport of long-chain fatty acids into the cell (Ramsay and Zammit, 2004). For these reasons, many clinical trials have been conducted. Improvement in insulin resistance has been documented by oral supplementation of LC (Giancaterini et al., 2000; Mingrone, 2004). The first report by Giancaterini et al. (2000) studied 18 patients with type 2 DM by giving them ALC in comparison to placebo. They found that tissue glucose uptake increased in a dose-dependent manner due to increasing glucose storage. In a double-blind clinical trial of prediabetic patients, 3 g per day of ALC improved HbA1c and fasting blood glucose in comparison to placebo (Bloomer et al., 2009). Chronic administration of ALC for 24 weeks at a dose of 2 g per day has shown improvement in the glucose tolerance and systolic blood pressure (Ruggenenti et al., 2009). In addition to improving glucose intolerance, chronic administration of PLC in rats led to decrease in adiposity and insulin concentration (Mingorance et al., 2009).

2.2 The Effect of LC Derivatives on Lipids

As mentioned earlier, LC has significant effects on fatty acid transfer into the mitochondria. This has led to studies evaluating the effect of LC derivatives on lipids. In rat models with DM, LC treatment led to reduction of plasma glucose and lipids in comparison to the controls (Rodrigues et al., 1988). Lipoprotein (a) (La) is an important atherogenic lipid. Derosa et al. (2003) showed reduction in the La level by 29.9% after oral supplementation of 2 g of LC for 6 months. Similar effect to a lesser degree was found by Sirtori et al. (2000) This effect was confirmed in a randomized clinical trial after 3 months of LC treatment in patients with dialysis, but without any effect on the triglycerides or other lipoproteins (Shojaei et al., 2011). In another study of 28 patients who were on chronic hemodialysis receiving LC at the doses of 5 mg kg^{-1} body weight intravenously 3 times per week for a mean period of 25 months, LC did not modify most of the serum lipid levels. However, a significant decrease in the serum triglycerides was noticed in hypertriglyceridemic patients (Elisaf et al., 1998).

2.3 The Role of LC and its Derivatives on Oxidative Stress

Improvement in the fatty acid oxidation by LC was thought to have a positive effect on oxidative stress. LC treatment has been shown to inhibit oxidation and nitration of plasma protein in vitro (Kolodziejczyk et al., 2011) Higher level of reactive oxygen species (RoS) plays an important role in the pathogenesis of hypertension. PLC administration has been shown to restore the effect of impaired glutathione peroxidase and superoxide dismutase and reduce lipid peroxidation in hypertensive rat models (Gomez-Amores et al., 2006, 2007). PLC has been shown to prevent structural injury and deterioration of renal function induced by reperfusion in rat kidney, suggesting reduction in free radical generation (Mister et al., 2002). In rats, PLC has been shown to prevent cisplatin-induced cardiomyopathy, renal injury, and hepatotoxicity (Aleisa et al., 2007; Al-Majed, 2007; Al-Majed et al., 2006a,b).

3. THE EFFECT OF LC AND ITS DERIVATIVES ON PATIENTS WITH ATHEROSCLEROSIS

The vascular endothelial surface has many important homeostatic functions, including preventing intravascular coagulation and inflammation through regulation of vascular tone. Its regulatory activity is important for postexercise vasodilatation in order to increase supply due to higher oxygen and energy demand. This is mediated through production of nitric oxide and other vasoactive molecules. Atherosclerosis initially causes endothelial dysfunction and later leads to ischemia due to narrowing of the arterial supply. This leads to oxygen supply/demand mismatch during exercise or at rest if narrowing is severe. As mentioned earlier, many risk factors contribute to the development of atherosclerosis, including age, smoking, DM, hypertension, sedentary life style, and hyperlipidemia. The effect of LC on some of the important risk factors for atherosclerosis, such as DM or lipids, has already been discussed. As a substance that is important for fatty acid transfer into the mitochondria, LC has gained special interest in the treatment of conditions that lead to reduction in the energy supply, such as atherosclerosis. The aim of this chapter is to review the effect of LC and its derivates in patients with atherosclerotic cardiovascular disease.

3.1 Coronary Artery Disease

Coronary artery disease is one of the leading causes of death in the United States. It can lead to myocardial infarction by sudden narrowing or occlusion of coronary arteries or to chronic ischemia due to narrowing of the coronary tree, leading to angina or myocardial dysfunction and heart failure. In the early phase of coronary arteriosclerosis, endothelial dysfunction can occur that can trigger vasospasm without significant flow-limiting lesions. As the majority of myocardial energy is produced by fatty acid oxidation, LC and its derivatives play an important role in the production of myocardial energy. Furthermore, postmortem examination of patients who died of myocardial infarction has shown reduced carnitine concentration in the myocardial cells, supporting the important role of carnitine in the ischemic heart.

3.1.1 PLC and cardioprotection during coronary ischemia

Experimental data suggests that the PL derivative PLC exerts a protective effect during myocardial ischemia. In earlier studies in rat models on isolated healthy hearts, PLC was found to improve the imbalance between energy production and utilization (Bertelli et al., 1991). Cardioprotective effects of PLC appear to be more prominent during ischemia. Chronic treatment with PLC has shown to improve exercise tolerance and infarct size, with improvement in the cardiac function (Koh et al., 2003; Leasure and Kordenat, 1991; Sethi et al., 2004). Isolated ischemic reperfused hearts have been shown to have enhanced myocardial recovery after PLC administration (Ferrari et al., 1989; Paulson et al., 1986).

One of the reasons for the positive effect of PLC during ischemia was thought to be secondary to the replacement of LC loss that occurs during ischemia (Broderick et al., 1995; Martin et al., 2000), as low LC myocardial content can lead to vulnerability of the myocardial cell during ischemia (Broderick, 2006). Another explanation for the positive effect of LC in ischemic myocardium appears to be related to the antioxidant activity of LC (Ferrari et al., 1991; Reznick et al., 1992; Shug et al., 1991). As an important fatty acid transfer molecule for transport into the mitochondria, PLC leads to improvement in mitochondrial function (Di Lisa et al., 1989; Ferrari et al., 1991), with enhancement in the ATP level during reperfusion (Ferrari et al., 1991; Packer et al., 1991; Shug et al., 1991). Although fatty acids are the most important energy source for the heart, increase in glucose oxidation by PLC has also been documented (Loster et al., 1999). This effect appears to be mostly seen by PLC administration (Ferrari et al., 1989). In addition to improving energy supply, LC has been shown to reduce ischemia and reperfusion–induced arrhythmias in the isolated rat hearts. Interestingly, this effect could be reversed using etomoxir, suggesting that the efficacy of LC is related to mitochondrial action (Najafi et al., 2008).

3.1.2 Clinical trials in patients with coronary artery disease

One of the earliest studies evaluating the effect of 15 mg kg^{-1} of PLC administered intravenously in 16 patients vs. placebo showed acute improvement in the myocardial contractility in patients with coronary artery disease and increased the lactate uptake by 42% (Bartels et al., 1992). In 31 patients with coronary artery disease, the ejection fraction increased by 8% in the PLC-treated arms in comparison to placebo, without affecting myocardial oxygen supply–demand ratio (Bartels et al., 1994).

Furthermore, PLC reduced ST-segment depression during exercise but could not increase the time to onset of angina (Bartels et al., 1996). In another double-blind placebo-controlled study of patients with stable angina, PLC administration was able to increase workload, reduce ST-segment depression, and enhance exercise time (Lagioia et al., 1992). The anti–ischemic effect of oral 1.5 mg per day of PLC in 18 patients suffering from stable angina was studied in a randomized double-blind crossover study, showing an increase in the time for the occurrence of 1 mm ST-segment depression and the maximal exercise time (Cherchi et al., 1990).

The effect of LC during coronary bypass surgery has been studied in two trials. Sixty-eight patients with DM undergoing coronary bypass surgery were randomized to receive PLC vs. placebo intravenously. The patients on LC had a higher cardiac index after the surgery (3.30 vs. 2.9). Furthermore, mean pulmonary artery pressure was lower in LC-treated patients accompanied by reduced transcardiac endothelin intravenously and rapid hypoxanthine washout during reperfusion (Lango et al., 2005). The second was a placebo-controlled trial that assessed the effect of LC on the cardiac performance of 38 patients undergoing cardiac surgery. Five grams of LC was given intravenously over

2 h and orally twice daily for 5 days. Furthermore, 10 g of LC was added to 1500 ml cardioplegia. They found no differences in respect to all clinical parameters of cardiac performance after cardiopulmonary bypass in the treated patients, despite higher serum carnitine levels in the treated cohort. In patients undergoing mitral valve surgery, LC therapy was associated with significantly higher concentrations of ATP, pyruvate, and creatine phosphate in the papillary muscles. Myocardial ultrastructures obtained from septal biopsies showed better preservation scores for all in the treated patients (Pastoris et al., 1998). The largest randomized double-blind placebo-controlled trial evaluating the effects of LC at an oral dose of 2 g per day for 28 days in 51 patients with suspected acute myocardial infarction in comparison to a control group revealed a reduction in the infarct size in the LC-treated group assessed by cardiac enzymes (Singh et al., 1996). Furthermore, angina occurred in 17.6% of LC-treated patients vs. 36% in the control arm. The incidence of heart failure and left ventricular enlargement was also lower in the test cohort. Total major cardiac events such as cardiac death and nonfatal infarction were also lower in the LC group (15.6 vs. 26.0%) (Singh et al., 1996).

Based on these trials, LC and its derivatives appear to have a positive effect on patients presenting with coronary artery disease. However, these trails are limited due to small number of patients, with the largest enrolling number of 101 conducted by Singh et al. (1996) Furthermore, longer outcome data are lacking. Based on these positive studies, larger randomized controlled trials with longer duration should be conducted before LC treatment can be routinely recommended to patients with coronary artery disease.

3.2 Peripheral Vascular Disease

Due to theoretical improvement in energy production by enhancing mitochondrial fatty acid transfer, LC has been studied in patients with peripheral vascular disease (PVD). PVD is caused by atherosclerosis of peripheral arteries, leading to poor limb circulation and ischemia. This leads to increase in inflammation and oxidative stress (Silvestro et al., 2003). The beneficial effects of PLC on PVD patients have been shown in several clinical trials. PLC has led to improvement in the ankle/brachial index as well as the maximal walking distance and distance to the onset of claudication (Brevetti et al., 1995, 1997; Hiatt et al., 2001; Santo et al., 2006). This has improved the quality of life in this population (Brevetti et al., 1995; Hiatt et al., 2001). The underlying mechanism of PLC in patients with PVD is not clear. There are some studies suggesting improvement in the hemodynamic flow (Dal Lago et al., 1999; Loffredo et al., 2007; Signorelli et al., 2006a,b) while others could not find significant increases in the flow (Bolognesi et al., 1995; Cittanti et al., 1997). Many trials have shown reduction in the oxidative stress with restoration of vascular function (Loffredo et al., 2006, 2007; Signorelli et al., 2006a,b) and enhancement of nitric oxide availability (Loffredo et al., 2006, 2007). PLC in patients with PVD appears to increase maximal mitochondrial activity for

ATP synthesis in the lower limbs, with improvement in the walking distance (Taylor et al., 1996) and enhancement in the mitochondrial integrity in the skeletal muscle of patients with PVD (Cittanti et al., 1997). Many animal models have confirmed the beneficial effects of LC on PVD. PLC injection enhances rabbit limb postischemic blood flow recovery with restoration of vascular function by improving endothelial function (Stasi et al., 2010) Research in rat models using PLC has shown restoration of normal ATP level in ischemic muscles with increasing mitochondrial activities and integrities, providing another reason for PLC to be beneficial in patients with PVD (Corsico et al., 1993).

The hemodynamic effect of intravenous PLC was evaluated in a double-blind randomized crossover study of 12 men with PVD. PLC administration significantly reduced the halftime and the total time of hyperemia after exercise and ischemia, consistent with previous studies (Corsi et al., 1995). In another double-blind, crossover study evaluating LC treatment in patients with PVD, 20 patients were randomized to LC at the oral dose of 2 g twice daily vs. placebo for a period of 3 weeks, with crossover to the other treatment for an additional 3 weeks. Walking distance at the end of each treatment period was measured by treadmill test. Absolute walking distance rose significantly from 174 ± 63 m in placebo to 306 ± 122 m in the LC-treated arm. The main limitations of these studies are the small number of patients enrolled and the lack of long-term outcome data.

3.3 Cerebral Ischemia

ALC as an important LC derivate has a preferential effect on the brain tissue. For this reason, ALC is the drug of choice when studying the effect of LC on brain ischemia. In an animal study, PLC was used in a rat model of forebrain ischemia. In a total of 105 adult male rats, forebrain ischemia was attenuated by intravenous PLC assessed by a greater number of intact neurons (Al-Majed et al., 2006a,b). Other experimental studies evaluating the effect of ALC on cerebral ischemia have showed that ALC improved neurological outcomes (Calvani and Arrigoni-Martelli, 1999), prevented free radical formation (Rosenthal et al., 1992), and reduced the infarct size induced in rat models (Jalal et al., 2010). In one study involving humans with brain ischemia, ten male patients were studied using regional cerebral blood flow (rCBF) measurement. After 1 h of intravenous infusion of 1500 mg ALC, beneficial effects of the drug were seen in 8 patients (Rosadini et al., 1990). Based on positive animal data and this small clinical study, larger randomized clinical trials are warranted for the treatment of brain ischemia, which could be promising.

4. THE EFFECT OF LC AND ITS DERIVATIVES ON PATIENTS WITH CONGESTIVE HEART FAILURE/CARDIOMYOPATHY

Patients with heart failure suffer from many abnormal conditions leading to mismatch in oxygen supply and demand, triggering heart failure. This usually occurs when cardiac output fails to supply tissue demand. This could be secondary to the heart itself or not related to the myocardial function such as decrease in preload (bleeding, dehydration, sepsis, etc.) or afterload (sepsis, fistulas, etc.). The so-called secondary heart failure needs to be distinguished from primary heart failure due to failure of the heart itself to supply organs with required circulation. This failure could be primarily mechanic (valvular disease or myocardial muscle weakness, the so-called systolic heart failure) or due to abnormal relaxation leading to inability to increase output despite normal or near normal contractility (the so-called diastolic heart failure). There is a considerable overlap between different causes of heart failure. LC as an important molecule for fatty acid transport into the mitochondria plays an important role in myocardial energy production. Therefore, it is feasible that LC supplementation could prove to be beneficial in this population. The known fact that severe LC deficiency can lead to cardiomyopathy further elaborates the importance of LC for proper cardiac function (Paulson, 1998). The aim of this chapter is to review the effect of LC and its derivatives in patients with primary heart failure. The following sections discuss studies evaluating the effects of LC on systolic and diastolic heart failures.

4.1 Systolic Heart Failure

An adequate LC level in the myocardial tissue is an important requirement for normal functioning and energy metabolism of the heart for fatty acid oxidation (Rebouche and Paulson, 1986). This fact explains the occurrence of systolic heart failure and cardiomyopathy in some patients with carnitine deficiency (Christensen, 1989; Scholte et al., 1990; Vikre-Jorgensen, 1993) with reversal of cardiomyopathy after LC supplementation (Bennett et al., 1996; Waber et al., 1982; Zales and Benson, 1995). Therefore, LC and its derivatives have been tested in patients with congestive heart failure or cardiomyopathy. PLC has a high affinity to the muscular carnitine transferase, making it an ideal candidate for heart failure trials. In many experimental animal models of heart failure, PLC has shown to improve cardiac contractility (Pasini et al., 1992; Pierce et al., 1990; Yang et al., 1992). For example, repeated administration of PLC in comparison to saline in rats with pressure-overload cardiac hypertrophy and low myocardial carnitine levels showed improvement in cardiac function and relaxation (Yang et al., 1992). Use of PLC in cardiac hypertrophy induced by pressure overload in rats has shown improvement in the maximal rate of ventricular relaxation and an increase in the end-diastolic pressure at increasing balloon volume. Furthermore, it showed correlation with higher level of total adenine nucleotides and ATPs (Motterlini et al., 1992). In a large animal model, intravenous PLC has been investigated in anesthetized dogs. PLC administration showed dose-dependent short-lasting improvement of cardiac output in both open- and closed-chest conditions (Cevese et al., 1991).

The results of phase 2 clinical trials have also shown some clinical benefit. Anand et al. (1998) evaluated the effect of PLC administration at a dose of 1.5 g per day on hemodynamics and oxygen consumption in patients with mild to moderate heart failure. They could not find any significant hemodynamics or neurohormonal changes, but they demonstrated a reduction in pulmonary artery pressure and an increase in exercise capacity, suggesting a possible improvement in peripheral muscle metabolism. In another clinical study involving 16 patients with dilated cardiomyopathy, PLC supplementation increased pyruvate influx into the Krebs cycle and reduced lactate production in the skeletal muscle (Opasich et al., 1997). In a phase 2 double-blind randomized placebo-controlled study, 50 patients with ejection fraction of <45% and symptomatic NYHA class II heart failure on maximal medical therapy were enrolled. The treatment group received 1.5 g of PLC for 6 months. Bicycle exercise test, Doppler echocardiography, and clinical evaluation showed a statistically significant difference in the mean value of exercise time with improvement in the left ventricular ejection fraction, stroke volume index, and cardiac index in comparison to the placebo (Caponnetto et al., 1994). Similar benefits were seen in a double-blind phase II study of PLC in 60 patients with mild to moderate congestive heart failure. The treatment group received 500 mg of PLC 3 times a day. Maximum exercise time after 1 month of treatment showed significant increases in the values of the exercise time in the treatment group. Ejection fraction was also increased by 8.4, 11.6, and 13.6%, respectively (Mancini et al., 1992). In another study of double-blind placebo-controlled study, the effect of LC treatment on vasodilator function and blood pressure was studied for 8 weeks in 36 subjects with coronary artery disease. The LC-treated cohort had increased brachial artery diameter by 2.3%, and a significant effect was observed in the subgroup of subjects with blood pressure above the median and in the subgroup with the metabolic syndrome (McMackin et al., 2007).

ALC has been studied in 115 patients with circulatory and septic shock by administering it for 12 h intravenously. They found that ALC improved blood oxygenation during the course of sepsis and heart failure. Furthermore, they documented a decrease in the heart rate as well as right atrial pressure in patients with cardiogenic shock. Furthermore, ALC treatment increased systolic and mean arterial pressures in septic patients (Gasparetto et al., 1991). LC has been tested in a randomized double-blind trial of 472 patients with a first acute myocardial infarction vs. placebo. Intravenous LC was given at a dose of 9 g per day for the first 5 days and then orally at a dose of 6 g per day for the next 12 months. Left ventricular volumes and ejection fraction were evaluated serially up to 12 months after the first acute myocardial infarction. They found a significant attenuation in the left ventricular dilation in patients treated with LC with reduction in the end-diastolic and end-systolic volumes from the time of admission to after 3, 6, and 12 months. Ejection fraction did not change over time with similar prevalence of combined death and congestive heart failure after discharge and ischemic events during follow-up (Iliceto et al., 1995). In the largest phase III double-blind randomized multicenter study of 537 patients with mild to moderate heart failure, the effect of PLC was evaluated on the maximal exercise duration using a bicycle exercise test. The results showed only a trend in the maximal exercise duration in the PLC-treated cohort. However, a secondary analysis showed a statistically significant difference in the maximal exercise duration in favor of the PLC-treated patients with higher ejection fractions (30–40%) (Anon, 1999b). In a longest survival study, the efficacy of LC for the treatment of heart failure secondary to dilated cardiomyopathy has been studied. Seventy patients with moderate to severe heart failure after a period of stable cardiac function, up to 3 months, were randomly assigned to receive either LC at a dose of 2 g per day orally or placebo. There were no statistical differences between the two groups at baseline clinical or hemodynamic parameters (ejection fraction, Weber classification, maximal time of cardiopulmonary exercise test, peak VO_2 consumption, arterial and pulmonary blood pressures or cardiac output). After a mean follow-up period of 33.7 ± 11.8 months, 6 deaths occurred in the placebo group vs. 1 death in the LC cohort. Kaplan–Meier Survival Analysis showed that survival was statistically improved in the LC-treated patients ($P < 0.04$) (Rizos, 2000). This is the first study evaluating the long-term outcome involving patients with heart failure and it showed a positive and encouraging result. However, this study enrolled only small number of patients, requiring confirmation in larger clinical trials.

In summary, based on the current clinical data, LC and its derivatives appear to have a positive effect on patients with cardiomyopathy, including improved mortality. However, large randomized long-term clinical trials are not available, to recommend routine

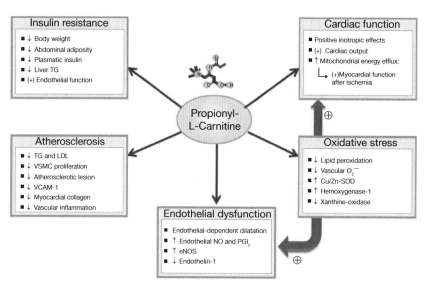

Figure 23.1 Pharmacological effects of propionyl-L-carnitine (eNOS, endothelial nitric oxide synthase; LDL, low-density lipoprotein; NO, nitric oxide; PGI2, prostacyclin; SOD, superoxide dismutase; TG, triglycerides; VCAM-1, vascular cell adhesion molecule-1; VSMC, vascular smooth muscle cells, with permission from International life science institute. *Reproduced from Mingorance, C. et al. 2011. Pharmacological effects and clinical applications of propionyl-L-carnitine. Nutrition Reviews 69, 279–290*

LC treatment in patients with heart failure. Hopefully, future studies can give us more answers in this regard.

4.2 Diastolic Heart Failure/Dysfunction

Diastolic heart failure accounts for a significant number of patients presenting with heart failure (Movahed et al., 2005; Redfield et al., 2003). In patients with diastolic heart failure, despite normal contractility, cardiac output cannot increase without a compensatory elevation of ventricular filling pressure due to impaired relaxation. Relaxation is a highly energy-dependent process requiring ATP. As an important component of fatty acid transfer into the mitochondria for β-oxidation and ATP production, LC plays an important role during diastolic relaxation. LC has shown to have a positive and dose-dependent effect on improving left ventricular compliance and myocardial relaxation in postischemic dogs (Silverman et al., 1985). In rat models of left ventricular hypertrophy as

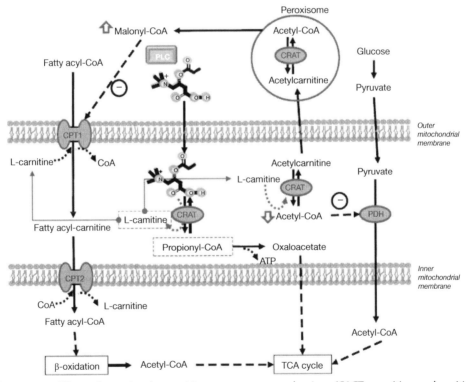

Figure 23.2 Effect of propionyl-L-carnitine on energy mechanism (CACT, carnitine-acylcarnitine translocase; CoA, coenzyme A; CPT, carnitine palmitoyl transferase; CRAT, acylcarnitine transferase; PDH, pyruvate dehydrogenase; PLC, phospholipase C; TCA, tricarboxylic acid, with permission from International life science institute. *Reproduced from Mingorance, C. et al. 2011. Pharmacological effects and clinical applications of propionyl-L-carnitine. Nutrition Reviews 69, 279–290*

a surrogate of diastolic dysfunction, the maximal rate of ventricular relaxation was increased in PLC-treated rats in comparison to controls (Motterlini et al., 1992).

The beneficial effects of LC were also reported in vivo in isolated working hearts in rats with DM. LC treatment protected diabetic rats from impaired contractility and abnormal relaxation (Rodrigues et al., 1988).

There is only one randomized double-blind clinical trial in humans evaluating the effect of oral LC in patients with isolated diastolic heart failure (Serati et al., 2010). In this study, 60 patients with mild symptomatic diastolic heart failure were randomized to oral LC supplementation at a dose of 1.5 g per day vs. placebo. Significant improvement in the diastolic parameters and symptoms was found in the treated patients vs. placebo arm (Serati et al., 2010). Improved diastolic parameters were assessed using echocardiographic examination after 3 months of treatment. Systolic heart failure and coronary artery diseases were excluded. LC supplementation showed improvement in the left atrial size, septal and lateral mitral E' velocities, and isovolumic relaxation. This study is very encouraging and should trigger larger randomized clinical trials in patients with diastolic heart failure (Figures 23.1 and 23.2).

REFERENCES

Adams, S.H., Hoppel, C.L., et al., 2009. Plasma acylcarnitine profiles suggest incomplete long-chain fatty acid beta-oxidation and altered tricarboxylic acid cycle activity in type 2 diabetic African-American women. The Journal of Nutrition 139 (6), 1073–1081.

Aleisa, A.M., Al-Majed, A.A., et al., 2007. Reversal of cisplatin-induced carnitine deficiency and energy starvation by propionyl-L-carnitine in rat kidney tissues. Clinical and Experimental Pharmacology & Physiology 34 (12), 1252–1259.

Al-Majed, A.A., 2007. Carnitine deficiency provokes cisplatin-induced hepatotoxicity in rats. Basic & Clinical Pharmacology & Toxicology 100 (3), 145–150.

Al-Majed, A.A., Sayed-Ahmed, M.M., et al., 2006a. Carnitine esters prevent oxidative stress damage and energy depletion following transient forebrain ischaemia in the rat hippocampus. Clinical and Experimental Pharmacology & Physiology 33 (8), 725–733.

Al-Majed, A.A., Sayed-Ahmed, M.M., et al., 2006b. Propionyl-L-carnitine prevents the progression of cisplatin-induced cardiomyopathy in a carnitine-depleted rat model. Pharmacological Research 53 (3), 278–286.

Anand, I., Chandrashekhan, Y., et al., 1998. Acute and chronic effects of propionyl-L-carnitine on the hemodynamics, exercise capacity, and hormones in patients with congestive heart failure. Cardiovascular Drugs and Therapy 12 (3), 291–299.

Anon, 1999a. Diabetes mellitus: a major risk factor for cardiovascular disease. A joint editorial statement by the American Diabetes Association; The National Heart, Lung, and Blood Institute; The Juvenile Diabetes Foundation International; The National Institute of Diabetes and Digestive and Kidney Diseases and The American Heart Association. Circulation 100 (10), 1132–1133.

Anon, 1999b. Study on propionyl-L-carnitine in chronic heart failure. European Heart Journal 20 (1), 70–76.

Bartels, G.L., Remme, W.J., et al., 1992. Acute improvement of cardiac function with intravenous L-propionylcarnitine in humans. Journal of Cardiovascular Pharmacology 20 (1), 157–164.

Bartels, G.L., Remme, W.J., et al., 1994. Effects of L-propionylcarnitine on ischemia-induced myocardial dysfunction in men with angina pectoris. The American Journal of Cardiology 74 (2), 125–130.

Bartels, G.L., Remme, W.J., et al., 1996. Anti-ischaemic efficacy of L-propionylcarnitine–a promising novel metabolic approach to ischaemia?. European Heart Journal 17 (3), 414–420.

Bennett, M.J., Hale, D.E., et al., 1996. Endocardial fibroelastosis and primary carnitine deficiency due to a defect in the plasma membrane carnitine transporter. Clinical Cardiology 19 (3), 243–246.

Bertelli, A., Conte, A., et al., 1991. Effect of propionyl carnitine on cardiac energy metabolism evaluated by the release of purine catabolites. Drugs Under Experimental and Clinical Research 17 (2), 115–118.

Bloomer, R.J., Fisher-Wellman, K.H., et al., 2009. Effect of oral acetyl L-carnitine arginate on resting and postprandial blood biomarkers in pre-diabetics. Nutrition and Metabolism (London) 6, 25.

Bolognesi, M., Amodio, P., et al., 1995. Effect of 8-day therapy with propionyl-L-carnitine on muscular and subcutaneous blood flow of the lower limbs in patients with peripheral arterial disease. Clinical Physiology 15 (5), 417–423.

Brevetti, G., Perna, S., et al., 1995. Propionyl-L-carnitine in intermittent claudication: Double-blind, placebo-controlled, dose titration, multicenter study. Journal of the American College of Cardiology 26 (6), 1411–1416.

Brevetti, G., Perna, S., et al., 1997. Effect of propionyl-L-carnitine on quality of life in intermittent claudication. The American Journal of Cardiology 79 (6), 777–780.

Broderick, T.L., 2006. Hypocarnitinaemia induced by sodium pivalate in the rat is associated with left ventricular dysfunction and impaired energy metabolism. Drugs in R&D 7 (3), 153–161.

Broderick, T.L., Quinney, H.A., et al., 1992. Carnitine stimulation of glucose oxidation in the fatty acid perfused isolated working rat heart. The Journal of Biological Chemistry 267 (6), 3758–3763.

Broderick, T.L., Quinney, H.A., et al., 1995. L-carnitine increases glucose metabolism and mechanical function following ischaemia in diabetic rat heart. Cardiovascular Research 29 (3), 373–378.

Calvani, M., Arrigoni-Martelli, E., 1999. Attenuation by acetyl-L-carnitine of neurological damage and biochemical derangement following brain ischemia and reperfusion. International Journal of Tissue Reactions 21 (1), 1–6.

Caponnetto, S., Canale, C., et al., 1994. Efficacy of L-propionylcarnitine treatment in patients with left ventricular dysfunction. European Heart Journal 15 (9), 1267–1273.

Cevese, A., Schena, F., et al., 1991. Short-term hemodynamic effects of intravenous propionyl-L-carnitine in anesthetized dogs. Cardiovascular Drugs and Therapy 5 (Suppl 1), 45–56.

Chapela, S.P., Kriguer, N., et al., 2009. Involvement of L-carnitine in cellular metabolism: Beyond Acyl-CoA transport. Mini Reviews in Medicinal Chemistry 9 (13), 1518–1526.

Cherchi, A., Lai, C., et al., 1990. Propionyl carnitine in stable effort angina. Cardiovascular Drugs and Therapy 4 (2), 481–486.

Christensen, E., 1989. Cardiomyopathy and abnormal carnitine metabolism. The Journal of Pediatrics 114 (5), 903.

Cittanti, C., Colamussi, P., et al., 1997. Technetium-99m sestamibi leg scintigraphy for non-invasive assessment of propionyl-L-carnitine induced changes in skeletal muscle metabolism. European Journal of Nuclear Medicine 24 (7), 762–766.

Corsi, C., Pollastri, M., et al., 1995. L-propionylcarnitine effect on postexercise and postischemic hyperemia in patients affected by peripheral vascular disease. Angiology 46 (8), 705–713.

Corsico, N., Nardone, A., et al., 1993. Effect of propionyl-L-carnitine in a rat model of peripheral arteriopathy: A functional, histologic, and NMR spectroscopic study. Cardiovascular Drugs and Therapy 7 (2), 241–251.

Dal Lago, A., De Martini, D., et al., 1999. Effects of propionyl-L-carnitine on peripheral arterial obliterative disease of the lower limbs: A double-blind clinical trial. Drugs under Experimental and Clinical Research 25 (1), 29–36.

Derosa, G., Cicero, A.F., et al., 2003. The effect of L-carnitine on plasma lipoprotein(a) levels in hypercholesterolemic patients with type 2 diabetes mellitus. Clinical Therapeutics 25 (5), 1429–1439.

Di Lisa, F., Menabo, R., et al., 1989. L-propionyl-carnitine protection of mitochondria in ischemic rat hearts. Molecular and Cellular Biochemistry 88 (1–2), 169–173.

Elisaf, M., Bairaktari, E., et al., 1998. Effect of L-carnitine supplementation on lipid parameters in hemodialysis patients. American Journal of Nephrology 18 (5), 416–421.

Ferrari, R., Ceconi, C., et al., 1989. Protective effect of propionyl-L-carnitine against ischaemia and reperfusion-damage. Molecular and Cellular Biochemistry 88 (1–2), 161–168.

Ferrari, R., Ceconi, C., et al., 1991. The effect of propionyl-L-carnitine on the ischemic and reperfused intact myocardium and on their derived mitochondria. Cardiovascular Drugs and Therapy 5 (Suppl 1), 57–65.

Gasparetto, A., Corbucci, G.G., et al., 1991. Influence of acetyl-L-carnitine infusion on haemodynamic parameters and survival of circulatory-shock patients. International Journal of Clinical Pharmacology Research 11 (2), 83–92.

Giancaterini, A., De Gaetano, A., et al., 2000. Acetyl-L-carnitine infusion increases glucose disposal in type 2 diabetic patients. Metabolism 49 (6), 704–708.

Gomez-Amores, L., Mate, A., et al., 2006. Antioxidant activity of propionyl-L-carnitine in liver and heart of spontaneously hypertensive rats. Life Sciences 78 (17), 1945–1952.

Gomez-Amores, L., Mate, A., et al., 2007. L-carnitine attenuates oxidative stress in hypertensive rats. The Journal of Nutritional Biochemistry 18 (8), 533–540.

Hiatt, W.R., Regensteiner, J.G., et al., 2001. Propionyl-L-carnitine improves exercise performance and functional status in patients with claudication. The American Journal of Medicine 110 (8), 616–622.

Iliceto, S., Scrutinio, D., et al., 1995. Effects of L-carnitine administration on left ventricular remodeling after acute anterior myocardial infarction: The L-carnitine Ecocardiografia Digitalizzata Infarto Miocardico (CEDIM) Trial. Journal of the American College of Cardiology 26 (2), 380–387.

Jalal, F.Y., Bohlke, M., et al., 2010. Acetyl-L-carnitine reduces the infarct size and striatal glutamate outflow following focal cerebral ischemia in rats. Annals of the New York Academy of Sciences 1199, 95–104.

Koh, S.G., Brenner, D.A., et al., 2003. Exercise intolerance during post-MI heart failure in rats: Prevention with supplemental dietary propionyl-L-carnitine. Cardiovascular Drugs and Therapy 17 (1), 7–14.

Kolodziejczyk, J., Saluk-Juszczak, J., et al., 2011. L-carnitine protects plasma components against oxidative alterations. Nutrition 27 (6), 693–699.

Lagioia, R., Scrutinio, D., et al., 1992. Propionyl-L-carnitine: a new compound in the metabolic approach to the treatment of effort angina. International Journal of Cardiology 34 (2), 167–172.

Lango, R., Smolenski, R.T., et al., 2005. Propionyl-L-carnitine improves hemodynamics and metabolic markers of cardiac perfusion during coronary surgery in diabetic patients. Cardiovascular Drugs and Therapy 19 (4), 267–275.

Leasure, J.E., Kordenat, K., 1991. Effect of propionyl-L-carnitine on experimental myocardial infarction in dogs. Cardiovascular Drugs and Therapy 5 (Suppl 1), 85–95.

Loffredo, L., Marcoccia, A., et al., 2007. Oxidative-stress-mediated arterial dysfunction in patients with peripheral arterial disease. European Heart Journal 28 (5), 608–612.

Loffredo, L., Pignatelli, P., et al., 2006. Imbalance between nitric oxide generation and oxidative stress in patients with peripheral arterial disease: Effect of an antioxidant treatment. Journal of Vascular Surgery 44 (3), 525–530.

Loster, H., Keller, T., et al., 1999. Effects of L-carnitine and its acetyl and propionyl esters on ATP and PCr levels of isolated rat hearts perfused without fatty acids and investigated by means of 31P-NMR spectroscopy. Molecular and Cellular Biochemistry 200 (1–2), 93–102.

Lysiak, W., Lilly, K., et al., 1988. Quantitation of the effect of L-carnitine on the levels of acid-soluble short-chain acyl-CoA and CoASH in rat heart and liver mitochondria. The Journal of Biological Chemistry 263 (3), 1151–1156.

Mancini, M., Rengo, F., et al., 1992. Controlled study on the therapeutic efficacy of propionyl-L-carnitine in patients with congestive heart failure. Arzneimittel-Forschung 42 (9), 1101–1104.

Martin, M.A., Gomez, M.A., et al., 2000. Myocardial carnitine and carnitine palmitoyltransferase deficiencies in patients with severe heart failure. Biochimica et Biophysica Acta 1502 (3), 330–336.

McMackin, C.J., Widlansky, M.E., et al., 2007. Effect of combined treatment with alpha-Lipoic acid and acetyl-L-carnitine on vascular function and blood pressure in patients with coronary artery disease. Journal of Clinical Hypertension (Greenwich, Conn.) 9 (4), 249–255.

Mingorance, C., Gonzalez del Pozo, M., et al., 2009. Oral supplementation of propionyl-L-carnitine reduces body weight and hyperinsulinaemia in obese Zucker rats. The British Journal of Nutrition 102 (8), 1145–1153.

Mingrone, G., 2004. Carnitine in type 2 diabetes. Annals of the New York Academy of Sciences 1033, 99–107.

Mister, M., Noris, M., et al., 2002. Propionyl-L-carnitine prevents renal function deterioration due to ischemia/reperfusion. Kidney International 61 (3), 1064–1078.

Motterlini, R., Samaja, M., et al., 1992. Functional and metabolic effects of propionyl-L-carnitine in the isolated perfused hypertrophied rat heart. Molecular and Cellular Biochemistry 116 (1–2), 139–145.

Movahed, M.R., Ahmadi-Kashani, M., et al., 2005. Prevalence of suspected diastolic dysfunction in patients with a clinical diagnosis of congestive heart failure. Heart Failure Reviews 10 (4), 263–264.

Najafi, M., Garjani, A., et al., 2008. Antiarrhythmic and arrhythmogenic effects of L-carnitine in ischemia and reperfusion. Bulletin of Experimental Biology and Medicine 146 (2), 210–213.

Neely, J.R., Morgan, H.E., 1974. Relationship between carbohydrate and lipid metabolism and the energy balance of heart muscle. Annual Review of Physiology 36, 413–459.

Opasich, C., Pasini, E., et al., 1997. Skeletal muscle function at low work level as a model for daily activities in patients with chronic heart failure. European Heart Journal 18 (10), 1626–1631.

Packer, L., Valenza, M., et al., 1991. Free radical scavenging is involved in the protective effect of L-propionyl-carnitine against ischemia-reperfusion injury of the heart. Archives of Biochemistry and Biophysics 288 (2), 533–537.

Pasini, E., Cargnoni, A., et al., 1992. Effect of prolonged treatment with propionyl-L-carnitine on erucic acid-induced myocardial dysfunction in rats. Molecular and Cellular Biochemistry 112 (2), 117–123.

Pastoris, O., Dossena, M., et al., 1998. Effect of L-carnitine on myocardial metabolism: Results of a balanced, placebo-controlled, double-blind study in patients undergoing open heart surgery. Pharmacological Research 37 (2), 115–122.

Paulson, D.J., 1998. Carnitine deficiency-induced cardiomyopathy. Molecular and Cellular Biochemistry 180 (1–2), 33–41.

Paulson, D.J., Traxler, J., et al., 1986. Protection of the ischaemic myocardium by L-propionylcarnitine: effects on the recovery of cardiac output after ischaemia and reperfusion, carnitine transport, and fatty acid oxidation. Cardiovascular Research 20 (7), 536–541.

Pierce, G.N., Ramjiawan, B., et al., 1990. Na(+)-H+ exchange in cardiac sarcolemmal vesicles isolated from diabetic rats. The American Journal of Physiology 258 (1 Pt 2), H255–H261.

Ramsay, R.R., Zammit, V.A., 2004. Carnitine acyltransferases and their influence on CoA pools in health and disease. Molecular Aspects of Medicine 25 (5–6), 475–493.

Rebouche, C.J., Paulson, D.J., 1986. Carnitine metabolism and function in humans. Annual Review of Nutrition 6, 41–66.

Redfield, M.M., Jacobsen, S.J., et al., 2003. Burden of systolic and diastolic ventricular dysfunction in the community: Appreciating the scope of the heart failure epidemic. JAMA: The Journal of the American Medical Association 289 (2), 194–202.

Reznick, A.Z., Kagan, V.E., et al., 1992. Antiradical effects in L-propionyl carnitine protection of the heart against ischemia-reperfusion injury: The possible role of iron chelation. Archives of Biochemistry and Biophysics 296 (2), 394–401.

Rizos, I., 2000. Three-year survival of patients with heart failure caused by dilated cardiomyopathy and L-carnitine administration. American Heart Journal 139 (2 Pt 3), S120–S123.

Rodrigues, B., Xiang, H., et al., 1988. Effect of L-carnitine treatment on lipid metabolism and cardiac performance in chronically diabetic rats. Diabetes 37 (10), 1358–1364.

Rosadini, G., Marenco, S., et al., 1990. Acute effects of acetyl-L-carnitine on regional cerebral blood flow in patients with brain ischaemia. International Journal of Clinical Pharmacology Research 10 (1–2), 123–128.

Rosenthal, R.E., Williams, R., et al., 1992. Prevention of postischemic canine neurological injury through potentiation of brain energy metabolism by acetyl-L-carnitine. Stroke 23 (9), 1312–1317 Discussion 1317–1318.

Ruggenenti, P., Cattaneo, D., et al., 2009. Ameliorating hypertension and insulin resistance in subjects at increased cardiovascular risk: Effects of acetyl-L-carnitine therapy. Hypertension 54 (3), 567–574.

Santo, S.S., Sergio, N., et al., 2006. Effect of PLC on functional parameters and oxidative profile in type 2 diabetes-associated PAD. Diabetes Research and Clinical Practice 72 (3), 231–237.

Scholte, H.R., Rodrigues Pereira, R., et al., 1990. Primary carnitine deficiency. Journal of Clinical Chemistry and Clinical Biochemistry 28 (5), 351–357.

Serati, A.R., Motamedi, M.R., et al., 2010. L-carnitine treatment in patients with mild diastolic heart failure is associated with improvement in diastolic function and symptoms. Cardiology 116 (3), 178–182.

Sethi, R., Wang, X., et al., 2004. Improvement of cardiac function and beta-adrenergic signal transduction by propionyl L-carnitine in congestive heart failure due to myocardial infarction. Coronary Artery Disease 15 (1), 65–71.

Shojaei, M., Djalali, M., et al., 2011. Effects of carnitine and coenzyme Q10 on lipid profile and serum levels of lipoprotein(a) in maintenance hemodialysis patients on statin therapy. Iranian Journal of Kidney Diseases 5 (2), 114–118.

Shug, A., Paulson, D., et al., 1991. Protective effects of propionyl-L-carnitine during ischemia and reperfusion. Cardiovascular Drugs and Therapy 5 (Suppl 1), 77–83.

Signorelli, S.S., Fatuzzo, P., et al., 2006a. Propionyl-L-carnitine therapy: Effects on endothelin-1 and homocysteine levels in patients with peripheral arterial disease and end-stage renal disease. Kidney & Blood Pressure Research 29 (2), 100–107.

Signorelli, S.S., Fatuzzo, P., et al., 2006b. A randomised, controlled clinical trial evaluating changes in therapeutic efficacy and oxidative parameters after treatment with propionyl L-carnitine in patients with peripheral arterial disease requiring haemodialysis. Drugs & Aging 23 (3), 263–270.

Siliprandi, N., Di Lisa, F., et al., 1991. Propionyl-L-carnitine: Biochemical significance and possible role in cardiac metabolism. Cardiovascular Drugs and Therapy 5 (Suppl 1), 11–15.

Silverman, N.A., Schmitt, G., et al., 1985. Effect of carnitine on myocardial function and metabolism following global ischemia. The Annals of Thoracic Surgery 40 (1), 20–24.

Silvestro, A., Scopacasa, F., et al., 2003. Inflammatory status and endothelial function in asymptomatic and symptomatic peripheral arterial disease. Vascular Medicine 8 (4), 225–232.

Singh, R.B., Niaz, M.A., et al., 1996. A randomised, double-blind, placebo-controlled trial of L-carnitine in suspected acute myocardial infarction. Postgraduate Medical Journal 72 (843), 45–50.

Sirtori, C.R., Calabresi, L., et al., 2000. L-carnitine reduces plasma lipoprotein(a) levels in patients with hyper Lp(a). Nutrition, Metabolism, and Cardiovascular Diseases 10 (5), 247–251.

Stasi, M.A., Scioli, M.G., et al., 2010. Propionyl-L-carnitine improves postischemic blood flow recovery and arteriogenetic revascularization and reduces endothelial NADPH-oxidase 4-mediated superoxide production. Arteriosclerosis, Thrombosis, and Vascular Biology 30 (3), 426–435.

Taylor, D.J., Amato, A., et al., 1996. Changes in energy metabolism of calf muscle in patients with intermittent claudication assessed by 31P magnetic resonance spectroscopy: A phase II open study. Vascular Medicine 1 (4), 241–245.

Vikre-Jorgensen, J., 1993. Cardiomyopathy caused by carnitine deficiency. Ugeskrift for Laeger 155 (42), 3390–3392.

Waber, L.J., Valle, D., et al., 1982. Carnitine deficiency presenting as familial cardiomyopathy: A treatable defect in carnitine transport. Journal of Pediatrics 101 (5), 700–705.

Yang, X.P., Samaja, M., et al., 1992. Hemodynamic and metabolic activities of propionyl-L-carnitine in rats with pressure-overload cardiac hypertrophy. Journal of Cardiovascular Pharmacology 20 (1), 88–98.

Zales, V.R., Benson Jr., D.W., 1995. Reversible cardiomyopathy due to carnitine deficiency from renal tubular wasting. Pediatric Cardiology 16 (2), 76–78.

Zammit, V.A., 1999. Carnitine acyltransferases: Functional significance of subcellular distribution and membrane topology. Progress in Lipid Research 38 (3), 199–224.

Zhang, L., Keung, W., et al., 2010. Role of fatty acid uptake and fatty acid beta-oxidation in mediating insulin resistance in heart and skeletal muscle. Biochimica et Biophysica Acta 1801, 1–22.

CHAPTER 24

Dietary Blueberry Supplementation as a Means of Lowering High Blood Pressure

M.I. Sweeney*, J.E. Slemmer*,†

*Department of Biology, University of Prince Edward Island, Charlottetown, PE, Canada
†Department of Applied Human Sciences, University of Prince Edward Island, Charlottetown, PE, Canada

ABBREVIATIONS

ACE Angiotensin-converting enzyme
BP Blood pressure
CVD Cardiovascular disease
DASH Dietary approaches to stop hypertension
GSH Glutathione
NO Nitric oxide
NOS Nitric oxide synthase
RAA Renin–angiotensin–aldosterone
ROS Reactive oxygen species
SHRSP Spontaneously hypertensive stroke-prone rats
SOD Superoxide dismutase

1. HYPERTENSION

1.1 What Is Hypertension?

Hypertension is defined as persistently high blood pressure (BP), a condition whereby systolic/diastolic pressure is greater than 140/90 mmHg (Hackam et al., 2010; Savica et al., 2010; see Table 24.1). Elevated BP places unnecessary strain on blood vessels and circulation and, over time, causes or exacerbates cardiovascular diseases (CVD) such as atherosclerosis, heart attack, and stroke. Currently one in three adults in the western world have some form of CVD – The World Health Organization estimates that this is also a problem for the developing world, with CVD accounting for 30% of global deaths (Tourlouki et al., 2009). Hypertension is also the leading cause of chronic renal failure and, thus, is considered a major risk for death (Kearney et al., 2005). It is often referred to as the 'silent killer' as many affected people are completely unaware of their hypertension. Regular screening for hypertension is necessary as a means of reducing the risk of developing CVD; prevention, treatment, and management of hypertension is a top priority (Hackam et al., 2010).

Bioactive Food as Dietary Interventions for Cardiovascular Disease
http://dx.doi.org/10.1016/B978-0-12-396485-4.00022-0
© 2013 Elsevier Inc.
All rights reserved.

Table 24.1 Blood Pressure Classifications in Adults

Blood pressure classification	Systolic blood pressure		Diastolic blood pressure	Drug therapy
Normal	Under 120 mmHg	and	Under 80 mmHg	No drug therapy
Prehypertension	120–139 mmHg	or	80–89 mmHg	Lifestyle modifications; no drugs
Stage 1 hypertension	140–159 mmHg	or	90–99 mmHg	Lifestyle modifications; anti-hypertensive drugs
Stage 2 hypertension	160 mmHg or greater	or	100 mmHg or greater	

Source: Chobanian, A.V., Bakris, G.L., Black, H.R., et al., 2003. The Seventh Report of the Joint National Committee on Prevention, Detection, Evaluation, Treatment of High Blood Pressure: The JNC 7 report. JAMA 289, 2560–2572.

There are two major classes of hypertension. 'Secondary hypertension' arises from another disease state, such as adrenal gland tumors or renal failure. By contrast, the etiology of 'essential hypertension,' which accounts for 90–95% of high BP cases, is not caused by another ailment. The exact causes of essential hypertension are often unclear, and so treatment is usually pharmacological in nature. In this review, we focus first on traditional pharmacotherapeutic methods to reduce hypertension, followed by health benefits obtained from lifestyle modifications, especially dietary changes containing blueberries.

1.2 Epidemiology and Cost of Hypertension

CVD accounts for 21–37% of deaths in western countries, with the United States topping that list (Thom et al., 2006). In 2005–06, the estimated annual cost of treating CVD in terms of physician services, drugs, and other hospital costs, as well as decreased productivity and lost wages to the patient, was over $400 billion in the United States (Muszbek et al., 2008). Much of the preventative care aimed at reducing the incidence of CVD is focused on controlling-related conditions such as diabetes, atherosclerosis, and hypertension (Muszbek et al., 2008).

Hypertension has a worldwide prevalence of ~26% of adults, representing almost one billion people (Savica et al., 2010), but this incidence is even higher (29% of adults, 50 million people) when only the rates of high BP in America are considered (Hedayati et al., 2011; Thom et al., 2006). In 1999–2000, 31% of adults were pre-hypertensive, which refers to BP between 120/80 and 140/90 mmHg (Table 24.1), and 29% were fully hypertensive, with only 39% of adults being classified as normotensive. Hypertension is more prevalent in men than in women when matched for age (Thom et al., 2006). The costs, both direct and indirect, for high BP in the United States were estimated to be $63.5 billion in 2006 (Thom et al., 2006).

1.3 Mechanisms of Essential Hypertension

Homeostatic regulation of normal BP is maintained through cardiac output (the volume of blood that the heart pumps every minute) as well as resistance of arterioles to blood flow. Cardiac output is affected by heart rate, primarily controlled by the autonomic nervous system, and stroke volume, which is proportional to circulating blood volume, among other things. Vascular resistance and BP are decreased when arterioles dilate, stimulated by many mechanisms including nitric oxide (NO). NO is made via the action of nitric oxide synthase (NOS) and subsequently released from the vascular endothelium. By analogy, resistance, and thus BP, is increased when arterioles are constricted through several different means, such as increased sympathetic nervous activity or by the vasoconstrictor angiotensin II produced through the renin–angiotensin–aldosterone (RAA) pathway (Figure 24.1). In short, renin is released from the kidneys in response to low BP; it cleaves the inactive protein angiotensinogen into the active angiotensin I. Angiotensin-converting enzyme (ACE), made predominantly in the lungs, then converts angiotensin I into angiotensin II (Figure 24.1). Angiotensin II binds to its receptor, inducing a range of physiological responses, including vasoconstriction of arterioles (increasing vascular resistance) and release of vasopressin and aldosterone (which increases Na^+ and water reabsorption and, thus, blood volume).

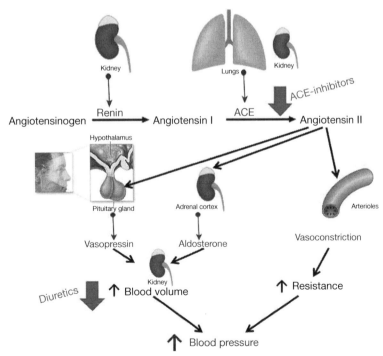

Figure 24.1 Flow chart demonstrating the physiology of the renin–angiotensin–aldosterone (RAA) system and where various anti-hypertensive drugs act. *Modified from http://www.ourmed.org.*

The genetic basis of human essential hypertension has been widely studied. It is a complex genetic trait influenced by polymorphisms of multiple genes, such as those involved in the RAA, adrenergic receptors, vascular endothelial NOS, and inflammatory cytokines (Puddu et al., 2007). It has become increasingly evident that oxidative stress and inflammation play a role in the development of progression of hypertension. Reactive oxygen species (ROS) are generated in blood vessels and cause oxidative damage to the endothelium; this restricts its ability to release NO (Papaharalambus and Griendling, 2007). The loss of NO in blood vessels leads to vasoconstriction, contributing to the development and progression of elevated BP (Figure 24.1). More damage occurs to arterial walls as hypertension progresses, leading to a vicious cycle of oxidative stress (Papaharalambus and Griendling, 2007). ROS are also generated in the kidneys by many cell types such as fibroblasts, renal tubular cells, and inflammatory cells (see Shaughnessy et al., 2009). Since endogenous antioxidant systems like superoxide dismutase (SOD) and reduced glutathione (GSH) tend to be down-regulated in hypertension, ROS accumulate and damage renal cellular machinery, leading to kidney failure and contributing to the pathophysiology of hypertension (Vaziri, 2004).

2. CONVENTIONAL TREATMENT OF HYPERTENSION

2.1 Current Medications for High BP

Pharmaceutical treatment options for hypertension have one common aim – lowering BP. As indicated in Table 24.1, all adults presenting with Stages 1 and 2 of hypertension are recommended for anti-hypertensive drug treatment. Since blood volume has a direct effect on BP, many hypertensive patients can be treated with diuretics, which promote a net loss of body fluids (Figure 24.1). Diuretics are the first-line drugs in many forms of hypertension, such as isolated systolic hypertension or hypertension with diabetes or renal disease (Hackam et al., 2010).

Interference with the RAA pathway is another key way to reduce BP (Figure 24.1). This includes the use of (1) renin blockers, such as aliskiren, (2) angiotensin receptor blockers, also called angiotensin receptor antagonists, such as losartan, and (3) ACE-inhibiting drugs, such as captopril. Like diuretics, ACE inhibitors and angiotensin receptor blockers are first-line drugs in the treatment of elevated BP (Hackam et al., 2010).

Other classes of drugs block adrenergic receptors: alpha-blockers (e.g., prazosin) antagonize $\alpha1$-receptors in vascular smooth muscle to prevent vasoconstriction, while beta-blockers (e.g., propranolol) block cardiac $\beta1$-receptors, reducing heart rate, which reduces cardiac output and thus BP. Calcium-channel blockers (e.g., verapamil) are another popular class of anti-hypertensive drugs. They block Ca^{2+} channels in cardiac and smooth muscle cells, reducing vascular resistance, heart rate, and the force of contraction. Together, this inhibition of Ca^{2+} reduces BP (Crawford, 2003).

2.2 Pharmacotherapy Versus Lifestyle Change

Many of the pharmaceutics listed above have adverse side effects. As a result of increased urination with diuretics and ACE inhibitors, patients may become dehydrated and depleted of K^+, leading to muscle weakness or mental confusion. When coupled with the economic burden of sustaining drug treatment for a lifetime and poor compliance with drug regimens (Hackam et al., 2010), this has encouraged researchers to investigate alternative means of treating hypertension. Indeed, the efficacy of anti-hypertensive medications can be greatly enhanced when they are paired with certain changes in lifestyle (Padwal et al., 2005). Many hypertensive individuals have found that these lifestyle changes are very effective in managing high BP, even without prescribed medications. Adults presenting with prehypertension are not suitable candidates for anti-hypertensive drugs; instead, it is suggested that these individuals manage their high BP through lifestyle modifications only (Table 24.1). Adults with Stages 1 and 2 of hypertension are recommended to make lifestyle changes in addition to being prescribed medications (Hackam et al., 2010; Hedayati et al., 2011; Savica et al., 2010).

2.2.1 Lifestyle change: Diet

Modifications to diet appear to have the biggest impact on BP (Hedayati et al., 2011; Savica et al., 2010). It is recommended that hypertensive individuals limit their dietary Na^+ since high levels of serum Na^+ require more water to be retained in the blood. Half the individuals with high BP are 'salt sensitive,' where high Na^+ diets exacerbate hypertension (Savica et al., 2010). A group of hypertensive individuals followed a DASH (dietary approaches to stop hypertension) diet, which is high in whole grains, fruits, and vegetables (see Table 24.2), for 4 months. On this DASH diet, an average lowering of 11.2/7.5 mmHg was observed (reviewed in Hedayati et al., 2011), returning some patients back to normal BP. The benefits of specific foods and beverages will be outlined in more detail in Section 3. Excess alcohol consumption causes an acute increase in BP and should be avoided (Savica et al., 2010), but alcohol in moderation (one or two drinks per day for women and men, respectively) can actually decrease BP (Savica et al., 2010) and the overall risk for coronary heart disease (Crawford, 2003). Increasing one's levels of K^+, Ca^{2+}, and Mg^{2+} can reduce the risk of high BP, especially when hypertensive individuals continue to maintain a high Na^+ diet (Hackam et al., 2010; Hedayati et al., 2011; Savica et al., 2010) (see Table 24.2 for recommended intakes of these cations).

2.2.2 Lifestyle change: Physical activity and weight loss

Other highly effective lifestyle changes are weight loss and increased physical activity: 45 min of moderate exercise per day, three to five times per week, has been shown to reduce diastolic BP by as much as 10 mmHg (Crawford, 2003; Savica et al., 2010). When a low-calorie diet was combined with a DASH diet, BP fell by 16.1/9.9 mmHg; weight loss

Table 24.2 Dietary Approaches to Stop Hypertension (DASH) Diet

Recommended Food Group and preparation[a]	Recommended numbers of daily servings[a]	Recommended daily nutrient intakes (cf. western diet)[b]
Whole grains, for example, whole wheat bread and oatmeal	7–8	31 g fiber (9 g)
Vegetables and fruits, especially a variety of richly colored, for example,	8–10	
— Spinach and broccoli (green)		
— Carrots, oranges (yellow/orange)		4700 mg K$^+$ (1700 mg)
— Tomatoes, strawberries (red)		
— Blueberries, grapes (blue/purple)		
— Bananas, grapefruit (white, mixed)		
Meats, poultry, fish: lean and skinless cuts, cooked without frying, for example, steam, broil or bake	Up to 2	Protein, 18% of kcal (15%)
Meat alternatives: beans, for example, lentils, nuts (walnuts and almonds are especially heart-healthy), and seeds (sunflower seeds have omega fatty acids)	~1 (4–5 per week)	
Dairy: no fat (skimmed) or low fat (1%) milk or yogurt; avoid cheese	2–3	1240 mg Ca^{2+} (450 mg)
Fats and oils: choose soft spreads, olive oil, peanut butter, low fat mayonnaise, fat free condiments like mustard	2–3	Fat, 27% of kcal (37%)
Sweets: jams and jellies, candy, ice cream, baked desserts	~1 (4–5 per week)	Sugars and starches, 24 g (39 g)

[a] Modified from: Hackam, D.G., et al., 2010. The 2010 Canadian Hypertension Education Program recommendations for the management of hypertension: part 2 – therapy. Canadian Journal of Cardiology 26, 249–258.
[b] Modified from: Savica, V., et al., 2010. The effect of nutrition on blood pressure. Annual Review of Nutrition 30, 365–401. Numbers in brackets represent the current average intake in a western diet.

over 9 weeks lowered BP by 9.5/5.3 mmHg when combined with a low Na$^+$ DASH diet (Hedayati et al., 2011). Obesity, characterized by body weight more than 20% above ideal, is a risk factor for hypertension since RAA and sympathetic nervous systems are overactive in obese patients (Savica et al., 2010). Hypertensive individuals can expect a decreased diastolic BP of 2 mmHg for every kilogram of body weight lost (Crawford, 2003).

2.2.3 Other lifestyle changes

There are other recommendations for hypertensive individuals (Hackam et al., 2010). They should stop smoking, as inhaling cigarette smoke increases vasoconstriction, which further compounds the problem of high BP. Chronic stress should be avoided – any stressors, which stimulate the sympathetic nervous system, induce a variety of systemic effects, many of which lead to increased BP.

Regardless of the behavioral changes recommended to hypertensive patients and the documented benefits to heart health and general wellness, patient compliance is an ongoing battle (Hedayati et al., 2011; Savica et al., 2010).

3. TREATMENT OF HYPERTENSION THROUGH FUNCTIONAL FOODS AND PHYTOCHEMICALS

3.1 Foods and Beverages with Anti-Hypertensive Effects

Diets containing fruits and vegetables, as well as functional foods and nutraceuticals, play a role in the treatment and prevention of hypertension and CVD (reviewed by Perez-Vizcaino et al., 2009; Savica et al., 2010; Tourlouki et al., 2009). Vegetarians have lower incidence of CVD and hypertension, possibly linked to lower rates of obesity (Fraser, 2009; Perez-Vizcaino et al., 2009). It is now well established that the DASH diet helps to manage and prevent hypertension (Hackam et al., 2010; Hedayati et al., 2011; Savica et al., 2010). This diet is rich in plant-based foods, and low in oils and sweets (Table 24.2), and is similar to dietary patterns in Mediterranean countries. For many years, researchers have evaluated the so-called Mediterranean diet in terms of its ability to maintain normal body weight, and prevent dyslipidemia and hypertension (Tourlouki et al., 2009), possibly due to its profile of 'good oils' such as olive oil. Polyunsaturated fatty acids at high doses can lower BP (Savica et al., 2010). Also well studied is the 'French Paradox,' where people in France in particular have lower incidence of CVD, likely due to red wine consumption (Wallace, 2011). Consuming small amounts of alcohol, as well as teas (green and black), and in some cases even coffee, has been linked to promoting cardiovascular health, including lowering BP (Savica et al., 2010).

Although the link between diet and hypertension is not completely clear, it was originally thought that the high level of antioxidant compounds in vegetables, fruits, and some beverages contributed to their effects on CVD. Indeed, treatments with SOD mimetics, which act as antioxidants, have been shown to be hypotensive (Papaharalambus and Griendling, 2007; Vaziri, 2004). Pharmacological doses of antioxidant vitamins, especially vitamin C, have been shown to vasodilate arteries, improve vascular function, and lower BP, although results from multiple studies have been inconclusive or disappointing (Papaharalambus and Griendling, 2007). Thus, there is insufficient support for the anti-hypertensive role for vitamin C. Plants contain thousands of different phytochemicals, and it is estimated that the daily intake of vitamins A, C, and E is actually 10–20 times lower than that of other bioactive compounds from plants (Wallace, 2011).

3.2 Polyphenols as Anti-Hypertensive Agents

Epidemiologic studies have suggested that one benefit of plant-based diets on cardiovascular health is their high content of polyphenolic phytochemicals (Ghosh and Scheepens, 2009). There are many types of polyphenols, of which flavonoids make up the majority consumed in the diet. Approximately one-third of polyphenol intake is in the form of phenolic acids, and the remainder of polyphenol classes includes stilbenes, tannins, and lignans. Daily intakes of polyphenols are quite high ($\sim$1,000 mg per day), as compared to less than 100 mg daily of vitamin C (Wallace, 2011).

3.2.1 Flavonols

Quercetin is a highly abundant flavonoid in fruits (e.g., apples) and vegetables (e.g., onions), representing more than half of the average dietary intake of flavonols, a sub-class of flavonoids. It is also available as a nutraceutical (Perez-Vizcaino et al., 2009). Quercetin has potent and long-lasting anti-hypertensive effects in several animal models of hypertension, as well as in humans. BP-lowering effects of quercetin have been seen after single oral doses given daily to animals before the onset of hypertension, as well as after hypertension is established. Quercetin has also been shown to prevent elevation of BP induced by NOS inhibitors (Perez-Vizcaino et al., 2009).

In spontaneously hypertensive stroke-prone rats (SHRSP), a model of salt-sensitive human stroke and essential hypertension, flavonols from tea (catechins) lower BP and prolong life span (see Shaughnessy et al., 2009, for references). Green tea flavonols are good vasodilators, but studies on the efficacy of tea as a BP-lowering food in humans are inconclusive (Savica et al., 2010). Phenolics, such as those from rice bran, also lowered systolic BP in SHRSP, and phytoestrogens, a form of flavones, have been shown to protect arterial endothelium in SHRSP (see Shaughnessy et al., 2009).

3.2.2 Anthocyanins and flavanols

Anthocyanins are another commonly ingested flavonoid; daily intakes are estimated to be around 200 mg per day, compared to 25 mg per day for quercetin (Wallace, 2011). They also have beneficial effects on BP, likely due to beneficial effects on endothelial NO and on reducing oxidative stress (Wallace, 2011). Foods rich in flavanols and procyanidins, such as cocoa, lower BP (Ghosh and Scheepens, 2009; Savica et al., 2010). A seven-day randomized, cross-over study fed dark chocolate to 20 patients with Stage 1 of hypertension. There was a significant reduction in both systolic and diastolic BP (11.9 ± 9.7 and 8.1 ± 5 mmHg, respectively) (Savica et al., 2010).

3.3 Blueberry Diets as a means of Treating Hypertension
3.3.1 Flavonoid profile of blueberries

The antioxidant capacity of blueberries, in particular the lowbush variety (*Vaccinium angustifolium* Aiton), is very high relative to other fruits. Blueberries contain anthocyanins predominantly, with lower levels of flavonol glycosides (such as quercetin) and even lower amounts of catechins, proanthocyanidins, and chlorogenic acid (Neto, 2007).

3.3.2 Early studies with blueberries

Blueberry feeding has been shown to be beneficial to the brain, reducing its vulnerability to oxidative stress during cerebral ischemia (Sweeney et al., 2002; Wang et al., 2005; Yasuhara et al., 2008) and aging (reviewed in Joseph et al., 2009). Effects of blueberries on the cardiovascular system, and more specifically BP, are less well studied, although blueberries appear to decrease CVD mortality and various risk factors (Basu et al., 2010; Wallace, 2011). There is preliminary evidence that 3 months of feeding blueberry diets to rodents protects cardiac muscle from ischemic damage (Ahmet et al., 2009). Blueberry feeding to SHRSP enhances relaxation of the aorta by acetylcholine, suggested to be due to an interaction of blueberries with NO (Kalea et al., 2010), actions that would decrease vascular resistance and lower BP. We have been determining directly whether blueberry diets have any effects on BP.

3.3.3 Blueberries lower systolic BP in rats

In the first experiments, we fed 3% blueberry-enriched diets, with 4% added NaCl, to SHRSP. Systolic BP was monitored weekly using the tail cuff method. There was no effect of blueberry diets in the first 3 weeks of feeding, but then systolic BP was 19% lower after 4 weeks and 30% lower after 6 weeks in blueberry-fed rats. The maximum systolic BP was 216 ± 11 mmHg in hypertensive rats consuming control diet at week 7 of the trial versus only 178 ± 15 mmHg in the blueberry-fed group at the same time point. Thus, inclusion of blueberries in the diet slows the progression of hypertension (Shaughnessy et al., 2009). SHRSP excreted twice as much F2-isoprostanes in their urine as compared to normotensive rats, but blueberry feeding had no effect on F2-isoprostane excretion. F2-isoprostanes are produced from the non-specific oxidation of unsaturated fatty acids and are a marker of oxidative stress. Thus, it is not likely that a systemic antioxidant effect of blueberries is responsible for the BP-lowering effects. In this same study, blueberry-fed rats had reduced proteinuria, suggesting that blueberry diets protect the kidneys from damage (Shaughnessy et al., 2009).

3.3.4 Blueberries prevent oxidative renal damage in rats

A follow-up study evaluated more directly renal damage in hypertensive rats fed blueberries. SHRSP were fed control or 3% blueberry-enriched food (with 4% NaCl) and then one kidney was analyzed for GSH while the other kidney was fixed in paraformaldedye and then paraffin sections were examined for multiple histological parameters by a blinded examination. There was no renal damage in normotensive rats but significant renal damage in hypertensive rats, specifically those fed a control diet (Figure 24.2(a)). Blueberry feeding reduced some of the damage associated with hypertension, such as glomerular sclerosis, Bowman's capsule thickening, arcuate artery myointimal hyperplasia, and presence of tubular protein but had no effect on other kidney pathologies such as vascular thrombosis and renal artery myointimal hyperplasia (Sweeney et al.,

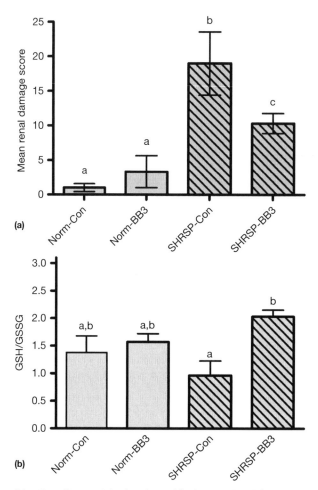

Figure 24.2 Effect of feeding diets enriched with 3% blueberries (BB3) for 16 weeks on kidneys from spontaneously hypertensive stroke-prone rats (SHRSP) or normotensive control rats (Norm). Both strains of rats were also fed control blueberry-free diets (Con). Kidneys were either fixed in formalin and the damage was assessed histologically and assigned a damage score of 0–3 (a) or were frozen and later assayed for glutathione (GSH/GSSG) using spectrophotometric kits from Cayman Chemical Company (b). Values in bars represent means ± standard errors of the means for $N = 4$. Letters denote statistically significant differences (one-way ANOVA with Tukey's post-hoc analysis)

unpublished data; see Figure 24.2(a)). Blueberry diets more than doubled the ratio of reduced to oxidized GSH in the kidney (Figure 24.2(b)). Depletion of GSH and a decreased GSH/GSSG ratio in tissues are indicators of oxidative stress; thus, blueberries improve the redox state of kidneys and reduce renal oxidative stress. Together, these results suggest that blueberries reduce early hypertensive changes to the kidneys.

3.3.5 Blueberries inhibit ACE in rats

ACE inhibitors are first-line drugs in the treatment of elevated BP, with or without other comorbidities, such as diabetes and renal disease (Hackam et al., 2010). As discussed above, ACE leads to the formation of angiotensin II, a potent stimulator of BP (Figure 24.1). Polyphenols and foods rich in them have been shown to inhibit ACE activity (see Wiseman et al., 2011, for references). We have shown recently that blueberries inhibit ACE activity in blood but not in tissues such as lung and kidney. After 2 weeks on control diet, hypertensive rats had 56% higher levels of soluble ACE activity as compared to normotensive rats; feeding a 3% blueberry diet for 2 weeks inhibited ACE activity. ACE was no longer inhibited at 4 weeks; hence, the results suggest that dietary blueberries may be effective in managing early stages of hypertension (Wiseman et al., 2011).

4. CONCLUSION

Elevated BP, or hypertension, is a global crisis: it affects one in three adults and is a precursor to heart attack, stroke, and renal disease. BP is proportional to blood volume and vascular resistance. Drugs or lifestyle choices that lower either of these physiologic variables will manage hypertension. A low Na^+ DASH is effective at lowering blood volume via decreasing Na^+ load and promoting vasodilation. Vegetables, fruits, and beverages containing flavonoids also lower BP by relaxing the vasculature, among other actions. Our work with experimental animals that develop hypertension suggests that blueberries lower systolic BP after 4–7 weeks of feeding. The mechanism for the antihypertensive effect of blueberries is partially due to an early inhibition of ACE activity, seen after only 2 weeks of diet intervention. The phytochemical(s) in blueberries that are responsible for inhibiting ACE is not known, but it may be anthocyanins or other flavonoids. Long-term blueberry feeding protected the kidneys of SHRSP from oxidative damage. Together, these effects slow the progression of, but do not completely prevent, hypertension.

GLOSSARY

dyslipidemia abnormally elevated blood lipids
oxidative stress a state where cellular proteins, lipids and DNA become oxidized and thus damaged
proteinuria protein in the urine, an abnormal clinical finding
RAA physiologic pathway for generating angiotensin II to regulate blood pressure

REFERENCES

Ahmet, I., Spangler, E., Shukitt-Hale, B., et al., 2009. Blueberry-enriched diet protects rat heart from ischemic damage. Public Library of Science One 4, e5954.
Basu, A., Du, M., Leyva, M.J., et al., 2010. Blueberries decrease cardiovascular risk factors in obese men and women with metabolic syndrome. Journal of Nutrition 140, 1582–1587.

Crawford, M.H., 2003. Current Diagnosis & Treatment in Cardiology, second ed. McGraw Hill, New York, NY.

Fraser, G.E., 2009. Vegetarian diets: what do we know of their effects on common chronic diseases? American Journal of Clinical Nutrition 89, 1607S–1612S.

Ghosh, D., Scheepens, A., 2009. Vascular action of polyphenols. Molecular Nutrition and Food Research 53, 322–331.

Hackam, D.G., et al., 2010. The 2010 Canadian Hypertension Education Program recommendations for the management of hypertension: part 2 – therapy. Canadian Journal of Cardiology 26, 249–258.

Hedayati, S.S., Elsayed, E.F., Reilly, R.F., 2011. Non-pharmacological aspects of blood pressure management: what are the data? Kidney International 79 (10), 1061–1070.

Joseph, J.A., Shukitt-Hale, B., Willis, L.M., 2009. Grape juice, berries, and walnuts affect brain aging and behavior. Journal of Nutrition 139, 1813S–1817S.

Kalea, A.Z., Clark, K., Schuschke, D.A., Kristo, A.S., Klimis-Zacas, D.J., 2010. Dietary enrichment with wild blueberries (*Vaccinium angustifolium*) affects the vascular reactivity in the aorta of young spontaneously hypertensive rats. Journal of Nutritional Biochemistry 21, 14–22.

Kearney, P.M., Whelton, M., Reynolds, K., et al., 2005. Global burden of hypertension: analysis of worldwide data. Lancet 365, 217–223.

Muszbek, N., Brixner, D., Benedict, A., Keskinaslan, A., Khan, Z., 2008. The economic consequences of noncompliance in cardiovascular disease and related conditions: a literature review. International Journal of Clinical Practice 62, 338–351.

Neto, C., 2007. Cranberry and blueberry: evidence for protective effects against cancer and vascular diseases. Molecular Nutrition and Food Research 51, 652–664.

Padwal, R., Campbell, N., Touyz, R., 2005. Applying the 2005 Canadian Hypertension Education Program recommendations: 3. Lifestyle modifications to prevent and treat hypertension. Canadian Medical Association Journal 173, 749–751.

Papaharalambus, C.A., Griendling, K.K., 2007. Basic mechanisms of oxidative stress and reactive oxygen species in cardiovascular injury. Trends in Cardiovascular Medicine 17, 48–54.

Perez-Vizcaino, F., Duarte, J., Jimenez, R., Santos-Buelga, C., Osuna, A., 2009. Anti-hypertensive effects of the flavonoid quercetin. Pharmacological Reports 61, 67–75.

Puddu, P., Puddu, G.M., Cravero, E., Ferrari, E., Muscari, A., 2007. The genetic basis of essential hypertension. Acta Cardiologia 62, 281–293.

Savica, V., Bellinghieri, G., Kopple, J.D., 2010. The effect of nutrition on blood pressure. Annual Review of Nutrition 30, 365–401.

Shaughnessy, K.S., Boswall, I.A., Scanlan, A.P., Gottschall-Pass, K.T., Sweeney, M.I., 2009. Diets containing blueberry extract lower blood pressure in spontaneously hypertensive stroke-prone rats. Nutrition Research 29, 130–138.

Sweeney, M.I., Kalt, W., MacKinnon, S.L., Ashby, J., Gottschall-Pass, K.T., 2002. Feeding of diets enriched in lowbush blueberries (*Vaccinium angustifolium*) for six weeks decreases stroke severity in rats. Nutritional Neuroscience 5, 427–431.

Thom, T., Haase, N., Rosamond, W., et al., 2006. Heart disease and stroke statistics – 2006 update: a report from the American Heart Association Statistics Committee and Stroke Statistics Subcommittee. Circulation 113, e85–e151.

Tourlouki, E., Matalas, A.L., Panagiotakos, D.B., 2009. Dietary habits and cardiovascular disease risk in middle-aged and elderly populations: a review of evidence. Clinical Interventions in Aging 4, 319–330.

Vaziri, N.D., 2004. Roles of oxidative stress and antioxidant therapy in chronic kidney disease and hypertension. Current Opinion in Nephrology and Hypertension 13, 93–99.

Wallace, T.C., 2011. Anthocyanins in cardiovascular disease. Advances in Nutrition 2, 1–7.

Wang, Y., Chang, C.F., Chou, J., et al., 2005. Dietary supplementation with blueberries, spinach, or spirulina reduces ischemic brain damage. Experimental Neurology 193, 75–84.

Wiseman, W., Egan, J.M., Slemmer, J.E., et al., 2011. Feeding blueberry diets inhibits angiotensin II converting enzyme (ACE) activity in spontaneously hypertensive stroke-prone rats. Canadian Journal of Physiology and Pharmacology 89, 67–71.

Yasuhara, T., Hara, K., Maki, M., et al., 2008. Dietary supplementation exerts neuroprotective effects in ischemic stroke model. Rejuvenation Research 11, 201–214.

FURTHER READING

Actis-Goretta, L., Ottaviani, J., Fraga, C., 2006. Inhibition of angiotensin converting enzyme activity by flavanol-rich foods. Journal of Agricultural Food Chemistry 54, 229–234.

Chobanian, A.V., Bakris, G.L., Black, H.R., et al., 2003. Seventh Report of the Joint National Committee on Prevention, Detection, Evaluation, Treatment of High Blood Pressure: the JNC 7 Report (2003). Journal of the American Medical Association 289, 2560–2572.

de Pascual-Teresa, S., Moreno, D.A., García-Viguera, C., 2010. Flavanols and anthocyanins in cardiovascular health: a review of current evidence. International Journal of Molecular Sciences 11, 1679–1703.

Klabunde, R., 2005. Cardiovascular Physiology Concepts. Lippincott Williams & Wilkins, Baltimore, MD.

RELEVANT WEBSITES

Canadian Hypertension Education Program publications. http://hypertension.ca/chep/educational-resources/publications/.

DASH eating plan. http://www.nhlbi.nih.gov/health/public/heart/hbp/dash/new_dash.pdf.

World Health Organization global statistics. http://www.who.int/mediacentre/factsheets/fs317/en/.

CHAPTER 25

Vitamin D and Cardiometabolic Risks

F.R. Pérez-López*, A.M. Fernández-Alonso[†], P. Chedraui[‡], T. Simoncini[§]
*Universidad de Zaragoza, Zaragoza, Spain
[†]Hospital Torrecárdenas, Almeria, Spain
[‡]Universidad Católica de Santiago de Guayaquil, Guayaquil, Ecuador
[§]University of Pisa, Pisa, Italy

ABBREVIATIONS

1,25(OH)$_2$D 1,25-dihydroxy-vitamin D or calcitriol
25(OH)D 25-hydroxyvitamin D or calcidiol
BMI Body mass index
CVD Cardiovascular disease
HDL-C High-density lipoprotein cholesterol
HOMA-IR Homeostasis model assessment of insulin resistance
IR Insulin resistance
LDL-C Low-density lipoprotein cholesterol
NHANES-III Third US National Health and Nutrition Examination Survey
T2DM Type 2 diabetes mellitus

1. INTRODUCTION

Vitamin D shares properties of both vitamins and hormones. It is acquired both by successive synthesis at the skin, liver, and kidneys or digestive absorption in the upper part of the small intestine through the actions of bile salts. Vitamin D from both sources is stored in the adipose tissue. Although its regulatory actions on calcium and bone metabolism are the most well-known functions, other pleiotropic effects are not less important, including actions over the cardiovascular system. Vitamin D receptors are present in endothelial cells, vascular smooth muscle cells, and cardiomyocytes. The vitamin is capable of affecting inflammation, proliferation, and differentiation. In addition, nongenomic actions are also operative in many cell types (Pérez-López, 2009; Pérez-López et al., 2011).

Basic, experimental, and clinical evidence support the association between vitamin D and cardiovascular risk factors. Thus, hypovitaminosis D is linked to alterations in glucose and lipoprotein metabolism, diabetes, hypertension, and obesity. Endogenous vitamin D status is generally determined by plasma levels of 25-hydroxyvitamin D [25(OH)D] or calcidiol, although the bioactive compound is the one–alpha hydroxylated derivative with a shorter half life: 1,25-dihydroxy-vitamin D [1,25(OH)2D] or calcitriol. Serum

Bioactive Food as Dietary Interventions for Cardiovascular Disease
http://dx.doi.org/10.1016/B978-0-12-396485-4.00023-2

© 2013 Elsevier Inc.
All rights reserved.

25(OH)D levels are expressed as ng ml^{-1} or nmol l^{-1}, being the equivalence of 1 ng ml^{-1} = 2.5 nmol l^{-1}.

This chapter reviews relevant aspects concerning the effects of low plasma vitamin D on the metabolic syndrome (METS) and cardiovascular-related risks.

2. THE METABOLIC SYNDROME

METS is a cluster of metabolic alterations including abdominal adiposity, hypertension, insulin resistance (IR), dyslipidemia, proinflammatory status, and increased thrombosis risk. The syndrome is linked to type 2 diabetes mellitus (T2DM), cardiovascular disease (CVD), and overall mortality. It is suspected that visceral fat secretes several inflammatory adipokines that precipitate both IR and an inflammatory status (Elks and Francis, 2010). In diabetic and nondiabetic individuals low plasma vitamin D levels have been linked to inflammatory endothelial dysfunction (Yiu et al., 2011). Despite this, the etiology of the METS is complex and includes genetic, metabolic, and lifestyle factors.

The third US National Health and Nutrition Examination Survey (NHANES-III) found that mean serum 25(OH)D levels were significantly lower among individuals with the METS as compared with those without the syndrome (67.1 vs. 75.9 nmol l^{-1}; Ford et al., 2005). Individuals with 25(OH)D levels below 20 ng ml^{-1} had a higher prevalence of the METS components (Chiu et al., 2004). In general, it seems there is an inverse correlation between serum 25(OH)D levels and the METS prevalence, suggesting that the vitamin has some degree of protective effect (Kayaniyil et al., 2011).

An association between serum 25(OH)D levels and components of the METS has been reported in nonobese young individuals. Serum 25(OH)D is inversely correlated with body mass index (BMI), systolic blood pressure, waist circumference, fasting glucose and insulin levels, and the homeostasis model assessment of insulin resistance (HOMA-IR), whereas positively correlated with adiponectin and high-density lipoprotein cholesterol (HDL-C) levels (Gannagé-Yared et al., 2009). These observations seem in some way the initial status of what could be the outcome in older individuals. Despite this, further studies are required.

3. IR, DIABETES, AND VITAMIN D

Epidemiological evidence supports the fact that hypovitaminosis D increases IR, with associations observed between serum 25(OH)D levels and glycemia, insulin secretion, and T2DM prevalence. The prevalence of low serum 25(OH)D levels ($\leq$37.5 nmol l^{-1}) is 34% among adults with T2DM as compared to nondiabetics. In addition, diabetic patients with low vitamin D levels have increased thickening of the common carotid medial intima (indirect marker of atherosclerosis) as compared to diabetics with normal vitamin D levels (Targher et al., 2006).

The value of serum 25(OH)D levels in predicting future glycemic status and IR has been studied in nondiabetic subjects 40–69 years followed up for 10 years. Baseline 25(OH)D levels were inversely associated to a 10-year risk for hyperglycemia, IR, and METS (Forouhi et al., 2008).

Associations between plasma 25(OH)D levels and indirect markers of IR have been studied in nondiabetic subjects of the Framingham Offspring Study. After adjusting for confounding factors, plasma 25(OH)D levels were inversely associated to HOMA-IR and fasting glucose and insulin plasma levels. When subjects were stratified by 25(OH)D tertiles, those in the highest tertile group had lower glucose (1.6%), insulin (9.8%), and HOMA-IR (12.7%) levels. In addition, plasma 25(OH)D levels were associated to the insulin sensitivity index, adiponectin, and HDL-C and inversely to plasma triacylglycerol levels. However, these associations were no longer significant after further adjustment for BMI, waist circumference, and current smoking status. No association has been observed between serum 25(OH)D and 2-h postoral glucose tolerance test values (Liu et al., 2009).

The influence of metabolic and anthropometric variables and lifestyle over 25(OH)D levels have been assessed in native Americans without type 1 diabetes or T2DM from Cree communities (South Canada). Multiple regression analysis determined that serum 25(OH)D (per 10 nmol l^{-1} increment) was inversely associated to HOMA-IR and β-cell function. However, when adjustments for age, sex, physical activity, education, alcohol consumption, and smoking were carried out, associations disappeared (Del Gobbo et al., 2011). Further studies are needed in other populations to better delineate the effect of cofactors influencing the relationship between pancreatic function and vitamin D metabolism.

It has been suggested that vitamin D and calcium supplements may be important in the prevention of T2DM. A recent meta-analysis of heterogeneous studies reported that three of six analyses showed a lower diabetes risk in the highest compared to the lowest vitamin D status groups, and eight trials found no effect of vitamin D supplementation over glucose levels or incident diabetes (Pittas et al., 2010). The oral administration of a 100 000 IU of cholecalciferol (2 weeks apart) in nondiabetic subjects with low serum 25(OH)D levels ($\leq$50 nmol l^{-1}) increased vitamin D levels from a mean of 39.9 to 90.3 $\pm$ 4.3 nmol l^{-1}, with no changes observed in mean blood glucose or insulin concentrations (including insulin sensitivity; Tai et al., 2008).

4. OVERWEIGHT, OBESITY, AND VITAMIN D

Although abdominal adiposity mass has a pivotal role in the development of the METS, adipose tissue dysfunction may be more relevant to IR and other metabolic changes (associated to METS and cardiovascular risk) than to the amount of fat mass per se (Chandalia and Abate, 2007). Vitamin D is a group of fat soluble compounds with a tropism for the adipose tissue. Functions within this tissue are to date unknown.

Administration of pharmacological doses of vitamin D increases the fraction of circulating free vitamin D, and its metabolites accumulate in adipose tissue and muscle (Vieth, 1999). After prolonged sunlight exposure blood vitamin D levels increase and may saturate the capacity of its binding protein. Consequently, excessive free vitamin D is stored in the adipose tissue. In relation to this, many studies have reported that low serum 25(OH)D levels are more prevalent among overweight and obese subjects. Therefore, adipose tissue may serve as a buffer when vitamin D acquisition is high and produce its slow release during fasting conditions.

Increased body weight is linked to hypertension and lipid abnormalities, and cardiovascular risk independent of hyperinsulinemia. Low plasma vitamin D levels have been reported in obese patients. However, it is unlikely that the inverse associations found between BMI and serum 25(OH)D and 1,25(OH)D levels contribute to obesity development (Parikh et al., 2004).

Reports have linked low 25(OH)D levels and obesity (BMI or waist circumference defined). It has been estimated that vitamin D decreases 0.74 and 0.29 nmol l^{-1} for every increase in 1 kg m^{-2} for BMI and 1 cm increase in waist, respectively (McGill et al., 2008). Fat excess makes vitamin D less available for body use. Many obese subjects have disturbances in body imaging and low self esteem and therefore minimize sunlight exposure. However, sun exposure habits do not differ according to adiposity, and do not explain low 25(OH)D with increasing body fat mass. In addition, body fat composition and vitamin D relationship is influenced by skin characteristics.

Metabolic status in the presence of excess body fat mass is quite complex and influenced by different hormones. The relevance of vitamin D status in relation to cardiovascular risk remains to be determined. Nevertheless, it seems reasonable that obese individuals receive vitamin D supplements to prevent the long-term consequences of hypovitaminosis.

5. LIPOPROTEINS AND VITAMIN D

Studies of healthy men and women from several ethnic groups have found that low vitamin D status adversely affects total cholesterol and low-density lipoprotein cholesterol (LDL-C) concentrations (Pérez-López, 2009; Pérez-López et al., 2011). In mid-aged Finish men who are not receiving antidiabetic treatment, low 1,25(OH)2D levels were associated to low HDL-C, whereas low serum 25(OH)D levels correlated to high total cholesterol, LDL-C and triglyceride levels (Karhapää et al., 2010). This lipid profiling increases cardiovascular risk. The Tromsø University cohort of nearly 8000 subjects followed for more than 14 years reported an association between 25(OH)D and lipoproteins which may explain the link between vitamin D status and cardiovascular mortality. Serum total cholesterol, HDL-C, and LDL-C levels significantly increased and LDL-C/HDL-C ratio and triacylglycerol levels decreased with increasing 25(OH)D levels expressed as quartiles (Jorde et al., 2010).

6. HYPERTENSION

There is experimental, epidemiological, and clinical evidence linking low vitamin D status and hypertension. Impaired vascular health in correlation with lower vitamin D levels would contribute to hypertension and CVD risk. The results from the NHANES-III, carried out during 1988–94, reported an inverse association between serum 25(OH)D and blood pressure levels that was evident even after adjusting for several cofactors such as age, gender, ethnicity, and physical activity. In addition, when subjects were classified into 25(OH)D quintiles, those in highest quintile as compared to those in the lowest displayed lower mean systolic and diastolic blood pressures (3.0 and 1.6 mmHg, respectively) (Scragg et al., 2007). In a more recent analysis of the same cohort, overall serum 25(OH)D levels were lower in 2000–04 than in 1988–94 which were justified by measurement methods, but also due to changes in relation to BMI, milk intake, sun protection that contribute to a real descent in vitamin D status (Looker et al., 2008).

The association between blood pressure and vitamin D status is contradictory in general due to methodological gaps. Other explanations include that low vitamin D levels probably increase blood pressure via inhibiting the renin–angiotensin system. In this regard, low vitamin D should be below a certain threshold that produces renin increases. Therefore, it would be unlikely that vitamin D supplementation produce any blood pressure decrease in normotensive subjects because renin levels are normal.

7. CVD AND VITAMIN D

The large cohort of the Intermountain Heart Collaborative Study Group reported a relationship between vitamin D levels and cardiovascular risk factors, disease status and incidental events. Low vitamin D status was associated with significant increases in the prevalence of diabetes, hypertension, hyperlipidemia, and peripheral vascular disease. In addition, vitamin D was also associated to coronary artery disease, myocardial infarction, heart failure, and stroke (Anderson et al., 2010).

Serum 25(OH)D status is an independent risk factor for CVD. In the NHANES-III cohort CVD prevalence was higher in individuals with 25(OH)D levels below 20 ng ml^{-1} as compared to those with higher levels (Kendrick et al., 2009). After adjusting for a long list of cofactors related to CVD, a strong and independent association emerged between 25(OH)D and CVD prevalence. After a 14-year follow up another recent NHANES-III report found that among Caucasians but not blacks fatal stroke was linked to low vitamin D levels (Michos, 2010).

Serum 25(OH)D levels were measured in acute myocardial infarction patients enrolled in a 20-hospital US prospective registry. Serum 25(OH)D deficiency (≤ 20 ng ml^{-1}) was more common among non-Caucasian patients, and those with lower social support, no insurance, diabetes, and less physical activity. Thus, vitamin D deficiency is present in almost all acute myocardial infarction patients (Lee et al., 2011).

Reports indicate that low serum vitamin D levels may increase mortality risk due to CVD, cancer and other chronic diseases. It has been postulated, although not proven, that high endogenous vitamin D status could increase longevity (Pérez-López et al., 2011). A meta-analysis reported that vitamin D (300–2000 IU day^{-1}; mean dose 528 IU) supplementation for an average of 5 or more years decreased risk for all-cause death by 7% (Autier and Gandini, 2007). The systematic review of prospective studies and randomized trials regarding calcium and/or vitamin D supplementation and subsequent cardiovascular events showed that vitamin D supplementation produces a non-significant reduction in CVD risk, whereas calcium or the vitamin D plus calcium supplementation had no effect (Wang et al., 2010).

8. FINAL REMARKS

A significant proportion of the world population has low serum vitamin D levels which may negatively affect components of the METS and CVD associated conditions. The molecular mechanisms of these associations remain incompletely understood. Low sun exposure, use of sunscreens, changes in lifestyle, dietary habits, obesity, and other environmental factors contribute to hypovitaminosis D. The controversial puzzling results are due to complex metabolic mechanisms acting on the cardiocirculatory tree. Although vitamin D is not the health panacea, optimal vitamin D status should be a major task in order to improve health in the present generation. A traditional lifestyle with a vitamin D enriched natural diet, exposure to sunlight in a responsible manner and regular outdoor activities should be highly recommended.

'Normal' vitamin D levels required for optimal cell functioning are still unknown. In addition, causes of death may be confounded or poorly specified and hence result in bias. Nevertheless, low 25(OH)D levels do seem to be a marker of poor health. The ongoing *Vitamin D and Omega-3 Trial* (VITAL) will provide answers to many questions and hopefully confirm the benefits of vitamin D.

GLOSSARY

Metabolic syndrome A cluster of metabolic risk factors including abdominal obesity, hypertension, insulin resistance, dyslipidemia, proinflammatory status, and increased thrombosis risk.
Vitamin D A group of fat soluble secosteroids that exerts actions through both specific receptor and nongenomic mechanisms.
Vitamin D receptor Cell structure that specifically binds vitamin D to initiate molecular changes.

REFERENCES

Anderson, J.L., May, H.T., Horne, B.D., et al., 2010. Intermountain Heart Collaborative (IHC) Study Group. Relation of vitamin D deficiency to cardiovascular risk factors, disease status, and incident events in a general healthcare population. The American Journal of Cardiology 106, 963–968.

Autier, P., Gandini, S., 2007. Vitamin D supplementation and total mortality: a meta-analysis of randomized controlled trials. Archives of Internal Medicine 167, 1730–1737.

Chandalia, M., Abate, N., 2007. Metabolic complications of obesity: inflated or inflamed? Journal of Diabetes and its Complications 21, 128–136.

Chiu, K.C., Chu, A., Go, V.L., Saad, M.F., 2004. Hypovitaminosis D is associated with insulin resistance and beta cell dysfunction. American Journal of Clinical Nutrition 79, 820–825.

Del Gobbo, L.C., Song, Y., Dannenbaum, D.A., Dewailly, E., Egeland, G.M., 2011. Serum 25-hydroxyvitamin D is not associated with insulin resistance or beta cell function in Canadian Cree. Journal of Nutrition 141, 290–295.

Elks, C.M., Francis, J., 2010. Central adiposity, systemic inflammation, and the metabolic syndrome. Current Hypertension Reports 12, 99–104.

Ford, E.S., Ajani, U.A., McGuire, L.C., Liu, S., 2005. Concentrations of serum vitamin D and the metabolic syndrome among U.S. adults. Diabetes Care 28, 1228–1230.

Forouhi, N.G., Luan, J., Cooper, A., Boucher, B.J., Wareham, N.J., 2008. Baseline serum 25-hydroxy vitamin D is predictive of future glycemic status and insulin resistance: the Medical Research Council Ely Prospective Study 1990–2000. Diabetes 57, 2619–2625.

Gannagé-Yared, M.H., Chedid, R., Khalife, S., et al., 2009. Vitamin D in relation to metabolic risk factors, insulin sensitivity and adiponectin in a young Middle-Eastern population. European Journal of Endocrinology 160, 965–971.

Jorde, R., Figenschau, Y., Hutchinson, M., Emaus, N., Grimnes, G., 2010. High serum 25-hydroxyvitamin D concentrations are associated with a favorable serum lipid profile. European Journal of Clinical Nutrition 64, 1457–1464.

Karhapää, P., Pihlajamäki, J., Pörsti, I., et al., 2010. Diverse associations of 25-hydroxyvitamin D and 1,25-dihydroxy-vitamin D with dyslipidaemias. Journal of Internal Medicine 268, 604–610.

Kayaniyil, S., Vieth, R., Harris, S.B., et al., 2011. Association of 25(OH)D and PTH with metabolic syndrome and its traditional and nontraditional components. Journal of Clinical Endocrinology and Metabolism 96, 168–175.

Kendrick, J., Targher, G., Smits, G., Chonchol, M., 2009. 25-Hydroxyvitamin D deficiency is independently associated with cardiovascular disease in the Third National Health and Nutrition Examination Survey. Atherosclerosis 205, 255–260.

Lee, J.H., Gadi, R., Spertus, J.A., Tang, F., O' Keefe, J.H., 2011. Prevalence of vitamin D deficiency in patients with acute myocardial infarction. The American Journal of Cardiology 107 (11), 1636–1638.

Liu, E., Meigs, J.B., Pittas, A.G., et al., 2009. Plasma 25-hydroxyvitamin D is associated with markers of the insulin resistant phenotype in nondiabetic adults. Journal of Nutrition 139, 329–334.

Looker, A.C., Pfeiffer, C.M., Lacher, D.A., et al., 2008. Serum 25-hydroxyvitamin D status of the US population: 1988–1994 compared with 2000–2004. American Journal of Clinical Nutrition 88, 1519–1527.

McGill, A.T., Stewart, J.M., Lithander, F.E., Strik, C.M., Poppitt, S.D., 2008. Relationships of low serum vitamin D3 with anthropometry and markers of the metabolic syndrome and diabetes in overweight and obesity. Nutrition Journal 7, 4.

Michos, E., 2010. Vitamin-D deficiency linked to fatal stroke in whites but not blacks. Risk of fatal stroke associated with vitamin-D deficiency (25[OH]D <15 ng/mL) in white vs black participants. Available from: http://www.theheart.org/article/1149285.do (accessed 30 March 2011).

Parikh, S.J., Edelman, M., Uwaifo, G.I., et al., 2004. The relationship between obesity and serum 1,25-dihydroxy vitamin D concentrations in healthy adults. Journal of Clinical Endocrinology and Metabolism 89, 1196–1199.

Pérez-López, F.R., 2009. Vitamin D metabolism and cardiovascular risk factors in postmenopausal women. Maturitas 62, 248–262.

Pérez-López, F.R., Chedraui, P., Fernández-Alonso, A.M., 2011. Vitamin D and aging: beyond calcium and bone metabolism. Maturitas 69, 27–36.

Pittas, A.G., Chung, M., Trikalinos, T., et al., 2010. Systematic review: vitamin D and cardiometabolic outcomes. Annals of Internal Medicine 152, 307–314.

Scragg, R., Sowers, M., Bell, C., 2007. Serum 25-hydroxyvitamin D, ethnicity, and blood pressure in the Third National Health and Nutrition Examination Survey. American Journal of Hypertension 20, 713–719.

Tai, K., Need, A.G., Horowitz, M., Chapman, I.M., 2008. Glucose tolerance and vitamin D: effects of treating vitamin D deficiency. Nutrition 24, 950–956.

Targher, G., Bertolini, L., Padovani, R., et al., 2006. Serum 25-hydroxyvitamin D3 concentrations and carotid artery intima-media thickness among type 2 diabetic patients. Clinical Endocrinology 65, 593–597.

Vieth, R., 1999. Vitamin D supplementation, 25-hydroxyvitamin D concentrations, and safety. American Journal of Clinical Nutrition 69, 842–856.

Wang, L., Manson, J.E., Song, Y., Sesso, H.D., 2010. Systematic review: vitamin D and calcium supplementation in prevention of cardiovascular events. Annals of Internal Medicine 152, 315–323.

Yiu, Y.F., Chan, Y.H., Yiu, K.H., et al., 2011. Vitamin D deficiency is associated with depletion of circulating endothelial progenitor cells and endothelial dysfunction in patients with type 2 diabetes. Journal of Clinical Endocrinology and Metabolism 8 (1), 47–52.

FURTHER READING

Bischoff-Ferrari, H.A., Shao, A., Dawson-Hughes, B., 2010. Benefit-risk assessment of vitamin D supplementation. Osteoporosis International 21, 1121–1132.http://www.ncbi.nlm.nih.gov/pmc/articles/PMC3062161/pdf/nihms-280261.pdf.

Grant, W.B., 2009. In defense of the sun: an estimate of changes in mortality rates in the United States if mean serum 25-hydroxyvitamin D levels were raised to 45 ng/mL by solar ultraviolet-B irradiance. Dermatoendocrinol 1, 207–214.

Kulie, T., Groff, A., Redmer, J., Hounshell, J., Schrager, S., 2009. Vitamin D: an evidence-based review. Journal of the American Board of Family Medicine 22, 698–706.http://www.jabfm.org/cgi/pmidlookup?view=long&pmid=19897699.

Manson, J.E., 2010. Vitamin D and the heart: why we need large-scale clinical trials. Cleveland Clinic Journal of Medicine 77, 903–910.http://www.ccjm.org/content/77/12/903.full.pdf+html.

Ross, A.C., Manson, J.E., Abrams, S.A., et al., 2011. The 2011 report on dietary reference intakes for calcium and vitamin D from the Institute of Medicine: what clinicians need to know. Journal of Clinical Endocrinology and Metabolism 96, 53–58.http://www.ncbi.nlm.nih.gov/pmc/articles/PMC3046611/?tool=pubmed.

Relevant Websites

http://www.iom.edu/Reports/2010/Dietary-Reference-Intakes-for-Calcium-and-Vitamin-D.aspx – Institute of Medicine. Dietary reference intakes for calcium and vitamin D.

http://ods.od.nih.gov/factsheets/vitamind/ – National Institutes of health. Office of Dietary Supplements. Vitamin D.

http://www.naturaldatabase.com – Natural Medicines. Comprehensive database. Vitamin D.

http://www.vitamindsociety.org/ – The Vitamin D Society.

http://www.vitamindcouncil.org/ – Vitamin D council.

CHAPTER 26

Phytosterols and Micronutrients for Heart Health

V. Spitzer, S. Maggini
Bayer Consumer Care AG, Basel, Switzerland

ABBREVIATIONS

ATP Adenosine triphosphate
EFSA European Food Safety Authority
FDA Food and Drug Administration
HDL High-density lipoprotein
IU International units
LDL Low-density lipoprotein

1. INTRODUCTION

Every day, the heart pumps about 8000 l of blood through the blood vessels and supplies the organs with vital nutrients and oxygen. To accomplish this enormous pumping activity, the cardiovascular system depends on a powerful heart muscle, an adequate energy supply, the right blood pressure, and healthy blood vessels. A number of micronutrients play a crucial role in supporting the cardiovascular system. Many vitamins and minerals are essential to support the energy generation in the heart and have antioxidant and antiinflammatory properties. They also play a role at the blood vessel level by maintaining normal endothelial function, and controlling vasodilation, blood pressure, blood clotting, and atherosclerotic lesion formation. Therefore, many public health initiatives have been started to provide information on the benefits of high-quality nutrition. However, theory is not practice, and marginal micronutrient deficiencies are a reality in the Western world too (Huskisson et al., 2007a,b; Maggini et al., 2008).

Later in life, many people suffer from atherosclerotic deposits in the blood vessels, which lead to reduced or blocked blood flow. One of the major risk factors for atherosclerosis is oxidized low-density lipoprotein (LDL) cholesterol. This prevalent oxidation hypothesis implies that the antioxidant micronutrients, which inhibit oxidation of LDL, should be effective in suppressing atherosclerosis. There is also emerging evidence that antioxidants possess functions of gene regulation and signal transduction that may have beneficial effects against atherosclerosis as well. Many *in vitro* and *in vivo* studies support

Bioactive Food as Dietary Interventions for Cardiovascular Disease
http://dx.doi.org/10.1016/B978-0-12-396485-4.00024-4

© 2013 Elsevier Inc.
All rights reserved.

the involvement of LDL oxidation in the pathogenesis of atherosclerosis and also the beneficial effects of antioxidants. However, intervention studies have not always shown consistency in the efficacy of antioxidants against atherosclerosis (Niki, 2004).

Instead of preventing the oxidation of LDL, other dietary and pharmacological approaches have been proposed to control cholesterol. High blood cholesterol levels (hypercholesterolemia) are also a well-established risk factor for cardiovascular disease (CVD). Currently, most clinical attention is focused on limiting the biosynthesis of cholesterol using statin drugs. However, the absorption of dietary cholesterol from the intestine is another critical component of cholesterol homeostasis that has been addressed. Phytosterols, also being part of the food chain, have been shown to successfully reduce blood cholesterol levels.

In this chapter, the role of phytosterols and other micronutrients for heart health are discussed in detail.

2. MICRONUTRIENTS

2.1 Deficiencies

A sufficient and balanced diet should cover the overall micronutrient requirements. However, many population segments in both developing and industrialized countries do not get adequate amounts of essential vitamins and minerals through the diet. There are various reasons why dietary recommendations are not met even in countries where food availability and supply would be expected to be sufficient. These include economic reasons (e.g., inflation rates, unemployment, and working poor), illnesses, dietary habits, particular life stages, and/or lifestyle, which either limit intakes or increase micronutrient requirements (Huskisson et al., 2007a,b; Maggini et al., 2008). Even otherwise 'healthy' individuals in industrialized countries can be at risk due to lifestyle-related factors. They are typically young to middle-aged adults with high occupational pressure or the double burden of family and work, for whom time is always in short supply. Examples include people on a diet or eating an unbalanced diet, people facing demanding periods such as extensive physical exercise or in situations of occupational, emotional, and physiological stress and demanding cognitive tasks, frequent travel (Huskisson et al., 2007a,b; Maggini et al., 2008). Furthermore, during the past 50 years, in developed countries, there have been many changes in the way fruits, vegetables, and other crops are grown, stored, transported, and distributed. These changes have resulted in lower micronutrient contents and densities (e.g., calcium, iron, vitamins B_2 and C) in many foods (Davis et al., 2004). On the other hand, countries still less affected by such changes experienced a significant decline in fruit intake due to dietary and habit changes. In Brazil, for instance, the annual per capita fruit intake was halved in only 16 years (from 48 kg year^{-1} in 1987 to only 24.5 kg year^{-1} in 2003) (IBGE, 2004).

2.2 Antioxidants

Antioxidants are needed by the human body for protection of cell tissues and membranes against free-radical-induced damage. Although oxidation reactions are crucial for life, they can also be damaging; hence, plants and animals maintain complex systems of multiple types of antioxidants, such as glutathione (GSH), vitamin C, and vitamin E, as well as enzymes often requiring trace elements as cofactors such as catalase, superoxide dismutase, and various peroxidases. Oxidative stress is associated with chronic diseases mainly because inflammatory responses have an oxidative stress component. Thus, decreasing oxidative stress by increasing antioxidant intakes should decrease cellular damage caused by reactive oxygen species created during inflammatory reactions, thereby protecting tissues against injury and thus, hypothetically, reducing the incidence of chronic diseases such as CVD.

2.2.1 Vitamin C

Vitamin C is a cofactor for several enzymes involved in the biosynthesis of collagen, carnitine, and neurotransmitters. It is also a highly effective antioxidant protecting indispensable molecules in the body, such as proteins, lipids, carbohydrates, and nucleic acids. Vitamin C is also able to regenerate other antioxidants such as vitamin E and is involved in maintenance of enzyme thiols in a reduced state and sparing of GSH (Carr and Frei, 1999).

A number of mechanisms may explain why vitamin C lowers heart disease risk (Ginter, 2007; Li and Schellhorn, 2007). Vitamin C acts as the first line of antioxidant defense in plasma (Frei et al., 1989); it effectively inhibits LDL oxidation (Retsky et al., 1993) and thus, potentially, atherosclerotic lesion formation (Carr and Frei, 1999). Furthermore, vitamin C has been shown to play a pivotal role in maintaining normal endothelial function. In particular, endothelial synthesis of nitric oxide is impaired in patients with coronary heart disease (CHD) or coronary risk factors, and nitric oxide is known to cause vasodilation and inhibit platelet aggregation and thrombus formation, thus inhibiting clinical expression of coronary heart diseases (Gewaltig and Kojda, 2002).

The outcome of most population-based studies indicated that low or deficient intakes of vitamin C were associated with an increased risk of CVDs and that modest dietary intakes of about 100 mg day^{-1} were sufficient for maximum reduction of CVD risk among nonsmoking men and women (Carr and Frei, 1999). However, some studies (Osganian et al., 2003) have shown that vitamin C intake from diet alone, in contrast to vitamin C supplements, was not associated with a reduced CHD rate. A vitamin C intake of ca. 400 mg day^{-1} from both diet and supplements was needed for a 27–28% risk reduction. Indeed, the results of the pooled analysis of prospective cohort studies suggested that maximum reduction of CHD risk required vitamin C intakes of around 400–500 mg day^{-1}, high enough to saturate plasma and circulating cells, and thus the vitamin

C body pool (Frei, 2003). On the other hand, the association between vitamin C and heart health has not been consistently shown in intervention and randomized clinical trials (see, e.g., Li and Schellhorn, 2007; Mente et al., 2009). These types of studies, while considered the 'gold standard' for establishing the safety and efficacy of pharmaceutical drugs, suffer from numerous limitations when applied to micronutrients. For example, dose and duration of supplementation, baseline micronutrient levels and oxidative stress status of study participants, inter-individual differences in micronutrient absorption and metabolism, and nutrient–nutrient and nutrient–drug interactions may render the design of randomized clinical trials and the interpretation of their results problematic.

Another heart-protecting property of vitamin C is its ability to modulate blood lipid levels. A meta-analysis of 13 randomized clinical trials that included 405 subjects (average age 58.9 years) with high cholesterol levels analyzed data on subjects receiving vitamin C supplements of at least 500 mg day^{-1} for a period of 3–24 weeks (McRae, 2008). Supplementation with vitamin C, for a minimum of 4 weeks, resulted in a significant decrease in serum LDL cholesterol (-7.9 mg dl^{-1}) and triglyceride (-20 mg dl^{-1}) concentrations. In addition, there was a nonsignificant elevation of serum high-density lipoprotein (HDL) cholesterol. Although the changes were modest, any small change can have beneficial effects on the incidence of CHD, especially in light of the low cost and safety of vitamin C.

2.2.2 Vitamin E

The term vitamin E describes a family of eight antioxidants: four tocopherols (alpha-, beta-, gamma-, and delta-) and four tocotrienols (alpha-, beta-, gamma-, and delta-). Alpha-tocopherol is the only form of vitamin E that is actively maintained in the human body; therefore, it is the form of vitamin E found in the largest quantities in blood and tissues (Traber, 2007). The main function of alpha-tocopherol in humans appears to be that of an antioxidant necessary to prevent propagation of lipid peroxidation (Traber, 2007). The results of large observational studies suggest that increased vitamin E consumption is associated with decreased risk of heart attack or death from heart disease in men and in women. Subjects consuming more than 7 mg of dietary alpha-tocopherol were only $\sim$35% as likely to die from heart disease as those consuming less than 3–5 mg of alpha-tocopherol (Knekt et al., 1994; Kushi et al., 1996). Two other large studies found a significant reduction in the risk of heart disease only in women and men taking alpha-tocopherol supplements of at least 100 international units (IU) (67 mg of alpha-tocopherol) daily (Rimm et al., 1993; Stampfer et al., 1993). Furthermore, plasma or red blood cell alpha-tocopherol levels were shown to be inversely associated with the presence or severity of carotid atherosclerosis (Cherubini et al., 2001; Gale et al., 2001; McQuillan et al., 2001; Simon et al., 2001). The Women's Health Study (Lee et al., 2005) investigated the efficacy of vitamin E supplements in preventing heart disease or cancer in healthy women. Vitamin E (600 IU or 400 mg alpha-tocopherol) or placebo administered every other day for 10 years in about 40 000 women aged 45 years and older was tested. Overall, vitamin E had no effect on incidence of cancer, cardiovascular events, or total mortality; however, vitamin E decreased cardiovascular-related deaths by 24% (Lee et al., 2005). In a subgroup analyses, a significant 26% reduction in major cardio-vascular events was observed among women aged at least 65 years assigned to vitamin E along with a 49% reduction in cardiovascular death. Decrease in cardiovascular death was attributed to a decrease in sudden death (Traber et al., 2008). Further analysis of data from the Women's Health Study showed that women receiving vitamin E experienced a 21% reduction in risk of venous thromboembolism (Glynn et al., 2007). Recent re-views have discussed the benefits of vitamin E supplementation in chronic disease pre-vention (Traber et al., 2008). A critical piece of information emerged from recent investigations indicating that serum alpha-tocopherol concentrations of 13–14 mg l^{-1} (30–33 µmol l^{-1}) optimally reduce mortality due to chronic disease (Traber, 2006; Wright et al., 2006).

Despite these positive findings in the area of prevention, the results of clinical trials using vitamin E for the treatment of heart disease have been inconsistent. A recent and highly criticized (Blumberg and Frei, 2007; Traber, 2007) meta-analysis that combined the results of 19 clinical trials of vitamin E supplementation for various diseases, including heart disease, reported that adults who took high-dose supplements of 400 IU day^{-1} or more were 6% more likely to die from any cause than those who did not take vitamin E supplements (Miller et al., 2005). However, further breakdown of the risk by vitamin E dose and adjustment for other vitamin and mineral supplements revealed that the increased risk of death was statistically significant only at a dose of 2000 IU day^{-1}, which is higher than the upper level for adults (Institute of Medicine, 2000). Furthermore, three other meta-analyses that combined the results of randomized controlled trials designed to evaluate the efficacy of vitamin E supplementation for the prevention or treatment of CVD found no evidence that vitamin E supplementation up to 800 IU day^{-1} signifi-cantly increased CVD mortality or all-cause mortality (Eidelman et al., 2004; Shekelle et al., 2004; Vivekananthan et al., 2003). To date, no vitamin E related mechanisms for increased heart failure have been described. On the other hand, the decreased sudden death and thromboembolism observed in clinical studies may arise from vitamin E's abil-ity to decrease clot formation (Traber et al., 2008). Supplementation of the diet with vi-tamin E to meet the recommended dietary allowance may be a necessary option considering the widespread deficiency of this vitamin. It has been reported for instance that more than 90% of the U.S. population does not consume an amount (15 mg or 22 IU) known to decrease chronic disease risk (Traber et al., 2008).

2.2.3 Selenium

Selenium is another antioxidant that helps to prevent the accumulation of free radicals, thus protecting cell membranes in all organs, including the heart (Foster and Sumar,

1997; Rayman, 2000; Sunde, 2001). In contrast to vitamins C and E, which act directly as antioxidants, selenium functions largely through an association with proteins, known as selenoproteins, including selenium-dependent GSH peroxidases. The known biological functions of selenium comprise, besides defense against oxidative stress, regulation of thyroid hormone action and regulation of the redox status of vitamin C and other molecules (Boosalis, 2008; Foster and Sumar, 1997; Rayman, 2000). Some epidemiological evidence suggests that low levels of selenium may increase the risk of CVDs; however, definitive evidence regarding the role of selenium in preventing CVDs will require controlled clinical trials (Boosalis, 2008). Maintenance of adequate selenium nutriture and, at minimum, the prevention of selenium deficiency is advisable for all individuals to maintain heart health (Boosalis, 2008).

2.3 B-Vitamins

The heart muscle is constantly active and, therefore, relies on continuous energy supply and transformation. Heart function depends on a fine equilibrium between the work the heart has to perform to meet the requirements of the body and the energy that it is able to synthesize and transfer in the form of energy-rich phosphate bonds to sustain excitation–contraction coupling. Heart muscle is a highly oxidative tissue that produces more than 90% of its energy from mitochondrial respiration (Mootha et al., 1997). The role of B-vitamins in energy metabolism is well-established (Huskisson et al., 2007b). A recent study (Huss et al., 2007) revealed that impaired energy production in heart muscle may underlie heart failure in some hypertensive patients. This study showed for the first time that changes in the ability of the heart to produce energy lead to heart failure in some cases. Although the study did not involve vitamin micronutrients, it seems prudent to recommend adequate dietary intake of B-vitamins required for energy transformation in human cells including the heart muscle (Huskisson et al., 2007b). Indeed, micronutrient deficiencies, including B-vitamins, have been recently identified as an unmet need in heart failure (Keith et al., 2009; Soukoulis et al., 2009). It is also well-known that severe vitamin B1 deficiency can cause cardiac failure (clinically referred to as wet beriberi) and muscle weakness among other symptoms (Soukoulis et al., 2009).

In 1969, McCully was the first to suggest that homocysteine may be involved in the pathophysiology of the atherosclerotic process (McCully, 1969). Since then, numerous observational studies have associated hyperhomocysteinemia with cardiovascular risk and have established homocysteine as an independent risk factor (Gerhard and Duell, 1999; Homocysteine Studies Collaboration, 2002). Adverse effects of homocysteine on blood clotting, arterial vasodilation, and thickening of arterial walls are among the mechanism by which homocysteine may increase cardiovascular risk (Seshadri and Robinson, 2000). Folic acid and vitamins B12 and B6 are important cofactors in the metabolism of homocysteine and have been shown to reduce elevated homocysteine levels effectively (see, e.g., Clarke et al., 2007). It was suggested, therefore, that supplementation with these vitamins might decrease cardiovascular mortality substantially – the 'homocysteine hypothesis.' However, several large clinical trials designed to test this theory have yielded inconsistent results. Therefore, there is still significant controversy over the possibility that B-vitamin supplementation contributes to the prevention of CVD via homocysteine lowering (Ntaios et al., 2009). However, in view of the crucial role of B-vitamins in energy metabolism and maintenance of cardiac function, supplementation of the diet to reach the recommended dietary intake of vitamin B is advised in individuals with marginal deficiencies.

2.4 Vitamin D

Vitamin D, the sunshine vitamin, has been recognized for more than a century as essential for the normal development and mineralization of a healthy skeleton. However, the pioneering work of Holick and other researchers has opened a wide field of investigation that has now linked vitamin D deficiency to increased risk of cancer, CVDs, autoimmune diseases, and infectious diseases (Holick, 2004, 2006, 2008). These observations are particularly worrisome, because it is estimated that up to 50–60% of the general population worldwide is vitamin D deficient (Gilsanz et al., 2010). The figures are even worse for vulnerable target groups such as the elderly (Holick, 2004, 2006, 2008).

It has been reported that CVD risk is elevated at higher latitudes and increases in incidence during the winter months. This pattern is consistent with an adverse effect of vitamin D deficiency (Zittermann and Gummert, 2010). Accordingly, epidemiological studies indicate an inverse association between vitamin D deficiency and the prevalence of CVD and heart failure, as well as individual cardiometabolic risk factors, such as hypertension (through the renin–angiotensin system), diabetes, dyslipidemia, and the metabolic syndrome. Vitamin D deficiency has also been implicated in the atherosclerotic process. In addition, direct effects of vitamin D on the cardiovascular system may also be involved. Vitamin D receptors are expressed in a variety of tissues, including cardiomyocytes, vascular smooth muscle cells, and endothelial cells, and vitamin D has been shown to affect inflammation and cell proliferation and differentiation (Anagnostis et al., 2010; Giovannucci, 2009; Gouni-Berthold et al., 2009; Kilkkinen et al., 2009; Lee and Kang, 2010; Nemerovski et al., 2009). The active vitamin D metabolite, 1,25-dihydroxyvitamin D, which is synthesized from its precursor 25-hydroxyvitamin D, downregulates several negative and upregulates various protective pathways in the heart and vasculature. The first randomized trials demonstrate that vitamin D supplementation leads to vasodilatation and suppresses cardiovascular risk markers, such as triglycerides, and the inflammation marker, tumor necrosis factor-alpha (Zittermann and Gummert, 2010).

In conclusion, there is accumulating evidence that vitamin D deficiency is a nonclassical risk factor for CVD. Experimental and epidemiological evidence supports a plausible role for improving vitamin D status in CVD prevention and maintenance of heart health in the population at large. Nevertheless, further randomized clinical trials are required to evaluate whether vitamin D is effective with respect to primary, secondary, and/or tertiary prevention of CVD.

2.5 Calcium and Magnesium

Calcium plays a role in mediating the constriction and relaxation of blood vessels (vasoconstriction and vasodilation), nerve impulse transmission, muscle contraction, and the secretion of hormones like insulin (Institute of Medicine, 1997). Magnesium is required for the active transport of ions like potassium and calcium across cell membranes. Through its role in ion transport systems, magnesium affects the conduction of nerve impulses, muscle contraction, and normal heart rhythm (Institute of Medicine, 1997).

The heart muscle is constantly active and, therefore, requires a strong energy signaling pathway to ensure a close match between oxygen consumption and energy utilization. At present, the nature and function of such signals are still under debate; however, one of the candidates for coupling aerobic metabolism and cardiac work is calcium. Calcium regulates myosin and sarcoplasmic reticulum ATPases directly linked to heart muscle contraction on the one hand and the major mitochondrial dehydrogenases and F0/F1-ATPase on the other (Balaban, 2002).

Furthermore, large epidemiological studies suggest a positive effect of both calcium (Appel et al., 1997; Griffith et al., 1999; Miller et al., 2000; van Mierlo et al., 2006) and magnesium intake (Ascherio et al., 1996, 1992; Peacock et al., 1999) on blood pressure.

Table 26.1 summarizes the functions of the micronutrients described here and of phytosterols and their main roles in supporting heart health.

3. PHYTOSTEROLS

More than 50 years ago, phytosterols had already been described as a group of natural compounds able to reduce the absorption of cholesterol (Best et al., 1954). Since then, a number of products containing phytosterols have been marketed as a nonprescription approach to manage cholesterol. In the year 2000, the U.S. Food and Drug Administration (FDA) issued an official health claim for reducing the risk of CHD for foods that contain phytosterols and are low in saturated fat and cholesterol. Many other international health organizations followed suit to consider phytosterols as a nutritional option to address cholesterol problems. In 2009, European Food Safety Authority (EFSA) experts also concluded that certain foods containing phytosterols can reduce blood cholesterol levels.

Table 26.1 Micronutrients and Phytosterols: Functions and Main Roles in Heart Health

Vitamin	Functions	Main roles in heart health
Vitamin C	• Enzyme cofactor and water-soluble antioxidant • Needed for synthesis of collagen, carnitine, neurotransmitters	• Protection from oxidative stress and regeneration of other antioxidants • Inhibition of LDL oxidation and potentially of atherosclerotic lesion formation • Pivotal role in maintaining normal endothelial function • Supplementation decreases LDL cholesterol and triglycerides
Vitamin E	• Fat-soluble nonspecific chain-breaking antioxidant • Prevents propagation of free-radical reactions	• Protection from oxidative stress • Able to decrease clot formation • Plasma levels inversely associated with presence/severity of carotid atherosclerosis • Supplementation leads to reduction in risk of venous thromboembolism
Selenium	• Functions through association with selenoproteins, e.g., selenium-dependent glutathione peroxidases • Important for defense against oxidative stress, regulation of thyroid hormone action and of the redox status of vitamin C and other molecules	• Antioxidant helping to prevent the accumulation of free radicals • Epidemiological evidence suggests that low levels of selenium may increase risk of cardiovascular diseases
B-Vitamins	• Coenzymes and cofactors in metabolism of carbohydrates, fats, and proteins and in energy production • Needed for neurotransmitter synthesis • Folate, vitamins B6 and B12 are involved in homocysteine metabolism	• Support energy production in the heart muscle • Deficiency of B-vitamins recently identified as an unmet need in heart failure • B1 deficiency causes cardiac failure • Folate, vitamins B6 and B12 reduce elevated homocysteine levels effectively
Vitamin D	• Classical function (mediated through its metabolites) is the maintenance of calcium and phosphorous homeostasis by regulating their intestinal absorption • Essential for bone formation and resorption	• Epidemiological data indicate an inverse association between deficiency and prevalence of cardiovascular disease and heart failure • Epidemiological data show an inverse association between deficiency and risk factors such as hypertension (through the renin-angiotensin system), diabetes,

Continued

Table 26.1 Micronutrients and Phytosterols: Functions and Main Roles in Heart Health—cont'd

Vitamin	Functions	Main roles in heart health
		dyslipidemia, and the metabolic syndrome • Deficiency has been implicated in the atherosclerotic process • Vitamin D receptors are found in cardiomyocytes, vascular smooth muscle cells, and endothelial cells
Calcium and magnesium	• Calcium mediates vascular contraction and vasodilation, muscle contraction, nerve transmission, etc. • Ionized calcium is the most common signal transduction element in cells. Ninety-nine percent of body calcium is in teeth and bones • Magnesium is a required cofactor for over 300 enzyme systems • It is required for both anaerobic and aerobic energy generation	• Calcium is linked to heart muscle contraction via its second messenger role • Magnesium affects the conduction of nerve impulses, muscle contraction, and normal heart rhythm • Epidemiological studies suggest a positive effect of both calcium and magnesium intakes on blood pressure
Phytosterols	• The role of dietary amounts of phytosterols has not yet been studied in detail	• Supplemental phytosterols reduce the absorption of dietary cholesterol and also lower blood cholesterol levels

The collective term 'phytosterols' describes plant-derived sterols and stanols with a similar structure and biological function as cholesterol (Figure 26.1). Stanols are different from sterols as they have no double bond in the B-ring of the steroid skeleton. This small structural difference has obviously no influence in terms of clinical effectiveness (Hallikainen et al., 2000). In general, stanols are of less importance as they comprise only

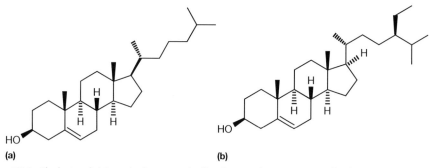

Figure 26.1 Cholesterol (a) and phytosterols (b, sitosterol as an example) have similar chemical structures. In stanol derivatives, the double bond at position 5 in ring B is reduced.

about 10% of total dietary phytosterols. Interestingly, the human diet contains approximately equal amounts of cholesterol and phytosterols. However, usually about 50% of dietary cholesterol is retained and more than 95% of dietary phytosterols undergo direct fecal excretion. This suggests that the human body is able to discriminate between cholesterol and non-cholesterol phytosterols (Lu et al., 2001). Interestingly, the early human diet was richer in phytosterols compared to the modern diet. Our ancestors consumed as much as 1 g day^{-1} of phytosterols while the typical Western diet today delivers only about 300 mg day^{-1}.

Until now, hundreds of phytosterol structures have been identified, but the main constituents are typically sitosterol, campesterol, and stigmasterol. As their structures are quite similar, it is difficult to obtain these sterols as single substances on an industrial scale. Commercially, phytosterols are isolated from vegetable oils [e.g., soybean oil, rapeseed (canola) oil, sunflower oil, and corn oil].

Foods with the highest content of phytosterols are vegetable oils, breads or cereals, and nuts. Most fruits and vegetables do not contain significant amounts of phytosterols. Many naturally occurring phytosterols are glycosylated, and it is not known whether these phytosterol glycosides are bioactive in humans. Most of the clinical studies have been done with free phytosterols or phytosterols esterified with fatty acids.

3.1 How Phytosterols Lower Blood Cholesterol Levels

Until now, the mechanism by which these natural compounds lower cholesterol levels has not been fully determined. However, a number of theories have been proposed, and three distinct features have been elaborated:
- Effects at the absorption site
- Physico-chemical effects
- Effects on intracellular trafficking of sterols

After a fat-containing meal is consumed, dietary cholesterol is usually incorporated into mixed micelles consisting of mixtures of bile salts/lecithin. This takes place in the small intestine and is a necessary step to bring cholesterol into the right format to get absorbed by the enterocytes in the intestine. Phytosterols are able to compete for cholesterol in these mixed bile salt/lecithin micelles, which leads to a decreased solubilization of cholesterol (Ostlund and Lin, 2006). As the affinity of phytosterols for micelles exceeds that of cholesterol, the latter is excluded from the absorption process in the duodenum. In its free form, cholesterol cannot be absorbed by the body and is excreted with the feces. Another explanation for how phytosterols inhibit cholesterol absorption involves their co-crystallization with cholesterol to form insoluble mixed crystals that are unable to pass across the intestinal barrier (Mel'nikov et al., 2004). However, this mechanism seems to be of less importance.

Usually, about 50–60% of dietary cholesterol is absorbed. By contrast, the net systemic absorption of phytosterols is below 5%. As a consequence, serum phytosterol levels are usually several hundred times lower than serum cholesterol concentrations in humans (Ostlund et al., 2002). The very low absorption rate of phytosterols may lead to the conclusion that its activity is limited to the intestinal lumen. However, recent evidence suggests that these compounds may regulate proteins implicated in cholesterol metabolism both in enterocytes and hepatocytes.

Recent studies suggest that both cholesterol and phytosterols are taken up by the enterocytes by the Niemann-Pick C1L1 transporter (Davis and Altmann, 2009). Inside the enterocytes, phytosterols induce the expression of adenosine triphosphate (ATP)-binding cassette proteins. These ABC transporters utilize the energy of ATP hydrolysis to translocate cholesterol and phytosterols across membranes. An increased activity of ATP-binding cassette transporter A1 (ABCA1) and ABCG5/G8 heterodimer has been proposed as a mechanism underlying the hypocholesterolemic effect of phytosterols. ABCA1 and ABCG5/G8 heterodimer secrete phytosterols and free cholesterol from the enterocytes back into the intestinal lumen (Calpe-Berdiel et al., 2009). Here, the competition between cholesterol and phytosterols to get into the mixed bile salt/lecithin micelles to be prepared for the absorption within the enterocytes starts again.

As the secretion rate is much greater for phytosterols than for cholesterol, the systemic absorption of dietary phytosterols is much lower.

In the enterocytes, the phytosterols are also not as readily esterified as cholesterol. As a consequence, they are incorporated into chylomicrons at much lower concentrations. Chylomicrons are a class of lipoproteins that transport dietary cholesterol (and triglycerides) from the small intestine to tissues. That part of the phytosterols finally ending up in the circulation is taken up by the liver and rapidly secreted into bile by hepatic ABCG5/G8 transporters. The secretion rate to the bile of phytosterols exceeds that of cholesterol (Sudhop and von Bergmann, 2002). Overall, the decreased intestinal absorption and increased excretion into bile explains the low serum concentrations of phytosterols relative to cholesterol. About 1000 mg of cholesterol is excreted to the bile every day; of which 60% is reabsorbed and the rest is excreted. The displacement of cholesterol by the phytosterols decreases also the reabsorption of cholesterol through the bile.

Due to the overall decreased cholesterol absorption induced by phytosterols, the body is confronted with a 'cholesterol deficiency.' Therefore, the tissue LDL–receptor expression is increased, resulting in increased clearance of circulating LDL. As a disadvantage, the decreased cholesterol absorption can lead to an increased endogenous cholesterol synthesis in the liver. However, the net result is still a reduction in serum LDL cholesterol concentration (Ostlund, 2007).

3.2 Clinical Evidence for Phytosterols

More than 150 clinical trials showed that phytosterols significantly decrease LDL cholesterol and total cholesterol in treatment groups compared with control groups in a dose-dependent manner (Demonty et al., 2009; Wu et al., 2009). A number of meta-analyses demonstrated that an average of about 2–3.4 g day^{-1} of phytosterols lowered serum LDL cholesterol concentrations by 9–15% (Chen et al., 2005; Demonty et al., 2009; Katan et al., 2003; Law, 2000). Doses higher than 2 g day^{-1} did not substantially improve the cholesterol-lowering effects of phytosterols. Serum concentrations of HDL cholesterol usually remain unaffected by this natural compound. As an overall rule, it has been elaborated that phytosterol esters dissolved in food fat reduce LDL cholesterol by 10% at a maximum effective dose of 2 g day^{-1} (Ostlund, 2004). It has been suggested that such a 10% reduction in LDL cholesterol could decrease the risk of CHD by as much as 20% (Anonymous, 2002). Therefore, the U.S. National Cholesterol Education Program Adult Treatment Panel III has included the use of phytosterols at a dose of 2 g day^{-1} as a component of a dietary therapy for elevated LDL cholesterol. Although there is no direct evidence yet available that could link this cholesterol-lowering ability with a lower risk of CVDs, a positive relationship is probable. Further prospective studies need to be done.

In some other trials, doses lower than 2 g day^{-1} of phytosterols have been tested over periods of several weeks to 1 year. It was concluded that a dose range of 0.8–1.0 g day^{-1} still results in clinically significant LDL cholesterol reductions of about 5–10% (Hendriks et al., 1999; Miettinen and Vanhanen, 1994; Pelletier et al., 1995; Sierksma et al., 1999; Volpe et al., 2001).

The clinical efficacy of phytosterol products is probably related to individuals' baseline LDL levels, phytosterol carriers, and frequency and time of intake. Some data revealed that reductions in LDL levels were greater in individuals with high baseline LDL levels compared with those with normal-to-borderline baseline LDL levels (Abumweis et al., 2008). Also, the formulations of the used phytosterol products is of importance as the reductions in LDL were greater when plant sterols were incorporated into fat spreads, mayonnaise and salad dressing, milk and yoghurt compared with other food products such as croissants and muffins, orange juice, non-fat beverages, cereal bars, and chocolate (Abumweis et al., 2008). Others did not find significant differences between fat-based or non-fat-based and dairy or non-dairy food formats, but did observe a larger effect for solid foods compared to liquid foods at phytosterol doses of over 2 g day^{-1} (Demonty et al., 2009). Present data also indicate that to obtain optimal cholesterol-lowering impact, phytosterols should be consumed as smaller doses given more often, rather than one large dose (AbuMweis et al., 2009). Plant sterols consumed as a single morning dose did not have a significant effect on LDL cholesterol levels (Abumweis et al., 2008).

The overwhelming clinical evidence has clearly proven that phytosterols have an important role in controlling cholesterol intake. However, they must be clearly distinguished from pharmacological interventions, such as statins, that are needed in case of more serious hypercholesterolemia. Typical target group for phytosterols are people with mild hypercholesterolemia or people who want to maintain normal cholesterol levels. Phytosterols are also recommended as an adjunct to drug treatment.

3.3 Sources of Phytosterols

Although the typical modern diet contains about 150–400 mg day^{-1} of phytosterols (Ostlund, 2002), this cannot be related to any desired cholesterol-lowering effects. To obtain efficacious doses of phytosterols, functional foods enriched with these compounds or specific dietary supplements are available. As a key concept, it is important that these compounds must be dissolved in other complex lipids or digested together with fatty meals. Taking crystalline phytosterols alone would not be effective at all as they are very stable and would not interact with the cholesterol absorption. Free phytosterols are also not well soluble in lipids such as triglycerides; therefore, in many applications, phytosterol esters (esterfied with fatty acids) are used showing increased solubility. Also, aqueous dispersions can provide a good bioavailability for phytosterols. In most cases, they are combined with an emulsifying agent (Ostlund and Lin, 2006). Nowadays, a number of phytosterol formulations are available that have led to the successful development of cholesterol-lowering products such as dietary supplements in combination with vitamins, margarine, mayonnaise, vegetable oils, low-fat yogurt, low-fat milk, low-fat cheese, dark chocolate, snack bars, and even orange juice.

Functional foods containing phytosterols are convenient for some consumers, but they also have a number of obvious disadvantages. Many of them contain a high level of dietary fat (e.g., margarine). Some products in the market combine a healthy phytosterol dose with foodstuff having an unfavorable nutrient profile. Phytosterol-enriched croissants would be such an example. From a medical point of view, this is cause for concern as suddenly more critical foods may be considered as 'healthy' by their consumers. This is probably not the right educational message for people who want or need to control their cholesterol and fat intake. In addition, the daily dose of phytosterols cannot be effectively controlled in an easy way in most of the functional foods. Both, too low or too high doses of phytosterols can be ingested by using functional foods. Most of the functional foods need also cooling and cannot be taken to work or during travel.

By contrast, dietary supplements containing phytosterols have the advantage that the daily dose can be exactly managed. In addition, they may be combined with other micronutrients supporting health and well-being. They are typically available in portable formats, do not need refrigeration, and can hence be easily transported. This is of special importance for phytosterols as they have to be combined together with the main meal many working people nowadays have during lunch in a restaurant. As it has been recommended, the daily dose should be divided into at least two portions, which can be easily done with a dietary supplement without adding unnecessary calories. In contrast to a functional food with a dietary supplement, consumption of phytosterols by other persons within the household, such as pregnant women, can also be avoided (see Section 3.4).

3.4 Safety of Phytosterols

Due to their broad use in functional foods and dietary supplements as a functional ingredient, phytosterols and their safety profiles have been reviewed by major health authorities. More than 80 studies have been conducted with this group of natural compounds, and no major adverse effects have been reported. Positive approvals have been obtained in the European Union (EU), Australia, Switzerland, Norway, Iceland, Brazil, South Africa, Japan, Turkey, and Israel. Also, the U.S. FDA has recognized phytosterol esters as safe ingredients after a 'self-GRAS' (GRAS = Generally Recognized As Safe) procedure has been followed (FDA, 2003). The Scientific Committee on Food (now EFSA) in Europe concluded that a numerical upper safe level for the total daily intake of phytosterols could not be established on the basis of the available data. In consideration of the dosages found to be effective for cholesterol lowering, it was recommended that plant sterol intakes exceeding 3 g day^{-1} be avoided as they did not show additional benefits (SCF, 2003).

Phytosterols are very well tolerated even when consumed daily for many months. Trials with people who consumed a phytosterol-enriched spread providing 1.6–2.6 g day^{-1} did not report any more adverse effects than those consuming a control spread for up to 1 year. Even consumption of up to 8.6 g day^{-1} of phytosterols for 3–4 weeks was well tolerated. Importantly, the intestinal bacteria and female hormone levels also remained unaffected by phytosterols. As minor side effects, mild gastrointestinal discomfort including gas, diarrhea, and constipation have been reported in rare cases (St-Onge and Jones, 2003).

Some concern has been expressed regarding patients suffering from sitosterolemia or 'phytosterolemia.' This is a very rare genetic disorder that is caused by mutations in the genes encoding the ABCG5 and ABCG8 cholesterol transport proteins. It is characterized by increased absorption of both phytosterols and cholesterol and linked to an increased CHD risk (Patel and Thompson, 2006). However, studies with the more common heterozygous carriers of the mutation showed that no abnormally elevated serum phytosterols could be observed after consumption of 3 g day^{-1} of phytosterols for 4 weeks and 2.2 g day^{-1} of phytosterols for 6–12 weeks. As the disease is rare and involves defective cholesterol as well as phytosterol transport, it may not be directly relevant to phytosterol feeding (Kwiterovich et al., 2003).

For pregnant or breast-feeding women, supplemental phytosterols are not recommended as no related safety studies are available yet.

3.5 Interaction with Drugs and Other Micronutrients

3.5.1 Interaction with statins

The most prominent group of drugs that are prescribed to manage high cholesterol levels are statins. This class of drugs lowers the level of cholesterol in the blood by reducing the endogenous production of cholesterol by the liver. Statins block hydroxy-methylglutaryl–coenzyme A reductase, a key enzyme in cholesterol biosynthesis (Stancu and Sima, 2001). As their mode of action is different from that of phytosterols, a synergistic effect is to be expected when both agents are taken together. Clinical studies have proven that the consumption of $2–3$ g day^{-1} of phytosterols on top of a statin therapy can result in an additional $7–11\%$ reduction in LDL cholesterol. This is a level of reduction similar to that obtained by doubling the statin dose (Normen et al., 2005). Consequently, phytosterol supplements, when taken with a statin drug, can help in further reducing cholesterol levels. This is a very positive aspect as statins have also an unwanted side effect that is based on their mode of action. As coenzyme Q10 (CoQ10) and cholesterol are both synthesized from the same substance, mevalonate, statin drugs also inhibit the body's synthesis of CoQ10. In fact, the use of statins can decrease the body's synthesis of CoQ10 by as much as 40% (Ghirlanda et al., 1993).

3.5.2 Interaction with vitamins and carotenoids

Some research has shown that phytosterols can slightly lower concentrations of fat-soluble vitamins, but other studies did not show such effect. Plasma vitamin A did not drop after consumption of phytosterols for up to 1 year (Hendriks et al., 2003). For vitamin D, only one study showed that after 1 year of 1.6 g day^{-1} of phytosterol esters, a small (7%), but statistically significant, decrease in plasma 25-hydroxyvitamin D3 concentrations could be observed (Hendriks et al., 2003). For vitamin K, there is no significant evidence that phytosterols may influence plasma levels negatively (Raeini-Sarjaz et al., 2002). Vitamin E levels have been affected slightly by phytosterols but those decreases disappear when plasma alpha-tocopherol concentrations are standardized to LDL cholesterol concentrations (Hendriks et al., 2003).

Another group of essential fat-soluble micronutrients are carotenoids that are also transported by lipoproteins. Some studies revealed that phytosterols may lead to a $10–20\%$ reduction in plasma carotenoids. This is true even after standardizing the carotenoid levels to LDL cholesterol concentrations. In this case, it looks like the phytosterols are affecting the proper absorption of compounds such as alpha-carotene, beta-carotene, lycopene, lutein, and zeaxanthin. At this time, it is not known if this causes any health risks. However, it could be shown that the reduced absorption of carotenoids can be prevented by increasing the intake of fruits and vegetables (Ntanios and Duchateau, 2002).

4. CONCLUSION

Micronutrients play a central role in supporting heart metabolism and in maintaining the blood vessel system. Selected vitamins and minerals as well as phytosterols are important for an adequate energy stream of the heart muscle, a healthy blood pressure, and 'clean' blood vessels. Therefore, an adequate intake of these compounds in nutritional amounts is desired, but excess should be avoided. Single micronutrient deficiency states are comparatively easy to detect and treat. However, marginal micronutrient deficiencies are often multiple deficiencies and occur frequently in otherwise healthy populations. These are much more difficult to recognize and good nutrition is highly recommended for prevention activities. As endorsed by scientists from Harvard University, a daily multivitamin is a great nutrition insurance policy to top a healthy, nutritious diet (Anonymous, 2010). Phytosterols – no longer part of a modern diet at the right dose level – are a safe and effective possibility to control blood cholesterol levels in order to prevent later atherosclerotic developments. Lower levels of phytosterols (e.g., 800 mg day^{-1}) are probably recommendable for preventive approaches, while intake of higher levels (e.g., 2 g day^{-1}) is useful to lower cholesterol at borderline levels. In combination with cholesterol-lowering drugs such as statins, phytosterols can act synergistically in a natural way. The available evidence strongly suggests that a combination of selected micronutrients and phytosterols may be beneficial to heart health. In cases when dietary intakes are insufficient, supplementation with a combination of micronutrients and phytosterols may be an advisable option. However, more clinical trials with good clinical outcomes are required to optimize intake recommendations for both prevention and treatment of diseases.

REFERENCES

Abumweis, S.S., Barake, R., Jones, P.J., 2008. Plant sterols/stanols as cholesterol lowering agents: a meta-analysis of randomized controlled trials. Food & Nutrition Research 52.

Abumweis, S.S., Vanstone, C.A., Lichtenstein, A.H., Jones, P.J., 2009. Plant sterol consumption frequency affects plasma lipid levels and cholesterol kinetics in humans. European Journal of Clinical Nutrition 63, 747–755.

Anagnostis, P., Athyros, V.G., Adamidou, F., Florentin, M., Karagiannis, A., 2010. Vitamin D and cardiovascular disease: a novel agent for reducing cardiovascular risk? Current Vascular Pharmacology 8 (5), 720–730.

Anonymous, 2002. National Cholesterol Education Program. Third Report of the National Cholesterol Education Program Expert Panel on Detection, Evaluation, and Treatment of High Blood Cholesterol in Adults (Adult Treatment Panel III) National Heart Lung and Blood Institute, National Institutes of Health.

Anonymous, 2010. Harvard University, The Nutrition Source Healthy Eating Pyramid. http://www.hsph.harvard.edu/nutritionsource/what-should-you-eat/pyramid/.

Appel, L.J., Moore, T.J., Obarzanek, E., et al., 1997. A clinical trial of the effects of dietary patterns on blood pressure. DASH Collaborative Research Group. The New England Journal of Medicine 336, 1117–1124.

Ascherio, A., Rimm, E.B., Giovannucci, E.L., et al., 1992. A prospective study of nutritional factors and hypertension among US men. Circulation 86, 1475–1484.

Ascherio, A., Hennekens, C., Willett, W.C., et al., 1996. Prospective study of nutritional factors, blood pressure, and hypertension among US women. Hypertension 27, 1065–1072.

Balaban, R.S., 2002. Cardiac energy metabolism homeostasis: role of cytosolic calcium. Journal of Molecular and Cellular Cardiology 34, 1259–1271.

Best, M.M., Duncan, C.H., Van Loon, E.J., Wathen, J.D., 1954. Lowering of serum cholesterol by the administration of a plant sterol. Circulation 10, 201–206.

Blumberg, J.B., Frei, B., 2007. Why clinical trials of vitamin E and cardiovascular diseases may be fatally flawed. Commentary on "The relationship between dose of vitamin E and suppression of oxidative stress in humans" Free Radical Biology & Medicine 43, 1374–1376.

Boosalis, M.G., 2008. The role of selenium in chronic disease. Nutrition in Clinical Practice 23, 152–160.

Calpe-Berdiel, L., Escola-Gil, J.C., Blanco-Vaca, F., 2009. New insights into the molecular actions of plant sterols and stanols in cholesterol metabolism. Atherosclerosis 203, 18–31.

Carr, A.C., Frei, B., 1999. Toward a new recommended dietary allowance for vitamin C based on antioxidant and health effects in humans. The American Journal of Clinical Nutrition 69, 1086–1107.

Chen, J.T., Wesley, R., Shamburek, R.D., Pucino, F., Csako, G., 2005. Meta-analysis of natural therapies for hyperlipidemia: plant sterols and stanols versus policosanol. Pharmacotherapy 25, 171–183.

Cherubini, A., Zuliani, G., Costantini, F., et al., 2001. High vitamin E plasma levels and low low-density lipoprotein oxidation are associated with the with the absence of atherosclerosis in octogenarians. Journal of the American Geriatrics Society 49, 651–654.

Clarke, R., Lewington, S., Sherliker, P., Armitage, J., 2007. Effects of B-vitamins on plasma homocysteine concentrations and on risk of cardiovascular disease and dementia. Current Opinion in Clinical Nutrition and Metabolic Care 10, 32–39.

Davis Jr., H.R., Altmann, S.W., 2009. Niemann–Pick C1 Like 1 (NPC1L1) an intestinal sterol transporter. Biochimica et Biophysica Acta 1791, 679–683.

Davis, D.R., Epp, M.D., Riordan, H.D., 2004. Changes in USDA food composition data for 43 garden crops, 1950 to 1999. Journal of the American College of Nutrition 23, 669–682.

Demonty, I., Ras, R.T., Van Der Knaap, H.C., et al., 2009. Continuous dose-response relationship of the LDL-cholesterol-lowering effect of phytosterol intake. The Journal of Nutrition 139, 271–284.

Eidelman, R.S., Hollar, D., Hebert, P.R., Lamas, G.A., Hennekens, C.H., 2004. Randomized trials of vitamin E in the treatment and prevention of cardiovascular disease. Archives of Internal Medicine 164, 1552–1556.

FDA, 2003. Food and Drug Administration. GRAS Notice No. GRN 000112. http://www.cfsan.fda.gov/rdb/opa-g112.html.

Foster, L.H., Sumar, S., 1997. Selenium in health and disease: a review. Critical Reviews in Food Science and Nutrition 37, 211–228.

Frei, B., 2003. To C or not to C, that is the question!. Journal of the American College of Cardiology 42, 253–255.

Frei, B., England, L., Ames, B.N., 1989. Ascorbate is an outstanding antioxidant in human blood plasma. Proceedings of the National Academy of Sciences of the United States of America 86, 6377–6381.

Gale, C.R., Ashurst, H.E., Powers, H.J., Martyn, C.N., 2001. Antioxidant vitamin status and carotid atherosclerosis in the elderly. The American Journal of Clinical Nutrition 74, 402–408.

Gerhard, G.T., Duell, P.B., 1999. Homocysteine and atherosclerosis. Current Opinion in Lipidology 10, 417–428.

Gewaltig, M.T., Kojda, G., 2002. Vasoprotection by nitric oxide: mechanisms and therapeutic potential. Cardiovascular Research 55, 250–260.

Ghirlanda, G., Oradei, A., Manto, A., et al., 1993. Evidence of plasma CoQ10-lowering effect by HMG-CoA reductase inhibitors: a double-blind, placebo-controlled study. The Journal of Clinical Pharmacology 33, 226–229.

Gilsanz, V., Kremer, A., Mo, A.O., Wren, T.A., Kremer, R., 2010. Vitamin D status and its relation to muscle mass and muscle fat in young women. The Journal of Clinical Endocrinology and Metabolism 95 (4), 1595–1601.

Ginter, E., 2007. Chronic vitamin C deficiency increases the risk of cardiovascular diseases. Bratislavské Lekárske Listy 108, 417–421.

Giovannucci, E., 2009. Vitamin D and cardiovascular disease. Current Atherosclerosis Reports 11, 456–461.

Glynn, R.J., Ridker, P.M., Goldhaber, S.Z., Zee, R.Y.L., Buring, J.E., 2007. Effects of random allocation to vitamin E supplementation on the occurrence of venous thromboembolism – report from the Women's Health Study. Circulation 116, 1497–1503.

Gouni-Berthold, I., Krone, W., Berthold, H.K., 2009. Vitamin D and cardiovascular disease. Current Vascular Pharmacology 7, 414–422.

Griffith, L.E., Guyatt, G.H., Cook, R.J., Bucher, H.C., Cook, D.J., 1999. The influence of dietary and nondietary calcium supplementation on blood pressure: an updated metaanalysis of randomized controlled trials. American Journal of Hypertension 12, 84–92.

Hallikainen, M.A., Sarkkinen, E.S., Gylling, H., Erkkila, A.T., Uusitupa, M.I., 2000. Comparison of the effects of plant sterol ester and plant stanol ester-enriched margarines in lowering serum cholesterol concentrations in hypercholesterolaemic subjects on a low-fat diet. European Journal of Clinical Nutrition 54, 715–725.

Hendriks, H.F., Weststrate, J.A., Van Vliet, T., Meijer, G.W., 1999. Spreads enriched with three different levels of vegetable oil sterols and the degree of cholesterol lowering in normocholesterolaemic and mildly hypercholesterolaemic subjects. European Journal of Clinical Nutrition 53, 319–327.

Hendriks, H.F., Brink, E.J., Meijer, G.W., Princen, H.M., Ntanios, F.Y., 2003. Safety of long-term consumption of plant sterol esters-enriched spread. European Journal of Clinical Nutrition 57, 681–692.

Holick, M.F., 2004. Sunlight and vitamin D for bone health and prevention of autoimmune diseases, cancers, and cardiovascular disease. The American Journal of Clinical Nutrition 80, 1678S–1688S.

Holick, M.F., 2006. High prevalence of vitamin D inadequacy and implications for health. Mayo Clinic Proceedings 81, 353–373.

Holick, M.F., 2008. Vitamin D: a D-Lightful health perspective. Nutrition Reviews 66, S182–S194.

Homocysteine Studies Collaboration, 2002. Homocysteine and risk of ischemic heart disease and stroke: a meta-analysis. Journal of the American Medical Association 288, 2015–2022.

Huskisson, E., Maggini, S., Ruf, M., 2007a. The influence of micronutrients on cognitive function and performance. The Journal of International Medical Research 35, 1–19.

Huskisson, E., Maggini, S., Ruf, M., 2007b. The role of vitamins and minerals in energy metabolism and well-being. The Journal of International Medical Research 35, 277–289.

Huss, J.M., Imahashi, K., Dufour, C.R., et al., 2007. The nuclear receptor ERRalpha is required for the bioenergetic and functional adaptation to cardiac pressure overload. Cell Metabolism 6, 25–37.

IBGE, 2004. Pesquisa de Orçamentos Familiares 2002–2003. Análise da Disponibilidade Domiciliar de Alimentos e do Estado Nutricional no Brasil. IBGE, Coordenação de Índices de Preços. IBGE, Rio de Janeiro.

Institute of Medicine, 1997. DRI Dietary Reference Intakes for Calcium, Phosphorus, Magnesium, Vitamin D, and Fluoride. The National Academies Press, Washington, DC.

Institute of Medicine, 2000. DRI Dietary Reference Intakes for Vitamin C, Vitamin E, Selenium and Carotenoids. A Report of the Panel on Dietary Antioxidants and Related Compounds. The National Academies Press, Washington, DC.

Katan, M.B., Grundy, S.M., Jones, P., Law, M., Miettinen, T., Paoletti, R., 2003. Efficacy and safety of plant stanols and sterols in the management of blood cholesterol levels. Mayo Clinic Proceedings 78, 965–978.

Keith, M.E., Walsh, N.A., Darling, P.B., et al., 2009. B-vitamin deficiency in hospitalized patients with heart failure. Journal of the American Dietetic Association 109, 1406–1410.

Kilkkinen, A., Knekt, P., Aro, A., et al., 2009. Vitamin D status and the risk of cardiovascular disease death. American Journal of Epidemiology 170, 1032–1039.

Knekt, P., Reunanen, A., Jarvinen, R., Seppanen, R., Heliovaara, M., Aromaa, A., 1994. Antioxidant vitamin intake and coronary mortality in a longitudinal population study. American Journal of Epidemiology 139, 1180–1189.

Kushi, L.H., Folsom, A.R., Prineas, R.J., Mink, P.J., Wu, Y., Bostick, R.M., 1996. Dietary antioxidant vitamins and death from coronary heart disease in postmenopausal women. The New England Journal of Medicine 334, 1156–1162.

Kwiterovich Jr., P.O., Chen, S.C., Virgil, D.G., Schweitzer, A., Arnold, D.R., Kratz, L.E., 2003. Response of obligate heterozygotes for phytosterolemia to a low-fat diet and to a plant sterol ester dietary challenge. Journal of Lipid Research 44, 1143–1155.

Law, M.R., 2000. Plant sterol and stanol margarines and health. The Western Journal of Medicine 173, 43–47.

Lee, W., Kang, P.M., 2010. Vitamin D deficiency and cardiovascular disease: is there a role for vitamin D therapy in heart failure? Current Opinion in Investigational Drugs 11, 309–314.

Lee, I.M., Cook, N.R., Gaziano, J.M., et al., 2005. Vitamin E in the primary prevention of cardiovascular disease and cancer – the Women's Health Study: a randomized controlled trial. Journal of the American Medical Association 294, 56–65.

Li, Y., Schellhorn, H.E., 2007. New developments and novel therapeutic perspectives for vitamin C. The Journal of Nutrition 137, 2171–2184.

Lu, K., Lee, M.H., Patel, S.B., 2001. Dietary cholesterol absorption; more than just bile. Trends in Endocrinology and Metabolism 12, 314–320.

Maggini, S., Beveridge, S., Sorbara, P.J.P., Senatore, G., 2008. Feeding the immune system: the role of micronutrients in restoring resistance to infections. CAB Reviews: Perspectives in Agriculture, Veterinary Science, Nutrition and Natural Resources 3, 1–21.

Mccully, K.S., 1969. Vascular pathology of homocysteinemia: implications for the pathogenesis of arteriosclerosis. The American Journal of Pathology 56, 111–128.

Mcquillan, B.M., Hung, J., Beilby, J.P., Nidorf, M., Thompson, P.L., 2001. Antioxidant vitamins and the risk of carotid atherosclerosis. The Perth Carotid Ultrasound Disease Assessment study (CUDAS). Journal of the American College of Cardiology 38, 1788–1794.

Mcrae, M.P., 2008. Vitamin C supplementation lowers serum low-density lipoprotein cholesterol and triglycerides: a meta-analysis of 13 randomized controlled trials. Journal of Chiropractic Medicine 7, 48–58.

Mel'nikov, S.M., Seijen Ten Hoorn, J.W.M., Bertrand, B., 2004. Can cholesterol absorption be reduced by phytosterols and phytostanols via a cocrystallization mechanism? Chemistry and Physics of Lipids 127, 15–33.

Mente, A., De Koning, L., Shannon, H.S., Anand, S.S., 2009. A systematic review of the evidence supporting a causal link between dietary factors and coronary heart disease. Archives of Internal Medicine 169, 659–669.

Miettinen, T.A., Vanhanen, H., 1994. Dietary sitostanol related to absorption, synthesis and serum level of cholesterol in different apolipoprotein E phenotypes. Atherosclerosis 105, 217–226.

Miller, G.D., Dirienzo, D.D., Reusser, M.E., Mccarron, D.A., 2000. Benefits of dairy product consumption on blood pressure in humans: a summary of the biomedical literature. Journal of the American College of Nutrition 19, 147S–164S.

Miller, E.R., Pastor-Barriuso, R., Dalal, D., Riemersma, R.A., Appel, L.J., Guallar, E., 2005. Meta-analysis: high-dosage vitamin E supplementation may increase all-cause mortality. Annals of Internal Medicine 142, 37–46.

Mootha, V.K., Arai, A.E., Balaban, R.S., 1997. Maximum oxidative phosphorylation capacity of the mammalian heart. The American Journal of Physiology 272, H769–H775.

Nemerovski, C.W., Dorsch, M.P., Aaronson, K.D., Bleske, B.E., Simpson, R.U., Bone, H.G., 2009. Vitamin D and cardiovascular disease. Pharmacotherapy 29, 691–708.

Niki, E., 2004. Antioxidants and atherosclerosis. Biochemical Society Transactions 32, 156–159.

Normen, L., Holmes, D., Frohlich, J., 2005. Plant sterols and their role in combined use with statins for lipid lowering. Current Opinion in Investigational Drugs 6, 307–316.

Ntaios, G., Savopoulos, C., Grekas, D., Hatzitolios, A., 2009. The controversial role of B-vitamins in cardiovascular risk: an update. Archives of Cardiovascular Diseases 102, 847–854.

Ntanios, F.Y., Duchateau, G.S., 2002. A healthy diet rich in carotenoids is effective in maintaining normal blood carotenoid levels during the daily use of plant sterol-enriched spreads. International Journal for Vitamin and Nutrition Research 72, 32–39.

Osganian, S.K., Stampfer, M.J., Rimm, E., et al., 2003. Vitamin C and risk of coronary heart disease in women. Journal of the American College of Cardiology 42, 246–252.

Ostlund Jr., R.E., 2002. Phytosterols in human nutrition. Annual Review of Nutrition 22, 533–549.

Ostlund Jr., R.E., 2004. Phytosterols and cholesterol metabolism. Current Opinion in Lipidology 15, 37–41.

Ostlund Jr., R.E., 2007. Phytosterols, cholesterol absorption and healthy diets. Lipids 42, 41–45.

Ostlund Jr., R.E., Lin, X., 2006. Regulation of cholesterol absorption by phytosterols. Current Atherosclerosis Reports 8, 487–491.

Ostlund Jr., R.E., Mcgill, J.B., Zeng, C.M., et al., 2002. Gastrointestinal absorption and plasma kinetics of soy delta(5)-phytosterols and phytostanols in humans. American Journal of Physiology, Endocrinology and Metabolism 282, E911–E916.

Patel, M.D., Thompson, P.D., 2006. Phytosterols and vascular disease. Atherosclerosis 186, 12–19.

Peacock, J.M., Folsom, A.R., Arnett, D.K., Eckfeldt, J.H., Szklo, M., 1999. Relationship of serum and dietary magnesium to incident hypertension: the Atherosclerosis Risk in Communities (ARIC) Study. Annals of Epidemiology 9, 159–165.

Pelletier, X., Belbraouet, S., Mirabel, D., et al., 1995. A diet moderately enriched in phytosterols lowers plasma cholesterol concentrations in normocholesterolemic humans. Annals of Nutrition & Metabolism 39, 291–295.

Raeini-Sarjaz, M., Ntanios, F.Y., Vanstone, C.A., Jones, P.J., 2002. No changes in serum fat-soluble vitamin and carotenoid concentrations with the intake of plant sterol/stanol esters in the context of a controlled diet. Metabolism 51, 652–656.

Rayman, M.P., 2000. The importance of selenium to human health. Lancet 356, 233–241.

Retsky, K.L., Freeman, M.W., Frei, B., 1993. Ascorbic acid oxidation product(s) protect human low density lipoprotein against atherogenic modification. Anti-rather than prooxidant activity of vitamin C in the presence of transition metal ions. Journal Biological Chemistry 268 (2), 1304–1309.

Rimm, E.B., Stampfer, M.J., Ascherio, A., Giovannucci, E., Colditz, G.A., Willett, W.C., 1993. Vitamin E consumption and the risk of coronary heart disease in men. The New England Journal of Medicine 328, 1450–1456.

SCF, 2003. Scientific Committee on Food. Opinion on Applications for Approval of a Variety of Plant Sterol-Enriched Foods. http://europa.eu.int/comm/food/fs/sc/scf/out174_en.pdf.

Seshadri, N., Robinson, K., 2000. Homocysteine, B vitamins, and coronary artery disease. The Medical Clinics of North America 84, 215–237.

Shekelle, P.G., Morton, S.C., Jungvig, L.K., et al., 2004. Effect of supplemental vitamin E for the prevention and treatment of cardiovascular disease. Journal of General Internal Medicine 19 (4), 380–389.

Sierksma, A., Weststrate, J.A., Meijer, G.W., 1999. Spreads enriched with plant sterols, either esterified 4,4-dimethylsterols or free 4-desmethylsterols, and plasma total- and LDL-cholesterol concentrations. The British Journal of Nutrition 82, 273–282.

Simon, E., Gariepy, J., Cogny, A., Moatti, N., Simon, A., Paul, J.L., 2001. Erythrocyte, but not plasma, vitamin E concentration is associated with carotid intima–media thickening in asymptomatic men at risk for cardiovascular disease. Atherosclerosis 159, 193–200.

Soukoulis, V., Dihu, J.B., Sole, M., et al., 2009. Micronutrient deficiencies an unmet need in heart failure. Journal of the American College of Cardiology 54, 1660–1673.

Stampfer, M.J., Hennekens, C.H., Manson, J.E., Colditz, G.A., Rosner, B., Willett, W.C., 1993. Vitamin E consumption and the risk of coronary disease in women. The New England Journal of Medicine 328, 1444–1449.

Stancu, C., Sima, A., 2001. Statins: mechanism of action and effects. Journal of Cellular and Molecular Medicine 5, 378–387.

St-Onge, M.P., Jones, P.J., 2003. Phytosterols and human lipid metabolism: efficacy, safety, and novel foods. Lipids 38, 367–375.

Sudhop, T., Von Bergmann, K., 2002. Cholesterol absorption inhibitors for the treatment of hypercholesterolaemia. Drugs 62, 2333–2347.

Sunde, R.A., 2001. Selenium. In: Bowman, B.A., Russel, R.M. (Eds.), Present Knowledge in Nutrition. eighth ed. ILSI Press, Washington, DC.

Traber, M.G., 2006. How much vitamin E? . . . just enough!. The American Journal of Clinical Nutrition 84, 959–960.

Traber, M.G., 2007. Vitamin E regulatory mechanisms. Annual Review of Nutrition 27, 347–362.

Traber, M.G., Frei, B., Beckman, J.S., 2008. Vitamin E revisited: do new data validate benefits for chronic disease prevention? Current Opinion in Lipidology 19, 30–38.

Van Mierlo, L.A., Arends, L.R., Streppel, M.T., et al., 2006. Blood pressure response to calcium supplementation: a meta-analysis of randomized controlled trials. Journal of Human Hypertension 20, 571–580.

Vivekananthan, D.P., Penn, M.S., Sapp, S.K., Hsu, A., Topol, E.J., 2003. Use of antioxidant vitamins for the prevention of cardiovascular disease: meta-analysis of randomised trials. Lancet 361, 2017–2023.

Volpe, R., Niittynen, L., Korpela, R., et al., 2001. Effects of yoghurt enriched with plant sterols on serum lipids in patients with moderate hypercholesterolaemia. The British Journal of Nutrition 86, 233–239.

Wright, M.E., Lawson, K.A., Weinstein, S.J., et al., 2006. Higher baseline serum concentrations of vitamin E are associated with lower total and cause-specific mortality in the Alpha-Tocopherol, Beta-Carotene Cancer Prevention Study. The American Journal of Clinical Nutrition 84, 1200–1207.

Wu, T., Fu, J., Yang, Y., Zhang, L., Han, J., 2009. The effects of phytosterols/stanols on blood lipid profiles: a systematic review with meta-analysis. Asia Pacific Journal of Clinical Nutrition 18, 179–186.

Zittermann, A., Gummert, J.F., 2010. Sun, vitamin D, and cardiovascular disease. Journal of Photochemistry and Photobiology B 101 (2), 124–129.

CHAPTER 27

Protection by Plant Flavonoids Against Myocardial Ischemia–Reperfusion Injury

M. Akhlaghi*, B. Bandy[†]
*Shiraz University of Medical Sciences, Shiraz, Iran
[†]University of Saskatchewan, Saskatoon, SK, Canada

ABBREVIATIONS

AP-1 Activator protein-1
ATP Adenosine triphosphate
EGCG Epigallocatechin gallate
iNOS Inducible nitric oxide synthase
IR Ischemia–reperfusion
NF-κB Nuclear factor-κB

1. INTRODUCTION

Flavonoids are a vast group of phytochemicals, common in the core phenyl-benzopyran structure (Figure 27.1). They are divided into several classes, including flavonols, flavanols, flavanones, flavones, isoflavones, and anthocyanins. Flavonoids within each class have similarities in chemical structure, plant sources, and perhaps biological effects.

Knowledge of the salubrious effects of flavonoids on ischemic hearts is dated to the 1980s. Since then, extensive investigations have engrossed many researchers and evoked enthusiastic views on the issue. Now, after a decade in the new millennium, still many unsolved dilemmas remain from nutritional and mechanistic perspectives concerning the effects of flavonoids on the heart during ischemia–reperfusion (IR). This chapter endeavors to describe what is known to date of the biological effects of flavonoids from different classes on ischemic–reperfused myocardium and to delineate some of the mechanisms involved. So far, almost all of the research publications in this area (i.e., effect of flavonoids on myocardial IR) have been performed on animals (with some on cell models that are not included in this chapter) and, in most, the Langendorff model has been used for the induction of IR. Various protocols regarding the time point, course, dosage, and the manner of the administration of flavonoids have been employed. Here, we have quoted major findings presented in the field and expounded in some parts to details of

Bioactive Food as Dietary Interventions for Cardiovascular Disease
http://dx.doi.org/10.1016/B978-0-12-396485-4.00025-6
© 2013 Elsevier Inc.
All rights reserved.

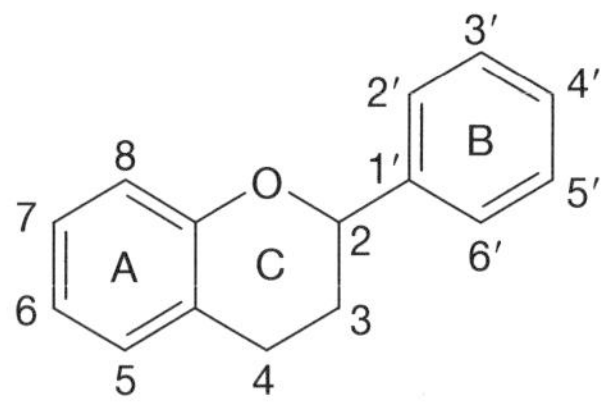

Figure 27.1 General structure of and numbering system of flavonoids.

study and treatment design. In a recent review, we focused in detail on potential mechanisms of cardioprotection (Akhlaghi and Bandy, 2009). Here, we review recent research on each class of flavonoid, to reveal similarities and differences between them.

2. FLAVONOLS

Flavonols are one of the most important groups of flavonoids owing to a structure in the C-ring (described later) that endows them good antioxidant capacity. Some flavonols have been examined in the course of myocardial IR injury. Quercetin, the most investigated flavonol, demonstrated the improvement of hemodynamic parameters in hearts when delivered either intragastrically (Brookes et al., 2002; Ikizler et al., 2007) or *in vitro* in the perfusate (Barteková et al., 2010; Scarabelli et al., 2009; Yamashiro et al., 2003) before ischemia and/or during reperfusion. The improvements included, for instance, higher systolic pressure, lower end-diastolic pressure, higher left ventricular developed pressure, and better left ventricular contractility. In one study comparing preischemic treatments, the alterations were more pronounced in prolonged (7 days) rather than short-term (30 min) treatment, showing that chronic treatment is more effective than an acute treatment before ischemia (Ikizler et al., 2007). The functional recovery of the heart after ischemia has also been reported with administration of other flavonols, including rutin (Lebeau et al., 2001), myricetin (Scarabelli et al., 2009), kaempferol (Kim et al., 2008), and hyperin (Wang et al., 1996).

The improvement of cardiac functional recovery after ischemia may be the result of preserving cell integrity and inhibition of cell death. When delivered to isolated rat hearts *in vitro*, quercetin and myricetin limited the infarction area (Barteková et al., 2010; Scarabelli et al., 2009). Accordingly, quercetin and myricetin also lowered biochemical markers of cell death, for instance, postischemic release of lactate dehydrogenase and creatine kinase in the heart effluents, and caspase-3 activity and DNA fragmentation (TUNEL examination) in the myocardium (Scarabelli et al., 2009). However, differences exist between quercetin and myricetin protection; myricetin had the ability to prevent the activation of caspases-3, -8, and -9, while quercetin was unable to prevent activation of caspase-8 (involving extrinsic cell death pathways), but retained ability to inhibit caspase-9 (involving intrinsic mitochondrial cell death pathways; Scarabelli et al., 2009).

The difference between quercetin and myricetin in inhibiting various death pathways suggests that their mechanism of action is probably divergent, and this occurs only because of the substitution of a hydrogen in quercetin with a hydroxyl group in myricetin (Figure 27.2). Prevention of cell death by flavonols may also result from alteration of death/survival proteins. Kaempferol, administered to isolated rat hearts *in vitro*, increased expression of antiapoptotic protein Bcl-2 and reduced the expression of proapoptotic protein Bax and endoplasmic reticulum stress proteins CHOP and GRP78 (Kim et al., 2008).

Flavonol protection of myocardial cells against IR injury and cell death may be a consequence of attenuation of oxidative stress. Flavonols possess good antioxidant activity because of the structural traits of a 3-OH group (or 3-OR), a 2–3 double bond, and a 4-oxo group, all in the C-ring, and a fully conjugated structure (Figure 27.2). Administered *in vivo* or *in vitro*, quercetin (Ikizler et al., 2007; Scarabelli et al., 2009; Yamashiro et al., 2003), myricetin (Scarabelli et al., 2009), and hyperin (Wang et al., 1996) inhibited postischemic elevation of malondialdehyde in the myocardium. Quercetin also elevated glutathione (Ikizler et al., 2007), which is inversely related with the extent of oxidative stress. Furthermore, quercetin reduced the expression of nicotinamide adenine dinucleotide phosphate oxidases that are activated during IR and on activation produce superoxide radicals and augment oxidative stress (Wan et al., 2009).

Failure in restoring blood flow in the myocardium is not unusual after reperfusion, resulting in the no-reflow phenomenon. Hence, dilation of coronary arteries can improve blood circulation in the myocardium. Quercetin has shown a vasodilatory effect on ischemic hearts. Quercetin retained coronary wall integrity, abated clot generation in the coronary vasculature, and improved blood circulation in hearts 24 h after coronary artery occlusion in dogs (Kolchin et al., 1991). Administered to isolated rat hearts in the perfusate, quercetin increased coronary flow when treated during reperfusion but not when administered for 15 min before ischemia (Barteková et al., 2010). In another study, however, quercetin elevated nitrite, an indicator of the vasodilator nitric oxide, when given chronically by oral administration to rats for 7 days before ischemia and less

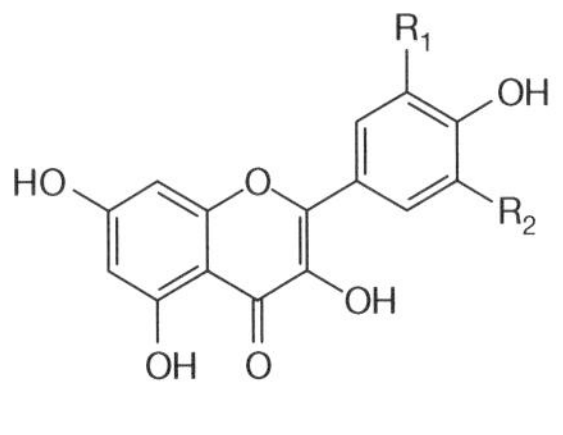

Kaemferol: R_1 = H, R_2 = H
Quercetin: R_1 = OH, R_2 = H
Myricetin: R_1 = OH, R_2 = OH

Figure 27.2 Chemical structure of some flavonols.

effectively when administered *in vitro* during reperfusion (Ikizler et al., 2007). Together the results suggest that quercetin can acutely improve vasodilation if present during reperfusion, and also produce changes that improve vasodilation when delivered chronically before ischemia.

While nitric oxide is an important vasodilator with antiplatelet and anti–inflammatory properties, massive production of nitric oxide by inducible nitric oxide synthase (iNOS), which is induced after IR, leads to oxidative stress and inflammation as a consequence of peroxynitrite formation. Intravenous injection of quercetin 5 min before coronary artery ligation reduced the IR–induced mRNA and protein expression of iNOS and endothelium nitric oxide synthase in rabbit ischemic–reperfused hearts (Wan et al., 2009).

Quercetin can also help preserve energy in myocardial cells during ischemia, as evidenced by higher cellular adenosine triphosphate (ATP) and creatine phosphate and lower Pi when quercetin was present in the perfusate during reperfusion of isolated rat hearts (Yamashiro et al., 2003). Depletion of cellular ATP produces ischemic contracture and subsequent tissue injury. Quercetin prolonged the time to onset of ischemic contracture when delivered in the perfusate (Yamashiro et al., 2003) or when delivered orally for 4 days before IR (Brookes et al., 2002).

It is of interest that quercetin and rutin have also shown benefits on hearts of diabetic rats, which are more susceptible to IR injury. These two flavonols delivered by intraperitoneal injection limited infarct damage, improved heart rate, and prevented lipid peroxidation after ischemia induced by coronary artery ligation in both normal and diabetic rats (Annapurna et al., 2009).

3. FLAVANOLS

Many of beneficial effects of flavanols (catechins and catechin gallates) on myocardial IR injury are similar to flavonols. The most frequently investigated flavanols are catechin, epicatechin, epigallocatechin, and epigallocatechin gallate (EGCG; Figure 27.3), as well as proanthocyanidins (polymeric catechins). As green tea is a dominant dietary source of catechins, some investigators choose green tea for the examination of biological effects of catechins.

Improvements of heart functional recovery following ischemia have been demonstrated by pure catechins or green tea extract in both dietary (Modun et al., 2003; Potenza et al., 2007; Townsend et al., 2004; Yanagi et al., 2011) and nondietary treatments (Aneja et al., 2004; Hirai et al., 2007; Kim et al., 2010; Modun et al., 2003). Interestingly, 3 weeks treatment with EGCG not only reduced systolic blood pressure in spontaneously hypertensive rats (SHR) but also lowered left ventricular end-diastolic pressure and raised left ventricular developed pressure in hearts of SHR rats subjected to IR *ex vivo* (Potenza et al., 2007), showing an effect on the heart tissue. Moreover, both short and prolonged dietary treatments and *in vitro* administration of catechin effectively reduced the incidence

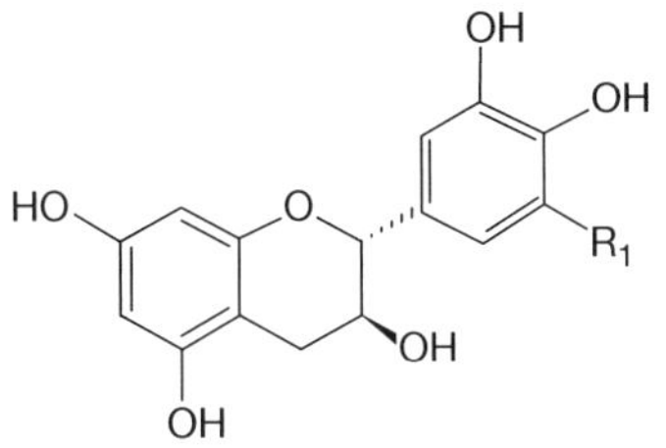

(+)-Catechin: R_1 = H
(+)-Gallocatechin: R_1 = OH

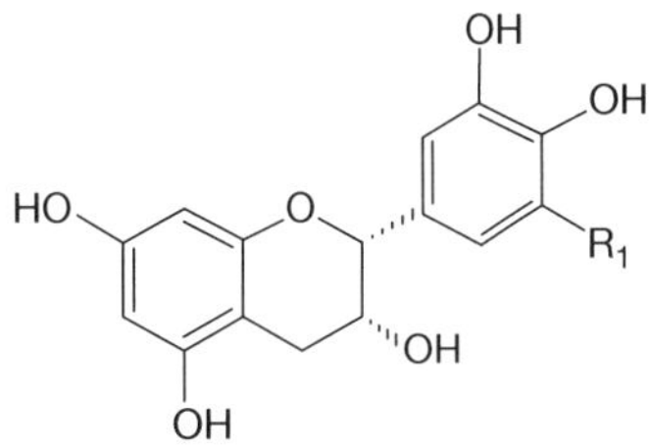

(–)-Epicatechin: R_1 = H
(–)-Epigallocatechin: R_1 = OH

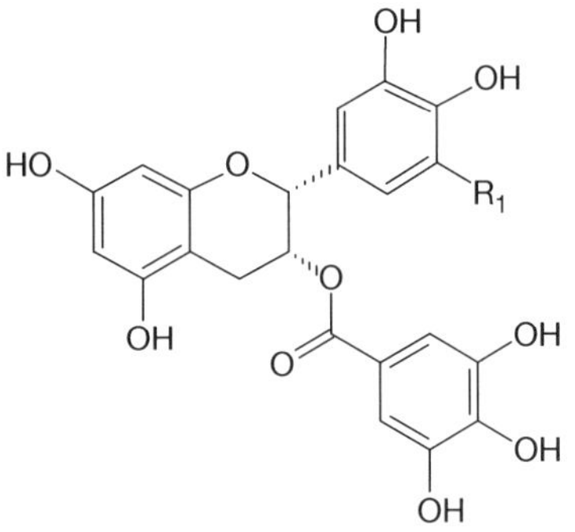

(–)-Epicatechin gallate: R_1 = H
(–)-Epigallocatechin gallate: R_1 = OH

Figure 27.3 Chemical structures of some catechins.

as well as duration of ventricular fibrillation after 30 min of global ischemia (Modun et al., 2003). Furthermore, catechin in all three aforementioned treatment protocols improved relative cardiac efficiency as defined by the product of heart rate and left ventricular developed pressure divided by the amount of oxygen consumed (Modun et al., 2003). However, exceptions existed in one study using 1 mg kg^{-1} body weight per day oral epicatechin (Yamazaki et al., 2008) and another with EGCG added to perfusate (Song et al., 2010), which revealed no impact on hemodynamic and functional measurements, such as systolic and diastolic pressures, although benefits were seen in limiting oxidative damage and infarct size. A low dosage of administered epicatechin and a short length of perfusion with EGCG could be reasons of the ineffectiveness of treatments on hemodynamic parameters.

All published studies on catechins reported reductions of infarct area (Kim et al., 2010; Potenza et al., 2007; Song et al., 2010; Yamazaki et al., 2008), tissue necrosis (Aneja et al., 2004) and indices of cell death, including caspase-3 activity (Akhlaghi and Bandy, 2010;

Hirai et al., 2007; Townsend et al., 2004; Yanagi et al., 2011), extracellular lactate dehydrogenase (Modun et al., 2003), and extracellular creatine phosphokinase (Aneja et al., 2004). However, although 10 days oral pretreatment with epicatechin reduced infarct zone by almost 50%, 2 days of the same treatment did not significantly limit the infarct area (Yamazaki et al., 2008), showing that prolonged treatment is probably needed. The 10 days treatment with epicatechin also lowered activity of matrix metalloproteinase-9 (but not matrix metalloproteinase-2) in the infarct area of the left ventricle in days following 45 min of coronary artery occlusion (Yamazaki et al., 2008). Similarly, suppression of metalloproteinase-2 and -9 by prolonged (28 days) oral administration of tea catechins has been documented as a possible mechanism of attenuation of infarct size and tissue fibrosis in an *in vivo* model of focal ischemia (Suzuki et al., 2007). Activation of matrix metalloproteinases occurs as a consequence of IR-induced cell death, which leads to ventricular thinning and remodeling. Hence, lower metalloproteinase activity will be accompanied with diminished cardiac structural damage. Reduction of infarct size and apoptosis by green tea extract has also been associated with decreased activation of cell death signaling pathways (Townsend et al., 2004). Pure EGCG mimicked the changes seen with green tea extract, suggesting that beneficial effects of green tea extract may be mainly because of EGCG (Townsend et al., 2004). Similar to the results of Yamazaki and colleagues' study, dietary treatment with green tea extract for 10 days protected isolated rat hearts from IR-induced cell death (Akhlaghi and Bandy, 2010). The protection was accompanied by preserved activity of the phase-2 enzymes, glutamate cysteine ligase and quinone reductase, suggesting that these enzymes may play a role in the protection (Akhlaghi and Bandy, 2010).

Flavanols show strong antioxidant potential during IR. In isolated rat hearts subjected to IR *ex vivo*, 2 weeks dietary pretreatment with green tea catechins (Miwa et al., 2004) or EGCG (Yanagi et al., 2011) inhibited DNA oxidation assessed by 8-hydroxy-deoxyguanosine production. In another study, as a result of attenuation of oxidative stress, intravenous infusion of EGCG inhibited activation of proinflammatory nuclear factor-κB (NF-κB) as well as the transcription factor activator protein-1 (AP-1) (Aneja et al., 2004). As a consequence of blockade of NF-κB and AP-1 pathways, EGCG prevented interleukin-6 release from infarcted region and therefore neutrophil infiltration into the infarct zone (Aneja et al., 2004). In agreement with these results for EGCG, daily oral delivery of tea catechins gave antioxidant and anti-inflammatory effects through inhibition of NF-κB and AP-1 activation in myocardium of rats subjected to 4 weeks coronary artery ligation (Suzuki et al., 2007). Both *in vitro* administration and either short- or long-term dietary treatment with catechin also prevented formation of lipid peroxides in isolated ischemic-reperfused hearts (Modun et al., 2003). Ten-day feeding of epicatechin similarly inhibited elevation of oxidized to reduced glutathione ratio in an *in vivo* IR situation (Yamazaki et al., 2008). However, epicatechin in this dietary treatment did not completely attenuate oxidative stress, as it did not significantly prevent neutrophil infiltration into ischemic myocardium (Yamazaki et al., 2008), which was probably due to the low dose of epicatechin. The antioxidant effects of flavanols may extend to mitochondria. EGCG and gallocatechin gallate added to the perfusate preserved cellular ATP and phosphocreatine in isolated guinea pig hearts following IR (Hirai et al., 2007). Further, anti–infarct effects of EGCG was accompanied with opening of mitochondrial K_{ATP} channels (Song et al., 2010), which on opening are known to reduce mitochondrial calcium overload during IR conditions.

Vasodilatory effects of flavanols have also been reported. Perfusing hearts with EGCG and gallocatechin gallate 4 min before ischemia and throughout reperfusion improved postischemic coronary flow, with more remarkable flow seen with longer treatments (Hirai et al., 2007). Furthermore, in hypertensive rats, 3 weeks dietary treatment with EGCG enhanced postischemic coronary flow to a degree even higher than nonischemic controls (Potenza et al., 2007). It was shown that the vasodilatory effect of EGCG and gallocatechin gallate is nitric oxide-dependent (Hirai et al., 2007; Potenza et al., 2007). Catechin (100 μM) added to the perfusate of isolated rat hearts for short periods also increased coronary flow and was able to keep this effect after removal from the perfusate (Modun et al., 2003). In contrast, either short or prolonged dietary treatment with catechin did not change the flow rate, but it helped preserve cardiac efficiency to a greater extent than when delivered *in vitro* (Modun et al., 2003). These results suggest that at relatively high levels in the perfusate catechin can improve coronary flow, but that loading through the diet produces other changes to the heart that provides protection.

4. PROANTHOCYANIDINS

Proanthocyanidins are in fact oligomers and polymers of catechins (Figure 27.4). Several investigators have examined the effects of grape seed proanthocyanidins on heart IR injury. Delivered orally, grape seed proanthocyanidins showed better preservation of left ventricular developed pressure after IR of rat hearts, lower incidence of tachycardia and fibrillation, and higher coronary and/or aortic flow (Facino et al., 1999; Pataki et al., 2002; Sato et al., 1999; Zhao et al., 2010). Augmentation of blood flow could result from production of a vasorelaxation agent such as prostacyclin, which was elevated by grape seed proanthocyanidins in nonischemic and IR conditions (Maffei Facino et al., 1999). The antioxidant capacity of grape seed proanthocyanidins after oral delivery may be involved in their protection against IR as evidenced by inhibition of hydroxyl radical formation (Pataki et al., 2002) and lower production of malondialdehyde (Sato et al., 1999) in hearts subjected to IR *ex vivo*, as well as enhancement of total plasma antioxidant capacity and plasma ascorbic acid reserve (Facino et al., 1999). The loss of Na^+/K^+ ATPase activity is a consequence of ATP depletion following IR, and it is an important contributor to calcium overload, which is one of the main causes of reperfusion injury. Zhao and colleagues (2010) reported that grape seed proanthocyanidins delivered

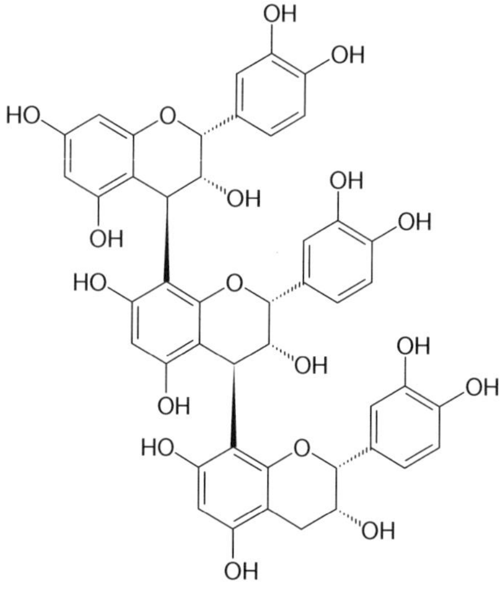

Procyanidin trimer

Figure 27.4 Chemical structure of proanthocyanidins.

intragastrically may act to prevent suppression of heart Na^+/K^+ ATPase activity following IR. Among the flavonoids in red wine, the cardioprotection elicited by the proanthocyanidin-rich fraction when administered (at 30 mgl^{-1}) to isolated rat heart *in vitro* was as potent as red wine extract (at 50 mgl^{-1}; Fantinelli et al., 2005). Fractions rich in anthocyanins, flavonols, and resveratrol in concentrations present in red wine were either weaker or ineffective (Fantinelli et al., 2005). As several of the studies have observed the benefits of proanthocyanidins delivered orally, it seems that proanthocyanidins are sufficiently bioavailable to exert cardioprotective effects.

5. FLAVANONES

Information on the effect of flavanones on myocardial IR is sparse. Gandhi et al. (2009) reported that 15 days oral treatment of rats with 100 mgkg^{-1} day^{-1} hesperidin (but not 100 mgkg^{-1}day^{-1} vitamin E) improved hemodynamic parameters, reduced cardiac arrhythmias, inhibited oxidative stress and inflammation, and reduced infarct area in an *in vivo* coronary artery ligation model of heart IR.

6. FLAVONES

Flavones have chemical structures very similar to flavonols except that they do not have an −OH (−OR) attachment at the C3 position (Figure 27.5). Although it still needs more

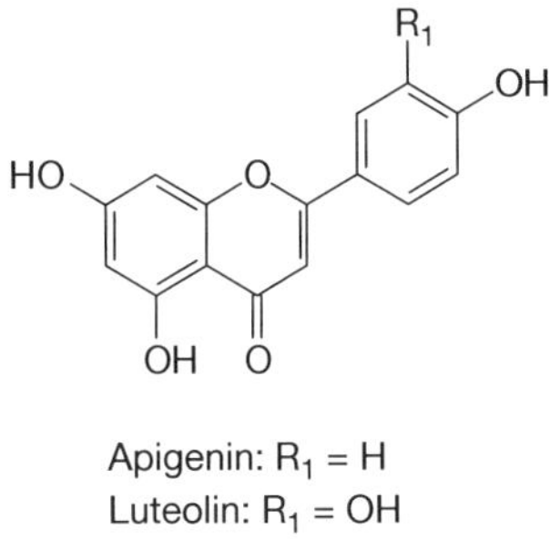

Apigenin: R$_1$ = H
Luteolin: R$_1$ = OH

Figure 27.5 Chemical structure of flavones.

studies, like other flavonoids flavones have shown cardioprotection in IR-exposed hearts. Perfusing hearts with luteolin-7-glucoside during regional ischemia and reperfusion elevated left ventricular pressure and improved global coronary flow in isolated ischemic rabbit hearts (Rump et al., 1995). However, it did not alter end-diastolic pressure. Luteolin-7-glucoside also strongly reduced the ischemic area (as measured from NADH fluorescence). The anti-ischemic effect of luteolin-7-glucoside may not be only correlated to its antioxidant activity, as superoxide dismutase did not decrease the ischemic area except when administered before ischemia, while luteolin-7-glucoside or the phosphodiesterase inhibitor amrinone decreased the affected area when administered either during ischemia or minutes after initiation of reperfusion. The results suggested that the cyclic nucleotide phosphodiesterase inhibitory effect of lueolin-7-glucoside may be important. In a canine model of regional ischemia, intravenous pretreatment with 10–30 mg kg^{-1} flavone, likewise helped resume cardiac functional parameters after ischemia and was associated with lower oxidative injury (Maulik et al., 1999).

7. ISOFLAVONES

As their name indicates, isoflavones are isomers of flavones, with the phenolic B ring attached at the 3-position (Figure 27.6). Isoflavones have been of interest for years because of their similar spatial structure to estrogens, imparting them activity as 'phytoestrogens.'

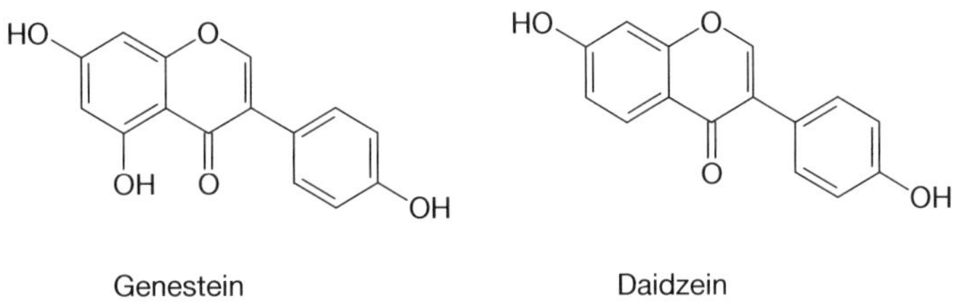

Genestein   Daidzein

Figure 27.6 Chemical structure of isoflavones.

Like other flavonoids, one of the effects of isoflavones on ischemic hearts is restoration of cardiac function after ischemia. Two days subcutaneous injection of 250-mg kg^{-1} genistein to rats before subjecting the isolated hearts to IR gave elevated postischemic heart rate and cardiac contractility and output (Al-Nakkash et al., 2009). Similarly, higher left ventricular contractility was observed in ischemic–reperfused hearts following consumption of a high-phytoestrogen diet, containing chiefly genistein and daidzein, for 3 months (Zhai et al., 2001) or intravenous injection of genistein 5 min before ischemia (Ji et al., 2004). Interestingly, intravenous injection of 1 mg kg^{-1} genistein to rats only 5 min after coronary occlusion was powerful enough to restore left ventricular contractility and prevent arrhythmias (Deodato et al., 1999).

The protective effect of isoflavones on myocardium during IR may be partially due to maintenance of coronary flow which in turn could result from increased production of nitric oxide or inhibition of its reaction with superoxide (Zhai et al., 2001). Nevertheless, the results of human studies are contradictory, although a vasorelaxant effect of supplemental genistein has been reported in postmenopausal women (Squadrito et al., 2003), an epidemiological study found a negative association between blood levels of genistein and coronary microvascular function in a mostly postmenopausal women population (Pepine et al., 2007).

It is not clear whether an antioxidant effect of isoflavones is involved in their protection of hearts against IR injury. However, tumor necrosis factor-α, which is expressed under oxidative stress circumstances including IR, was diminished in serum and macrophages following administration of genistein, and as a consequence expression of intercellular adhesion molecule-1 and accumulation of leukocytes decreased in the ischemic myocardium (Deodato et al., 1999). These results show a beneficial effect of isoflavones against inflammation.

Some studies show protective effects of isoflavones against cell death induced by myocardial IR. Genistein administered intravenously shortly before *in vivo* coronary occlusion decreased infarct size and suppressed apoptosis (Ji et al., 2004). The alleviation of apoptosis was accompanied by suppressed expression of death-associated proteins Fas and Bax and elevated expression of survival protein Bcl-2. In another set of studies, intravenous genistein (1 mg kg^{-1}) lowered necrosis along with reducing infarct area in the heart of rats subjected to coronary artery occlusion (Deodato et al., 1999). In addition, dietary soy isoflavones were observed to preserve normal myofibril and mitochondrion ultrastructure in rat myocardium subjected to IR *ex vivo* (Zhai et al., 2001). The protection by phytoestrogens of myocyte integrity may be in part due to prevention of calcium accumulation in the cytosol and mitochondria (Zhai et al., 2001).

It is worthy to note that in spite of much evidence pertaining to the beneficial effects of genistein on cardiac IR there exist contrary reports. For instance, Sbarouni and colleagues (2006) found no effect of subcutaneous genistein on infarct size or oxidative stress caused by coronary artery ligation and reperfusion in rabbits. The low dosage of genistein

$(0.2 \, \text{mg kg}^{-1} \, \text{day}^{-1}$ subcutaneously for 4 weeks) could be a reason for the genistein futility in this study. Moreover, intraperitoneal delivery of $1 \, \text{mg kg}^{-1}\text{day}^{-1}$ genistein to rats for 6 days before subjecting isolated hearts to IR with and without episodes of preconditioning was shown to abolish the protection afforded by ischemia preconditioning (Benter et al., 2004). Genistein is a nonspecific inhibitor of tyrosine kinases, which are important mediators of ischemia preconditioning (Benter et al., 2005). Thus, administration of genistein may block protection initiated by preconditioning. However, inhibition by genistein of tyrosine kinases that activate phospholipase C may induce cardiac protection, as genestein was observed to block Fas-mediated mechanical dysfunction and apoptosis in cultured cardiomyocytes exposed to a period of hypoxia followed by normoxia (Binah et al., 2004).

8. ANTHOCYANINS

Anthocyanins have unique structures among flavonoids because of a difference in charge and conjugation in the pyran (i.e., C) ring (Figure 27.7). With the prevalence of anthocyanins in red and purple fruits, and their good antioxidant capacity, a few studies to date have examined the effect of anthocyanins on myocardial IR. As with other flavonoids, the anthocyanin delphinidin delivered at $10 \, \mu M$ in the perfusate of isolated rat hearts subjected to IR was able to reduce infarct size, attenuate both apoptotic and necrotic cell death, and ameliorate postischemic functional recovery of the left ventricle (Scarabelli et al., 2009). The protection was greater than that of quercetin and similar to that of myricetin. Delphinidin also inhibited production of lipid peroxides and activation of STAT1, which is associated with cardiac cell apoptosis and IR injury (Scarabelli et al., 2009). Similarly, 10 or $30 \, \mu M$ cyanidin-3-O-β-glucopyranoside in the perfusate of isolated

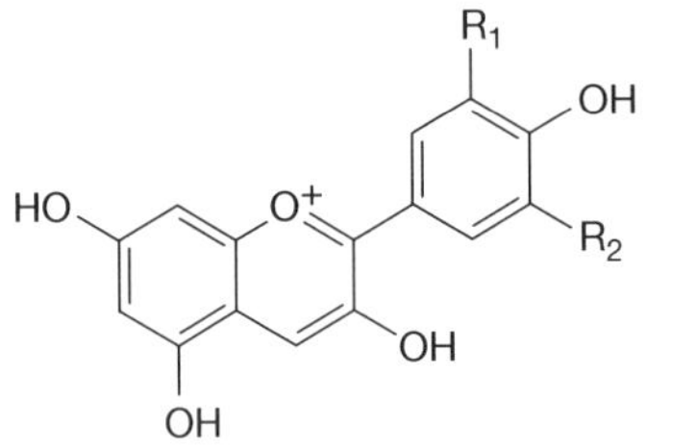

Pelargonidin: $R_1 = H$, $R_2 = H$
Cyanidin: $R_1 = OH$, $R_2 = H$
Delphinidin: $R_1 = OH$, $R_2 = OH$
Petunidin: $R_1 = OCH_3$, $R_2 = OH$
Delphinidin: $R_1 = OCH_3$, $R_2 = OCH_3$

Figure 27.7 Chemical structure of anthocyanins.

rat hearts subjected to IR was able to greatly diminish lipid peroxidation and preserve ATP levels (Amorini et al., 2003). One of the major questions and concerns regarding the biomedical effects of anthocyanins is whether they can pass the enteral barrier and approach the body tissues in sufficient quantity to exert their effects. Three dietary studies have diminished such concerns. Toufektsian and colleagues (2008) detected anthocyanins in blood and urine of rats following 2 months consumption of anthocyanin-rich maize kernels. Such a diet was effective in protecting the heart against IR as evidenced by limited infarct size and preservation of glutathione levels after coronary artery occlusion *in vivo* and *ex vivo* (Toufektsian et al., 2008). Likewise, Falchi et al. (2006) reported lower infarct size and better heart functional recovery of rat hearts subjected to global IR after 1 month consumption of 5 mg kg^{-1} day^{-1} of anthocyanin-rich skins of red grapes, although consumption of the grape flesh that does not contain anthocyanins was equally protective. These diets also decreased lipid peroxidation in IR heart tissues. Similarly, a dose-dependent decrease in infarct area was observed in isolated rat hearts subjected to global IR *ex vivo* 24 h following oral delivery of 25–100 mg kg^{-1} of an anthocyanin-rich extract from soybean seed coat (Kim et al., 2006). In an attempt to determine the effect of polyphenols in human beings, Sumner et al. (2005) found that 3 months consumption of pomegranate juice, which contains a mixture of polyphenols, tannins, and anthocyanins, by patients with a history of coronary heart disease or myocardial infarction improved myocardial perfusion and may reduce the risk of heart ischemia.

9. CONCLUSIONS

Although flavonoids from individual classes are different in chemical structure and dietary sources, the studies done so far indicate that they possess similar properties and exhibit similar protective effects against IR injury. Flavonoids are good antioxidants; however, there is evidence that some of their effects may be delivered through properties other than as antioxidants, such as by affecting gene expression and enzyme activities. Among flavonoids, catechins and catechin derivatives have received the most attention, followed by flavonols, especially quercetin. The IR model itself produces variabilities between studies, which make interpretation and comparison of the results difficult. Nevertheless, it seems that agreements outweigh controversies. Overall, for results relevant to functional food or nutraceutical therapy for ischemic heart disease, dietary treatments, and *in vivo* IR models are preferable. Using dietary approaches, including issues of absorption and metabolism in the intestine and liver, and employing *in vivo* IR conditions invokes effects of blood factors, such as platelets, red and white blood cells, and cytokines. Situations *in vitro*, where flavonoids are applied to isolated hearts, often have a drawback of delivering relatively high concentrations of flavonoids and do not account for absorption and metabolism obstacles. Nonetheless such *in vitro* studies have relevance to acute situations such as coronary bypass surgery or heart transplantation, where flavonoids can be applied directly to the blood or cardioplegic solution. Very few studies, *in vitro* or *in vivo*, have compared different flavonoids in the same experimental protocol to determine which are more potent protectors. Future research needs to shed more light on these and other mechanistic questions.

REFERENCES

Akhlaghi, M., Bandy, B., 2009. Mechanisms of flavonoid protection against myocardial ischemia–reperfusion injury. Journal of Molecular and Cellular Cardiology 46, 309–317.

Akhlaghi, M., Bandy, B., 2010. Dietary green tea extract increases phase 2 enzyme activities in protecting against myocardial ischemia–reperfusion. Nutrition Research 30, 32–39.

Al-Nakkash, L., Markus, B., Bowden, K., et al., 2009. Effects of acute and 2-day genistein treatment on cardiac function and ischemic tolerance in ovariectomized rats. Gender Medicine 6, 488–497.

Amorini, A.M., Lazzarino, G., Galvano, F., et al., 2003. Cyanidin-3-O-beta-glucopyranoside protects myocardium and erythrocytes from oxygen radical-mediated damages. Free Radical Research 37, 453–460.

Aneja, R., Hake, P.W., Burroughs, T.J., et al., 2004. Epigallocatechin, a green tea polyphenol, attenuates myocardial ischemia reperfusion injury in rats. Molecular Medicine 10, 55–62.

Annapurna, A., Reddy, C.S., Akondi, R.B., Rao, S.R., 2009. Cardioprotective actions of two bioflavonoids, quercetin and rutin, in experimental myocardial infarction in both normal and streptozotocin-induced type I diabetic rats. The Journal of Pharmacy and Pharmacology 61, 1365–1374.

Barteková, M., Carnická, S., Pancza, D., et al., 2010. Acute treatment with polyphenol quercetin improves postischemic recovery of isolated perfused rat hearts after global ischemia. Canadian Journal of Physiology and Pharmacology 88, 465–471.

Benter, I.F., Juggi, J.S., Khan, I., Akhtar, S., 2004. Inhibition of Ras-GTPase, but not tyrosine kinases or Ca^{2+}/calmodulin–dependent protein kinase II, improves recovery of cardiac function in the globally ischemic heart. Molecular and Cellular Biochemistry 259, 35–42.

Benter, I.F., Juggi, J.S., Khan, I., et al., 2005. Signal transduction mechanisms involved in cardiac preconditioning: role of Ras-GTPase, Ca^{2+}/calmodulin–dependent protein kinase II and epidermal growth factor receptor. Molecular and Cellular Biochemistry 268, 175–183.

Binah, O., Shilkrut, M., Yaniv, G., Larisch, S., 2004. The Fas receptor-1,4,5-IP3 cascade: a potential target for treating heart failure and arrhythmias. Annals of the New York Academy of Sciences 1015, 338–350.

Brookes, P.S., Digerness, S.B., Parks, D.A., Darley-Usmar, V., 2002. Mitochondrial function in response to cardiac ischemia–reperfusion after oral treatment with quercetin. Free Radical Biology & Medicine 32, 1220–1228.

Deodato, B., Altavilla, D., Squadrito, G., et al., 1999. Cardioprotection by the phytoestrogen genistein in experimental myocardial ischaemia–reperfusion injury. British Journal of Pharmacology 128, 1683–1690.

Facino, R., Carini, M., Aldini, G., et al., 1999. Diet enriched with procyanidins enhances antioxidant activity and reduces myocardial post-ischaemic damage in rats. Life Sciences 64, 627–642.

Falchi, M., Bertelli, A., Lo Scalzo, R., et al., 2006. Comparison of cardioprotective abilities between the flesh and skin of grapes. Journal of Agricultural and Food Chemistry 54, 6613–6622.

Fantinelli, J.C., Schinella, G., Cingolani, H.E., Mosca, S.M., 2005. Effects of different fractions of a red wine non-alcoholic extract on ischemia–reperfusion injury. Life Sciences 76, 2721–2733.

Gandhi, C., Upaganalawar, A., Balaraman, R., 2009. Protection against in vivo focal myocardial ischemia/reperfusion injury-induced arrhythmias and apoptosis by hesperidin. Free Radical Research 43, 817–827.

Hirai, M., Hotta, Y., Ishikawa, N., et al., 2007. Protective effects of EGCg or GCg, a green tea catechin epimer, against postischemic myocardial dysfunction in guinea-pig hearts. Life Sciences 80, 1020–1032.

Ikizler, M., Erkasap, N., Dernek, S., Kural, T., Kaygisiz, Z., 2007. Dietary polyphenol quercetin protects rat hearts during reperfusion: enhanced antioxidant capacity with chronic treatment. Anadolu Kardiyoloji Dergici 7, 404–410.

Ji, E.S., Yue, H., Wu, Y.M., He, R.R., 2004. Effects of phytoestrogen genistein on myocardial ischemia/reperfusion injury and apoptosis in rabbits. Acta Pharmacologica Sinica 25, 306–312.

Kim, D.S., Ha, K.C., Kwon, D.Y., et al., 2008. Kaempferol protects ischemia/reperfusion-induced cardiac damage through the regulation of endoplasmic reticulum stress. Immunopharmacology and Immunotoxicology 30, 257–270.

Kim, C.J., Kim, J.M., Lee, S.R., et al., 2010. Polyphenol (−)-epigallocatechin gallate targeting myocardial reperfusion limits infarct size and improves cardiac function. Korean Journal of Anesthesiology 58, 169–175.

Kim, H.J., Tsoy, I., Park, J.M., et al., 2006. Anthocyanins from soybean seed coat inhibit the expression of TNF-alpha-induced genes associated with ischemia/reperfusion in endothelial cell by NF-kappaB-dependent pathway and reduce rat myocardial damages incurred by ischemia and reperfusion in vivo. FEBS Letters 580, 1391–1397.

Kolchin, Iu.N., Maksiutina, N.P., Balanda, P.P., et al., 1991. The cardioprotective action of quercetin in experimental occlusion and reperfusion of the coronary artery in dogs. Farmakologiia i Toksikologiia 54, 20–23.

Lebeau, J., Neviere, R., Cotelle, N., 2001. Beneficial effects of different flavonoids, on functional recovery after ischemia and reperfusion in isolated rat heart. Bioorganic & Medicinal Chemistry Letters 11, 23–27.

Maulik, S.K., Kumari, R., Maulik, M., Reddy, K.S., Seth, S.D., 1999. Effect of flavone in a canine model of myocardial stunning. Indian Journal of Experimental Biology 37, 965–970.

Miwa, S., Yamazaki, K., Hyon, S.H., Komeda, M., 2004. A novel method of 'preparative' myocardial protection using green tea polyphenol in oral uptake. Interactive Cardiovascular and Thoracic Surgery 3, 612–615.

Modun, D., Music, I., Katalinic, V., Salamunic, I., Boban, M., 2003. Comparison of protective effects of catechin applied in vitro and in vivo on ischemia–reperfusion injury in the isolated rat hearts. Croatian Medical Journal 44, 690–696.

Pataki, T., Bak, I., Kovacs, P., et al., 2002. Grape seed proanthocyanidins improved cardiac recovery during reperfusion after ischemia in isolated rat hearts. The American Journal of Clinical Nutrition 75, 894–899.

Pepine, C.J., von Mering, G.O., Kerensky, R.A., et al., 2007. Phytoestrogens and coronary microvascular function in women with suspected myocardial ischemia: a report from the Women's Ischemia Syndrome Evaluation (WISE) Study. Journal of Womens Health (Larchmt) 16, 481–488.

Potenza, M.A., Marasciulo, F.L., Tarquinio, M., et al., 2007. EGCG, a green tea polyphenol, improves endothelial function and insulin sensitivity, reduces blood pressure, and protects against myocardial I/R injury in SHR. American Journal of Physiology, Endocrinology and Metabolism 292, E1378–E1387.

Rump, A.F., Schüssler, M., Acar, D., et al., 1995. Effects of different inotropes with antioxidant properties on acute regional myocardial ischemia in isolated rabbit hearts. General Pharmacology 26, 603–611.

Sato, M., Maulik, G., Ray, P.S., Bagchi, D., Das, D.K., 1999. Cardioprotective effects of grape seed proanthocyanidin against ischemic reperfusion injury. Journal of Molecular and Cellular Cardiology 31, 1289–1297.

Sbarouni, E., Iliodromitis, E.K., Zoga, A., et al., 2006. The effect of the phytoestrogen genistein on myocardial protection, preconditioning and oxidative stress. Cardiovascular Drugs and Therapy 20, 253–258.

Scarabelli, T.M., Mariotto, S., Abdel-Azeim, S., et al., 2009. Targeting STAT1 by myricetin and delphinidin provides efficient protection of the heart from ischemia/reperfusion-induced injury. FEBS Letters 583, 531–541.

Song, D.K., Jang, Y., Kim, J.H., et al., 2010. Polyphenol (−)-epigallocatechin gallate during ischemia limits infarct size via mitochondrial K(ATP) channel activation in isolated rat hearts. Journal of Korean Medical Science 25, 380–386.

Squadrito, F., Altavilla, D., Crisafulli, A., et al., 2003. Effect of genistein on endothelial function in post-menopausal women: a randomized, double-blind, controlled study. American Journal of Medicine 114, 470–476.

Sumner, M.D., Elliott-Eller, M., Weidner, G., et al., 2005. Effects of pomegranate juice consumption on myocardial perfusion in patients with coronary heart disease. The American Journal of Cardiology 96, 810–814.

Suzuki, J., Ogawa, M., Maejima, Y., et al., 2007. Tea catechins attenuate chronic ventricular remodeling after myocardial ischemia in rats. Journal of Molecular and Cellular Cardiology 42, 432–440.

Toufektsian, M.C., de Lorgeril, M., Nagy, N., et al., 2008. Chronic dietary intake of plant-derived anthocyanins protects the rat heart against ischemia–reperfusion injury. Journal of Nutrition 138, 747–752.

Townsend, P.A., Scarabelli, T.M., Pasini, E., et al., 2004. Epigallocatechin-3-gallate inhibits STAT-1 activation and protects cardiac myocytes from ischemia/reperfusion-induced apoptosis. The FASEB Journal 18, 1621–1623.

Wan, L.L., Xia, J., Ye, D., et al., 2009. Effects of quercetin on gene and protein expression of NOX and NOS after myocardial ischemia and reperfusion in rabbit. Cardiovascular Therapeutics 27, 28–33.

Wang, W.Q., Ma, C.G., Xu, S.Y., 1996. Protective effect of hyperin against myocardial ischemia and reperfusion injury. Acta Pharmacologica Sinica 17, 341–344.

Yamashiro, S., Noguchi, K., Matsuzaki, T., et al., 2003. Cardioprotective effects of extracts from *Psidium guajava* L and *Limonium wrightii*, Okinawan medicinal plants, against ischemia–reperfusion injury in perfused rat hearts. Pharmacology 67, 128–135.

Yamazaki, K.G., Romero-Perez, D., Barraza-Hidalgo, M., et al., 2008. Short- and long-term effects of (−)-epicatechin on myocardial ischemia–reperfusion injury. American Journal of Physiology. Heart and Circulatory Physiology 295, H761–H767.

Yanagi, S., Matsumura, K., Marui, A., et al., 2011. Oral pretreatment with a green tea polyphenol for cardioprotection against ischemia–reperfusion injury in an isolated rat heart model. The Journal of Thoracic and Cardiovascular Surgery 141, 511–517.

Zhai, P., Eurell, T.E., Cotthaus, R.P., et al., 2001. Effects of dietary phytoestrogen on global myocardial ischemia–reperfusion injury in isolated female rat hearts. American Journal of Physiology. Heart and Circulatory Physiology 281, H1223–H1232.

Zhao, G., Gao, H., Qiu, J., Lu, W., Wei, X., 2010. The molecular mechanism of protective effects of grape seed proanthocyanidin extract on reperfusion arrhythmias in rats *in vivo*. Biological & Pharmaceutical Bulletin 33, 759–767.

CHAPTER 28

Bioactive Compounds in Heart Disease

S.N. Batchu, K.R. Chaudhary, G.J. Wiebe, J.M. Seubert
University of Alberta, Edmonton, AB, Canada

1. INTRODUCTION

Our daily intake of food ideally provides enough essential nutrients for us to survive and function. Specific dietary patterns, apart from being a source of energy, can provide protection against various chronic and degenerative diseases. Heart disease and stroke are major causes of illness, disability, and death in both developed and developing countries; as such, they impose a great burden on societies worldwide (Patil et al., 2009; Shukla et al., 2010). As populations increase in age and comorbidities such as obesity and diabetes become more prevalent, both the human cost and economic burden from cardiovascular disease (CVD) will have a significantly increased impact in the coming years (Kris-Etherton et al., 2002; Patil et al., 2009). While extensive research has produced numerous medications to treat CVD, there has been limited success in preventing or curtailing the progression of related pathological conditions. In this context, development of preventive measures that can limit the progression of pathological conditions is necessary to lower the incidence of morbidity and mortality. As a result, there is a strong interest in determining the role of food-based bioactive compounds in reducing the risk of CVD.

There exist many different dietary patterns across cultures, each composed of various nutrient profiles (Patil et al., 2009; Shukla et al., 2010). Some promote health and others increase the risk of disease. Bioactive compounds are considered 'extra-nutritional' constituents that typically occur in plant products and lipid-rich foods. Epidemiological evidence consistently suggests a strong correlation between individuals who consume higher amounts of fruits, vegetables, whole grains, and fish, and lower rates of CVD (Geleijnse et al., 2002; Hertog et al., 1993; Joshipura et al., 1999; Kris-Etherton et al., 2002). Plant-based foods such as fruits, vegetables, and nuts have been shown to contain certain chemical compounds called phytochemicals. The most important of these bioactive compounds are flavonoids, carotenoids, organosulfur compounds, resveratrol, and $n-3/n-6$ polyunsaturated fatty acids (PUFAs). Interest in natural products as an adjunct to conventional therapy in chronic disease continues to grow. In this chapter, the ways in which some bioactive compounds are thought to help in the regulation or prevention of CVD are discussed (Table 28.1).

Bioactive Food as Dietary Interventions for Cardiovascular Disease
http://dx.doi.org/10.1016/B978-0-12-396485-4.00026-8

© 2013 Elsevier Inc.
All rights reserved.

Table 28.1 General Summary of Key Bioactive Compounds and Their Biological Effects Related to Cardiovascular Disease

Bioactive compounds	Example	Source	Biological effects
Flavonols	Quercetin, catechin, epicatechin, epigallocatechin	Onion, tea, berries, red wine, cocoa, citrus fruits	Antioxidant, ↓ platelet aggregation, ↓ eicosanoid synthesis, ↓ inflammation
Flavonone	Hespertein		↓ LDL oxidation, regulates vascular tone
Isoflavones	Genistein, daidzein	Soybeans, legumes	Antioxidant, ↓ platelet aggregation, ↓ LDL, ↑ HDL, inhibits ACE enzyme
β-Carotenoids	Lycopene	Tomatoes, apricots, grapefruit, guava, watermelon, and papaya	Antioxidant, hypocholestrolemic, ↓ LDL, ↓ LDL oxidation, ↑ HDL
Resveratrol		Grapes, berries, jackfruit, peanut, butterfly orchid, lily, eucalyptus	↓ LDL, ↓ LDL oxidation, ↑ HDL, antioxidant, ↓ platelet aggregation, ↓ cytokines, ↓ endothelin-1, ↑ NO, ↓ angiotensin-II secretion
Organosulfur compounds	Allicin-diallyl sulfide, diallyl disulfide, allyl mercaptan	Garlic, onion	↓ Systolic blood pressure, antioxidant, ↓ inflammation, ↓ platelet aggregation, allycysetine ↓ LDL oxidation, ↓ LDL levels
$n-3$ PUFA	α-Lenoleic acid, EPA, DHA, ecosatrienoic acids, ecosatetraenoic acids, stearidonic acid, docosapentaenoic acids, tetracosapentaenoic acids, tetracosahexaenoic acids	Green leaves, rapeseed oil, soybean oil, flaxseed, nuts, and oily fish	Antioxidant, antiarrhythmic, ↓ platelet aggregation, ↓ LDL levels, ↓ TG levels ↓ inflammation, ↓ blood pressure, antiatherogenic, ↓ arterial cholesterol
$n-6$ PUFA	LA, arachidonic acid	Liquid vegetable oils, including soybean, corn, sunflower, safflower oil, cotton seed oils	↓ Ischemia–reperfusion injury, ↓ inflammation, ↓ hypertrophy, ↓ LDL-C, ↓ total cholesterol, ↓ BP, ↓ platelet aggregation

LDL, low-density lipoprotein; HDL, high-density lipoprotein; PUFA, polyunsaturated fatty acid.

2. FLAVONOIDS

Flavonoids are phenolic compounds present in almost all plants, most commonly in berries, onions, citrus fruits, red wine, tea, and cocoa. Of the different types of flavonoids, the most common are flavones, flavonones, flavonols, and isoflavonones (Patil et al., 2009; Shukla et al., 2010). It has been shown that a diet rich in flavonoids renders protection against oxidative stress-mediated diseases. Many epidemiologic studies have reported that increased consumption of flavonoids reduces the rate of mortality from CVDs, indicating a prospective role for flavonoids as potential agents in preventing or decreasing the risk of CVDs (Liu, 2003).

In recent years, many efforts have been made toward elucidating the cardioprotective role of flavonoids, particularly the flavonones and flavonols found in onions, apples, grapes, wine, nuts, and tea. One of the first studies to suggest the protective role of flavonoids was the Zutphen Elderly study from the Netherlands (Hertog et al., 1993). In this study, the relationship between the development of coronary heart disease, myocardial infarction, and the incidence of mortality was assessed in 805 men, aged 65–84 years, over a five-year period, based on their intake of flavonoids, both flavonols quercetin, kaempferol, and myricetin; and flavones apigenin and luteolin. The results demonstrated an inverse correlation between high intake of flavonoids and the incidence of development of coronary heart diseases and myocardial infarction, suggesting that intake of food rich in flavonoids such as tea, onions, and apples reduces the risk of death from coronary artery disease (CAD) in elderly men. Similarly, the Rotterdam study demonstrated a reduction in the relative risk of adverse outcomes associated with CAD, notably myocardial infarction, in a cohort of 4807 individuals aged 55 years following a high flavonoid intake from tea. These and many other studies demonstrate the positive effect of flavonoids; their increased consumption decreases the risk of CVD and reduces mortality (Geleijnse et al., 2002).

The exact protective mechanism(s) of flavonoids has not been fully elucidated, but much evidence suggests that the decreased development of CVD can be attributed to antioxidant properties. Structure–activity experiments demonstrate that flavonoids can scavenge free radicals, notably superoxides. Flavonoids have been shown to inhibit the reactive oxygen species (ROS)-mediated pathological conditions, stimulating effects such as oxidation of low-density lipoproteins (LDL) (Patil et al., 2009; Shukla et al., 2010). Additional evidence suggests that flavonoids can increase endothelial flow-mediated dilation, thereby regulating vessel function by enhancing the bioavailability of basal and stimulated nitric oxide (NO) and increasing the resistance to contraction caused by elevated Ca^{2+} levels under certain pathological conditions (Woodman and Chan, 2004). Other evidence demonstrates flavonoids, such as rutin and quercetin, possess anti-inflammatory activity reducing both acute and chronic inflammation. Generally, flavonoid-rich foods can provide compounds that improve vessel function and increase vasodilatation response in CVD patients (Liu, 2003).

3. PHYTOESTROGENS

Phytoestrogens are naturally occurring estrogenic compounds present in plants; they are divided into three main classes: isoflavones, coumestans, and lignans. They are largely found in plants from the leguminosae family, such as beans, lentils, lupins, peas, peanuts, and soybeans (Kris-Etherton et al., 2002; Shukla et al., 2010). Isoflavones, the most extensively studied phytoestrogens with regards to CVD, are diphenolic compounds structurally similar to human estrogen; as such, their biological effect predominately involves interaction with estrogen receptors. However, the specific mechanism(s) of action is still not fully elucidated as they can also produce effects independent of estrogen receptors. Isoflavones are reported to decrease atherosclerotic lesion formation, reduce LDL oxidation, and decrease platelet aggregation, which work to inhibit or slow the development of atherosclerosis and its complications. The genistein and daidzen isoflavones are bioactive compounds thought to account for the protective effects of soy protein (Shukla et al., 2010). Various studies demonstrate that individuals with a higher intake of soybean (rich in genistein) in their diet tend to have reduced platelet aggregation and decreased levels of cholesterol and LDL lipoprotein. However, it has also been reported that genistein does not affect the plasma cholesterol levels in healthy individuals with normal cholesterol levels. The antihypertensive properties of genistein are demonstrated by studies showing that increased soy protein intake triggers vasorelaxation and a modest decrease in blood pressure (Kris-Etherton et al., 2002; Patil et al., 2009). Moreover, animal studies have demonstrated that genistein inhibits the angiotensin converting enzyme (ACE) and can enhance a hypotensive response of bradykinin; however, this effect is still to be verified in humans (Guang and Phillips, 2009; Montenegro et al., 2009). Research to date indicates multiple beneficial effects of isoflavones in general, but more studies are required to elucidate the biological effects of individual isoflavones on CVD risk.

These beneficial effects in CVD notwithstanding, higher dietary levels of phytoestrogens are known to have detrimental effects. It has been reported that in human males, it can cause decreased sperm production, and in females, it can lead to fewer or smaller offspring (Cederroth et al., 2010). Thus, while the beneficial effects appear to be promising, further studies are needed to study the mechanisms through which these effects are rendered and also how to reconcile the adverse effects of isoflavones.

4. RESVERATROL

Resveratrol (3,5,4′-trihydroxy-trans-stilbene) is a naturally occurring plant polyphenolic phytoalexin. While it has been identified in over 100 different kinds of plants, the richest source is the roots of *Polygonum cuspidatum* (Japanese knotweed). Resveratrol has been found most notably in both the skin and seeds of grapes and as such is believed to be responsible for the cardioprotective properties of red wine. In addition to grapes, resveratrol is also present in a large variety of other fruits, mainly berries such as cranberries, mulberries, lingonberries, and blueberries, jackfruit, peanuts, as well as in a wide variety of flowers and leaves including the butterfly orchid, lily, and eucalyptus (Das and Maulik, 2006; Leifert and Abeywardena, 2008). In plants, resveratrol is inducibly synthesized to protect the plant in times of stress and pathogen-induced injury. In humans, resveratrol is known to function as an antioxidant, anti-inflammatory, and antimicrobial agent and has long been used in Japanese and Chinese traditional medicine to treat fungal infections, skin inflammations, and liver disease.

Anecdotal evidence from historical medicine records described the use of grape juice or red wine for therapeutic purposes. Renewed interest in resveratrol as a cardioprotective agent comes from epidemiological studies correlating mild-to-moderate alcohol consumption with reduced morbidity and mortality from coronary heart disease. As stated by Dr. Serge Renaud, there exists a "French Paradox," that is, despite the typical French diet, rich in cheese and fat, the incidence of CVD-mediated mortality is much less than would be expected (Leifert and Abeywardena, 2008). Subsequent research investigating resveratrol's protective effects has revealed that it can decrease the risk of CVDs via numerous different effects, which include limiting ischemia–reperfusion injury; promoting vascular relaxation; maintaining endothelial cell function; decreasing arrhythmias; inhibiting apoptosis; stimulating angiogenesis; inhibiting LDL peroxidation; reducing oxidative stress; limiting atherosclerosis formation; and curtailing hypertension development (Das and Maulik, 2006; Leifert and Abeywardena, 2008).

Although resveratrol has been demonstrated to protect against numerous adverse consequences associated with CVD, the specific mechanism(s) of action is still ambiguous. Overall, resveratrol demonstrates a 'preconditioning effect' whereby it increases various endogenous defense mechanisms that provide protection against injury. Consistent with this effect, resveratrol activates many well-defined molecular survival signaling events. Experimental data demonstrate that resveratrol can activate prosurvival signaling through various kinases, such as phosphoinositol-3 kinase (PI3K), protein kinase C (PKC), and mitogen-activated protein kinase (MAPK), ion channels such as the ATP-sensitive potassium channel, receptors such as adenosine receptors, and NO via inducible nitric oxide synthase (iNOS) and nitric oxide synthase (eNOS). While the vast array of prosurvival pathways activated by resveratrol protects cells from adverse effects related to CVD and potentially slows the progression of a pathological state, evidence suggests a dichotomy in resveratrol action (Das and Maulik, 2006). Some examples of the differing responses reflect a wide range of effects; for example, it can activate prosurvival signaling to protect heart cells, but it can selectively kill cancer cells by inhibiting antiapoptotic pathways; at low concentrations, it has antioxidant properties, but at higher concentrations, it is a pro-oxidant; or, at low concentrations, it stimulates angiogenesis, but at higher concentrations, it blocks the angiogenic response. Important differences in resveratrol pharmacokinetics and pharmacodynamic properties that impact its bioavailability need to be addressed. Clearly, resveratrol is an important compound that possesses multi-target bioactivity that can have significant protective effects toward CVD (Das and Maulik, 2006; Leifert and Abeywardena, 2008).

5. CAROTENOIDS

Carotenoids are fat-soluble pigments present in plants, algae, and microorganisms efficient in quenching singlet oxygen. These are divided into two classes based on their chemical composition, carotenes and xanthophylls. Carotenes include α-carotene, β-carotene, and lycopene, and xanthophylls include lutein, zeaxanthin, and astaxanthin. Lycopene is the most common carotenoid expressed in many regular vegetables and fruits (Riccioni, 2009). Tomatoes and processed tomato products such as sauce, ketchup, and soup are rich sources of lycopene. Fruits such as apricots, grapefruit, guava, watermelon, and papaya are also known to contain lycopene (Shukla et al., 2010). Similar to other phytochemicals, lycopene is also known to lower the risk of CVD. Several large epidemiologic studies, such as the Physicians' Health Study and the EURAMIC study, have confirmed that individuals with high plasma lycopene levels have a lower risk of CVD compared to individuals with lower plasma lycopene levels. The 1991–92 EURAMIC study was a multicenter case-control study looking at the role of antioxidants, vitamin E, and β-carotene in protection against coronary heart disease. Results from 683 people with acute myocardial infarction and 727 controls suggested that the consumption of β-carotene-rich foods such as carrots and green-leaf vegetables may reduce the risk of myocardial infarction (Kris-Etherton et al., 2002).

Carotenoids are acyclic isomers consisting of numerous conjugated and nonconjugated double bonds arranged in a linear fashion with the ability to scavenge free super oxide radicals. Lycopenes in particular are known to have antioxidant properties and have also been shown to have hypocholesterolemic properties. It has been demonstrated that lycopene renders this effect by decreasing the cholesterol synthesis and LDL formation by inhibiting the 3-hydroxy-3-methylglutaryl-coenzyme A (HMG-CoA) reductase enzyme. Though the exact mechanism is not clear, data from the above-mentioned studies suggest that lycopene decreases the plasma LDL and cholesterol levels and prevents the oxidation of LDL, limiting the damage to critical cellular biomolecules, including lipids, lipoproteins, proteins, and DNA, leading to either inhibition or slowing of the development process of atherosclerosis and its mediated risk (Kris-Etherton et al., 2002; Patil et al., 2009; Riccioni, 2009).

6. ORGANOSULFUR COMPOUNDS

Organosulfur compounds can be derived from both plant and animal sources; sulfur is essential for life, and these compounds are abundant in nature. The most common source of sulfur for humans is through a diet composed of broccoli, cauliflower, cabbage, garlic, onion, meat, eggs, and fish (Sener et al., 2007; Vazquez-Prieto and Miatello, 2010). Organosulfur compounds can be classified based on the functional groups to which sulfur is attached. The allium genus of flowering plants, which includes garlic and onions, contains important compounds such as cysteine sulfoxides and γ-glutamylcysteines. The hydrolysis of cysteine sulfoxides accounts for the flavor and pungency of garlic and onions (Vazquez-Prieto and Miatello, 2010). The cysteine sulfoxides are of four types: alliin, methiin, propiin, and isoalliin. Onions are especially rich in isoallin, whereas garlic is rich in alliin. Alliin is converted into allicin by a hydrolyzing enzyme when garlic cells are crushed during chewing or cooking. Allicin is a very unstable compound that can be readily converted to more stable compounds depending on the conditions; for example, it is converted to dithiin when extracted with oil, ajoene when extracted with ethanol, and diallyl disulfide/diallyl trisulfide or S-allylcysetine/S-allylmercaptocysteine when extracted with aqueous solutions (Sener et al., 2007; Vazquez-Prieto and Miatello, 2010). Experimental evidence demonstrates that all allicin-derived compounds have similar antibiotic, antioxidant, antithrombic, and lipid-lowering properties. Indeed, these properties are thought to render protection against various chronic disease conditions such as hypertension, atherosclerosis, obesity, and related diseases (Sener et al., 2007; Vazquez-Prieto and Miatello, 2010).

Clinical studies suggest that supplementing diets with garlic to elevate blood allicin levels can significantly reduce systolic blood pressure in hypertensive patients (Kris-Etherton et al., 2002; Sener et al., 2007). Although the mechanism(s) of protection remains unknown, data strongly indicate that the main beneficial effect stems from its antioxidant property. Organosulfur compounds decrease ROS levels by inhibiting ROS generating systems, such as nicotinamide adenine dinucleotide phosphate (NADPH) oxidase, or preventing the degradation of antioxidant enzymes, such as glutathione S-transferase. Additionally, organosulfur compounds can increase the bioavailability of NO by increasing eNOS expression or preventing the formation of NO/peroxynitrite (ONOO$^-$; Kris-Etherton et al., 2002; Vazquez-Prieto and Miatello, 2010). Other evidence indicates that organosulfur compounds can inhibit ACE, which will increase vasodilation and decrease peripheral resistance, leading to decrease in blood pressure, and limit endothelial injury, demonstrating their antihypertensive properties. Finally, organosulfur compounds have also been shown to reduce the risk of acute vascular inflammation and atherosclerosis. Although the mechanism is not fully elucidated, *in vitro* models suggest that organosulfur compounds work to inhibit cyclooxygenase, HMG-CoA, and platelet aggregation (Vazquez-Prieto and Miatello, 2010).

7. POLYUNSATURATED FATTY ACIDS

Fatty acids are carboxylic acids consisting of a long aliphatic hydrocarbon chain that is either saturated or unsaturated. The unsaturated fatty acids can be $n-3$ or $n-6$ PUFAs based on the position of the double bonds present. $n-3$ PUFAs have a double bond at the third carbon atom from the terminal methyl, whereas $n-6$ PUFAs have the double bond at the sixth carbon atom. The role of fatty acids in structure and function of the cell is well defined. While fatty acids are known as integral components of cell and organelle membranes, they are also an important source of energy for the cell, especially for cardiac muscles, and play an important role in signal transduction, most importantly via $n-3$ and $n-6$ PUFAs. The effects of $n-3$ and $n-6$ PUFA on cardiovascular systems are discussed in the following section.

7.1 $n-3$ PUFA

α-Linolenic acid (18:3n3, ALA), ecosapentaenoic acid (20:5n3, EPA), and docosahexaenoic acid (22:6n3, DHA) are the most important of the $n-3$ PUFA not synthesized in the human body. ALA is a plant-derived PUFA that is essential in mammals and is the precursor for the synthesis of long chain $n-3$ PUFA. ALA gets converted to EPA or DHA in endoplasmic reticulum by the action of desaturase and elongase enzymes (Rodriguez-Leyva et al., 2010). Other members of this family include ecosatrienoic acids, ecosatetraenoic acids, stearidonic acid, docosapentaenoic acids, tetracosapentaenoic acids, and tetracosahexaenoic acids. Green leaves, canola oil, soybean oil, flaxseed, nuts, and oily fish are the main sources of ALA in the diet. Other common sources are food products enriched with $n-3$ (omega-3) PUFA, such as eggs, breads etc.

The importance of dietary $n-3$ PUFA in the reduction of CVD has been recognized for many years. Its protective role was first demonstrated in studies reporting lower CVD-mediated mortality in Greenland Inuits, who have a higher dietary fish oil intake compared to Americans and Danes (Dyerberg and Bang, 1979). Similarly, people living in Japan and Nunavik have a lower incidence of thrombotic events and mortality due to CVD (Yokoyama et al., 2007). The beneficial results are attributed to the effects of PUFA on the lipid profile. Fish oil consumption in the diet is therefore inversely related to coronary heart disease mortality. More recently, data from a randomized, double-blind, placebo-controlled trial, the 'GISSI-HF Trial,' demonstrated that $n-3$ PUFA supplementation was associated with reduced mortality and admission to hospital for cardiovascular reasons in patients receiving standard treatment for heart failure (Tavazzi et al., 2008). These results demonstrate the added advantage of $n-3$ PUFA supplements on current treatment of heart failure (Tavazzi et al., 2008). Positive results from these studies led to numerous subsequent studies investigating the cardioprotective effects of $n-3$ PUFA in animal models. Experimental studies have demonstrated a broad range of overlapping cardiovascular effects attributed to $n-3$ PUFA that account for the improved outcomes. Several mechanisms have been proposed to explain the cardioprotective effects of $n-3$ PUFA, most notably of EPA and DHA (Hirafuji et al., 2003). These include effects on resting heart rate, eicosanoid signaling and gene expression, antiarrhythmic properties, antiatherogenic effects, reduced blood pressure, increased blood clotting factor (fibrin), decreased plasma triacylglycerol, altered membrane microdomains, and arterial cholesterol levels (Egert and Stehle, 2011; Shukla et al., 2010).

However, not all studies have shown beneficial effects of $n-3$ PUFA in preventing overall risk of cardiac events. Some studies also report ineffectiveness of $n-3$ fatty acid supplements in prevention of CVD. For example, no significance was observed in any coronary heart disease including nonfatal myocardial infarction (MI), sudden cardiac death, coronary artery bypass grafting, or angioplasty in the Health Professionals' Follow-up Study (Ascherio et al., 1995). Other studies have also shown that there is marginal or no correlation between fish intake and reduced risk of fatal MI, nonsudden cardiac death, and total cardiovascular mortality (Marchioli et al., 2002). These differences may be partially attributed to the particular study design as some studies were performed in populations with a high baseline intake of $n-3$ PUFA and others in populations with lower doses of EPA and DHA. Many additional confounding factors include alcohol consumption, exercise habits, and misclassification of dietary saturated fatty acids or $n-6$ PUFA. Whether $n-3$ PUFAs are beneficial in preventing CVDs or not is still being debated; however, the majority of the literature strongly indicates that $n-3$ PUFAs are cardioprotective.

7.2 $n-6$ PUFA

Linoleic acid (18:2n6, LA) is the primary source of the essential $n-6$ PUFA. Dietary sources of $n-6$ fatty acids are abundantly present in liquid vegetable oils, including soybean, corn, sunflower, safflower, and cotton seed oils. LA is converted to arachidonic acid (20:4n6, AA) by desaturation and elongation via enzyme systems within the body. Importantly, both $n-6$ and $n-3$ PUFAs compete for the rate-limiting desaturase for conversion to longer chain PUFA. Therefore, an overabundance of LA will limit the conversion of ALA to EPA or DHA, thereby influencing physiological events.

Controversy exists in studies reporting the effects of $n-6$ PUFA on CVD. Early epidemiological studies demonstrated that a higher intake of LA reduced the risk of coronary heart diseases, while a lower dietary intake of LA was associated with a higher incidence of myocardial infarction (Roels, 1967). In the 1960s and again in the 1980s, Western countries recommended the replacing of saturated fatty acids with unsaturated fatty acids, which resulted in an increased intake of linoleic acid and a significant reduction in the mortality rates (Stephen and Wald, 1990). This has since been attributed to the $n-6$ PUFAs that are produced from cytochrome P450 (CYP) epoxygenases, reported to be cardioprotective in animal models (Seubert et al., 2006). CYP epoxygenase metabolites of AA, epoxyeicosatrienoic acids (EETs), are important components of many intracellular signaling pathways in both cardiac and extracardiac tissues (Spector and Norris, 2007). For example, EETs activate Ca^{2+}-sensitive K^+ channels (BKCa) in vascular smooth muscle cells resulting in hyperpolarization of the resting membrane potential and vasodilation of the coronary circulation (Seubert et al., 2007; Spector and Norris, 2007). EETs have been shown to have anti-inflammatory, thrombolytic, and angiogenic properties within the vasculature. Moreover, drugs that prevent degradation of EETs have been shown to reverse pathological cardiac hypertrophy in animal models (Imig and Hammock, 2009).

Contrary to the beneficial effects of CYP epoxygenase metabolites $n-6$ PUFA, a higher intake of LA has been associated with a high risk of heart disease by shifting the physiological state to a more pathogenic state (Haag, 2003). This is partially attributed to the metabolism of $n-6$ PUFA by cyclooxygenase and lipoxygenase enzymes that produce proinflammatory, prethrombotic, and proconstrictive eicosanoids (Haag, 2003). These eicosanoid products are biologically active in very small amounts and contribute to effects such as increased blood viscosity, thrombosis, vasospasm, vasoconstriction, and decreased bleeding time, which increases the risk of CVD (Simopoulos, 2008). Overall, the effect of $n-6$ PUFA on CVD depends on the individual metabolite.

7.3 $n-6$ to $n-3$ Ratio

The beneficial and detrimental outcomes of PUFA are ultimately dependent upon the ratio of $n-6/n-3$ PUFA (Simopoulos, 2006). As described earlier, an abundance of $n-6$ PUFA will limit the elongation of $n-3$ PUFA, thereby limiting the beneficial effects of $n-3$ PUFA. Humans evolved consuming a diet that contained roughly equal amounts of $n-3$ and $n-6$ PUFA (Simopoulos, 2006). However, over the last two centuries, there has been a dramatic increase in the consumption of vegetable oils, which has resulted in an increased intake of the $n-6$ fatty acids (Simopoulos, 2006, 2008). Today, in Western diets, the ratio of $n-6$ to $n-3$ fatty acids ranges from approximately 20–30:1 instead of the traditional range of 1–2:1 (Simopoulos, 2006). Studies indicate that a high intake of $n-6$ fatty acids shifts the physiologic state to one that is prothrombotic and proaggregatory, characterized by increase in blood viscosity, vasospasm, and vasoconstriction and decrease in bleeding time (Simopoulos, 2006). $n-3$ Fatty acids, however, have anti-inflammatory, antithrombotic, antiarrhythmic, hypolipidemic, and vasodilatory properties. These beneficial effects of $n-3$ fatty acids have been shown in the secondary prevention of CVD.

The balance between $n-3$ and $n-6$ PUFA can be achieved by replacing $n-6$-rich diets with $n-3$ rich food. To restore balance and receive the benefits of $n-3$ PUFA, the American Heart Association (AHA) recommends 1 g day^{-1} EPA + DHA for individuals with known coronary heart disease, and consumption of two meals per week of oily fish + oils rich in ALA for persons without known coronary heart disease. AHA also recommends 2–4 g day^{-1} of EPA and DHA in capsule form for individuals with hypertriglyceridemia. Recent recommendations suggest the intake of at least 250 mg day^{-1} of EPA and DHA as part of a management program for prevention of CVD.

8. CONCLUSION

Dietary patterns that include the consumption of fruit, vegetables, whole grains, and certain lipids are positively associated with beneficial health effects that reduce morbidity and mortality from CVD. The intent of this brief chapter is to highlight the emerging evidence suggesting how 'bioactive compounds' found in foods can have a favorable effect in the prevention of cardiovascular disorders. While epidemiological evidence suggests that they have beneficial effects, and the use of dietary supplements, functional foods and nutraceuticals is increasing, there remain many unanswered questions. For example, does a purified 'bioactive compound' have the same beneficial effect as bioactive compounds obtained from whole food sources? Our current level of understanding supports a balanced diet approach, which involves obtaining bioactive compounds from multiple food sources to achieve the nutritional dose necessary to maintain optimal health. Importantly, there remains a lack of evidence to support using many of these bioactive compounds at therapeutic dosing levels. A further understanding of efficacy and long-term safety of many bioactive compounds is required.

RELEVANT WEBSITE

http://www.heart.org – American Heart Association, Learn and Live.

REFERENCES

Ascherio, A., Rimm, E.B., Stampfer, M.J., Giovannucci, E.L., Willett, W.C., 1995. Dietary intake of marine N-3 fatty acids, fish intake, and the risk of coronary disease among men. The New England Journal of Medicine 332 (15), 977–982.

Cederroth, C.R., Zimmermann, C., Beny, J.L., et al., 2010. Potential detrimental effects of a phytoestrogen-rich diet on male fertility in mice. Molecular and Cellular Endocrinology 321 (2), 152–160.

Das, D.K., Maulik, N., 2006. Resveratrol in cardioprotection: a therapeutic promise of alternative medicine. Molecular Interventions 6 (1), 36–47.

Dyerberg, J., Bang, H.O., 1979. Lipid metabolism, atherogenesis, and haemostasis in Eskimos: the role of the prostaglandin-3 family. Haemostasis 8 (3–5), 227–233.

Egert, S., Stehle, P., 2011. Impact of N-3 fatty acids on endothelial function: results from human interventions studies. Current Opinion in Clinical Nutrition and Metabolic Care 14 (2), 121–131.

Geleijnse, J.M., Launer, L.J., Van der Kuip, D.A., Hofman, A., Witteman, J.C., 2002. Inverse association of tea and flavonoid intakes with incident myocardial infarction: the Rotterdam study. American Journal of Clinical Nutrition 75 (5), 880–886.

Guang, C., Phillips, R.D., 2009. Plant food-derived angiotensin I converting enzyme inhibitory peptides. Journal of Agricultural and Food Chemistry 57 (12), 5113–5120.

Haag, M., 2003. Essential fatty acids and the brain. Canadian Journal of Psychiatry 48 (3), 195–203.

Hertog, M.G., Feskens, E.J., Hollman, P.C., Katan, M.B., Kromhout, D., 1993. Dietary antioxidant flavonoids and risk of coronary heart disease: the Zutphen Elderly study. Lancet 342 (8878), 1007–1011.

Hirafuji, M., Machida, T., Hamaue, N., Minami, M., 2003. Cardiovascular protective effects of N-3 polyunsaturated fatty acids with special emphasis on docosahexaenoic acid. Journal of Pharmacological Sciences 92 (4), 308–316.

Imig, J.D., Hammock, B.D., 2009. Soluble epoxide hydrolase as a therapeutic target for cardiovascular diseases. Nature Reviews. Drug Discovery 8 (10), 794–805.

Joshipura, K.J., Ascherio, A., Manson, J.E., et al., 1999. Fruit and vegetable intake in relation to risk of ischemic stroke. Journal of the American Medical Association 282 (13), 1233–1239.

Kris Etherton, P.M., Hecker, K.D., Bonanome, A., et al., 2002. Bioactive compounds in foods: their role in the prevention of cardiovascular disease and cancer. American Journal of Medicine 113, 71S–88S Suppl. 9B.

Leifert, W.R., Abeywardena, M.Y., 2008. Cardioprotective actions of grape polyphenols. Nutrition Research 28 (11), 729–737.

Liu, R.H., 2003. Health benefits of fruit and vegetables are from additive and synergistic combinations of phytochemicals. American Journal of Clinical Nutrition 78 (Suppl. 3), 517S–520S.

Marchioli, R., Barzi, F., Bomba, E., et al., 2002. Early protection against sudden death by N-3 polyunsaturated fatty acids after myocardial infarction: time-course analysis of the results of the gruppo italiano per lo studio Della sopravvivenza nell'infarto miocardico (GISSI)-prevenzione. Circulation 105 (16), 1897–1903.

Montenegro, M.F., Pessa, L.R., Tanus-Santos, J.E., 2009. Isoflavone genistein inhibits the angiotensin-converting enzyme and alters the vascular responses to angiotensin I and bradykinin. European Journal of Pharmacology 607 (1–3), 173–177.

Patil, B.S., Jayaprakasha, G.K., Chidambara Murthy, K.N., Vikram, A., 2009. Bioactive compounds: historical perspectives, opportunities, and challenges. Journal of Agricultural and Food Chemistry 57 (18), 8142–8160.

Riccioni, G., 2009. Carotenoids and cardiovascular disease. Current Atherosclerosis Reports 11 (6), 434–439.

Rodriguez-Leyva, D., Dupasquier, C.M., McCullough, R., Pierce, G.N., 2010. The cardiovascular effects of flaxseed and its omega-3 fatty acid, alpha-linolenic acid. Canadian Journal of Cardiology 26 (9), 489–496.

Roels, O.A., 1967. Linolenic acid and coronary heart disease. Nutrition Reviews 25 (2), 37–39.

Sener, G., Sakarcan, A., Yegen, B.C., 2007. Role of garlic in the prevention of ischemia-reperfusion injury. Molecular Nutrition and Food Research 51 (11), 1345–1352.

Seubert, J.M., Sinal, C.J., Graves, J., et al., 2006. Role of soluble epoxide hydrolase in postischemic recovery of heart contractile function. Circulation Research 99 (4), 442–450.

Seubert, J.M., Zeldin, D.C., Nithipatikom, K., Gross, G.J., 2007. Role of epoxyeicosatrienoic acids in protecting the myocardium following ischemia/reperfusion injury. Prostaglandins and Other Lipid Mediators 82 (1–4), 50–59.

Shukla, S.K., Gupta, S., Ojha, S.K., Sharma, S.B., 2010. Cardiovascular friendly natural products: a promising approach in the management of CVD. Natural Product Research 24 (9), 873–898.

Simopoulos, A.P., 2006. Evolutionary aspects of diet, the omega-6/omega-3 ratio and genetic variation: nutritional implications for chronic diseases. Biomedicine and Pharmacotherapy 60 (9), 502–507.

Simopoulos, A.P., 2008. The omega-6/omega-3 fatty acid ratio, genetic variation, and cardiovascular disease. Asia Pacific Journal of Clinical Nutrition 17 (Suppl. 1), 131–134.

Spector, A.A., Norris, A.W., 2007. Action of epoxyeicosatrienoic acids on cellular function. American Journal of Physiology. Cell Physiology 292 (3), C996–C1012.

Stephen, A.M., Wald, N.J., 1990. Trends in individual consumption of dietary fat in the United States, 1920–1984. American Journal of Clinical Nutrition 52 (3), 457–469.

Tavazzi, L., Maggioni, A.P., Marchioli, R., et al., 2008. Effect of N-3 polyunsaturated fatty acids in patients with chronic heart failure (the GISSI-HF trial): a randomised, double-blind, placebo-controlled trial. Lancet 372 (9645), 1223–1230.

Vazquez-Prieto, M.A., Miatello, R.M., 2010. Organosulfur compounds and cardiovascular disease. Molecular Aspects of Medicine 31 (6), 540–545.

Woodman, O.L., Chan, E., 2004. Vascular and anti-oxidant actions of flavonols and flavones. Clinical and Experimental Pharmacology and Physiology 31 (11), 786–790.

Yokoyama, M., Origasa, H., Matsuzaki, M., et al., 2007. Effects of eicosapentaenoic acid on major coronary events in hypercholesterolaemic patients (JELIS): a randomised open-label, blinded-endpoint analysis. Lancet 369 (9567), 1090–1098.

CHAPTER 29

A Critical Appraisal of the Individual Constituents of Indian Diet in Modulating Cardiovascular Risk

P.L. Palatty*, A.R. Shivashankara*, J.J. Dsouza*, N. Mathew*, R. Haniadka*, B. Mathai†, M.S. Baliga*
*Father Muller Medical College, Mangalore, Karnataka, India
†St. John's Pharmacy College, Bangalore, Karnataka, India

1. INTRODUCTION

Information accrued from surveys conducted in the recent past suggests that cardiovascular diseases (CVD) is a major problem in India and contributes to nearly 27% of all deaths annually (Gupta et al., 2006). Additionally, reports also suggest that the incidence of CVD is increasing in both rural and urban populations and, more worryingly, in people of the younger age group (Gupta et al., 2006). Further, the increase in life expectancy, rapid urbanization, and affluence, changes in life style and dietary practice, and increase in the use of tobacco and alcohol are all factors contributing to CVD (Sivasankaran, 2010). Reports suggest major differences in CVD mortality rates in different Indian states and that they were the lowest in the underdeveloped Himalayan states of Nagaland, Meghalaya, Himachal Pradesh, and Sikkim, and high in the developed states of Andhra Pradesh, Tamil Nadu, Punjab, and Goa (Gupta et al., 2006). Critical analysis indicates that these differences in the mortality rates are due to the varied lifestyle and the diet of the respective areas.

2. THE INDIAN DIET AND CUISINE

The Indian cuisine is arguably the most diverse in the world. It is a blend of both vegetarian and nonvegetarian components and has been influenced over the centuries by the Arab and Chinese traders and by invaders such as the Greeks, Persians, Mongolians, Turks, British, French, and Portuguese. In today's India, nonvegetarians and vegetarians (in the form of semivegetarians, lacto-ovo vegetarians and vegans) are found in different proportions in each region. The typical Indian diet, which was predominantly vegetarian, was rich in fibers, and antioxidants, and low in calories. However, with the nutritional transition, today there is increased consumption of sugars, salt, high-fat dairy products, eggs, red meat, fast foods with trans fat, and heavy ghee (clarified

© 2013 Elsevier Inc.
All rights reserved.

butter)–based sweets containing oxidized cholesterol and hydrogenated fat. In the following section, the individual components of the Indian diet (cereals, pulses, fruits, vegetables, meat, fish, and oil) and their roles in CVD are critically addressed.

3. CEREALS

Cereals are an integral component of the Indian diet and contribute to around 30% of the total energy intake. The consumption of cereals differs from place to place and in accordance with availability. While wheat is the staple diet of the Northern and Western states of India, rice is the predominant cereal of the South and the Eastern regions. In addition to wheat and rice, other cereals such as millets, maize, corn, and barley are also consumed but in lesser proportions. Phytochemically, cereals are known to contain several nutrients reported to be effective in reducing the various risk factors for coronary heart disease (CHD). Cereals contain linoleic acid, fibers, vitamin E, selenium, folates, phytoestrogens, and phenolic acids, which have been shown to be effective in reducing CVD. They also contain polyunsaturated fatty acids and fibers, which lower the low–density lipoprotein cholesterol (LDL-C); vitamin E and selenium are effective antioxidants; and folic acid is effective in lowering plasma homocysteine. Phenolics, such as flavonoids, and ferulic acids; and carotenoids such as lutein, zeaxanthin, and β–cryptoxanthin possess antioxidant effects and contribute to the beneficial effects of cereals (Adom et al., 2003).

Studies have also shown that consumption of whole wheat and rice yields beneficial effects, while intake of the same amount of the refined grain products containing starch, but lesser amounts of dietary fiber, vitamins, minerals, essential fatty acids, phytochemicals and antioxidants, is not as beneficial in preventing CVD. Consumption of whole grain products, such as whole wheat breads, brown rice, oats and barley, results in a lower glycemic index than the consumption of refined grains because the loss of bran and pulverization of the endosperm in the latter facilitates faster digestion and absorption leading to a more rapid, and larger, increase in the concentrations of blood glucose and insulin (Hu et al., 2003; Harris and Kris-Etherton, 2010). Refining removes the bio-protective substances, such as linoleic acid, folate, and fibers that are reduced by half and the levels of selenium and vitamin E by more than three-fourths (Hu et al., 2003). Regular consumption of whole wheat is reported to reduce the plasma fasting cholesterol and LDL-C to reduce the blood glucose levels and blood pressure (Truswell, 2002; Harris and Kris-Etherton, 2010), while rice that contains hemicelluloses (soluble fiber), γ-oryzanol (fatty acid), tocotrienols, and ferulic acid has been shown to decrease the plasma total cholesterol and to bind bile acids (Truswell, 2002).

Studies have also shown that sparingly used grains, such as barley, to reduce the plasma total and LDL cholesterol (Truswell, 2002); maize to decrease the postprandial glycemic and to stimulate insulinemic responses (Adom et al., 2003); ragi (finger millet) to decrease the hypercholesterolemia and hyperglycemia associated with diabetes (Shobana et al.,

Table 29.1 Sources and Effects of Dietary Fibers

Compound	Sources	Effects
Soluble fiber: pectins and gums: fermented in GIT	Oat bran, oatmeal, beans, peas, rice bran, barley, citrus fruits, strawberries, fruit juices and apple pulp	When eaten regularly as part of a diet low in saturated fat, *trans* fat and cholesterol decreased risk of cardiovascular disease; modestly decreased LDL-C. Compared to insoluble fibers, less effective (American Heart Association; Lairon et al., 2005; Vasudevan et al., 2011)
Insoluble fiber: cellulose, hemicellulose, lignans; absorb water in the colon and are metabolically inert	whole-wheat breads, wheat cereals, wheat bran, rye, rice, barley, most other grains, cabbage, beets, carrots, Brussels sprouts, turnips, cauliflower and apple skin	Associated with decreased cardiovascular risk and slower progression of cardiovascular disease in high-risk individuals. Reduce serum cholesterol, prevent hyperglycemia and obesity, decrease homocysteine, TG, apo B (Lairon et al., 2005; Vasudevan et al., 2011)

2010); proso millet (common millet or white millet) to decrease plasma triglycerides (Lee et al., 2010) and to increase the plasma high-density lipoprotein (HDL) cholesterol (Lairon et al., 2005); and sorghum to improve HDL to non–HDL cholesterol equilibrium and to possess antithrombotic effects (Lairon et al., 2005). Grains also contain considerable amounts of dietary fibers, which reduce the risk of cardiovascular disease (Table 29.1). Dietary fibers from cereals have been shown to be associated with a lower body mass index, blood pressure, and homocysteine concentration (Lairon et al., 2005).

4. PULSES

Pulses are an integral part of the Indian diet and every course of meal contains at least one item prepared from pulses. Green gram, urad dal, chana dal, chickpea, green gram, and horse gram are some of the most commonly consumed pulses. Scientific studies have shown that *Phaseolus vulgaris* (the kidney beans) decreases serum triglycerides, free fatty acids, phospholipids, total cholesterol, and very-low-density lipoprotein (VLDL) and LDL cholesterol, and yields better antidiabetic effects than glibenclamide (Venkateswaran et al., 2002; Boualga et al., 2009). Regular consumption of chickpea and lentil is shown to decrease the levels of plasma VLDL and activity of adipose tissue lipoprotein lipase; they are also a rich source of dietary fibers that cause a reduction in serum total cholesterol (Pittaway, 2008). Soya beans, which are a recent inclusion in the Indian diet, are low in saturated fats and contain enormous amounts of dietary fibers and isoflavonoids, shown to be effective in decreasing serum cholesterol, and reducing hypertension, dyslipidemia, and insulin resistance factors, all of which contribute to the development of CHD (Pittaway, 2008).

Vicia faba (broad bean, fava bean) has also been shown to decrease the serum glucose, insulin, triglycerides, total cholesterol (TC), LDL-C, and VLDL-C values in hypercholesterolemic patients (Pittaway, 2008). The phytochemicals amoenin, quercetin, kaempferol present in *V. faba* have been shown to increase the fecal excretion of steroids, reduce hyperlipidemia and to increase the elasticity of the blood vessels (Pittaway, 2008). *Vigna mungo* (black gram) is reported to decrease the activity of HMG-CoA reductase, increase biliary excretion, decreased absorption of dietary cholesterol, and concomitantly reduce the serum TC, VLDL-C, LDL-C, and TG levels, which contributes to the cardioprotective effects of this pulse (Solanki and Jain, 2010). Studies have also shown that *Vigna angularis* (the azuki beans) contains polyphenols, such as proanthocyanidins, which are effective in increasing the production of NO and decreasing, blood pressure (Mukai and Sato, 2009).

5. NUTS

Contrary to existing beliefs, numerous studies have shown that a diet high in nuts (such as ground nuts (peanut), cashew, pistachio, almonds and walnuts) are good for the heart and protect against CVD (Lukito, 2001). Groundnut consumption is shown to increase polyunsaturated fatty acids (PUFAs) and mono-unsaturated fatty acids (MUFAs) and to decrease the value of saturated fatty acids (SFAs) in serum (Makni et al., 2010), to reduce postprandial glycemia and the TC/HDL-C and LDL-C/HDL-C ratios, and increase HDL and total antioxidant capacity (Ghadimi et al., 2010), which cumulatively reduces the risk of atherosclerosis. The phytochemicals, phytosterols, phenolic compounds, and resveratrol present in peanuts, have all been individually shown to possess cardioprotective properties (Stephens et al., 2010).

Nuts also contain high amounts of magnesium, copper, folic acid, potassium, fiber, and vitamin E and are known to possess cardioprotective effects (Hu et al., 2003). Nuts are also a rich source of the amino acid arginine, a precursor for the endothelium–derived relaxing factor, nitric oxide (NO). It is probable that the generation of NO may induce vasodilation and inhibit platelet adhesion and aggregation, thereby contributing to the cardioprotective effects (Hu et al., 2003). The ω–3 fatty acids and fiber present in nuts lower the LDL and total cholesterol levels without increasing the triglycerides levels (Makni et al., 2010)

Cashew nuts are reported to be good sources of unsaturated fatty acids, tocopherols, squalene, phytosterols and the phenolic constituents anacardic acid, cardol, cardanol, and 2-methylcardol compounds; they decrease the levels of total cholesterol, LDL, VLDL, TG, phospholipid, and free fatty acid, and increase HDL levels in diabetics (Jaya et al., 2010). Studies have also shown that almond decreases the levels of fasting glucose (Li, 2011), and improves insulin sensitivity (Wien et al., 2010). Almonds are reported to contain phytosterols, such as α and β-carotene, β-cryptoxanthin, lutein, and zeaxanthin, flavonoids, and proanthocyanidins, and these phenolic antioxidants are known to decrease the serum LDL-C, TC, and ApoB100 (Jalali-Khanabadi et al., 2010). Walnuts, which are a relatively less consumed nut are a rich source of PUFA and antioxidants; when consumed in high concentrations, they are reported to decrease the levels of TC and LDL-C (Mishra et al., 2010), to decrease the fasting blood glucose and glyco-sylated hemoglobin, and to increase the insulin level; they are also reported to possess antithrombotic and antiarrhythmic effects (Hu et al., 2003). Studies have also shown that pistachio, which is rich in tocopherols, vitamin C, trans–resveratrol, proanthocyanidins, and the isoflavones daidzein and genistein, decreases the TC/HDL-C and LDL-C/HDL-C ratios and improve endothelium–dependent vasodilatation (Sari et al., 2010).

6. DRY FRUITS

Dry fruits, especially the dates, figs, and raisins, are an integral part of the Indian diet and are used in many sweet dishes and cuisines. Raisins are a rich source of the isoflavones, daidzein and genistein, the antioxidants (vitamins A, C, E, folic acid, β-carotene, sele-nium, zinc), dietary fiber, and polyphenols, and their consumption has been shown to decrease the plasma total cholesterol, LDL-C, TG, and decrease the systolic blood pres-sure (Puglisi et al., 2008). Daily consumption of raisin is also shown to moderately in-crease the serum antioxidant levels and to decrease the serum markers of oxidative stress, thereby reducing the risk of cardiovascular disease (Rankin et al., 2008). Regular consumption of dry dates, rich in essential minerals such as selenium, copper, potassium, zinc, and magnesium; and the phytochemicals such as phenolics, sterols, carotenoids, anthocyanins, procyanidins, and flavonoids, is shown to increase free radical scavenging and to decrease hyperlipidemia (Baliga et al., 2011).

7. SPICES

Spices are an integral part of any Indian food cuisine and several kinds of herbs are added to impart organoleptic properties (flavor, color, and taste) and nutritional value to the food. In general, spices are the dried aromatic parts of the plant, such as the seeds, berries, roots, pods, and at times, the leaves (Lampe, 2003). Some of the most commonly used spices in Indian cooking include, turmeric, ginger, garlic, aniseed, asafetida, black cumin, black mus-tard, cardamom, cinnamon, cloves, coriander, cumin, curry leaf, fennel, fenugreek, Indian cassia, Indian dill or dill large cardamom, Kokum, lemon grass, dried raw mango, mustard, onion, saffron, tamarind, tulsi leaf, yellow mustard, and Xanthoxylum (Lampe, 2003).

Preclinical studies have shown that spices, such as turmeric, ginger, garlic, cardamom, cinnamon, coriander, cumin seeds, curry leaves, fenugreek, Malabar tamarind, black

Table 29.2 Protective Effects of Some of the Commonly Used Indian Spices Against CVD

Spice	Effect on CVD
Cardamon (Elaichi) (*Elattaria cardamomum*)	Antihypertensive, antiplatelet (Iyer et al., 2009)
Cinnamon (Dalchini) (*Cinnamomum verum*)	Antidiabetic, antihyperlipidemic, antihypertensive (Iyer et al., 2009)
Cumin seeds (Jeera) (*Cuminum cyminum*)	Antihyperglycemic, reduce AGE formation (Iyer et al., 2009)
Curry leaves (*Murraya korenigii*)	Antidiabetic, antihyperlipidemic (Iyer et al., 2009)
Coriander (*Coriandrum sativum*)	Antidiabetic, antihyperlipidemic (Iyer et al., 2009)
Garlic (*Allium sativum*)	Antihyperglycemic, antihyperlipidemic, antioxidant, antihypertensive, antiinflammatory, antiplatelet, fibrinolytic; preventing/reversing endothelial lesions (Iyer et al., 2009)
Ginger (*Zingiber officinale*)	Antihyperglycemic, antihyperlipidemic, antioxidant, antihypertensive, antiinflammatory, antiplatelet, fibrinolytic; preventing/reversing endothelial lesions (Iyer et al., 2009)
Fenugreek (Methi) (*Trigonella foenum*)	Antidiabetic, antihyperlipidemic (Iyer et al., 2009)
Tamarind (*Garcinia cambogia*)	Decreased insulin resistance, attenuation of obesity (Iyer et al., 2009)
Turmeric (*Curcuma longa*)	Amelioration of metabolic syndrome, antiatherogenic, antioxidant (Iyer et al., 2009)
Black pepper (*Piper nigrum*)	Antioxidant, attenuation of obesity (Iyer et al., 2009)
Black mustard (*Brassica nigra*)	Antihyperglycemic, beneficial effect of mucilage as dietary fiber (Iyer et al., 2009)
Nutmeg (*Myristica frgrans*)	Increases insulin sensitivity; antihyperlipidemic effect (Iyer et al., 2009)

mustard, black pepper, and nutmeg are useful in the treating multiple symptoms of the metabolic syndrome, such as insulin resistance, diabetes, obesity, altered lipid profile, and hypertension (Srinivasan, 2005). The cardioprotective effects of various Indian spices are summarized in Table 29.2.

8. FRUITS AND VEGETABLES

Vegetables and fruits are important components of the traditional Indian diet. Irrespective of the region, potatoes, onions, cabbages, gerkins, and egg plant are the most commonly used vegetables, while grapes, bananas, mangoes, apple, pomegranate, and oranges along with the native Indian fruits, like jamun, guava, and gooseberry are the most favored fruits. Chemical studies have shown that fruits and vegetables contain dietary fiber, folate, potassium, carotenoids, anthocyanins, flavonoids, sterols, phenol, sulfur-containing compounds, and antioxidant vitamins, all of which have been shown to reduce the risk of CVD (Dauchet et al., 2009). Fruits and vegetables are rich sources of fibers, which have cardioprotective effects (Table 29.1).

Clinical studies have also shown that diets rich in vegetables account for the lower risk of IHD among Indians (Devasagayam et al., 2004). Indigenous Indian fruits such as bael, amla, bimbli, and kokum, also possess medicinal properties and are scientifically reported to possess antioxidant, antidiabetic, antihyperlipidemic, anti-inflammatory, antiplatelet, antiatherogenic, and direct cardioprotective effects (Devasagayam et al., 2004). An interesting observation, which has implications for the incidence of CVD in India, is that the daily fruit and vegetable intake of South Asians (26%) is much lower when compared to the rest of the world (45%) (Goyal and Yusuf, 2006). Additionally, overcooking of vegetables has been a practice in many Indian kitchens and this has shown to reduce both the nutrient and protective contents (Goyal and Yusuf, 2006).

9. OILS AND FATS

Oils and fats are important dietary agents and the preference for visible oil is dependent on the region and community. Oils that are widely in use are coconut, palm, mustard, sesame, sunflower, safflower, corn, and ground nut oils, while dalda (vanaspati, hydrogenated fat), ghee, and butter are also in regular use. Coconut oil and palm oil are widely use in the coastal areas of South India; sunflower oil and safflower oil are used in the North and Northeastern parts of India, and also in some parts of South India (North Karnataka) and Gujarat (West); mustard oil has found wide use in the North and Northeastern parts of India; ground nut oil is used sparingly in parts of South India. Corn and sesame oils are not in common use.

An ideal diet should contain SFA, MUFA, and PUFA in the ratio of 1:1:1 (Vasudevan et al., 2011). The major SFAs present in oils are palmitic acid (C 16), stearic acid (C 18), myristic acid (C 14), and lauric acid (C 12). The unsaturated fatty acids belong to the ω-3, ω-6, or ω-9 series. The major MUFAs present in various oils are oleic acid (18:1, ω-9); linoleic acid (18:2, ω-6). The major PUFAs are α-linolenic acid (18:3, ω-3) (Benson and Devi, 2009).

The major ω-3 FA present in vegetarian oils is α-linolenic acid (ALA), which can form docosahexaenoic acid (DHA) and eicosapentanoic acid (EPA) in our body. Fatty acids of the ω-3 series are found to be effective in preventing CVD and in reducing mortality due to cardiovascular ailments. This has been attributed to their anti-inflammatory, antithrombotic, antiarrhythmic, hypolipidemic, and vasodilator properties, and decreased free radical generation. Most of the commonly used oils such as sunflower oil and safflower oil are rich in PUFA and which belong to the ω-6 series, which have beneficial effects in decreasing serum cholesterol level by inhibiting cholesterol biosynthesis and favoring clearance of cholesterol from circulation. However, ω-6 PUFA increase serum TG level, lead to formation of eicosanoids, which are inflammatory molecules, leading to formation of foam cells and thrombus (Benson and Devi, 2009; Kurup and Rajmohan, 1995). ω-6 PUFA are the molecules most vulnerable to oxidation by free radicals, propagating the chain reaction of lipid peroxidation, and they favor the oxidation of LDL, cause endothelial injury, develop insulin resistance, and are also found to be arrythmogenic. MUFA are much less easily oxidized and generate LDL particles, which are more resistant to oxidation. They also increase the rate of fibrinolysis, and substitution of SFA by MUFA causes a decrease in total LDL-C concentration but not in altering HDL-C (Benson and Devi, 2009; Kurup and Rajmohan, 1995).

There is widespread use of fast foods and baked items in the modern Indian diet, which is thus exposed to the transfats. The use of vanaspati (hydrogenated fat) in the preparation of commercially fried, processed, bakery, and ready-to-eat foods, has made Indians more vulnerable to dyslipidemia, endothelial dysfunction, prothrombotic shift, inflammation, obesity, and insulin resistance, thus leading to atherogenesis and cardiovascular diseases. SFAs are proposed to suppress the LDL receptor and decrease the clearance of cholesterol, to increase serum cholesterol and TG, and to enhance LDL, platelet aggregation (Kurup and Rajmohan, 1995).

The medium-chain fatty acids (lauric acid, myristic acid) predominant fatty acids of coconut oil, are found to have a metabolism different from that of LCSFA, and experimental evidence showing their atherogenic effect are lacking (Hostmark et al., 1980; Kurup and Rajmohan, 1995). More refined oils will have less antioxidant contents. Oils and fats also contain variable amounts of antioxidants (natural/added) and fibers, which influence the effects of oils (besides the FA) on cardiac risk factors and the atherogenesis process.

In India, fat is consumed in invisible and visible forms. Pulses, grains, milk, fish, meats, eggs, condiments, and spices, contribute to the invisible fat sources (Nigam, 2000). Estimates are that the invisible fat intake in the middle income group and lower income group is 8 and 6%, respectively, while that in the rural population is 8% (Nigam, 2000). The cholesterol phantom of the mid-1970s in the Indian kitchen has led to an increased consumption of ω-6 fatty acids in the form of sunflower and safflower oils, and a shift in the ω-6/ω-3 FA ratio, from 4:1 to 16:1, has been seen afterwards (Benson and Devi, 2009; Mitra and Bhattacharya, 2006). The fatty acid composition and effects of various oils and fats on CVD are presented in Table 29.3.

10. FISH AND FISH OILS

Fish is an important source of ω-3 fatty acids viz., DHA, EPA and ALA. The content of these FA in fish is significantly higher when compared to their content in plant oils. Many epidemiological studies have reported that men who ate at least some fish weekly had a lower incidence of CHD mortality rate than men who ate no fish (Kris-Etherton et al., 2002). The cardioprotective effects of fish have also been reported from India (Bulliyya, 2002).

Table 29.3 The Fatty Acid Composition and Effects of Various Oils and Fats on CVD

Type of oil/fat	Composition (% of total FA) (chemical composition of the oils may vary from one region to another and also with the plant variety)	Effects
Coconut	SFA: 86%; mainly lauric acid (C-12), myristic acid (C-14), palmitic acid (C-16), caprylic acid (C-8) and capric acid (C-10) MUFA: 12%; mainly oleic acid (18) PUFA: 2%; mainly linoleic acid (18:2; ω-6)	Rich in SFA. Coconut oil mainly contains medium-chain fatty acids whose metabolism is different from that of LCFA; may not lead to formation of atherosclerotic plaques. Lack of experimental evidence regarding harmful effects. A few authors reported that coconut oil does not increase serum cholesterol and is not atherogenic (Hostmark et al., 1980; Kurup and Rajmohan, 1995). Contradicting reports of increase in serum cholesterol, TG and LDL are also observed (Stucchi et al., 1991)
Palm	SFA: 42%; palmitic acid (C-16), stearic acid (C-18), myristic acid (C-14) MUFA: 52%; mainly oleic acid PUFA: 6%; mainly linoleic acid	Has almost equal percentage of SFA and UFA; scientific studies show that it is nonatherogenic and may be beneficial as an anticlotting agent and provide the benefits of the presence of vitamin E, the antioxidant (Berger, 1983; Tomeo et al., 1995; Truswell et al., 1992)
Mustard	SFA: 34% (stearic acid, palmitic acid) MUFA: 48%; mainly erucic acid = 45% of total oils (ω-9; 22:1) and also oleic acid PUFA: 18%; mainly α-linolenic acid (ω-3; 18:3)	Protective against cardiovascular diseases; reduces serum total and LDL cholesterol. It is rich in antioxidants and thus useful in preventing LDL oxidation (Rastogi et al., 2004)
Sesame	SFA: 12% MUFA: 48%; predominantly oleic acid (18:1; ω-9) PUFA: 40%; Mainly linoleic acid (18:2; ω-6), also traces of linolenic acid	Reduces serum cholesterol; has antihypertensive and antioxidant properties because of the presence of lignans, phenolics and vitamin E (Kita et al., 1995; Sankar et al., 2006)
Sunflower	SFA: 12% (palmitic acid, stearic acid) MUFA: 24% (predominantly oleic acid) PUFA: 64% (predominantly linoleic acid)	Due to high content of PUFA, sunflower oil known to decrease serum cholesterol, but because of the predominance of ω-6 FA, causes increased serum triglycerides and increased free radical generation, and decreased antioxidants (Benson and Devi, 2009; Henning et al., 1996)

Continued

Table 29.3 The Fatty Acid Composition and Effects of Various Oils and Fats on CVD—cont'd

Type of oil/fat	Composition (% of total FA) (chemical composition of the oils may vary from one region to another and also with the plant variety)	Effects
Safflower	SFA: 9% (Palmitic acid, stearic acid) MUFA: 12% (predominantly oleic acid) PUFA: 79% (predominantly linoleic acid)	Effects similar to sunflower oil. (there are two types of safflower that produce different kinds of oil: one high in monounsaturated fatty acid oleic acid, and the other high in polyunsaturated fatty acid linoleic acid) (Neschen et al., 2002; Sato et al., 2000)
Corn	SFA: 13% (predominantly palmitic acid) MUFA: 25% (99% of total MUFA is oleic acid) PUFA: 62% (98% of total PUFA is linoleic acid)	Reduces serum cholesterol, LDL cholesterol, VLDL and small dense LDL. (Leth-Espensen et al., 1988). The phytosterols present in this oil decrease cholesterol absorption, and account for the lowering of cholesterol in addition to the PUFA (Ostlund et al., 2002). Abundance of ω-6 linoleic acid makes it vulnerable to oxidation
Groundnut	SFA: 18% (palmitic acid, stearic acid, lignoceric acid, behenic acid) MUFA: 46% (oleic acid) PUFA: 36% (linoleic acid)	Presence of LCFAs, which raise serum cholesterol; PUFA have a cholesterol-lowering effect; marginal decrease in blood glucose, glycated Hb, cholesterol, LDL, TG, lipid peroxidation, and increase in HDL and antioxidants observed in diabetic animals (Ramesh et al., 2006). Contradicting reports are also available (Satchithanandam et al., 1999). However, absence of ω-3 FA is a drawback of this oil
Dalda (vanaspati; hydrogenated fat)	Transfatty acids+SFA = around 42–87% in Indian vanaspati marketed; abundance of trans fat (elaidic acid: 4–65% in different varieties), also oleic acid, stearic acid, palmitic acid	Observed to increase in risk of CVD (Abbé et al., 2009; Lichtenstein et al., 2003)
Butter	SFA: 75% (palmitic acid, myristic acid, stearic acid, and short chain volatile fatty acids such as butyric acid) MUFA: 20% (oleic acid, palmitoleic acid)	High content of SFA; excessive use is a risk factor for CVD; shown to increase LDL cholesterol and ratio of total cholesterol to HDL (Lichtenstein et al., 2003)

Continued

Table 29.3 The Fatty Acid Composition and Effects of Various Oils and Fats on CVD—cont'd

Type of oil/fat	Composition (% of total FA) (chemical composition of the oils may vary from one region to another and also with the plant variety)	Effects
Ghee (clarified butter)	PUFA: 5% (linoleic acid, linolenic acid) Also, about 280 mg cholesterol/100 g SFA: 75% (palmitic acid) MUFA: 20% (oleic acid) PUFA: 5% (linoleic acid) Also, about 310 mg cholesterol/100 g	High content of SFA; excessive use is a risk factor for CVD shown to increase LDL cholesterol and ratio of total cholesterol to HDL (Peterson, 1987; Singh et al., 1996)

Many randomized clinical trials have shown that consumption of fish or EPA and DHA, and ALA is beneficial and reduces the risk of CVD. ω-3 fatty acids exert their cardioprotective effects by reducing the susceptibility of the heart to ventricular arrhythmia, increasing antithrombogenic action, retarding the growth of atherosclerotic plaque by reducing the expression of adhesion molecules, reducing the platelet-derived growth factor and anti-inflammatory actions, and promoting nitric oxide-induced endothelial relaxation and hypotensive actions (Kris-Etherton et al., 2002).

Fish and fish oil are rich in PUFA, which makes them most vulnerable to oxidative attack. Many preclinical and a few clinical studies have shown increased lipid peroxidation in tissues after the patients were fed fish oil, and amelioration of this effect by vitamin E supplementation. Studies have also observed that fish oil supplementation or a habitual high-fish diet makes the LDL more vulnerable to oxidation (Turini et al., 2001). Authors proposing the beneficial effects of fish against oxidative stress highlight the presence of the natural enzymatic and nonenzymatic antioxidants in it (Jooyandeh and Aberoumand, 2011).

11. MILK AND DAIRY PRODUCTS

Milk and dairy products, such as cheese, paneer, buttermilk, lassi, curd (dahi), yogurt, butter, ghee, and ice cream prepared from milk are an integral part of the Indian diet. Buffalo's milk and cow's milk are the most preferred and prevalent, while yak, goat, and camel milk are also used in certain parts of India. Milk contains essential nutrients such as proteins, carbohydrates (lactose), and fats; minerals such as selenium, iodine, magnesium, potassium, calcium, and phosphorus; and vitamins such as biotin, pantothenic acid, riboflavin, thiamine, vitamin A, vitamin B12, vitamin D, and vitamin K. Milk contains about 33 g of lipid (fat) per liter, of which the triacylglycerols account for about 95%, and they are made up of fatty acids of different lengths (4–24 carbons), degrees of saturation, and positional specificity on the glycerol backbone; the diacylglycerol (about 2% of the lipid fraction), cholesterol ($<0.5\%$), phospholipids (about 1%) and free fatty acids ($<0.5\%$ of total milk lipids)and a variety of phospholipids derived from the mammary plasma membrane around each milk fat globule (German et al., 2009).

Although considered high cholesterol food, milk and dairy products may not be major contributors of dietary cholesterol, as whole milk contains 10–15 mg cholesterol per dl, while skimmed milk with 1% butterfat contains <8 mg dl^{-1} cholesterol. The presence of saturated fatty acids and cholesterol is presumed to be associated with a high risk of coronary heart disease, but scientific evidence is inconclusive (German et al., 2009) and some studies have shown that consumption of milk and dairy products (excluding ghee and butter) was inversely associated with the occurrence of one or several components of the metabolic syndrome (Pfeuffer and Schrezenmeir, 2007).

Whey proteins, amino acids, medium-chain fatty acids, and, in particular, calcium and other minerals may contribute to the beneficial effect of dairy products on both body weight and body fat. Studies have shown that the medium-chain fatty acids improve insulin sensitivity (Pfeuffer and Schrezenmeir, 2007; Phelan and Kerins, 2011). The peptides, calcium, and other minerals present in milk are known to reduce the blood pressure, and when given in a single meal, milk, and whey in specific are reported to possess insulinotropic effects (Pfeuffer and Schrezenmeir, 2007).

Fermented products, such as butter milk, yogurt and lassi, and the probiotic bacteria they contain are shown to decrease the absorption of cholesterol, sphingomyelin of cholesterol and fat, calcium of cholesterol, bile acids, and fat. Proteins, peptides, and bacteria may also reduce plasma cholesterol. Lactose, citrate, proteins, and peptides improve weight control, blood pressure, and plasma lipids indirectly, by improving calcium bioavailability. Furthermore, dairy consumption improves the bioavailability of folate and other secondary plant components (Pfeuffer and Schrezenmeir, 2007). However, recommendations are that the consumption of full fat milk should be reduced, and the quantity of skimmed milk and cheese increased as these are shown to reduce cholesterol and saturated fatty acid intake and to slow the progression of atherosclerosis (Pfeuffer and Schrezenmeir, 2007).

12. SWEETS AND DESSERTS

Depending on the area, community, and religion, various types of sweets are made in India. Most of the sweets are made of refined sugar. However, jaggery (brown sugar) and palm sugar are also used. Sweets are an integral part of the Indian cuisine, and in some communities, they are a necessary item on the breakfast, lunch, and dinner menu. The sweets may be either cooked in milk, water, etc. or fried in dalda, ghee, or oil. Based on the primary ingredients, the sweets can be broadly classified as milk-based, wheat based, rice based, fruit based, besan based, vegetable based, coconut based, and nut based. Ice creams, cakes and puddings, which are traditionally western food items are also popular. In most communities, consumption of sweets is high and the servings increase during the religious and happy occasions, and community events, such as festivals and celebrations. As most sweets contain high proportions of the refined sugar, oil, and fats, they contribute to atherogenesis, obesity, diabetes, and metabolic syndrome and also aggravate the medical conditions.

With regard to the correlation between consumption of sweets and cardiovascular diseases, there are contradicting reports. Some clinical studies have found that higher intake of sugar was associated with increased CVD (Parks and Hellerstein, 2000), while other studies have not found any relation between intake of sweets or desserts and the risk of CVD (Jacobs et al., 1998). Several studies have shown an inverse association between dietary sucrose and HDL cholesterol (Ernst et al., 1980). A diet high in sucrose is shown to be associated with an elevation of plasma triglyceride concentrations (Parks and Hellerstein, 2000). On the basis of overall data obtained from various studies it is recommended that high sugar intake should be avoided (refined sugars < 10% of total calories required), and that more quantity of complex carbohydrates should be included in the diet; foods with essential nutrients should not be replaced with foods high in refined sugars (Vasudevan et al., 2011).

13. MEAT AND MEAT PRODUCTS

India has a considerable population of non vegetarians, and chicken and mutton are the highly preferred meat. Pork, camel's meat, and beef are also consumed but the proportion of people favoring them is comparatively less. Meat-based diets tend to be higher in total fat, and studies have shown that compared to a vegetarian, a nonvegetarian has more chances of coronary heart disease, hypertension, obesity, type II diabetes, diet-related cancers, diverticular disease, constipation, and gall stones (Shiwani et al., 2007). Scientific studies have shown that when compared to the vegetarians the nonvegetarians have decreased cardiovascular fitness, and that consumption of meat increased cholesterol levels and the chances of heart disease (McAfee et al., 2010).

The nutritional composition of meat varies depending on breed, feeding regimen, season, and meat cut (Williams, 2007). Red meat has long been established as an important dietary source of protein and essential nutrients, including iron, zinc, and vitamin B12, but these nutritionally positive aspects are overshadowed by the adverse effects: red meat consumption has been linked to cardiovascular diseases. Table 29.4 represents the fatty acid composition of lean red meat. The meat exerts atherogenic effects mainly because of the high content of SFA and ω-6 FA. The cardiotoxic effects of meat are also attributed to its high content of heme-iron, which generates free radicals and causes oxidative damage. Both unprocessed and processed red meat increase the risk of coronary heart disease when compared to white meat, and processed red meat likely confers a greater risk (McAfee et al., 2010).

Table 29.4 Fatty Acid Composition of Lean Red Meat (Williams, 2007)

Type	SFA (% of total FA)	MUFA (% of total FA)	PUFA (% of total FA)	ω-3 to ω-6 FA ratio (ideal ratio = 1–1.5)
Beef	41	43	16	0.45
Lamb	39	46	15	0.37
Mutton	42	39	19	0.5
Pork	39	42	19	0.14
Chicken	33	47	20	0.13

Clinical studies have observed that consumption of red meat was associated with increased mortality from cardiovascular diseases (Sinha et al., 2009). Red meat consumption has been found to be associated with ischemic heart disease, acute coronary syndrome, stroke, and greater intima–media thickness (Kontogianni et al., 2007). Studies have indicated that higher consumption of total red meat, especially various processed meats, may increase the risk of type II diabetes in women (Song et al., 2004).

Epidemiological studies have also shown that over a period of 20 years, a 50% increase in the risk of CHD was observed in people who were nonvegetarians (Shiwani et al., 2007). Feeding vegetarians with beef, which is high in total fat and saturated fatty acids and cholesterol, caused a 19% increase in total plasma cholesterol because of the increase in LDL cholesterol, whereas HDL cholesterol levels stayed constant over a 2-week period (Knuiman and West, 1982). Studies have also shown that feeding normolipidemic nonvegetarians with a low fat, semi-vegetarian diet for 3 months decreased the total cholesterol, LDL cholesterol, and LDL:HDL ratios, while HDL level and plasma triglycerides stayed constant (Fisher et al., 1986).

Data from the National Sample Survey of India indicate that between 1988 and 2000, there was a 77% increase in animal product consumption in rural areas and a 45% increase in urban areas (Singh, 2011). Also, recent national consumption data indicate that between 2000 and 2006, broiler meat availability increased by about 10% per year (Singh, 2011). A study on young adult women in South India revealed a positive association between consumption of nonvegetarian (meat) food and risk of cardiovascular disease (Thilagamani and Mageshwari, 2010). North Indian nonvegetarian subjects accumulated more body fat and were more prone to diabetes mellitus (Nigam et al., 2007).

14. EGG AND EGG PRODUCTS

Chicken and duck eggs are the best and most affordable sources of proteins in India and the egg yolk is rich in fat (26%), proteins (16%), carbohydrates, vitamins, and minerals. The proportion of saturated and unsaturated fatty acids (as percentage of total FA) is 30 and 70% respectively; palmitic acid (23%), stearic acid (4%), and myristic acid (1%) are the major SFAs; oleic acid (47%) is the predominant MUFA; and linoleic acid (16%) and linolenic acid (2%) are the major PUFAs present. Egg yolk is a source of cholesterol (about 1000–1300 mg/100 g) and lecithin (600 mg/100 g) (Vasudevan et al., 2011). The yellow color is due to lutein and zeaxanthin, which are yellow or orange carotenoids known as xanthophylls. Egg white contains literally no fat and it is rich in proteins, vitamins, carbohydrates, and minerals (Fernandez and Calle, 2010).

An important feature of eggs, which is of interest to nutritionists and medical scientists, is its high cholesterol content. Clinical studies have observed that consumption of up to one egg per day is unlikely to have a substantial overall impact on the risk of CHD or stroke among healthy men and women, and there is an apparent increased risk of CHD associated with higher egg consumption among diabetic patients (Eckel, 2008). There are contradictory findings related to the cholesterol content of egg yolk and its impact on serum cholesterol levels, with some clinical studies reporting elevated cholesterol (Weggemans et al., 2001) and others reporting no adverse impact of egg consumption on cholesterol level (McNamara, 2000).

Studies have shown that the daily consumption of eggs is not associated with increased risk of coronary events after adjusting for other aspects of the diet (low fiber, more SFA, low ratio of ω-3 to ω-6 FA, less antioxidants, etc.) that may predispose toward coronary disease (Kritchevsky and Kritchevsky, 2000). A few Indian studies have observed that egg consumption per se does not have any significant effect on serum cholesterol and incidence of CVD (Chakrabarty et al., 2004). Egg intake has been shown to increase the number of both large LDL and HDL particles while decreasing the concentrations of small LDL subfractions (Mutungi et al., 2010). Increases in large HDL have been reported in adults consuming three eggs per day for 4 weeks (Ata et al., 2010), and in individuals following a weight loss intervention and consuming three eggs per day for 12 weeks (Mutungi et al., 2010).

Studies have demonstrated that hen egg yolk proteins potently inhibited collagen-induced human platelet aggregation in a dose-dependent manner, and that they had a synergistic effect on the inhibition of human platelet aggregation with inhibitors of cGMP-specific and cAMP-specific phosphodiesterases. The antiplatelet and fibrinolytic effects of egg yolk proteins are suggested to be protective against atherogenesis (Cho et al., 2003). Preclinical studies have shown that administration of egg white protein hydrolysates attenuated hypertension in rats (Miguel et al., 2010).

Eggs also contains lutein and zexanthin, two major carotenoids that have antioxidant action (Fernandez and Calle, 2010). Lutein protects against inflammation by decreasing C-reactive protein and other inflammatory markers (Fernandez and Calle, 2010). Eggs in combination with a low-carbohydrate diet have also been shown to decrease insulin resistance and leptin in overweight individuals (Fernandez and Calle, 2010). These findings indicate that eggs reduce the risk of CVD by mitigating the factors that predispose us to CVD.

15. CONSIDERATION OF HIGH SALT INTAKE IN INDIA

High salt intake is associated with a significantly increased risk of stroke and total cardio-vascular disease, mainly by hypertension. Indian meals are rich in salt and the food items such as pickles prepared from brined vegetables, fish, and prawns; and papads are high in salt concentration. Because of imprecision in measurement of salt intake, these effect sizes are likely to be underestimated. Reduction in salt intake has a substantial role in the prevention of cardiovascular disease. Sodium reduction in the diet is shown to reduce blood pressure and CVD (Morrison and Ness, 2011).

Epidemiological studies have shown that the intake of dietary salt in urban South India is higher than the currently recommended. Increasing salt intake is associated with increased risk for hypertension even after adjusting for potential confounders (Radhika et al., 2007). This necessitates recommending steps to reduce salt consumption among populations at high risk. Studies from other parts of India are in conformity with this observation (Haldiya et al., 2010).

16. MICRONUTRIENTS AND CARDIAC HEALTH

In addition to the much highlighted fats and cholesterol, there are other dietary components that play a crucial role in contributing to good health. They are vitamins and minerals. Iron and copper as prooxidants trigger free radical generation (Ford, 2000), while potassium, zinc, selenium, vitamin C, vitamin E, and β-carotenes and vitamin A, as protective antioxidants need to be given due importance in the Indian diet (refer Table 29.5).

17. CONCLUSIONS

A balanced dietary approach incorporating all the necessary nutrients is required to prevent CVD and reduce the risk factors for CVD in India. Diet is one of the chief modifiable risk factors of CVD. Indians mistakenly assume that CVD is the rich man's disease but in reality, it is not so. Easy, convenient, ready-to-eat fast foods (junk food) such as samosas, crisps, chips, pizzas, burgers, which are calorie rich and have poor nutritional value, have become the routine dietary components even in rural India. In particular, the younger age group is getting exposed to such junk food. Dietary habits change from region to region in India. However, the traditional Indian vegetarian diet has all the necessary beneficial ingredients such as antioxidants, minerals, proteins, vitamins, and fibers. No single dietary factor can be held responsible for cardiovascular disease; it is the summative effect of many lifestyle and genetic factors

The increased consumption of fast foods, affluence, and stress has led to the increas in CVD incidence in India. As a result of people migration from their native place to other

Table 29.5 Micronutrients Beneficial to the Heart

Micronutrient	Dietary sources	Effects
Potassium	Sugarcane, jaggery, banana, potato, dates, meat, green leafy vegetables	Antihypertensive (Mitra et al., 2009)
Zinc	Cereals, pulses, leafy vegetables, roots, tubers, nuts, beans	Decreases LDL and VLDL; antioxidant role (Mitra et al., 2009)
Selenium	Meat, milk, leafy vegetables, other plant sources	Antioxidant role (Vasudevan et al., 2011)
Copper	Meat, nuts	Contradictory reports; copper deficiency leads to CVD mainly due to its role in structural maturation of connective tissue (Klevay, 2000)
Vitamin E	Wheat germ oil, sunflower oil, safflower oil, cotton seed oil	Major antioxidant protecting PUFA in membranes (Mitra et al., 2009; Vasudevan et al., 2011)
Beta carotene	Carrots, mango, maize, lentils, dark green leaves, amaranth, spinach	Antioxidant (Vasudevan et al., 2011)
Vitamin C	Citrus fruits, amla, guava, green leafy vegetables	Most important extracellular front line antioxidant (Mitra et al., 2009; Vasudevan et al., 2011)
Niacin	Whole cereals, legumes, dried yeast, meat, fish	Hypolipidemic action (Mitra et al., 2009)
Vitamin B12, pyridoxine, folic acid	Cereals, pulses, egg, milk and milk products, leafy vegetables, yeast, meat	Prevent homocysteinemia (Mitra et al., 2009)
Magnesium	Cereals, beans, leafy vegetables, fish	Reduces LDL-C, antihypertensive effect, prevents hardening of endothelium preventing calcium deposition (Mitra et al., 2009)
Chromium	Yeast, nuts, cereals, green mango, gingelly seed	Antidiabetic; increases HDL (Mitra et al., 2009)

regions of the country (because of their jobs or for other reasons), dietary habits are now no longer traditional, but a confluence not confined to a region. The diet of Indian people is also influenced by attractive advertisements in media. Preventive measures for CVD are a need of the hour, as even children with a smaller body frame are succumbing to diabetes mellitus (DM), hyperlipidemia and hypertension. Proper labeling of food stuffs regarding their calorie content, and composition of nutrients should be made mandatory. Awareness should be created among the public regarding a 'Balanced diet' with emphasizing calorie restriction, reduction of salt intake, consumption of dietary fiber, and avoidance of junk food.

Studies have also shown that when compared to their western counterparts, Indians are predisposed to developing diabetes, hypertension, hyperlipidemia, and CVD and that this is influenced/governed by certain genes (Agarwal, 2001). Indians have a genetic predisposition toward sarcopenic obesity (i.e., having less muscle mass and more abdominal white fat for the same body mass index) and this is a major contributing factor to both metabolic syndrome and CVD (Sivasankaran, 2010; Shah and Mathur, 2010). In addition to genetic factors, changes in lifestyle and the nutritional transition toward a western diet has contributed to the rapid rise in the incidence of CVD. The observations of a positive correlation of cardiovascular disease mortality with prevalence of obesity, and dietary consumption of fats, sugars, milk and its products, and negative correlation with green leafy vegetable intake in Indian populations, validates the hypothesis that change in lifestyle and diet is indeed contributing to the rise in CVD (Gupta et al., 2006).

ACKNOWLEDGMENTS

The authors are grateful to Rev. Fr. Patrick Rodrigus (Director), Rev. Fr. Denis D'Sa (Administrator, Father Muller Medical College), and Dr. Jayaprakash Alva (Dean, Father Muller Medical College) for their unstinted support. Because of space constraints many of the published articles could not be quoted and we express our sincere regret to our esteemed colleagues.

REFERENCES

Abbé, M.R.L., Stender, S., Skeaff, C.M., Ghafoorunissa, T.M., 2009. Approaches to removing trans fats from the food supply in industrialized and developing countries. European Journal of Clinical Nutrition 63, S50–S67.

Adom, K.K., Sorrells, M.E., Liu, R.H., 2003. Phytochemical profiles and antioxidant activity of wheat varieties. Journal of Agricultural and Food Chemistry 51, 7825–7834.

Agarwal, D.P., 2001. Genetic predisposition to cardiovascular diseases. Indian Journal of Human Genetics 1, 233–241.

Ata, S., Barona, J., Kopec, R., Jones, J., Calle, M., Schwartz, S., et al., 2010. Consumption of either one egg or lutein-enriched egg per day increases HDL cholesterol, reduces apolipoprotein B while increasing plasma carotenoids and macular pigment density in adult subjects. The FASEB Journal 24, A92.4.

Baliga, M.S., Baliga, B.R.V., Kandathil, S.M., Bhat, H.P., Vayalil, P.R., 2011. A review of the chemistry and pharmacology of the date fruits (Phoneix dactylifera L.). Food Research International 44 (7), 1812–1822.

Benson, M.K., Devi, Kshama, 2009. Influence of ω-6/ω-3 rich oils on lipid profile and antioxidant enzymes in normal and stressed rats. Indian Journal of Experimental Biology 47, 98–103.

Berger, K.G., 1983. Palm oil. In: Chan Jr., H.T. (Ed.), Handbook of Tropical Oils. Marcel Dekker, New York, p. 445.

Boualga, A., Prost, J., Taleb-Senouci, D., et al., 2009. Purified chickpea or lentil proteins impair VLDL metabolism and lipoprotein lipase activity in epididymal fat, but not in muscle, compared to casein, in growing rats. European Journal of Nutrition 48, 162–169.

Bulliyya, G., 2002. Influence of fish consumption on the distribution of serum cholesterol in lipoprotein fractions: comparative study among fish-consuming and non-fish-consuming populations. Asia Pacific Journal of Clinical Nutrition 11, 104–111.

Chakrabarty, G., Manjunatha, S., Bijlani, R.L., Ray, R.B., Mahapatra, S.C., Mehta, N., et al., 2004. The effect of ingestion of egg on serum lipid profile of healthy young Indians. Indian Journal of Physiology and Pharmacology 48, 286–292.

Cho, H.J., Ham, H.S., Lee, D.S., Park, H.J., 2003. Effects of proteins from hen egg yolk on human platelet aggregation and blood coagulation. Biological and Pharmaceutical Bulletin 26, 1388–1392.

Dauchet, L., Amouyel, P., Dallongeville, J., 2009. Fruits, vegetables and coronary heart disease. Nature Reviews Cardiology 6, 599–608.

Devasagayam, T.P., Tilak, J.C., Boloor, K.K., Sane, K.S., Ghaskadbi, S.S., Lele, R.D., 2004. Free radicals and antioxidants in human health: current status and future prospects. The Journal of the Association of Physicians of India 52, 794–804.

Eckel, R.H., 2008. Egg consumption in relation to cardiovascular disease and mortality: the story gets more complex. American Journal of Clinical Nutrition 87, 799–800.

Ernst, N., Fisher, M., Smith, W., Gordon, T., Rifkind, B.M., Little, J.A., et al., 1980. The association of plasma high-density lipoprotein cholesterol with dietary intake and alcohol consumption. Circulation 62, IV41–IV52.

Fernandez, M.L., Calle, M.C., 2010. Revisiting dietary cholesterol recommendations: does the evidence support a 300 mg/d limit? Current Atherosclerosis Reports 12, 377–383.

Fisher, M., Levine, P.H., Weiner, B., Ockene, I.S., Johnson, B., Johnson, M.H., et al., 1986. The effect of vegetarian diets on plasma lipid and platelets levels. Archives of Internal Medicine 146, 1193–1197.

Ford, E.S., 2000. Serum copper concentration and coronary heart disease among US adults. American Journal of Epidemiology 151, 1182–1188.

German, J.B., Gibson, R.A., Krauss, R.M., Nestel, P., Lamarche, B., van Staveren, W.A., et al., 2009. A reappraisal of the impact of dairy foods and milk fat on cardiovascular disease risk. European Journal of Nutrition 48, 191–203.

Ghadimi, N.M., Kimiagar, M., Abadi, A., Mirzazadeh, M., Harrison, G., 2010. Peanut consumption and cardiovascular risk. Public Health Nutrition 13, 1581–1586.

Goyal, A., Yusuf, S., 2006. The burden of cardiovascular disease in the Indian subcontinent. Indian Journal of Medical Research 124, 235–244.

Gupta, R., Misra, A., Pais, P., Rastogi, P., Gupta, V.P., 2006. Correlation of regional cardiovascular disease mortality in India with lifestyle and nutritional factors. International Journal of Cardiology 108, 291–300.

Haldiya, K.R., Mathur, M.L., Sachdev, R., 2010. Lifestyle-related risk factors for cardiovascular disease in a desert population of India. Current Science 99, 25.

Harris, K.A., Kris-Etherton, P.M., 2010. Effects of whole grains on coronary heart disease risk. Current Atherosclerosis Reports 12, 368–376.

Henning, B., Toborek, M., McClain, C.J., Diana, J.N., 1996. Nutritional implications in vascular endothelial cell metabolism. Journal of the American College of Nutrition 15, 345–358.

Hostmark, A.T., Spydevold, O., Eilertsen, E., 1980. Plasma lipid concentration and liver output of lipoproteins in rats fed coconut fat or sunflower oil. Artery 7, 367–383.

Hu, F.B., 2003. Plant-based foods and prevention of cardiovascular disease: an overview. American Journal of Clinical Nutrition 78, 544S–551S.

Iyer, A., Panchal, S., Poudyal, H., Brown, L., 2009. Potential health benefits of Indian spices in the symptoms of the metabolic syndrome: a review. Indian Journal of Biochemistry & Biophysics 46, 467–481.

Jacobs Jr., D.R., Meyer, K.A., Kushi, L.H., Folsom, A.R., 1998. Whole-grain intake may reduce the risk of ischemic heart disease death in postmenopausal women: the Iowa Women's Health Study. American Journal of Clinical Nutrition 68, 248–257.

Jalali-Khanabadi, B.A., Mozaffari-Khosravi, H., Parsaeyan, N., 2010. Effects of almond dietary supplementation on coronary heart disease lipid risk factors and serum lipid oxidation parameters in men with mild hyperlipidemia. Journal of Alternative and Complementary Medicine 16, 1279–1283.

Jaya, A., Shanthi, P., Sachdanandam, P., 2010. Hypolipidemic activity of *Semecarpus anacardium* in streptozotocin induced diabetic rats. Endocrine 38, 11–17.

Jooyandeh, H., Aberoumand, A., 2011. A review on natural antioxidants in fish: stabilizing effect on sensitive nutrients. Middle East Journal of Scientific Research 7, 170–174.

Kita, S., Matsumura, Y., Morimoto, S., Akimoto, K., Furuya, M., Oka, N., et al., 1995. Antihypertensive effect of sesamin: II. Protection against two-kidney, oneclip renal hypertension and cardiovascular hypertrophy. Biological and Pharmaceutical Bulletin 18, 1283–1285.

Klevay, L.M., 2000. Trace element and mineral nutrition in disease: Ischemic heart disease. In: Clinical Nutrition of the Essential Trace Elements and Minerals: The Guide for Health Professionals, 1st edn, (eds. J.D. Bogden and L.M. Klevay), pp. 251–271, Humana Press Inc., Totowa, N.J.

Knuiman, J.T., West, C.E., 1982. The concentration of cholesterol in serum and in various serum lipopro-teins in microbiotics, vegetarian, and nonvegetarian man and boys. Atherosclerosis 43, 71–82.

Kontogianni, M.D., Panagiotakos, D.B., Pitsavos, C., Chrysohoou, C., Stefanadis, C., 2007. Relationship between meat intake and the development of acute coronary syndromes: the CARDIO2000 case–control study. European Journal of Clinical Nutrition 62, 171–177.

Kris-Etherton, P.M., Harris, W.S., Appel, L.J., 2002. Fish consumption, fish oil, omega-3 fatty acids, and cardiovascular disease. Circulation 106, 2747–2757.

Kritchevsky, S.B., Kritchevsky, D., 2000. Egg consumption and coronary heart disease: an epidemiologic overview. Journal of the American College of Nutrition 19 (90005), 549S–555S.

Kurup, P.A., Rajmohan, T., 1995. Consumption of coconut oil and coconut kernel and the incidence of ath-erosclerosis. In: Coconut and Coconut Oil in Human Nutrition, Proceedings. Symposium on Coconut and Coconut Oil in Human Nutrition. Coconut Development Board, Kochi, India, pp. 35–59.

Lairon, D., Arnault, N., Bertrais, S., Planells, R., Clero, E., Hercberg, S., Boutron-Ruault, M.C., 2005. Dietary fiber intake and risk factors for cardiovascular disease in French adults. American Journal of Clin-ical Nutrition 82 (6), 1185–1194.

Lampe, 2003. Spicing up a vegetarian diet: chemopreventive effects of phytochemicals. American Journal of Clinical Nutrition 78, 579S–583S.

Lee, S.H., Chung, I.M., Cha, Y.S., Park, Y., 2010. Millet consumption decreased serum concentration of triglyceride and C-reactive protein but not oxidative status in hyperlipidemic rats. Nutrition Research 30, 290–296.

Leth-Espensen, P., Stender, S., Ravn, H., Kjeldsen, K., 1988. Antiatherogenic effect of olive and corn oils in cholesterol-fed rabbits with the same plasma cholesterol levels. Arteriosclerosis, Thrombosis, and Vas-cular Biology 8, 281–287.

Li, S.C., Liu, Y.H., Liu, J.F., Chang, W.H, Chen, C.M., Chen, C.Y., 2011. Almond consumption im-proved glycemic control and lipid profiles in patients with type 2 diabetes mellitus. Metabolism 60 (4), 474–479.

Lichtenstein, A.H., Erkkilä, A.T., Lamarche, B., Schwab, U.S., Jalbert, S.M., Ausman, L.M., 2003. Influence of hydrogenated fat and butter on CVD risk factors: remnant-like particles, glucose and insulin, blood pressure and C-reactive protein. Atherosclerosis 171, 97–107.

Lukito, W., 2001. Candidate foods in the Asia-Pacific region for cardiovascular protection: nuts, soy, lentils and tempe. Asia Pacific Journal of Clinical Nutrition 10, 128–133.

Makni, M., Fetoui, H., Gargouri, N., Jaber, H., Boudawara, T., Zeghal, N., 2008. Hypolipidemic and hepa-toprotective effects of flaxseed and pumpkin seed mixture in ω-3 and ω-6 fatty acids in hypercholes-terolemic rats. Food and Chemical Toxicology 46, 3714–3720.

McAfee, A.J., McSorley, E.M., Cuskelly, G.J., Moss, B.W., Wallace, J.M., Bonham, M.P., et al., 2010. Red meat consumption: an overview of the risks and benefits. Meat Science 84, 1–13.

McNamara, D.J., 2000. Dietary cholesterol and atherosclerosis. Biochimica et Biophysica Acta 1529, 310–320.

Miguel, M., Galán, M., García-Redondo, A.B., Roque, F.R., López-Fandiño, R., Salaices, M., 2010. Effects of antihypertensive egg-derived peptides with in vitro ace-inhibitory activity in aorta from rats. Journal of Hypertension 28, e390–e391.

Mishra, N., Dubey, A., Mishra, R., Barik, N., 2010. Study on antioxidant activity of common dry fruits. Food and Chemical Toxicology 48 (12), 3316–3320.

Mitra, A., Bhattacharya, D., 2006. Ethical problems faced in villages of rural Bengal while conducting researches on chronic diseases like diabetes. Indian Journal of Medical Sciences 60, 475–484.

Mitra, A., Pradhan, R., Mukherjee, S., 2009. Importance of heart-healthy diet. Journal of Human Ecology 27, 53–61.

Morrison, A., Ness, R.B., 2011. Sodium intake and cardiovascular disease. Annual Review of Public Health 32, 71–90.

Mukai, Y., Sato, S., 2009. Polyphenol-containing azuki bean (*Vigna angularis*) extract attenuates blood pres-sure elevation and modulates nitric oxide synthase and caveolin-1 expressions in rats with hypertension. Nutrition, Metabolism, and Cardiovascular Diseases 19, 491–497.

Mutungi, G., Waters, D., Ratliff, J., Puglisi, M., Clark, R.M., Volek, J.S., Fernandez, M.L., 2010. Eggs distinctly modulate plasma carotenoid and lipoprotein subclasses in adult men following a carbohydrate-restricted diet. The Journal of Nutritional Biochemistry 21, 261–267.

Neschen, S., Moore, I., Regittning, W., Yu, C.L., Wang, Y., Pypaert, M., et al., 2002. Contrasting effects of fish oil and safflower oil on hepatic peroxisomal and tissue lipid content. American Journal of Physiology and Endocrinology 282, E395–401.

Nigam, A., 2000. Consumption of fat in Indian diet. International Journal of Diabetes in Developing Countries 20, 58–61.

Nigam, S., Koley, S., Sandhu, J.S., Yadav, V.S., Arora, P., 2007. A study on body composition components in vegetarian and non-vegetarian patients with diabetes mellitus. Journal of Human Ecology 22, 53–56.

Ostlund Jr., R.E., Racette, S.B., Okeke, A., Stenson, W.F., 2002. Phytosterols that are naturally present in commercial corn oil significantly reduce cholesterol absorption in humans. American Journal of Clinical Nutrition 75, 1000–1004.

Parks, E.J., Hellerstein, M.K., 2000. Carbohydrate-induced hypertriacylglycerolemia: historical perspective and review of biological mechanisms. American Journal of Clinical Nutrition 71, 412–433.

Peterson, D., 1987. Cholesterol, ghee, and atherosclerosis. Lancet 330 (8565), 970.

Pfeuffer, M., Schrezenmeir, J., 2007. Milk and the metabolic syndrome. Obesity Reviews 8, 109–118.

Phelan, M., Kerins, D., 2011. The potential role of milk-derived peptides in cardiovascular disease. Food & Function 2, 153–167.

Pittaway, J.K., Robertson, I.K., Ball, M.J., 2008. Chickpeas may influence fatty acid and fiber intake in an ad libitum diet, leading to small improvements in serum lipid profile and glycemic control. Journal of American Dietetic Association 108, 1009–1013.

Puglisi, M.J., Vaishnav, U., Shrestha, S., Torres-Gonzalez, M., Wood, R.J., Volek, J.S., et al., 2008. Raisins and additional walking have distinct effects on plasma lipids and inflammatory cytokines. Lipids in Health and Disease 7, 14–22.

Radhika, G., Sathya, R.M., Sudha, V., Ganesan, A., Mohan, V., 2007. Dietary salt intake and hypertension in an urban south Indian population – [CURES – 53]. The Journal of the Association of Physicians of India 55, 405–411.

Ramesh, B., Saravanan, R., Pugalendi, K.V., 2006. Effect of dietary substitution of groundnut oil on blood glucose, lipid profile, and redox status in streptozotocin-diabetic rats. The Yale Journal of Biology and Medicine 79, 9–17.

Rankin, J.W., Andreae, M.C., Oliver Chen, C.Y., O'Keefe, S.F., 2008. Effect of raisin consumption on oxidative stress and inflammation in obesity. Diabetes, Obesity & Metabolism 10 (11), 1086–1096.

Rastogi, T., Reddy, K.S., Vaz, M., Spiegelman, D., Prabhakaran, D., Willett, W.C., et al., 2004. Diet and risk of ischemic heart disease in India. American Journal of Clinical Nutrition 79, 582–592.

Sankar, D., Rao, M.R., Sambandam, G., Pugalendi, K.V., 2006. Effect of sesame oil on diuretics or ß-blockers in the modulation of blood pressure, anthropometry, lipid profile, and redox status. The Yale Journal of Biology and Medicine 79, 19–26.

Sari, I., Baltaci, Y., Bagci, C., Davutoglu, V., Erel, O., Celik, H., et al., 2010. Effect of pistachio diet on lipid parameters, endothelial function, inflammation, and oxidative status: A prospective study. Nutrition 26, 399–404.

Satchithanandam, S., Flynn, T.J., Calvert, R.J., Kritchevsky, D., 1999. Effect of peanut oil and randomized peanut oil on cholesterol and oleic acid absorption, transport, and distribution in the lymph of the rat. Lipids 34 (12), 1305–1311.

Sato, M., Yoshida, S., Nagao, K., Imaizumi, K., 2000. Superiority of dietary safflower oil over olive oil in lowering serum cholesterol and increasing hepatic mRnas for the LDL receptor and cholesterol 7alpha-hydroxylase in exogenously hypercholesterolemic (exHC) rats. Bioscience, Biotechnology, and Biochemistry 64, 1111–1117.

Shah, B., Mathur, P., 2010. Surveillance of cardiovascular disease risk factors in India: the need & scope. Indian Journal of Medical Research 132, 634–642.

Shiwani, A.H., Aziz, A., Hanif, S.M., 2007. Shall we become vegetarian to minimize the risk of coronary heart disease? The Journal of the Pakistan Medical Association 57, 46–48.

Shobana, S., Harsha, M.R., Platel, K., Srinivasan, K., Malleshi, N.G., 2010. Amelioration of hyperglycaemia and its associated complications by finger millet (*Eleusine coracana* L.) seed coat matter in streptozotocin-induced diabetic rats. British Journal of Nutrition 104 (12), 1787–1795.

Singh, P.N., 2011. Chronic disease burden in rural India attributable to diet, obesity, and tobacco use. Journal of Postgraduate Medicine 57, 1–2.

Singh, R.B., Niaz, M.A., Ghosh, S., Beegom, R., Rastogi, V., Sharma, J.P., et al., 1996. Association of trans fatty acids (vegetable ghee) and clarified butter (Indian ghee) intake with higher risk of coronary artery disease in rural and urban populations with low fat consumption. International Journal of Cardiology 56, 289–298.

Sinha, R., Cross, A.J., Graubard, B.I., Leitzmann, M.F., Schatzkin, A., 2009. Meat intake and mortality: a prospective study of over half a million people. Archives of Internal Medicine 169, 562–571.

Sivasankaran, S., 2010. The cardio-protective diet. Indian Journal of Medical Research 132, 608–616.

Solanki, Y.B., Jain, S.M., 2010. Antihyperlipidemic activity of *Clitoria ternatea* and *Vigna mungo* in rats. Pharmaceutical Biology 48, 915–923.

Song, Y., Manson, J.E., Buring, J.E., Liu, S., 2004. A prospective study of red meat consumption and type 2 diabetes in middle-aged and elderly women: the women's health study. Diabetes Care 27, 2108–2115.

Srinivasan, K., 2005. Plant foods in the management of diabetes mellitus: spices as beneficial antidiabetic food adjuncts. International Journal of Food Sciences and Nutrition 56, 399–414.

Stephens, A.M., Dean, L.L., Davis, J.P., Osborne, J.A., Sanders, T.H., 2010. Peanuts, peanut oil, and fat free peanut flour reduced cardiovascular disease risk factors and the development of atherosclerosis in Syrian golden hamsters. Journal of Food Science 75, H116–H122.

Stucchi, A.F., Hennessy, L.K., Vespna, D.B., Weiner, E.J., Osada, J., Ordovas, J.M., et al., 1991. Effect of corn and coconut oil-containing diets with and without cholesterol on high density lipoprotein apoprotein A-I metabolism and hepatic apoprotein A-I mRNA levels in cebus monkeys. Arteriosclerosis and Thrombosis 11, 1719–1729.

Thilagamani, S., Mageshwari, S.U., 2010. Risk appraisal for cardiovascular disease among selected young adult women in Coimbatore, India. Indian Journal of Science and Technology 3, 672–675.

Tomeo, A.C., Geller, M., Watkins, T.R., Gapor, A., Bierenbaum, M.L., 1995. Antioxidant effects of tocotrienols in patients with hyperlipidemia and carotid stenosis. Lipids 30 (12), 1179–1183.

Truswell, A.S., 2002. Cereal grains and coronary heart disease. European Journal of Clinical Nutrition 56, 1–14.

Truswell, A.S., Choudhury, N., Roberts, D.C.K., 1992. Double-blind comparison of plasma lipids in healthy subjects eating potato crisps fried in palm olein or canola oil. Nutrition Research 12, S34–S52.

Turini, M.E., Crozier, G.L., Donnet-Hughes, A., Richelle, M.A., 2001. Short-term fish oil supplementation improved innate immunity, but increased ex vivo oxidation of LDL in man – a pilot study. European Journal of Nutrition 40, 56–65.

Vasudevan, D.M., Sreekumari, S., Vaidyanathan, K., 2011. Textbook of Biochemistry for Medical Students, sixth ed. Jaypee Brothers, New Delhi p. 76, 436.

Venkateswaran, S., Pari, L., Saravanan, G., 2002. Effect of *Phaseolus vulgaris* on circulatory antioxidants and lipids in rats with streptozotocin-induced diabetes. Journal of Medicinal Food 5, 97–103.

Weggemans, R.M., Zock, P.L., Katan, M.B., 2001. Dietary cholesterol from eggs increases the ratio of total cholesterol to high-density lipoprotein cholesterol in humans: a meta-analysis. American Journal of Clinical Nutrition 73, 885–891.

Wien, M., Bleich, D., Raghuwanshi, M., Gould-Forgerite, S., Gomes, J., Monahan-Couch, L., et al., 2010. Almond consumption and cardiovascular risk factors in adults with prediabetes. Journal of the American College of Nutrition 29, 189–197.

Williams, P.G., 2007. Nutritional composition of red meat. http://ro.uow.edu.au/hbspapers/48.

CHAPTER 30

Omega-3 Fatty Acids in Prevention of Cardiovascular Disease in Humans: Chemistry, Dyslipidemia

R. Sharma

Amity University Uttar Pradesh, Noida, India
Florida State University, Tallahassee, FL, USA

1. INTRODUCTION

Two omega-3 fatty acids, docosaexaenoic acid (DHA) and eicosapentanoic acid (EPA) are found in cold-water fish such as mackerel, salmon, herring, trout, sardines, and tuna. Omega fatty acids have been shown to decrease the risk of sudden cardiac death in animal studies and in epidemiologic, metabolic, and small clinical trials(Adamsson et al., 2011; Albert et al., 2010; Bianconi et al., 2011; Brouwer et al., 2003, 2006; Christensen et al., 1999; Dall et al., 2009; Goldstein et al., 2011; Harris, 2009; Harris and Isley, 2001; Harris et al., 2004; Hathcock et al., 2006; Jones and Lau, 2002; Kris-Etherton et al., 2002, 2003; Leaf et al., 2003a,b; Lee et al., 2008; Lichtenstein et al., 2006; Marchioli et al., 2001, 2002, 2005, 2007, 2009, 2010; Mata Lopez et al., 2003; McLennan and Abeywardena, 2005; Mozaffarian, 2008; Okuyama et al., 2000; Rauch et al. 2006; Richter, 2003; Verboom, 2006; Zhao et al. 2009). Now omega-3 fatty acids with statins are under active consideration for approval from federal government agencies based on phase II and III trials (Archer et al., 1998, Daviglus et al., 1997; Genest et al., 2009; Finzi et al., 2011; Galan et al., 2010; Geleijnse et al., 2010; Gissi-HF Investigators et al., 2008; Harrison and Abhyankar, 2005; Heidarsdottir et al., 2010; Heidt et al., 2009; Kowey et al., 2010; Kromhout et al., 2010; Leaf et al., 2005; Macchia et al., 2009; Maresta et al., 1999; Oda et al., 2005; Pratt et al., 2009; Rauch et al., 2006; Savelieva et al., 2011, Tavazzi et al., 2004). These long-chain omega-3 fatty acids from fish oil have been reviewed and shown to reduce serum triglyceride levels and favorably affect platelet function, reduce heart arrhythmia, fibrillation in before and after cardiac injury (Aarsetøy et al., 2008; Bays et al., 2008; Calo et al., 2005; Cleland et al., 2004; Côté et al., 2004; de Roos et al., 2009; Geelen et al., 2005; Geppert et al., 2005; Grundt et al., 2003, 2004; Guallar et al., 1999; Hamaad et al., 2006; Harrison and Abhyankar, 2005; Johansen et al., 1999; Lindman et al. 2004; London et al., 2007; Madsen et al., 2007; Metcalf et al., 2008; Nilsen et al., 1991; O'Keefe et al., 2006; Raitt et al., 2005; Rajaram et al., 2009; Sanders et al., 2006; von Schacky et al., 1999, 2001; Walser and Stebbins, 2008). Different views and adverse reports on success of omega-3 fatty acids (Aarsetøy et al., 2008; Din et al.,

© 2013 Elsevier Inc.
All rights reserved.

2004; Kowey et al. 2010; Pratt et al., 2009; Saravanan et al. 2010) motivated us to contribute present state of art and prospects beyond omega fatty acid supplementation in CVD. Cardiovascular disease (CVD) includes all diseases that affect the heart and blood vessels, such as coronary heart disease (CHD), coronary artery disease, dyslipidemia, and hypertension (Van Horn et al., 2008). CVD remains the number one cause of death in the United States, and prevention of CVD is at the top of the public health agenda.

This chapter is divided into sections on chemistry, synthesis of omega fatty acids, mechanism of cardioprotection by omega fatty acids, and the 'Columbus concept' and futuristic approaches to omega fatty acid therapy. The authors propose the benefits of omega-3 fatty acid-rich foods in the prevention of CVD and revisit the available resources on omega fatty acids.

1.1 Chemistry of Omega Fatty Acids

Alpha-linolenic acid (ALA), a shorter chain omega-3 fatty acid, is the basic unit of a fatty acid. It is found in plant sources, including flaxseed, walnuts, canola oil, and soybeans. ALA may protect against CVD by interfering with the production of proinflammatory eicosanoids (Bistrian, 2004; de Lorgeril et al., 2002; Din et al., 2004; Russo, 2009; Simopoulos, 2009; Wilczynska-Kwiatek et al., 2010). ALA can be converted to omega fatty acids by substitution at the double bond at either the third carbon (called omega-3) or sixth carbon (called omega-6 fatty acid). ALA is converted to omega-3 fatty acid EPA, but only in small amounts (2–5%) in humans; even less is converted to omega-6 fatty acid DHA (<1%) (van Horn et al., 2008). There are many known omega-3 fatty acids (see Table 30.1 and Figure 30.1). The most common omega-3 fatty acids contain 18–22 carbons and a signature double bond at the third position from the methyl (or ω, or omega) end of the molecule. These fatty acids include: (1) omega-3 fatty acid, either plant-derived linolenic acid (ALA, 18:3ω-3), or fish-oil-derived eicosapentaenoic acid (EPA, C20:5ω-3) and docosahexaenoic acid (DHA, 22:6ω-3); and (2) omega-6 fatty acids mainly comprising of linoleic acid (LA, 18:2ω-6) and arachidonic acid (AA, 20:4ω-6). The essential fatty acid ALA cannot be synthesized by humans because they lack the enzymes to act on double bonds at omega-3 or 6 positions.

Table 30.1 Food Sources of Omega Polyunsaturatyed Fatty Acids (PUFA)

Omega-3 linolenic acid: canola oil, soybean products, walnuts, wheat germ, margerine

Omega-6 linoleic acid: leafy vegetables, seed, nuts, grains, safflower oil, sunflower oil, corn oil, soybean oil, cottonseed oil

Common sources: breast milk, fish oil (sardine, mackerel, anchovy, salmon, tuna, swordfish, shellfish)

PUFA (g/100 g): corn oil 56.2; olive oil 7.64; rapeseed oil 33.2; salmon 3.36; soybean oil 60.4; sunflower oil 63; walnuts 43.9

ω-3 PUFA(g/100 g) : corn oil 1.06; olive oil 0.56; rapeseed oil 11.1; salmon 3.01; soybean oil 6.88; sunflower oil 0; walnuts 7.46

ω-6 PUFA(g/100 g) : corn oil 55.2; olive oil 7.07; rapeseed oil 22.1; salmon 0.36; soybean oil 63.5; sunflower oil 63; walnuts 36.4

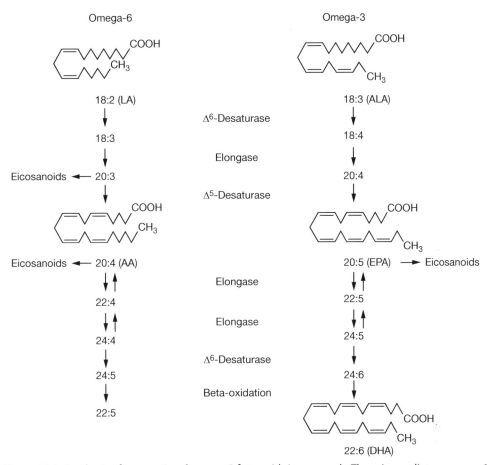

Figure 30.1 Synthesis of omega-6 and omega-3 fatty acids in mammals. The primary dietary omega-6 fatty acid is linoleic acid (LA) which has 18 carbons and 2 double bonds (18:2n-6). Alpha-linolenic acid (ALA) is a short-chain omega-3 fatty acid (18:3n-3) found in plant products such as flaxseed and soybean oils. The final step in the conversion of ALA to docosahexaenoic acid (DHA) is a β-oxidation step converting 24:6n-3 to 22:6n-3. Every day, 1–5% of ALA is converted to eicosapentaenoic acid (EPA), and conversion to DHA is very low (<0.1%) in human. The initial introduction of a double bond into ALA by α6-desaturase is the rate-limiting reaction of the pathway. Although the affinity of α-6-desaturase is higher for ALA than for LA, the typically higher cellular concentrations of LA result in greater net conversion of long-chain omega-6 fatty acids. Diets high in omega-6 fatty acids can reduce the conversion of ALA to EPA and DHA. *Reproduced from Harris, W.S., Sands, S.A., Windsor, S.L., et al., 2004. Omega-3 fatty acids in cardiac biopsies from heart transplantation patients. Circulation 110, 1645–1649, with permission.*

Chemically, omega–3 fatty acids are polyunsaturated fats in which the first double bond counting from the omega carbon is at position 3, hence the name omega–3 (or ω–3). The major omega–3 fatty acids include α-linolenic acid (ALA, 18:3ω–3), EPA (20:5ω–3), and DHA (22:6ω–3), and comprise one of the two classes of essential fatty acids. Preformed EPA and DHA are best obtained from fatty fish or fish–oil supplements.

1.2 Synthesis of Omega-3 Fatty Acids

ALA is converted to EPA and DHA and both are abundant in fish oil (see Figure 30.1).

In the following section, we describe two fatty acids abundant in fish oil. The activity of omega-3 fatty acids in beta-oxidation biochemical reactions and fatty acid transport in mitochondria occurs in a sequence of metabolic reactions.

1.3 Abundance

Essential fatty acids play a key role in many metabolic processes. Omega-3 fatty acids and their derivatives are active in lipid lowering. Omega-6 fatty acids and their derivatives play a role in the immune response and in thrombosis. Different sources are given in the following Table 30.1.

1.4 Digestion

After absorption, fatty acids are bound to triglycerides (TG) which have a glycerol backbone. Fatty acids also integrate into phospholipids and glycolipids in membranes. The cell membrane is made of cholesterol, phospholipids, and glycoproteins. About 70% of the cholesterol is circulated in plasma in the form of cholesteryl ester. In the membrane, the phospholipid bilayer has hydrophilic polar head groups, inside in an aqueous environment and the outside of the membrane has hydrophobic units, while the fatty acid chains are oriented toward the interior of the membrane to provide a water-impermeable barrier. In the membrane, a large variety of proteins (e.g., receptors, ion channels, signaling complexes) remain embedded between the phospholipid bilayer. The fluidity of the membrane depends on the multiple double bonds in the fatty acid content of the membrane phospholipids, which may partially account for their benefits in preventing cardiac arrhythmias and neurologic functions. Phospholipids form archidonic acid and eicosapentanoic acid by the enzyme action of phospholipase A2. Arachidonic acid forms prostaglandin series 2 and leukotriene series 4 products through the cyclooxygenase pathway. Eicosapentanoic acid forms prostacycline series 3 and leukotriene series 5 compounds. After digestion, 4% of the DHA fatty acid circulates in the bloodstream and 30% of the DHA fatty acid circulates in the brain and retina.

The final step in the conversion of ALA to DHA is a beta-oxidation step converting 24:6n-3 to 22:6n-3 in liver peroxisomes. Paroxysmal DHA deficient patients with a low fish intake show neurologic dysfunction and low phospholipid DHA. DHA appears to be important for central nervous system function (Simopoulos, 2011). Framingham Heart Study subjects who were in the highest quartile of plasma phospholipid DHA levels, consumed on average at least 180 mg of DHA per day and had a 50% reduction in neurological risk; progression of coronary atherosclerosis was slow in patients with higher levels of plasma DHA (Moyers et al., 2011). The next section is a discussion on dyslipidemia and the role of omega fatty acids in the prevention of CVD.

2. OMEGA FATTY ACIDS AND DYSLIPIDEMIA

2.1 Definition of Dyslipidemia

Dietary fat-intake and elevated blood lipids are considered risk factors for dyslipidemia and responsible for the development of atherosclerosis and diabetes. The elevated lipids are TG, lipoproteins (LDL-C), apolipoproteins (apo-B), non–HDL-C, TG, low HDL-C, and apo A-I in the blood. Lipid disorders are classified into seven dyslipidemia profiles.

- Elevated LDL-C (type IIa)
- Elevated LDL-C combined with high triglyceride (TG) (type IIb)
- Elevated TG (type IV)
- Low HDL-C (hypo-)
- Elevated LDL-C type IIa, type IIb, or type IV accompanied by low HDL-C
- Hyper-apobetalipoproteinemia (hyper-apoB), that is, elevated apolipoprotein B (apoB) but normal LDL-C
- Inherited lipoprotein disorders that often present in youth at high risk of future CVD include familial hypercholesterolemia (FH), familial combined hyperlipidemia (FCHL), hyper–apoB, familial hypoalphalipoproteinemia, apolipoprotein A-I mutations, common and rare variants in ABCA1 including Tangier disease, lecithin cholesterol acyl transferase (LCAT) deficiency, and hyper-TG associated with lipoprotein lipase (LPL) deficiency and defective apoC-II. The disorder of cholesteryl ester transfer protein (CETP) deficiency, often presents as high HDL-C, but its increased or reduced risk of CVD is not resolved (Zhang et al., 2012).

In the following section, the lipoproteins responsible for risk of CVD are described.

2.2 Lipids and Lipoproteins in Dyslipidemia

In blood, lipids are transported in almost all organs and remain in circulation to compensate the energy demands. The NCEP III guidelines state that non–HDL-C should be a secondary target if TG is >200 mg/dl. Atherogenic dyslipidemias (LDL-C, HDL-C, and TG) are interrelated and each component predicts the risk of CHD (Calder, 2004). Omega fatty acids bring dyslipidemia back to normal as shown in Table 30.2 and Figures 30.1–30.3b,c.

In the following section, we describe the individual lipoproteins.

2.2.1 Low-density lipoprotein cholesterol

Cholesterol is circulated in blood as free or cholesterol esters along with other lipoproteins in the form of LDL-C. LDL-C can be small density LDL particles or large intermediate density IDL particles in blood cholesterol. The size of lipoprotein LDL is a risk predictor of CVD (Azadbakht et al. 2007).

Table 30.2 Factors Involved in CHD that may be Affected by EPA and/or DHA

Factor	Effect
Serum TG	↓
Production of chemoattractants	↓
Production of growth factors	↓
Cell surface expression of adhesion molecules	↓
Production of inflammatory eicosanoids	↓
Blood pressure	↓
Endothelial relaxation	↑
Thrombosis	↓
Cardiac arrhythmias	↓
Heart rate variability	↑
Atherosclerotic plaque stability	↑

↑ = increase; ↓ = decrease.

2.2.2 High-density lipoprotein cholesterol

HDL is a high-density lipoprotein to transport cholesterol back to the liver. HDL-C is made of HDL particles with cholesterol ester inside. Low HDL-C is a risk factor for CHD (the golden rule is that every 1 mg/dl increase in HDL decreases the risk of CHD by 2–3%). Although the mechanism is not clear, it is believed that the antiatherogenic effect of HDL-C may be the result of reverse cholesterol transport (RCT), and the anti-oxidant and anti-inflammatory properties of HDL, as shown in Table 30.1. However, the small size of HDL-C particles and the action of CETP (cholesteryl ester transfer protein from liver) play an important role in making small HDL-C particles by exchanging more TG from VLDL particles and cholesterol esters from HDL-C. Smaller HDL-C particles are readily excreted from the kidneys to result in lower LDL-C levels.

2.2.3 Triglycerides

TG are circulated in blood in exchange with VLDL particles and constitute the small lipoproteins. The relationship of LDL and TG offers unique endpoints in evaluation of CHD. TG <150 mg/dl is considered to be a lower CHD risk in ACS patients. Omega-3 fatty acids are believed to decrease TG (Jacobson, 2008), and are described in the following section in detail.

2.3 How Much Lipid Lowering is Possible by Omega-3 Fatty Acids?

The elevated blood lipids or lipid disorder(s) in the body are mainly due to interrelated lipid metabolic changes in the liver, intestine, and adipose tissue at the cellular level of the membrane, mitochondria, and macrophages, as shown in Figure 30.2. Omega fatty acids act as the central regulatory pathways of cholesterol biosynthesis and its breakdown into bile acids. The first regulatory enzyme segment includes 3-hydroxy-3-methylglutaryl-coenzyme A (HMG-CoA) reductase (HMG-CoAR for cholesterol synthesis) and

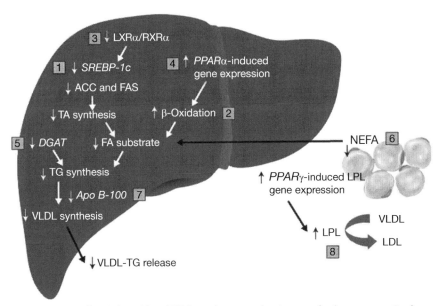

Figure 30.2 Potential triglyceride (TG)-lowering mechanisms of the omega-3 fatty acids eicosapentaenoic acid and docosahexaenoic acid. Reduced very-low-density lipoprotein cholesterol triglyceride (VLDL-TG) secretion may be due to decreased expression of sterol regulatory element-binding proteins (SREBP)-1c (1) or increased rates of mitochondrial and/or peroxisomal β-oxidation (2), leading to reduced substrate for TG synthesis. (3) Decreased SREBP-1c expression may be mediated by inhibition of liver X receptor (LXR) ligand binding to LXR/retinoid X receptor. Increased rates of peroxisomal beta-oxidation may be a consequence of peroxisome proliferator-activated receptor (PPAR)-α-induced increase in acyl-coenzyme A oxidase gene expression (4). Decreased activity of TG-synthesizing enzymes (5), decreased non-esterified fatty acid delivery from adipose tissue (6), and decreased availability of apo B (7) are potential mechanisms for reduced VLDL-TG release. In the periphery, increased lipoprotein lipase activity (8) may lead to increased VLDL-TG clearance, possibly due to increased PPAR-α and/or PPAR-α gene expression. *Adapted from Harris, W., Bulchandani, D., 2006. Why do omega-3 fatty acids lower serum triglycerides? Current Opinion in Lipidology 17, 387–93.*

cholesterol-7α hydroxylase (CHOL-H for cholesterol breakdown) to precursors. The ratio of HMG–CoAR:CHOL-H plays a significant role in controlling the lipids in the body. 'Lipid lowering' or cutting down cholesterol is the measure to bring back the elevated blood lipids in the body to normal lipid levels by using the HMG–CoAR inhibitors (mainly statins) or the CHOL-H stimulators (mainly bile acid sequesterants). Other means of lipid lowering include polyunsaturated fatty acids, dietary low fat intake to keep low supply of lipids or utilizing the stored lipids and fats (Step I and Step II diets). Lipid lowering by PUFA, diets or drugs also depends on several other body constitutional, age, heredity, socio–economic, and environmental factors.

The Japan EPA Lipid Intervention Study (JELIS) reported that the incidence of non-fatal coronary events was lower in hypercholesterolaemic Japanese patients with a 19%

decrease in plasma lipids in subjects who were given 1800 mg per day of the omega-3 fatty acid EPA compared with controls (Origasa et al., 2010; Vrablík et al., 2009; Yokoyama et al., 2007). Other studies indicated that the omega-3 fatty acids EPA and DHA reduce both lipids and the risk of cardiac death (Ishikawa et al., 2010; Kris-Etherton et al., 2002). However, EPA is not incorporated very efficiently into cell phospholipids of cardiac myocytes. Antiarrhythmic effects and the reduced cardiac mortality by intake of omega-3 fatty acids are related with heart phospholipids. EPA effectiveness is always lower than those of DHA (Harris et al., 2004; Mori and Woodman, 2006). EPA concentrations in plasma lipids increase after treatment (Itakura et al., 2011; Oikawa et al., 2009; Saito et al., 2008). After fish intake, conversion of EPA to DHA showed lower serum EPA in the presence of high levels of DHA (Burdge and Calder, 2005). EPA inhibits the production of proinflammatory eicosanoids to counter nonfatal inflammatory coronary events more efficiently than DHA. EPA competes with the omega-6 fatty acid (arachidonic acid) in a simultaneous reaction with oxygenases.

3. MECHANISM OF LIPID LOWERING AND CARDIOPROTECTION BY OMEGA-3 FATTY ACID INTAKE

EPA and DHA influence membranes, eicosanoid metabolism, and gene transcription at different levels. CVD includes all diseases that affect the heart and blood vessels, such as CHD, coronary artery disease, dyslipidemia, and hypertension. Omega-3 fatty acid rich fish oil intake was shown to be beneficial in primary or secondary prevention of CHD, which means low CVD risk and prevention of arrhythmias as well as lowering of heart rate and blood pressure, decrease in platelet aggregation and low triglyceride levels (Arnesen and Seljeflot, 2010; Das, 2000; Den Ruijter et al., 2008; Harrison and Abhyankar, 2005; McGuinness et al., 2006; Nair et al., 1997; Siddiqui et al., 2004; Terano et al., 1997; Xiao et al., 2004). High TG and low high-density lipoproteins (HDL) are considered major cardiovascular risks. Epidemiological evidence shows that omega-3 fatty acid can reduce CVD risk by LDL cholesterol lowering, but very limited data exists to validate this (Harris, 2007). The authors describe the lipid-lowering mechanisms of TG, VLDL-cholesterol, peroxisome proliferator-activated receptor, sterol regulatory element-binding proteins (SREBPs), phosphatidic acid phosphohydrolase (PAP) and acyl-CoA: diacylglycerol acyltransferase (DGAT), NEFAs, LPL, platelet aggregation, plaque stabilization, antiarrthymia by PUFA or combinatorial therapy in following sections mainly improving dyslipidemia back to normal to reduce cardiovascular occlusion and risk of CVD.

3.1 Omega-3 Fatty Acids: TG-Lowering Mechanisms

The liver plays a significant role in omega-3 fatty acid metabolism. Elevated TG levels may result from genetic or metabolic hypertriglyceridemia with increased atherogenic chylomicron and/or VLDL remnants in plasma. Hypertriglyceridemia associated with elevated VLDL can be due to various factors: overproduction of VLDL particles by the liver (as described in other chapter in detail); reduced intravascular lipolysis of VLDL-TG; and/or delayed clearance of small (remnant) VLDL particles from the plasma. VLDL particles are formed in the liver from Apo B, cholesterol, cholesteryl ester, phospholipids, and TG. TG derive from long-chain free fatty acids extracted from the plasma, recycled fatty acids, and/or de novo synthesis from acetyl co-enzyme A (Co-A) as shown in Figure 30.2.

Both EPA and DHA have similar TG-lowering effects. Treatment with 3.4 g/day of EPA and DHA for 4 months may increase EPA and DHA proportions in phospholipids two- to threefold from baseline levels. However, the molecular mechanisms by which EPA and DHA reduce serum TGs are not completely understood, as illustrated in Figure 30.2. It indicates that both fatty acids can modulate hepatic VLDL/TG synthesis and TG secretion to enhance TG clearance from chylomicrons and VLDL particles. Possibly, EPA and DHA are shunted into phospholipid synthesis pathways. Omega fatty acid-induced VLDL-TG synthesis is discussed in detail in the following section.

3.2 Reduced VLDL-TG Synthesis

Omega-3 fatty acids reduce serum TG concentration in humans. Two factors reduce serum TG: (1) inhibition of hepatic VLDL-TG secretion rates and (2) decreased synthesis of TG. So, reduced hepatic TG synthesis may lead to reduced production and secretion of VLDL (Harris and Bulchandani, 2006). Omega-3 EPA and/or DHA fatty acid-induced decrease in VLDL-TG synthesis may require decrease in transcription factors to control the enzyme expression responsible for TG assembly, increased intracellular degradation of apo B in hepatocytes and fatty-acid oxidation. Overall, the message is that EPA and/or DHA decrease hepatic lipogenesis (Harris and Bulchandani, 2006). The three regulatory proteins play roles in VLDL-TG synthesis, SREBPs, farnesoid X receptor (FXR), and PPAR-α-β-dependent protein (Horton, 1998).

One of the main molecular pathways for hepatic lipogenesis involves regulation of SREBP-1c expression and activation of the transcription factor SREBP-1c. STREBP-1c stimulates the synthesis of acetyl–CoA carboxylase-1 (ACC1), fatty-acid synthase (FAS), and lipogenic enzymes (Figure 30.2) (Horton, 1998; Horton et al., 2007). Fish-oil feeding was associated with a significant decrease in plasma TG levels; a marked decrease in the level of hepatic SREBP-1c mRNA (Le Jossic-Corcos et al., 2005) and its regulation by liver X receptor alpha/retinoid X receptor alpha (LXRα/RXRα) heterodimer; and expression of the SREBP-1c gene via two LXR–responsive elements (LXREs) in the SREBP-1c promoter. EPA and DHA showed inhibited binding of the LXRα/RXRα heterodimer with LXREs in the SREBP-1c promoter and suppressed SREBP-1c gene expression (Yoshikawa et al., 2002). As a result, suppression of SREBP-1c mRNA and the SREBP-1 protein decreased the TG synthesis or serum TGs (Zaima et al., 2006). Regulation of SREBP-1c expression may not be specific to only EPA and DHA and is controversial and efforts are in progress (Yu–Poth et al., 2005).

FXR plays a central role in lipid homeostasis (Edwards et al., 2002). FXR suppresses hepatic lipase and apo CIII gene expression to induce apo CII and VLDL-receptor gene expression, all of which may contribute to the TG-lowering action of FXR agonists (Davidson (2006)). DHA is a ligand for FXR and offers a mechanism for the TG-lowering effects of DHA and FXR-induced changes in gene expression (Davidson et al., 2007). PAP and acyl-CoA:DGAT are key enzymes in TG biosynthesis to catalyze the conversion of phosphatidate to diacylglycerol and diacylglycerol to TG, respectively. EPA and EPA plus DHA can inhibit the activities of DGAT and PAP in rat liver microsomes. Importantly, most of these studies used EPA or EPA and DHA at supraphysiological doses and employed different experimental conditions (Harris and Bulchandani, 2006).

Omega-3 fatty acids also lower circulating non-esterified fatty acid (NEFA) concentrations. NEFAs enter cells via fatty-acid transport proteins (Gimeno, 2007). NEFA are rapidly converted by acyl-CoA synthetases into fatty acyl-CoA thioesters that are potential substrates for TG synthesis (Jump, 2002). Human liver dataon intrahepatic processing of free EPA and DHA and TG-lowering effects are not available.

Fish oil-fed humans receiving dietary supplementation with 9 g of EPA+DHA per day showed faster rates of hepatic fatty-acid oxidation and slower formation of TG-rich VLDL (Dagnelie et al., 1994). However, the effect of increased β-oxidation in reducing the production of VLDL-TG in humans taking 3–4 g of EPA and DHA is not known. Overall, the message is that EPA and DHA reduce hepatic VLDL-TG synthesis by a less known mechanism. Perhaps, EPA and DHA modulate transcription factors involved in hepatic fatty-acid uptake, synthesis, β-oxidation, and VLDL-TG synthesis.

3.3 Enhanced TG Clearance

Chylomicrons and VLDL are main substrates for LPL, a TG hydrolase enzyme. EPA and DHA (4 g/day) intake showed a significantly increased rate of chylomicron clearance (see Figure 30.3a) (Park and Harris, 2003). Accelerated chylomicron TG clearance was associated with increased preheparin LPL activity in all omega-6/6 fed subjects (see Figure 30.3b). It reflects the possibility of insulin-induced high LPL activity and/or enhanced blood flow to adipose tissue and muscle, thereby exposing postprandial chylomicrons to tissues enriched with endothelial LPL (Jacobson, 2008). TG-lowering effects of EPA and DHA in atherogenic subjects were associated with increased LPL gene expression in adipose tissue (see Figure 30.2) and increased postheparin plasma LPL activity. EPA was shown to increase PPAR-α mRNA in isolated adipocytes (Chambrier

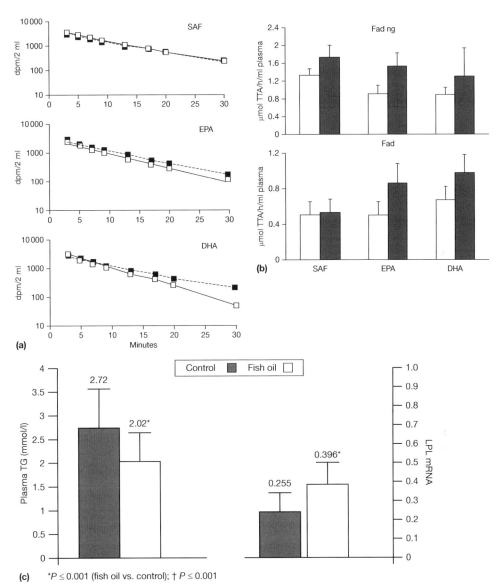

Figure 30.3 Effects of omega-3 acid ethyl esters (P-OM3, 4 g/day) and atorvastatin (singly and in combination) on apolipoprotein B-100 (apo B) kinetics. (a) Percentage change in the secretion rate of apo B-containing lipoproteins into the plasma. (b) Percentage change in the interconversion of apo B–containing lipoproteins. *$P < 0.01$ compared with placebo group. *Modified from Chan, D., Watts, G., Beilin, L., Redgrave, T., Mori, T., 2002. Regulatory effects of HMG CoA reductase inhibitor and fish oils on apolipoprotein B-100 kinetics in insulin-resistant obese male subjects with dyslipidemia. Diabetes 51, 2377–86.*

Continued

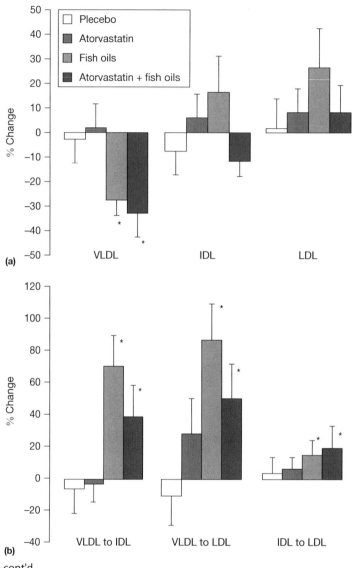

Figure 30.3—cont'd

Continued

et al., 2002), and correlated with plasma EPA concentrations in obese subjects. Most of the clinical studies do not support the catabolic rate of apo B particles and chylomicron remnants and the decrease in TG (Harris and Bulchandani, 2006). Possibly, omega-3 fatty acids activate LPL to remove TG from the VLDL and chylomicron particles in the circulation (Harris and Bulchandani, 2006).

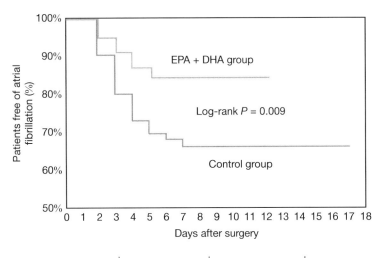

	Control (n = 81)	EPA + DHA (n = 79)	P
Post CABG AF	33%	15%	0.013
Hours of AF	24	16	0.12
Hospital length of stay after surgery	8.2 ± 2.6 days	7.3 ± 2.1 days	0.017

(c)

Figure 30.3—cont'd

3.4 The Combinatorial Effects of Omega-3 Fatty Acids and Statins

Statins (inhibitors of 3-hydroxy-3-methylglutaryl-CoA reductase) decrease LDL levels by increasing the number of LDL receptors and enhance the removal of LDL from plasma. The authors reported the side effects of statins and the urgency for combinatorial therapy to enhance cardiac capacity or reduce sudden cardiac death (Sharma et al., 2010). Omega-3 acid ethyl esters (P-OM3) decreased the rate of VLDL secretion and increased the conversion of VLDL to intermediate-density lipoprotein (IDL) and LDL (Figure 30.2). New clinical reports suggest omega-3 fatty acids in combination with statins as an ideal combinatorial approach in CVD subjects (Galan et al., 2003; Savelieva et al., 2011).

3.5 Cardiac Arrhythmia Suppression

Atrial fibrillation is the most common cardiac arrhythmia observed clinically and is the cause of costly cardiovascular morbidity (stroke and heart failure). The cardioprotective effects of fish oil have been attributed to the antiarrhythmic effects of EPA plus DHA (Brouwer et al., 2006; Christensen et al., 1997; Cleland et al., 2004; Leaf et al., 2005; London et al., 2007; Marchioli et al., 2005; Saravanan et al., 2010). Investigators indicated that several mechanisms may account for the antiarrhythmic action of omega-3 fatty acids. Some leading reports of the benefits of omega-3 fatty acids are cited in the following section.

- Lee et al. (2006) reported that omega-3 fatty acids incorporate into myocardial cell membranes and alter both eicosanoid production and ion-channel function in the membrane.
- Calo et al. (2005) demonstrated that administration of P-OM$_3$ (2 g/day) in patients undergoing coronary artery bypass graft surgery showed a substantially reduced incidence of postoperative atrial fibrillation (Figure 30.3). Omega-3 fatty acids may produce an antiarrhythmic action by preventing the cytosolic free calcium levels in cardiac myocytes from reaching toxic levels.
- Dhein and Michaelis (2005) showed the afterpotential discharges that accompany ischemia as an important mechanism underlying omega-3 fatty acid supplementation.

3.6 Decreased Platelet Aggregation

Greenlandic Eskimos consume large amounts of whale and seal meat. Omega-3 fatty acids showed antithrombotic potential in this population. However, omega-6 fatty acids and their derivatives showed enhanced thrombosis opposite with omega-3 fatty acids and their derivatives (Calder, 2004).

Two pathways control the process of atherogenesis. Arachidonic acid is the precursor of the two-series eicosanoids, thromboxane A2, and prostacyclin. Ecosanoids show a relationship with atherosclerosis in the following ways: (1) Thromboxane A2-stimulated platelet aggregation produces vasoconstriction, and 5-lipoxygenase metabolites (e.g., leukotrienes) attenuate inflammation and atherogenesis; and (2) arachidonic acid-derived prostacyclin is a potent vasodilator and counteracts platelet aggregation. Imbalance of essential metabolic functions of arachidonic acid metabolites may contribute to a proatherogenic state.

Consumption of EPA and DHA can lower tissue levels of arachidonic acid by inhibiting its synthesis and by taking its place in membrane phospholipids (Calder, 2004; Harris and Von Schacky, 2004, 2008). EPA-derived three-series eicosanoids are typically less vasoconstrictive and produce less platelet aggregation than those derived from arachidonic acid (Calder, 2004). Higher omega-3 fatty acid levels in cardiac tissue are thus antithrombotic. Although EPA plus DHA have been associated with modest increases in bleeding times, no published studies indicate clinically significant bleeding episodes among patients treated with antiplatelet drugs and relatively high doses (3–7 g/day) of EPA plus DHA (Harris, 2007; Kowey et al., 2010; Pratt et al., 2009).

3.7 Atherosclerotic Plaque Stabilization

Thies et al. (2003) demonstrated that atherosclerotic plaques from patients treated with fish oil were less heavily infiltrated with macrophages than those in the placebo group. Moreover, plaques from patients treated with fish oil were fibrous-cap atheromas (type IV plaque; considered more resistant to rupture), and less likely to be thin, inflamed-cap atheromas (type V plaque) compared to plaques from patients given placebo (Figure 30.4).

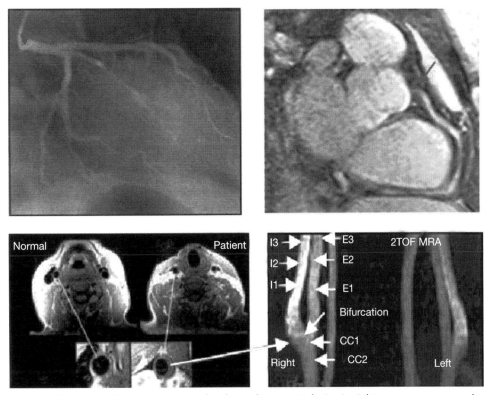

Figure 30.4 (On top) Coronary angiography showed a stenotic lesion in right coronary artery, and an intravascular magnetic resonance imaging showed a plaque with lipid core in this lesion (right, arrow). (At bottom) A comparison of atherosclerotic carotid artery wall with normal artery (shown in left panel) at different location (shown in right panel). *Reproduced from Sharma, R., Singh, R.B., Moffatt, R.J., Katz, J., 2010. Dietary fat intake: promotion of disease in carotid artery disease: Lipid lowering versus side effects of statins. In: Meester, F.D., Zibadi, S., Watson, R.R. (Eds.) Modern Dietary Fat Intakes in Disease Promotion, Nutrition and Health. Springer Science+Business Media, New York, pp. 151–185, with permission.*

3.8 Blood Pressure and Heart-Rate Reduction

A meta analysis of 36 randomized trials found that fish–oil intake (median dose 3.7 g/day EPA plus DHA) reduced systolic blood pressure by 2.1 mmHg ($P<0.01$) and diastolic blood pressure by 1.6 mmHg ($P<0.01$) in elderly populations with arterial stiffness and old subjects with microvascular dysfunction (Mori and Woodman, 2006). At least two mechanisms could account for this effect. First, incorporation of EPA and DHA into membrane phospholipids could increase systemic arterial compliance (Nestel et al., 2002). Second, EPA and DHA could improve endothelial function (Goodfellow et al., 2000). In addition, a metaanalysis of 30 randomized trials found that fish–oil intake (median dose 3.5 g/day EPA plus DHA) reduced heart rate by 1.6 bpm compared with placebo ($P=0.002$) (Mozaffarian et al. 2005; Mozaffarian, 2008).

3.9 Antioxidant Role of Omega-3 Fatty Acid in LDL Receptor and LDL Removal

Superoxide anion is formed by univalent reduction of molecular oxygen. Several enzymes are involved in the generation of superoxide anion, including xanthine oxidase, NADH/NADPH oxidase, lipoxygenase and nitric oxide synthase in mitochondrion (Chen et al., 2009; Radosinska et al., 2011). Superoxide anion is reduced to hydrogen peroxide. Transition metals such as iron or copper interact with hydrogen peroxide to produce highly toxic hydroxyl radicals. Omega-3 fatty acids decrease NOS expression (Shimojo et al., 2006; Yosefy et al., 2003). Reactive oxygen species (ROS) have detrimental effect on vascular function through several mechanisms. First, reactive hydroxyl radicals, injure cell membrane and nuclei. Second, ROS modulate vasomotion and the atherogenic process. Third, ROS combine with lipid components to form oxidized LDL as the key mediator of atherosclerosis. Oxidized LDL accumulates as cholesterol ester. Omega-3 fatty acids induce high LDL oxidation susceptibility in patients with CVD (Ziedén et al., 2002)

There are a number of clinical markers suggested to assess oxidative stress status (see Table 30.3). Oxidized LDL directly involve in the athelosclerosis process so they provide information regarding oxidative stress in atherosclerosis. Omega fatty acids act as anti-Ox-LDL in LDL oxidation at the level of tissues or cells (Ziedén et al., 2002). The titer of anti-Ox LDL is associated with short-term lesion progression or regression of atherosclerotic coronary artery disease as well as peripheral artery disease or higher in patients with ACS than in patients with stable angina.

3.10 Enzyme Modulation by Omega-3 Fatty Acids

The beneficial effects of fish oil are attributed to their n–3 polyunsaturated fatty acid contents. Dietary supplementation of DHA and EPA influences the fatty acid composition of plasma phospholipids that, in turn, may affect cardiac cell functions *in vivo*. Long-chain

Table 30.3 Oxidative Stress Markers Are Shown Active in Atherogenesis

Thiobarbituric acid reactive substance (TBARS)
Oxidized low density lipoprotein (LDL)
Malonic dialdehyde-modified LDL (MDA-LDL)
Oxidized LDL receptor (LOX-1)
8-Hydroxy-2-deoxyguanosine (8-OHdG)
8-iso prostaglandin F2α
Anti-oxidized LDL antibody
Oxidized α1-antitrypsin
Tetrahydrobiopterin (BH4)
Asymmetric di-methyl arginine (ADMA)

omega-3 fatty acids may exert beneficial effects by affecting a wide variety of cellular signaling mechanisms. Pathways involved in calcium homeostasis in the heart may be of particular importance. L-type calcium channels, the Na^+–Ca^{2+} exchanger and mobilization of calcium from intracellular stores are the most obvious key signaling pathways affecting the cardiovascular system. Recent studies suggest that other signaling pathways involving activation of phospholipases, synthesis of eicosanoids, regulation of receptor-associated enzymes and protein kinases also play very important roles in mediating n-3 PUFA effects on cardiovascular health (Siddiqui et al., 2004, 2008).

In present chapter, omega fatty acids are introduced as dietary fat. Role of omega-3 fatty acids is reviewed on lipid lowering in blood and regulation of lipoproteins at molecular level. A correlation is evidenced between influence of omega-3 fatty acids and prevention of CHD/CVD risk with mechanisms proposed in different clinical studies in support.

4. CONCLUSION

Omega fatty acids are basic lipids. Omega fatty acids are abundant in fish and probably modulate lipoprotein metabolism at molecular level. Several biochemical mechanisms such as triglyceride lowering, reduced VLDL–TG synthesis and enhanced TG clearance, show how dietary low fat intake or omega-3 fatty acid supplementation keeps down blood lipids to prevent CVD risk. Omega fatty acid-rich wild and traditional foods are believed to keep good health at low risk of dyslipidemia or CVDs. The major mechanisms of omega-3 fatty acid induced prevention of CHD/CVD are their action in suppression of cardiac *arrhythmia*, antioxidant activity, depleted platelet aggregation, atherosclerosis plaque stabilization and enzyme modulation. Strict medical treatment of dyslipidemia to completely cure CVD or heart disease causes more side effects. Recent clinical trials show clear benefits of omega-3 fatty acid therapy in management of dyslipidemia and reducing cardiac injury.

ACKNOWLEDGMENTS

The authors acknowledge the support of the Indian Council of Medical Research for postgraduate studies program in Applied Nutrition for providing training and the opportunity for patient data collection to the first author at National Institute of Nutrition, Hyderabad. Authors acknowledge the manuscript preparation at Department of Exercise, Food and Nutrition, Florida State University, Tallahassee and the discussions included in this chapter.

REFERENCES

Aarsetøy, H., Pönitz, V., Nilsen, O.B., Grundt, H., Harris, W.S., Nilsen, D.W., 2008. Low levels of cellular omega-3 increase the risk of ventricular fibrillation during the acute ischaemic phase of a myocardial infarction. Resuscitation 78 (3), 258–264.

Adamsson, V., Reumark, A., Fredriksson, I.B., et al., 2011. Effects of a healthy Nordic diet on cardiovascular risk factors in hypercholesterolaemic subjects: a randomized controlled trial (NORDIET). Journal of Internal Medicine 269 (2), 150–159.

Albert, C., Anderson, M., Nattel, S., 2010. Omega-3 oil: a fishy protection for the heart. Community corner. Nature Medicine 16 (11), 1192–1193.

Archer, S.L., Green, D., Chamberlain, M., Dyer, A.R., Liu, K., 1998. Association of dietary fish and n-3 fatty acid intake with hemostatic factors in the coronary artery risk development in young adults (CARDIA) study. Arteriosclerosis, Thrombosis, and Vascular Biology 18 (7), 1119–1123.

Arnesen, H., Seljeflot, I., 2010. Studies on very long chain marine n-3 fatty acids in patients with atherosclerotic heart disease with special focus on mechanisms, dosage and formulas of supplementation. Cellular and Molecular Biology (Noisy-le-Grand, France) 56 (1), 18–27.

Azadbakht, L., Mirmiran, P., Hedayati, M., Esmaillzadeh, A., Shiva, N., Azizi, F., 2007. Particle size of LDL is affected by the National Cholesterol Education Program (NCEP) step II diet in dyslipidaemic adolescents. British Journal of Nutrition 98 (1), 134–139.

Bays, H.E., et al., 2008. Prescription omega-3 fatty acids and their lipid effects: physiologic mechanisms of action and clinical implications. Expert Review of Cardiovascular Therapy 6 (3), 391–409.

Bianconi, L., Calò, L., Mennuni, M., et al., 2011. n-3 polyunsaturated fatty acids for the prevention of arrhythmia recurrence after electrical cardioversion of chronic persistent atrial fibrillation: a randomized, double-blind, multicentre study. Europace 13 (2), 174–181.

Bistrian, B.R., 2004. Practical recommendations of immune enhancing diets. Journal of Nutrition 134, 2868S–2872S.

Brouwer, I.A., Zock, P.L., Camm, A.J., et al., 2006. Effect of fish oil on ventricular tachyarrhythmia and death in patients with implantable cardioverter defibrillators: the Study on Omega-3 Fatty Acids and Ventricular Arrhythmia (SOFA) randomized trial. Journal of the American Medical Association 295 (22), 2613–2619.

Brouwer, I.A., Zock, P.L., Wever, E.F., et al., 2003. Rationale and design of a randomised controlled clinical trial on supplemental intake of n-3 fatty acids and incidence of cardiac arrhythmia: SOFA. European Journal of Clinical Nutrition 57 (10), 1323–1330.

Burdge, G.C., Calder, P.C., 2005. Conversion of alpha-linolenic acid to longer-chain polyunsaturated fatty acids in human adults. Reproduction Nutrition Development 45 (5), 581–597.

Calder, P.C., 2004. n-3 fatty acids and cardiovascular disease: evidence explained and mechanisms explored. Clinical Science 107, 1–11.

Calo, L., Bianconi, L., Colivicchi, F., et al., 2005. n-3 fatty acids for the prevention of atrial fibrillation after coronary artery bypass surgery: a randomized controlled trial. Journal of the American College of Cardiology 45, 1723–1728.

Chambrier, C., Bastard, J.P., Rieusset, J., et al., 2002. Eicosapentaenoic acid induces mRNA expression of peroxisome proliferator-activated receptor gamma. Obesity Research 10, 518–525.

Chen, H., Ren, J.Y., Xing, Y., et al., 2009. Short-term withdrawal of simvastatin induces endothelial dysfunction in patients with coronary artery disease: a dose-response effect dependent on endothelial nitric oxide synthase. International Journal of Cardiology 131 (3), 313–320.

Christensen, J.H., Dyerberg, J., Schmidt, E.B., 1999. n-3 fatty acids and the risk of sudden cardiac death assessed by 24-hour heart rate variability. Lipids 34 (Suppl), S197.

Christensen, J.H., Gustenhoff, P., Korup, E., et al., 1997. n-3 polyunsaturated fatty acids, heart rate variability and ventricular arrhythmias in post-AMI-patients. A clinical controlled trial. Ugeskr Laeger 159 (37), 5525–5529.

Cleland, J.G., Freemantle, N., Kaye, G., et al., 2004. Clinical trials update from the American Heart Association meeting: omega-3 fatty acids and arrhythmia risk in patients with an implantable defibrillator, ACTIV in CHF, VALIANT, the Hanover autologous bone marrow transplantation study, SPORTIF V, ORBIT and PAD and DEFINITE. European Journal of Heart Failure 6 (1), 109–115.

Côté, S., Dodin, S., Blanchet, C., et al., 2004. Very high concentrations of n-3 fatty acids in peri- and postmenopausal Inuit women from Greenland. International Journal of Circumpolar Health 63 (Suppl. 2), 298–301.

Dagnelie, P., Rietveld, T., Swart, G., Stijnen, T., van den Berg, J., 1994. Effect of dietary fish oil on blood levels of free fatty acids, ketone bodies and triacylglycerol in humans. Lipids 29, 41–45.

Dall, T.L., Bays, H., 2009. Addressing lipid treatment targets beyond cholesterol: a role for prescription omega-3 fatty acid therapy. Southern Medical Journal 102 (40), 390–396.

Das, U.N., 2000. Beneficial effect(s) of n-3 fatty acids in cardiovascular diseases: but, why and how? Prostaglandins, Leukotrienes, and Essential Fatty Acids 63 (6), 351–362.

Davidson, M., 2006. Mechanisms for the hypotriglyceridemic effect of marine omega-3 fatty acids. American Journal of Cardiology 98 (Suppl), 27i–33i.

Davidson, M.H., et al., 2007. Efficacy and tolerability of adding prescription omega-3 fatty acids 4 g/d to simvastatin 40 mg/d in hypertriglyceridemic patients: an 8-week, randomized, double-blind, placebo-controlled study. Clinical Therapeutics 29 (7), 1354–1367.

Daviglus, M.L., Stamler, J., Orencia, A.J., et al., 1997. Fish consumption and the 30-year risk of fatal myocardial infarction. The New England Journal of Medicine 336, 1046–1053.

de Lorgeril, M., Salen, P., Paillard, F., Laporte, F., Boucher, F., de Leiris, J., 2002. Mediterranean diet and the French paradox: two distinct biogeographic concepts for one consolidated scientific theory on the role of nutrition in coronary heart disease. Cardiovascular Research 54 (3), 503–515.

de Roos, B., Mavrommatis, Y., Brouwer, I.A., 2009. Long-chain n-3 polyunsaturated fatty acids: new insights into mechanisms relating to inflammation and coronary heart disease. British Journal of Pharmacology 158 (2), 413–428.

Den Ruijter, H.M., Berecki, G., Verkerk, A.O., et al., 2008. Acute administration of fish oil inhibits triggered activity in isolated myocytes from rabbits and patients with heart failure. Circulation 117 (4), 536–544.

Dhein, S., Michaelis, B., Mohr, F.W., 2005. Antiarrhythmic and electrophysiological effects of long-chain omega-3 polyunsaturated fatty acids. Naunyn-Schmiedeberg's Archives of Pharmacology 371, 202–211.

Din, J.N., Newby, D.E., Flapan, A.D., 2004. Omega 3 fatty acids and cardiovascular disease-fishing for a natural treatment. British Medical Journal 328 (7430), 30–35.

Edwards, P.A., Kast, H.R., Anisfeld, A.M., 2002. BAREing it all: the adoption of LXR and FXR and their roles in lipid homeostasis. Journal of Lipid Research 43, 2–12.

Finzi, A.A., Latini, R., Barlera, S., et al., 2011. Effects of n-3 polyunsaturated fatty acids on malignant ventricular arrhythmias in patients with chronic heart failure and implantable cardioverter-defibrillators: a substudy of the Gruppo Italiano per lo Studio della Sopravvivenza nell'Insufficienza Cardiaca (GISSI-HF) trial. American Heart Journal 161 (2), 338–343.e1.

Galan, P., de Bree, A., Mennen, L., et al., 2003. Background and rationale of the SU.FOL.OM3 study: double-blind randomized placebo-controlled secondary prevention trial to test the impact of supplementation with folate, vitamin B6 and B12 and/or omega-3 fatty acids on the prevention of recurrent ischemic events in subjects with atherosclerosis in the coronary or cerebral arteries. The Journal of Nutrition, Health and Aging 7 (6), 428–435.

Galan, P., Kesse-Guyot, E., Czernichow, S., et al., 2010. Effects of B vitamins and omega 3 fatty acids on cardiovascular diseases: a randomised placebo controlled trial. BMJ 341, c6273.

Geelen, A., Brouwer, I.A., Schouten, E.G., Maan, A.C., Katan, M.B., Zock, P.L., 2005. Effects of n-3 fatty acids from fish on premature ventricular complexes and heart rate in humans. American Journal of Clinical Nutrition 81 (2), 416–420.

Geleijnse, J.M., Giltay, E.J., Schouten, E.G., et al., 2010. Effect of low doses of n-3 fatty acids on cardio-vascular diseases in 4,837 post-myocardial infarction patients: design and baseline characteristics of the Alpha Omega Trial. American Heart Journal 159 (4), 539–546.e2.

Genest, J., McPherson, R., Frohlich, J., Anderson, T., Campbell, N., 2009. 2009 Canadian Cardiovascular Society/Canadian guidelines for the diagnosis and treatment of dyslipidemia and prevention of cardio-vascular disease in the adult – 2009 recommendations. Canadian Journal of Cardiology 25 (10), 567–579.

Geppert, J., Kraft, V., Demmelmair, H., Koletzko, B., 2005. Docosahexaenoic acid supplementation in veg-etarians effectively increases omega-3 index: a randomized trial. Lipids 40 (8), 807–814.

Gimeno, R.E., 2007. Fatty acid transport proteins. Current Opinion in Lipidology 18, 271–276.

Gissi-HF Investigators, Tavazzi, L., Maggioni, A.P., et al., 2008. Effect of n-3 polyunsaturated fatty acids in patients with chronic heart failure (the GISSI-HF trial): a randomised, double-blind, placebo-controlled trial. Lancet 372 (9645), 1223–1230.

Goldstein, L.B., Bushnell, C.D., Adams, R.J., et al., 2011. American Heart Association Stroke Council; Council on Cardiovascular Nursing; Council on Epidemiology and Prevention; Council for High Blood Pressure Research,; Council on Peripheral Vascular Disease, and Interdisciplinary Council on Quality of Care and Outcomes Research. Stroke 42 (2), 517–584.

Goodfellow, J., Bellamy, M.F., Ramsey, M.W., Jones, C.J., Lewis, M.J., 2000. Dietary supplementation with marine omega-3 fatty acids improve systemic large artery endothelial function in subjects with hy-percholesterolemia. Journal of the American College of Cardiology 35 (2), 265–270.

Grundt, H., Nilsen, D.W., Hetland, Ø., Mansoor, M.A., 2004. Clinical outcome and atherothrombogenic risk profile after prolonged wash-out following long-term treatment with high doses of n-3 PUFAs in patients with an acute myocardial infarction. Clinical Nutrition 23 (4), 491–500.

Grundt, H., Nilsen, D.W., Mansoor, M.A., Nordøy, A., 2003. Increased lipid peroxidation during long-term intervention with high doses of n-3 fatty acids (PUFAs) following an acute myocardial infarction. European Journal of Clinical Nutrition 57 (6), 793–800.

Guallar, E., Aro, A., Jiménez, F.J., et al., 1999. Omega-3 fatty acids in adipose tissue and risk of myocardial infarction: the EURAMIC study. Arteriosclerosis, Thrombosis, and Vascular Biology 19, 1111–1118.

Hamaad, A., Kaeng Lee, W., Lip, G.Y., MacFadyen, R.J., 2006. Oral omega n3-PUFA therapy (Omacor) has no impact on indices of heart rate variability in stable post myocardial infarction patients. Cardiovascular Drugs and Therapy 20 (5), 359–364.

Harris, W.S., 2007. Omega-3 fatty acids and cardiovascular disease: a case for omega-3 index as a new risk factor. Pharmacological Research 55 (3), 217–223.

Harris, W.S., 2009. Substudies of the Japan EPA Lipid Intervention Study (JELIS). Current Atherosclerosis Reports 11 (6), 399–400.

Harris, W., Bulchandani, D., 2006. Why do omega-3 fatty acids lower serum triglycerides? Current Opinion in Lipidology 17, 387–393.

Harris, W.S., Isley, W.L., 2001. Clinical trial evidence for the cardioprotective effects of omega-3 fatty acids. Current Atherosclerosis Reports 3 (2), 174–179.

Harris, W.S., Sands, S.A., Windsor, S.L., et al., 2004. Omega-3 fatty acids in cardiac biopsies from heart transplantation patients. Circulation 110, 1645–1649.

Harris, W.S., Von Schacky, C., 2004. The Omega-3 Index: a new risk factor for death from coronary heart disease? Preventive Medicine 39 (1), 212–220.

Harris, W.S., et al., 2008. Omega-3 fatty acids and coronary heart disease risk: clinical and mechanistic perspectives. Atherosclerosis 197 (1), 12–24.

Harrison, N., Abhyankar, B., 2005. The mechanism of action of omega-3 fatty acids in secondary prevention post-myocardial infarction. Current Medical Research and Opinion 21 (1), 95–100.

Hathcock, J., Richardson, D., Shao, A., Jennings, S., 2006. The Risk Assessment and Safety of Bioactive Substances in Food Supplements. IADSA, Brussels pp. 52–57.

Heidarsdottir, R., Arnar, D.O., Skuladottir, G.V., et al., 2010. Does treatment with n-3 polyunsaturated fatty acids prevent atrial fibrillation after open heart surgery? Europace 12 (3), 356–363.

Heidt, M.C., Vician, M., Stracke, S.K., et al., 2009. Beneficial effects of intravenously administered N-3 fatty acids for the prevention of atrial fibrillation after coronary artery bypass surgery: a prospective random-ized study. Thoracic and Cardiovascular Surgeon 57 (5), 276–280.

Horton, J., Bashmakov, Y., Shimomura, I., Shimano, H., 1998. Regulation of sterol regulatory element binding proteins in livers of fasted and refed mice. Proceedings of the National Academy of Sciences USA 95, 5987–5992.

Horton, J.D., Cohen, J.C., Hobbs, H.H., 2007. Molecular biology of PCSK9: its role in LDL metabolism. Trends in Biochemical Sciences 32, 71–77.

Ishikawa, Y., Yokoyama, M., Saito, Y., et al., 2010. Preventive effects of eicosapentaenoic acid on coronary artery disease in patients with peripheral artery disease. Circulation Journal 74 (7), 1451–1457.

Itakura, H., Yokoyama, M., Matsuzaki, M., et al., 2011. Relationships between plasma fatty acid composition and coronary artery disease. Journal of Atherosclerosis and Thrombosis 18 (2), 99–107.

Jacobson, T.A., 2008. Role of n-3 fatty acids in the treatment of hypertriglyceridemia and cardiovascular disease. American Journal of Clinical Nutrition 87 (6), 1981S–1990S.

Johansen, O., Brekke, M., Seljeflot, I., Abdelnoor, M., Arnesen, H., 1999. N-3 fatty acids do not prevent restenosis after coronary angioplasty: results from the CART study. Coronary angioplasty restenosis trial. Journal of the American College of Cardiology 33 (6), 1619–1626.

Jones, P.J., Lau, V.W., 2002. Effect of n-3 polyunsaturated fatty acids on risk reduction of sudden death. Nutrition Reviews 60 (12), 407–409.

Jump, D.B., 2002. The biochemistry of n-3 polyunsaturated fatty acids. Journal of Biological Chemistry 277, 8755–8758.

Kowey, P.R., Reiffel, J.A., Ellenbogen, K.A., Naccarelli, G.V., Pratt, C.M., 2010. Efficacy and safety of prescription omega-3 fatty acids for the prevention of recurrent symptomatic atrial fibrillation: a randomized controlled trial. Journal of the American Medical Association 304 (21), 2363–2372.

Kris-Etherton, P.M., Harris, W.S., Appel, L.J., 2003. Nutrition Committee. Fish consumption, fish oil, omega-3 fatty acids, and cardiovascular disease. Arteriosclerosis, Thrombosis, and Vascular Biology 23 (2), e20–e30.

Kris-Etherton, P.M., Harris, W.S., Appel, L.J., et al., 2002. Fish consumption, fish oil, omega-3 fatty acids, and cardiovascular disease. Circulation 106, 2747–2757.

Kromhout, D., Giltay, E.J., Geleijnse, J.M., 2010. Alpha Omega Trial Group. n-3 fatty acids and cardiovascular events after myocardial infarction. The New England Journal of Medicine 363 (21), 2015–2026.

Le Jossic-Corcos, C., Gonthier, C., Zaghini, I., et al., 2005. Hepatic farnesyl diphosphate synthase expression is suppressed by polyunsaturated fatty acids. Biochemical Journal 385, 787–794.

Leaf, A., Albert, C.M., Josephson, M., et al., 2005. Prevention of fatal arrhythmias in high-risk subjects by fish oil n-3 fatty acid intake. Circulation 112 (18), 2762–2768.

Leaf, A., Kang, J., Xiao, Y., Billman, G., 2003a. Clinical preservation of sudden cardiac death by n-3 polyunsaturated fatty acids and mechanism of prevention of arrhythmias by n-3 fish oils. Circulation 107, 2646–2652.

Leaf, A., Xiao, Y.F., Kang, J.X., Billman, G.E., 2003b. Prevention of sudden cardiac death by n-3 polyunsaturated fatty acids. Pharmacology and Therapeutics 98 (3), 355–377.

Lee, K.W., Blann, A.D., Lip, G.Y., 2006. Effects of omega-3 polyunsaturated fatty acids on plasma indices of thrombogenesis and inflammation in patients post-myocardial infarction. Thrombosis Research 118 (3), 305–312.

Lee, J.H., O'Keefe, J.H., Lavie, C.J., Marchioli, R., Harris, W.S., 2008. Omega-3 fatty acids for cardioprotection. Mayo Clinic Proceedings 83 (3), 324–332.

Lichtenstein, A.H., Appel, L.J., Brands, M., et al., 2006. Diet and lifestyle recommendations revision 2006: a scientific statement from the American Heart Association Nutrition Committee. Circulation 114, 82–96.

Lindman, A.S., Pedersen, J.I., Hjerkinn, E.M., et al., 2004. The effects of long-term diet and omega-3 fatty acid supplementation on coagulation factor VII and serum phospholipids with special emphasis on the R353Q polymorphism of the FVII gene. Thrombosis and Haemostasis 91 (6), 1097–1104.

London, B., Albert, C., Anderson, M.E., et al., 2007. Omega-3 fatty acids and cardiac arrhythmias: prior studies and recommendations for future research: a report from the National Heart, Lung, and Blood Institute and Office of Dietary Supplements Omega-3 Fatty Acids and their Role in Cardiac Arrhythmogenesis Workshop. Circulation 116 (10), e320–e335.

Macchia, A., Varini, S., Grancelli, H., et al., 2009. The rationale and design of the FORomegaARD Trial: a randomized, double-blind, placebo-controlled, independent study to test the efficacy of n-3 PUFA for the maintenance of normal sinus rhythm in patients with previous atrial fibrillation. American Heart Journal 157 (3), 423–427.

Madsen, T., Christensen, J.H., Schmidt, E.B., 2007. C-reactive protein and n-3 fatty acids in patients with a previous myocardial infarction: a placebo-controlled randomized study. European Journal of Nutrition 46 (7), 428–430.

Marchioli, R., Barzi, F., Bomba, E., et al., 2002. GISSI-Prevenzione Investigators. Early protection against sudden death by n-3 polyunsaturated fatty acids after myocardial infarction: time-course analysis of the results of the Gruppo Italiano per lo Studio della Sopravvivenza nell'Infarto Miocardico (GISSI)-Prevenzione. Circulation 105 (16), 1897–1903.

Marchioli, R., Levantesi, G., Macchia, A., et al., 2005. Antiarrhythmic mechanisms of n-3 PUFA and the results of the GISSI-Prevenzione trial. Journal of Membrane Biology 206 (2), 117–128.

Marchioli, R., Levantesi, G., Silletta, M.G., et al., 2009. Effect of n-3 polyunsaturated fatty acids and rosu-vastatin in patients with heart failure: results of the GISSI-HF trial. Expert Review of Cardiovascular Therapy 7 (7), 735–748.

Marchioli, R., Marfisi, R.M., Borrelli, G., et al., 2007. Efficacy of n-3 polyunsaturated fatty acids according to clinical characteristics of patients with recent myocardial infarction: insights from the GISSI-Prevenzione trial. Journal of Cardiovascular Medicine (Hagerstown, MD) 8 (Suppl. 1), S34–S37.

Marchioli, R., Schweiger, C., Tavazzi, L., Valagussa, F., 2001. Efficacy of n-3 polyunsaturated fatty acids after myocardial infarction: results of GISSI-Prevenzione trial. Gruppo Italiano per lo Studio della Sopravvivenza nell'Infarto Miocardico. Lipids 36 (Suppl), S119–S126.

Marchioli, R., Silletta, M.G., Levantesi, G., Pioggiarella, R., Tognoni, G., 2010. N-3 polyunsaturated fatty acids in heart failure: mechanisms and recent clinical evidence. Cellular and Molecular Biology (Noisy-le-Grand, France) 56 (1), 110–130.

Maresta, A., Balducelli, M., Varani, E., et al., 1999. Prevention in coronary postangioplasty restenosis with omega-3 fatty acids. Results of the Italian study on prevention of restenosis with esapent (ESPRIT). Cardiologia 44 (Suppl. 1(PtF 2)), 1751–1755.

Mata Lopez, P., Ortega, R.M., 2003. Omega-3 fatty acids in the prevention and control of cardiovascular disease. European Journal of Clinical Nutrition 57 (Suppl. 1), S22–S25.

McGuinness, J., Neilan, T.G., Sharkasi, A., Bouchier-Hayes, D., Redmond, J.M., 2006. Myocardial protection using an omega-3 fatty acid infusion: quantification and mechanism of action. The Journal of Thoracic and Cardiovascular Surgery 132 (1), 72–79.

McLennan, P.L., Abeywardena, M.Y., 2005. Membrane basis for fish oil effects on the heart: linking natural hibernators to prevention of human sudden cardiac death. Journal of Membrane Biology 206 (2), 85–102.

Metcalf, R.G., Sanders, P., James, M.J., Cleland, L.G., Young, G.D., 2008. Effect of dietary n-3 polyun-saturated fatty acids on the inducibility of ventricular tachycardia in patients with ischemic cardiomy-opathy. The American Journal of Cardiology 101 (6), 758–761.

Mori, T.A., Woodman, R.J., 2006. The independent effects of eicosapentaenoic acid and docosahexaenoic acid on cardiovascular risk factors in humans. Current Opinion in Clinical Nutrition and Metabolic Care 9, 95–104.

Moyers, B., Farzaneh-Far, R., Harris, W.S., Garg, S., Na, B., Whooley, M.A., 2011. Relation of whole blood n-3 fatty acid levels to exercise parameters in patients with stable coronary artery disease (from the Heart and Soul Study). The American Journal of Cardiology 107 (8), 1149–1154.

Mozaffarian, D., 2008. Fish and n-3 fatty acids for the prevention of fatal coronary heart disease and sudden cardiac death. American Journal of Clinical Nutrition 87 (6), 1991S–1996S.

Mozaffarian, D., Geelen, A., Brouwer, I., et al., 2005. Effect of fish oil on heart rate in humans: a meta-analysis of randomized controlled trials. Circulation 112, 1945–1952.

Nair, S.S., Leitch, J.W., Falconer, J., Garg, M.L., 1997. Prevention of cardiac arrhythmia by dietary (n-3) polyunsaturated fatty acids and their mechanism of action. Journal of Nutrition 127 (3), 383–393.

Nestel, P., Shige, H., Pomeroy, S., et al., 2002. The n-3 fatty acids eicosapentaenoic acid and docosahex-aenoic acid increase systemic arterial compliance in humans. American Journal of Clinical Nutrition 76, 326–330.

Nilsen, D.W., Dalaker, K., Nordøy, A., et al., 1991. Influence of a concentrated ethylester compound of n-3 fatty acids on lipids, platelets and coagulation in patients undergoing coronary bypass surgery. Thrombosis and Haemostasis 66 (2), 195–201.

Oda, E., Hatada, K., Katoh, K., Kodama, M., Nakamura, Y., Aizawa, Y., 2005. A case-control pilot study on n-3 polyunsaturated fatty acid as a negative risk factor for myocardial infarction. International Heart Journal 46 (4), 583–591.

Oikawa, S., Yokoyama, M., Origasa, H., et al., 2009. JELIS Investigators, Japan. Suppressive effect of EPA on the incidence of coronary events in hypercholesterolemia with impaired glucose metabolism: sub-analysis of the Japan EPA Lipid Intervention Study (JELIS). Atherosclerosis 206 (2), 535–539.

O'Keefe Jr., J.H., Abuissa, H., Sastre, A., Steinhaus, D.M., Harris, W.S., 2006. Effects of omega-3 fatty acids on resting heart rate, heart rate recovery after exercise, and heart rate variability in men with healed myocardial infarctions and depressed ejection fractions. The American Journal of Cardiology 97 (8), 1127–1130.

Okuyama, H., Fujii, Y., Ikemoto, A., 2000. N-6/N-3 ratio of dietary fatty acids rather than hypercholesterolemia as the major risk factor for atherosclerosis and coronary heart disease. Journal of Health Science 46 (3), 157.

Origasa, H., Yokoyama, M., Matsuzaki, M., Saito, Y., Matsuzawa, Y., 2010. Clinical importance of adherence to treatment with eicosapentaenoic acid by patients with hypercholesterolemia. Circulation Journal 74 (3), 510–517.

Park, Y., Harris, W.S., 2003. Omega-3 fatty acid supplementation accelerates chylomicron triglyceride clearance. Journal of Lipid Research 44, 455–463.

Pratt, C.M., Reiffel, J.A., Ellenbogen, K.A., Naccarelli, G.V., Kowey, P.R., 2009. Efficacy and safety of prescription omega-3-acid ethyl esters for the prevention of recurrent symptomatic atrial fibrillation: a prospective study. American Heart Journal 158 (2), 163–169.e1–3.

Radosinska, J., Bacova, B., Bernatova, I., et al., 2011. Myocardial NOS activity and connexin-43 expression in untreated and omega-3 fatty acids-treated spontaneously hypertensive and hereditary hypertriglyceridemic rats. Molecular and Cellular Biochemistry 347 (1–2), 163–173.

Raitt, M.H., Connor, W.E., Morris, C., et al., 2005. Fish oil supplementation and risk of ventricular tachycardia and ventricular fibrillation in patients with implantable defibrillators: a randomized controlled trial. Journal of the American Medical Association 293 (23), 2884–2891.

Rajaram, S., Haddad, E.H., Mejia, A., Sabaté, J., 2009. Walnuts and fatty fish influence different serum lipid fractions in normal to mildly hyperlipidemic individuals: a randomized controlled study. American Journal of Clinical Nutrition 89 (5), 1657S–1663S.

Rauch, B., Schiele, R., Schneider, S., et al., 2006. Highly purified omega-3 fatty acids for secondary prevention of sudden cardiac death after myocardial infarction-aims and methods of the OMEGA-study. Cardiovascular Drugs and Therapy 20 (5), 365–375.

Richter, W.O., 2003. Long-chain omega-3 fatty acids from fish reduce sudden cardiac death in patients with coronary heart disease. European Journal of Medical Research 8 (8), 332–336.

Russo, G.L., 2009. Dietary n-6 and n-3 polyunsaturated fatty acids: from biochemistry to clinical implications in cardiovascular prevention. Biochemical Pharmacology 77 (6), 937–946.

Saito, Y., Yokoyama, M., Origasa, H., et al., 2008. Effects of EPA on coronary artery disease in hypercholesterolemic patients with multiple risk factors: sub-analysis of primary prevention cases from the Japan EPA Lipid Intervention Study (JELIS). Atherosclerosis 200 (1), 135–140.

Sanders, T.A., Lewis, F., Slaughter, S., et al., 2006. Effect of varying the ratio of n-6 to n-3 fatty acids by increasing the dietary intake of alpha-linolenic acid, eicosapentaenoic and docosahexaenoic acid, or both on fibrinogen and clotting factors VII and XII in persons aged 45-70 y: the OPTILIP study. American Journal of Clinical Nutrition 84 (3), 513–522.

Saravanan, P., Bridgewater, B., West, A.L., O'Neill, S.C., Calder, P.C., Davidson, N.C., 2010. Omega-3 fatty acid supplementation does not reduce risk of atrial fibrillation after coronary artery bypass surgery: a randomized, double-blind, placebo-controlled clinical trial. Circulation: Arrhythmia and Electrophysiology 3 (1), 46–53.

Savelieva, I., Kakouros, N., Kourliouros, A., Camm, A.J., 2011. Upstream therapies for management of atrial fibrillation: review of clinical evidence and implications for European Society of Cardiology guidelines. Part I: primary prevention. Europace 13 (3), 308–328.

Sharma, R., Singh, R.B., Moffatt, R.J., Katz, J., 2010. Dietary fat intake: promotion of disease in carotid artery disease: lipid lowering versus side effects of statins. In: Meester, F.D., Zibadi, S., Watson, R.R. (Eds.), Modern Dietary Fat Intakes in Disease Promotion, Nutrition and Health. Springer Science+Business Media, New York, pp. 151–185.

Shimojo, N., Jesmin, S., Zaedi, S., et al., 2006. EPA effect on NOS gene expression and on NO level in endothelin-1-induced hypertrophied cardiomyocytes. Experimental Biology and Medicine (Maywood, NJ) 231 (6), 913–918.

Siddiqui, R.A., Harvey, K.A., Zaloga, G.P., 2008. Modulation of enzyme activities by n-polyunsaturated fatty acids to support cardiovascular health. The Journal of Nutritional Biochemistry 19 (7), 417–437.

Siddiqui, R.A., Shaikh, S.R., Sech, L.A., Yount, H.R., Stillwell, W., Zaloga, G.P., 2004. Omega-3 fatty acids: health benefits and cellular mechanisms of action. Mini Reviews in Medicinal Chemistry 4 (8), 859–871.

Simopoulos, A.P., 2009. Omega-6/omega-3 essential fatty acids: biological effects. World Review of Nutrition and Dietetics 99, 1–16.

Simopoulos, A.P., 2011. Evolutionary aspects of diet: the omega-6/omega-3 ratio and the brain. Molecular Neurobiology 44 (2), 203–215.

Tavazzi, L., Tognoni, G., Franzosi, M.G., et al., 2004. Rationale and design of the GISSI heart failure trial: a large trial to assess the effects of n-3 polyunsaturated fatty acids and rosuvastatin in symptomatic congestive heart failure. European Journal of Heart Failure 6 (5), 635–641.

Terano, T., Hirai, A., Shiina, T., Tamura, Y., Saitoh, Y., 1997. Mechanism of anti-proliferative action of eicosapentaenoic acid (EPA) in vascular cell growth: its effect on signal transduction system. Advances in Experimental Medicine and Biology 407, 399–404.

Thies, F., Garry, J., Yaqoob, P., et al., 2003. Association of n-3 polyunsaturated fatty acids with stability of atherosclerotic plaques: a randomised controlled trial. Lancet 361, 477–485.

Van Horn, L., McCoin, M., Kris-Etherton, P.M., et al., 2008. The evidence for dietary prevention and treatment of cardiovascular disease. Journal of the American Dietetic Association 108, 287–331.

Verboom, C.N., 2006. Critical analysis of GISSI-Prevenzione Trial. Highly purified omega-3 polyunsaturated fatty acids are effective as adjunct therapy for secondary prevention of myocardial infarction. Herz 31 (Suppl. 3), 49–59.

von Schacky, C., Angerer, P., Kothny, W., Theisen, K., Mudra, H., 1999. The effect of dietary omega-3 fatty acids on coronary atherosclerosis. A randomized, double-blind, placebo-controlled trial. Annals of Internal Medicine 130 (7), 554–562.

von Schacky, C., Baumann, K., Angerer, P., 2001. The effect of n-3 fatty acids on coronary atherosclerosis: results from SCIMO, an angiographic study, background and implications. Lipids 36 (Suppl), S99–S102.

Vrablík, M., Prusíková, M., Snejdrlová, M., Zlatohlávek, L., 2009. Omega-3 fatty acids and cardiovascular disease risk: do we understand the relationship? Physiological Research 58 (Suppl. 1), S19–S26.

Walser, B., Stebbins, C.L., 2008. Omega-3 fatty acid supplementation enhances stroke volume and cardiac output during dynamic exercise. European Journal of Applied Physiology 104 (3), 455–461.

Wilczynska-Kwiatek, A., Singh, R.B., De Meester, F., 2010. Nutrition and behavior: the role of ω3 fatty acids. The Open Nutrition Journal 3, 119–128.

Xiao, Y.F., Ke, Q., Chen, Y., Morgan, J.P., Leaf, A., 2004. Inhibitory effect of n-3 fish oil fatty acids on cardiac Na+/Ca2+ exchange currents in HEK293t cells. Biochemical and Biophysical Research Communications 321 (1), 116–123.

Yokoyama, M., Origasa, H., Matsuzaki, M., et al., 2007. Effects of eicosapentaenoic acid on major coronary events in hypercholesterolaemic patients (JELIS): a randomised open-label, blinded endpoint analysis. Lancet 369, 1090–1098.

Yosefy, C., Khalamizer, V., Viskoper, J.R., et al., 2003. Impaired nitric oxide production, brachial artery reactivity and fish oil in offspring of ischaemic heart disease patients. British Journal of Biomedical Science 60 (3), 144–148.

Yoshikawa, T., Shimano, H., Yahagi, N., et al., 2002. Polyunsaturated fatty acids suppress sterol regulatory element-binding protein 1c promoter activity by inhibition of liver X receptor (LXR) binding to LXR response elements. Journal of Biological Chemistry 277, 1705–1711.

Yu-Poth, S., Yin, D., Kris-Etherton, P.M., Zhao, G., Etherton, T.D., 2005. Long-chain polyunsaturated fatty acids upregulate LDL receptor protein expression in fibroblasts and HepG2 cells. Journal of Nutrition 135, 2541–2545.

Zaima, N., Sugawara, T., Goto, D., Hirata, T., 2006. Trans geometric isomers of EPA decrease LXRalpha-induced cellular triacylglycerol via suppression of SREBP-1c and PGC-1beta. Journal of Lipid Research 47, 2712–2717.

Zhang, L., Yan, F., Zhang, S., et al., 2012. Structural basis of transfer between lipoproteins by cholesteryl transfer protein. Nature Chemical Biology 8, 342–349.

Zhao, Y.T., Chen, Q., Sun, Y.X., et al., 2009. Prevention of sudden cardiac death with omega-3 fatty acids in patients with coronary heart disease: a meta-analysis of randomized controlled trials. Annals of Medicine 41 (4), 301–310.

Ziedén, B., Kaminskas, A., Kristenson, M., Olsson, A.G., Kucinskiene, Z., 2002. Long chain polyunsaturated fatty acids may account for higher low-density lipoprotein oxidation susceptibility in Lithuanian compared to Swedish men. Scandinavian Journal of Clinical and Laboratory Investigation 62 (4), 307–314.

CHAPTER 31

Herbal Supplements or Herbs in Heart Disease: Herbiceutical Formulation, Clinical Trials, Futuristic Developments

R. Sharma, R.J. Moffatt
Florida State University, Tallahassee, FL, USA

1. INTRODUCTION

In this chapter, readers are introduced to the emerging knowledge on the use of herbs in cardiac protection, the mechanism of dyslipidemia in development of heart disease, and the new technique of noninvasive microimaging of heart disease. The scope of herbal treatment is wider to manage initial dyslipidemia by lipid lowering and 'cardiac capacity' enhancing in cardioprotection and cardiac prevention. Prevention of disease includes prevention of hypertension, coronary heart disease (CHD), cerebrovascular disease, peripheral vascular disease, heart failure, rheumatic heart disease, congenital heart disease, and cardiomyopathy. This chapter is divided into different sections on present state of the art herbal formulas in cardioprotection, introduction to herbs in heart disease, biomarkers and biochemistry of herbal cardioprotective action, and herbiceutical formulas, and future prospects of herbiceuticals in cardioprotection with a comment on government policy.

2. HERBICEUTICAL FORMULA IN HEART DISEASE TREATMENT

In the following section, available herbiceuticals to treat CHD are described. The following description is modified from its original sources (Sheu and Shen, 2004).

2.1 Formula 1

San–Huang–Hsie–Hsin–Tang® is prepared from scutellaria (Radix Scutellariae):rhizome of coptis:root and rhizome of rhubarb (Radix et Rhizoma Rhei):Radix Ginseng (root of ginseng) in the ratio of 1–2:1–2:1–2:1–2 or 1:1:1:1 in 95% ethanol.

Scutellaria plant: All four ingredients are extracted, filtered, and mixed to form a herbal paste. This herbal paste can stabilize and lower blood pressure, and can prevent damage to endothelial cell by inhibiting iNOS activity, inhibiting COX-2 activity, reducing blood C-reactive protein (CRP) concentration, inhibiting smooth muscular cell proliferation,

Bioactive Food as Dietary Interventions for Cardiovascular Disease
http://dx.doi.org/10.1016/B978-0-12-396485-4.00178-X
© 2013 Elsevier Inc.
All rights reserved.

and reducing blood cholesterol level in people of all ages, and particularly the elderly. The mechanism of herbal paste in preventing heart disease can be described in four reactions: (1) Nitrogen monoxide (NO) produced in endothelium by eNOS is a potent vasodilator and inhibits platelet aggregation, smooth muscle cell proliferation, and monocyte adhesion and adhesion molecule expression, thus, maintaining the integrity of endothelial tissues. (2) Production of COX-dependent factors – prostanoids – and oxygen free radicals is due to endothelial dysfunction or vascular damage. Herbal-induced inhibition of COX may restore NO mediated vasodilation and anti-inflammatory utility. (3) Overexpression of iNOS leads to increased NO production and causes myocardial dysfunction, congestive heart failure (CHF), and cardiac arrest, while herbal formula suppresses iNOS expression; (4) CRP is formed in the inflammation process and atherosclerosis with prevalent CHD, stroke, and peripheral artery disease, while Scutellaria herbal SunTen® formula reduces C-reactive protein formation. Scutellaria has ingredients of baicalin, oroxylin, A-glucuronide, wogonin-7-O-glucuronide, baicalein, wogonin, and oroxylin A.

SunTen® cardiovascular drug is made from 20 g each of root of scutellaria, rhizome of coptis, and root/rhizome of rhubarb. All three are boiled, extracted, filtered, condensed, and reflexed in ethanol to make the dry powder containing the herbs and chemicals shown in Tables 31.1 and 31.2.

2.2 Formula 2

Mixture of four: Danshensu (*Salvia miltiorrhiza* Bge.) chemical formula D(+) β-(3,4-dihydroxyphenyl) lactic acid, Tanshinone IIA, matrine (*Sophorea flavescens* Ait.), and oxymatrine (Radix sophorae Flavescentis), puerarin (*Pueraria lobata* Phwi.). Fours herbs are mixed in the ratio of 1:1:1:1 to prepare a herbal mixture to treat atherosclerosis or obstructed blood supply to the heart. The mechanism of cardioprotection was invented to inhibit blood platelet accumulation and blood fibrin dissolution; for vasodilatation and relieving smooth muscle spasm in myocardium muscle; to improve myocardial muscle metabolism under anaerobic conditions and reducing ATP consumption as a protective measure; inhibiting peroxidation reaction or clearance of free radicals and fatty deposits; inhibiting blood platelets and improving cell membrane mobility; increasing cAMP in cardiac muscle to tolerate glucose and oxygen insufficiency; strengthening the immune system; and increasing vasodilation and blood flow. For details of cardiac protection outcome in experimental animals, readers are referred to read patents (Young, 2006) including herbal mixture testing by marker cardiac enzymes, ventricular function, right–left atrial driving force or anti-arrhythmicity, LVSD, and beta receptor of adenylate cyclase to prove the following:

1. The herbal mixture provides antimyocardial infarction protection of vascular epithelial tissue.
2. The herbal mixture reduces angina pectoris and endothelin (ET)-1 along with decalcification gene-related protoplasm (cGRP)-induced dilatation of blood vessels.

Table 31.1 A Herbal Content Analysis is Shown by HPLC for Different Components in San-Huang-Hsie-Hsin-Tang® Formula

Compound	Retention time	Maximum absorption wave length (nm)
Sennoside B	38	268
Sennoside A	46	269
Aloe–emodin	72	277
Rhein	87	257
Emodin	92.5	287
Chrysophenol	94	256
Baicalin	30	176
Orooxylin A–glucuronide	36	269
Wogonin-7-O-glucuronide	39	272
Baicalin	51	275
Wogonin	56	274
Oroxylin A	57	269
Berberstine	17	264; 357
Columnbamine	21	264; 345
Jatrorrhizine	21.5	264; 345
Epiberberine	22.5	267; 357
Coptisine	23.5	264; 358
Palmatine	26	272; 345
Berberine	27	263; 347
Gensenoside Rgl	23.5	204
Gensenoside Re	23.8	203
Gensenoside Rbl	38.5	203
6-Gingerol	17	230, 285
6-Shogol	26	230, 285

Source: Ref. [95].

Table 31.2 A Herbal Content Analysis is Shown by HPLC for Different Components in SunTen® Formula

Herbs of the present pharmaceutical composition

Pharmaceutical name	Botanical name	Family	Common description	Major ingredients
Radix Scutellariae	*Scutellaria baicalensis* Georgi	Labiatae	Scutellaria or scute	Baicalein, baicalin, wogonin, wogonin-7-O-glucuronide, neobaicalein, oroxylin A glucuronide, camphesterol, β-sitosterol, benzoic acid

Continued

Table 31.2 A Herbal Content Analysis is Shown by HPLC for Different Components in SunTen® Formula—cont'd

Herbs of the present pharmaceutical composition

Pharmaceutical name	Botanical name	Family	Common description	Major ingredients
Rhizoma Coptidis	*Coptis chinensis* Franch., *C. deltoidea* C. Y. Cheng, *C. omeiensis* (Chen) C. Y. Cheng, or *C. teetoides* C. Y. Cheng	Ranunculaceae	Coptis rhizome	Berberine, coptisine, worenine, palmatine, columbamine, obacunone, obaculactone, palmatine, jatrorrhizine, magnoflorine, ferulic acid
Radix et Rhizoma Rhei	*Rheum palmatum* L. or *R. tanguticum* Maxim. et Reg. (used in northChina) or *R. officinale* Baill. (used in south China)	Polygonaceae	Rhubarb root and rhizome	Derivatives of anthraquinone glycosides including chrysophanol, emodin, aloe-emodin, rhein, and physcion, rheum tannic acids, gallic acid, catechin, tetrarin, glucogallin, cinnamic acid, rheosmin, fatty acids, calcium oxalate, glucose, fructose, sennoside A, B, and C
Rhizoma Zingiberis	*Zingiber officinale* Roscoe	Zingiberaceae	Ginger, ginger rhizome	Gingerol, shogaol, and zingerone
Radix Panacis Quinquefolii	*Panax quinquefolium* L.	Araliaceae	American ginseng	Saponins, panaquilon
Radix Ginseng (Rubra)	*Panax ginseng* C. A. Mey	Araliaceae	Ginseng, red ginseng	Panaxatriol, panaxadiol, other panoxisides, panoquilon, panaxin, ginsenin, α-panaxin, protopanaxadiol, protopanaxtriol, panacene, panaxynol, panaenic acid, panose, dammarane, glucose, fructose, maltose, sucrose, nicotinic acid, riboflavin, thiamine

Source: Sheu, S.J., Shen, C.G., 2004. Herbal Pharmaceutical Composition for Prophylaxis and/or Treatment of Cardiovascular Diseases and the Method of Preparing the Same. US Patent US2004/0234627.

3. The herbal mixture reduces platelet agglutination and atheroma to resist myocardial infarction.
4. The following formula uses Radix Salviae Miltorrhizae and is a herbal extract described in its original source Berman et al. (2006).

2.3 Formula 3

Herbal pills (a mixture of 80.0–97.0% Radix Salviae Miltorrhizae, 1.0–19.0% Panax Notoginseng, and 0.1–1.0% Borneol) and its active ingredients were invented by the following steps: (a) obtaining an appropriate amount of smashed Radix Salviae Miltorrhizae and Panax Notoginseng; (b) extracting the obtained Radix Salviae Miltorrhizae and Panax Notoginseng in hot aqueous reflux at about 60–100 °C; (c) filtering and combining the extracts to form a combined extract; (d) concentrating the combined extract from step (c) into an appropriate ratio of the volume of the concentrated extract to the weight of the inputted herbal materials to form a concentrated extract; (e) adding ethanol to the concentrated extract from step (d) to about 50–85% final concentration of ethanol, performing ethanol precipitation and forming a precipitated resolution; (f) concentrating the supernatant liquid of the precipitate resulting from step (e) to form a plaster of about 1.15–1.45 in relative density; and (g) mixing the plaster from step (f) with an appropriate amount of Borneol, thereby producing the composition of herb extract of Radix Salviae Miltorrhizae, Panax Notoginseng, and Borneol. The active ingredient extracted from *Salvia miltiorrhiza* Beg. contains one or more ingredients selected from tanshinone, salvianolic acid, methyl tanshinonate, rosmarinic acid, methyl rosmarinate, danshexinkum, protocatechualdehyde, sodium 3′4-dihydroxyphenyllactate, and lithospermic acid. The ingredient extracted from Panax notoginseng or Ginseng contains one or more ingredients selected from notoginsenoside and ginsenoside. The ingredient extracted from Dryobalanops aromatica Geartu.F. or Cinnammon camphor. contains D-borneol or L-borneol or both of them. Herbal pill preparation was invented by (a) mixing the extracts of Panax Notoginseng, extracts of Radix Salviae Miltorrhizae, synthetic borneol, and polyethylene glycol 6000 in the ratio of 4.0:20.6:1.9:79.5; (b) melting the mixture; (c) manufacturing the melted mixture into pills using a dropping machine with the following characteristics: the temperature of the dropping pot is constantly 89–93 °C; the cooling solution is liquid paraffin, whose temperature is lower than 8 °C; the inner diameter of the dropping head is 1.8 mm; the outer diameter of the dropping head is 2.4 mm; the distance between the dropping head and the surface of the cooling solution is 15 cm; and (d) the pills are centrifuged at 800–1100 rpm for 15 min to remove oils.

The herbal pill ingredients were capable of increasing blood volume in the coronary artery; relaxing the smooth muscles of blood vessels; improving peripheral circulation; raising the oxygen content in veins, or significantly improving the acute myocardial ischemia or myocardial infarction; protecting the cells from damage by hypoxia or anoxia;

protecting cells suffering from myocardial ischemia; improving microcirculation; preventing arrhythmia, platelet aggregation, and thrombosis; dissolving fibrin; lowering blood viscosity; adjusting blood cholesterol or preventing atherosclerosis; raising tolerance to hypoxia or anoxia; preventing the oxidation of lipoprotein or removing the harmful free radicals; lowering plasma ET content; significantly improving liver, kidney, and pancreas function; preventing the occurrence or development of blood vessel or nerve diseases; enhancing the immune system; and regulating vascular nerve balance (Wei et al., 2004, 2005).

2.4 Treatment of CHD with Herbal Pill

The following is a description of the continuous trials in the direction of combinatorial therapy of CHD (Sheu and Shen, 2004; Wei et al., 2004; Young, 2006).

(1) Ordinary treatment of CHD

After herbal pills became available in the market in China, treatment that was basically similar to that of Isordil® was proposed and there is no significant difference between them statistically in the treatment of CHD (Chagan et al., 2005; Jia et al., 2001; Tam et al., 2009).

(2) Pain-killing effects of herbal pills on CHD were comparable to those of glyceryl trinitrate

(3) Effects of herbal pills on the onset of CHD, heart pain frequency

Herbal pills can reduce onset frequency and volume of glyceryl trinitrate. The pills can improve blood flow to the heart in addition to relieving pain (An and Yang, 2006).

(4) Improvement of blood pressure and cardiac function in patients with CHD

Herbal pills can reduce onset frequency and volume of glyceryl trinitrate. The pills can improve blood flow to the heart in addition to relieving pain.

(5) Effects of herbal pills on ECGs and blood flow in patients with CHD

No significant differences appeared on ECGs and average exercise testing standards to show improvement with herbal pills. The pills may control irregular blood flow, lower blood viscosity, reduce the occurrence of atherosclerosis, prevent thrombosis, and can be the first choice for the treatment of CHD (Gao et al., 2010).

(6) Effects of long-term herbal pill treatment on CHD

Long-term herbal pill results are stable. The herbal pill is a multilevel, multisubjected, and multimethod medicine, which improves cardiac muscle functionality; increases blood volume by blocking the chronic calcium route; stabilizes the myocardial membrane; removes free radicals; regulates myocardial cell metabolism; improves blood platelet aggregation; and lowers cholesterol and blood viscosity.

(7) Clinical research on the effects of herbal pills on unstable-type angina

The experiment showed that herbal pills can reduce oxygen consumption by cardiac muscles, improve blood flow in coronary arteries, and rebalance the oxygen demand-to-supply ratio in cardiac muscles (Gao et al., 2010).

(8) The effects of herbal pills on the treatment of exertion-type angina

Herbal pills can efficiently relieve pain and increase blood flow to the cardiac muscle. Herbal pills can also reduce oxygen consumption, improve blood flow to the coronary artery, rebalance oxygen demand and oxygen supply, and prevent atherosclerosis. It is reported to be an ideal medicine for the prevention or treatment of CHD, angina, and atherosclerosis (Tam et al., 2010).

3. HERBICEUTICAL TESTING

The following strategy is currently used in the development, testing, and approval of new herbal formulas.

- Preparation of herbal plant extraction: Herbs such as scutellaria, coptis, and rhubarb are extracted by using a solvent (water or organic solvent, 95% ethanol).
- Separation and filtration: Extracts are filtered. Individual herbal extracts are filtered and condensed under reduced pressure in a water bath at 50 °C to make herbal paste.
- Preparation of powders: American ginseng or ginger is prepared as a powder by extracting with solvent (cutting in pieces, grinding, and drying) and passing through a sieve.
- Herbal pharmaceutical mixture: Herb dry powders are mixed in herbal paste and dried to prepare as tablets, bolus, powders, capsules, and granules using binder, carrier, and filler.
- Experimental animal models: (A) Blood pressure lowering properties (BP, heart rate on multifunction recorder) were compared in spontaneous hypertensive rats, which were administered the herbal mixture through a catheter in the femoral artery, and also compared with captoril or nifedipine given in the same way. (B) In another set of animals, heart rate, systolic/diastolic BP, and mean arterial BP were compared in elderly animals. Isolated, perfused hearts with Kreb's Henseleit buffer containing the herbal mixture were used for measuring coronary flow and coronary perfusion pressure. (C) COX-2 and iNOS enzyme synthesis in mouse macrophage cells was induced by lipopolysaccharides and both COX-2 and iNOS were measured by ELISA. COX-2 and iNOS enzyme protein biosynthesis can be measured in excised tissues by antibody-based PAGE. (D) Herb-induced inhibition of iNOS gene expression was measured by tissue RNA extraction, mixing iNOS primer with cDNA, and amplifying DNA mixture by PCR and running DNA separation on agarose gel; (E) Herb-induced CRP reduction in hypertensive animals was measured by ELISA in blood after centrifugation (Figure 31.1).

3.1 Preclinical Trial

In animals, LD50 dosage determination; myocardial total ischemia burden (TIB), blood plasma ET, cGRP, NO, serum superoxide dismutase (SOD) and malonyl dialdehyde (MDA); plasma RT, NO, changes of TIBN.

- Vascular ET-1 release
- cGRP
- release of NO

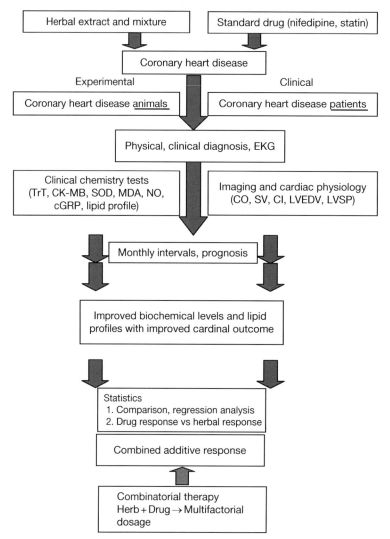

Figure 31.1 An algorithmic approach is shown to test cardiac response with herbal medicine and prepare it for combination herbal–chemotherapy treatment.

3.1.1 CHF: Experimental rat model

Symptoms:

- Palpitation, tightness in the chest, cough, pain in the front of the chest, shortness of breath, paroxysmal breathing difficulty at night, fatigue and weakness, upper body pain and discomfort, sweating, night sweating, cold phobia, and little urine.

- Physical manifestation: heart rate and heart rhythm, blood pressure, breathing, lip cyanosis, expanded cervical vein, wheezing lungs, thorax water stagnant, abdominal distension, enlarged liver, edema of lower limbs, head, and face dropsy.
- Improved cardial function index: heartbeat volume (SV), cardial output (CO), cardial index (CI), cardial emission fraction (EF), and left ventricle end diastole volume (LVEDV),
- Higher content of MDA, ANP-SOD, SOD, GSH-Px, and ANP after herbal treatment.
- Improved systolic capacity of cardial muscle by measuring left ventricle systole pressure value (LVSP), left ventricle maximum systole speed rate ($+dp/dt$), and left ventricle minimum systole speed rate ($-dp/dt$).
- With regard to animal experiments, pathological slice of animal model's heart shows hypertrophy of left ventricle myocardial cells; muscular tissue breaks; and inflammation by histology-MR microscopy.
- TIB

3.2 Clinical Trial: In Patients on WHO Criteria of Hypertrophic Cardiomyopathy with Angina Pectoris

- Confirmation by straight T wave improved strium and ventricular contraction; reduced ET-1 and rise in cGRP; high coagulation; or low platelet agglutination
- SOD activity and reduced MDA density
- Reduced ET-1
- Rise in cGRP comparison decalcification-related protoplasm (cGRP)
- Angina pectoris in A $\rightarrow$ D grades.
- Sex, age, disease course, angina pectoris types, and degree of seriousness of angina pectoris
- Irregular heart rhythm and diabetic complication
- Liver and renal function, electrocardiogram for tall T wave and suppressed ST section

3.3 Technique Development in Noninvasive Microimaging of Thrombosis and Measurement of Heart Disease

With the advancements in science, noninvasive imaging modalities are now in use to detect, measure, and monitor the prognosis and progress of heart disease condition before and after intervention. Coronary artery wall thickness and myocardium shape are the two major parameters in the assessment of heart disease burden. Magnetic resonance imaging and ultrasound scanning of heart are the choices to measure thrombosis and cardiac function, respectively. The cytomorphic and molecular markers of the heart have been established as measurable indices in different territories using magnetic resonance microscopy and nanoparticle-based molecular targeting to test cardioprotective herbal, nutraceutical, and pharmaceutical drugs. The new technique of drug testing includes multiple contrast *in vivo* heart MRI/MRA, *ex vivo* delayed ultrahigh magnetic field MRI, and histopathologic MRI correlation data, as reported previously. The major focus was to develop high diagnostic accuracy in noninvasive identification of plaque contents and heart territories by MR microscopy with structural details, as shown in Figures 31.2–31.5. For details, readers are referred to the original sources (Sharma, 2011; Sharma and Singh, 2004).

3.4 Strategy of Cardioprotection

Heart protection and preventive herbal action is described as antifibrillatory, antihypertensive, and antithrombotic, which essentially includes lumen space minimization, wall

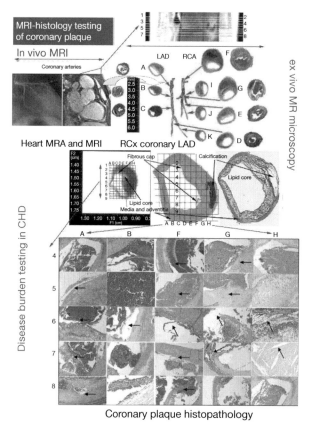

Figure 31.2 Schematics of coronary artery *in vivo* MRI and *ex vivo* MRI with corresponding histopathology at different locations to test and monitor the effect of drugs and herbs. *Reproduced from Sharma, R., Singh, R.B., 2004. Human coronary artery lesions: magnetic resonance imaging, NMR spectroscopy, histopathology and oxidative stress markers. World Heart Journal 1 (2), 179–184, with permission.*

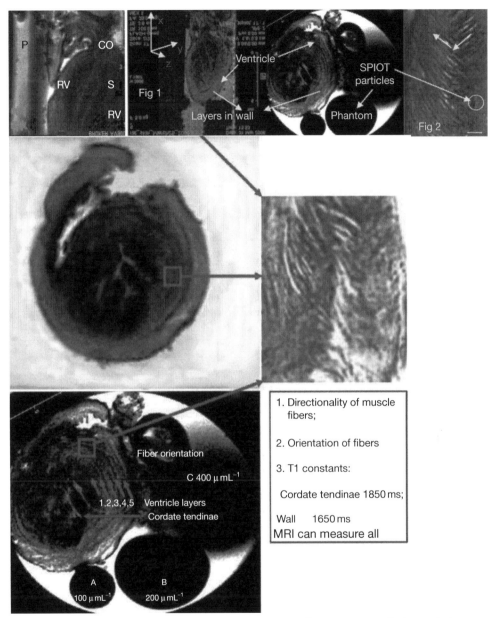

Figure 31.3 New nanoparticle-based NMR microscopy technique to test herbs and drugs on cardiac muscle structural–functional properties. *Reproduced from Sharma, R., 2011. Antibodies in nanomedicine and bioimaging. In: Pathak, Y., Benita, S. (Ed.), Antibody Mediated (mAB) Drug Delivery Systems (DDS): Concepts, Technology and Applications. John Willey and Sons, New York (Chapter 17), with permission.*

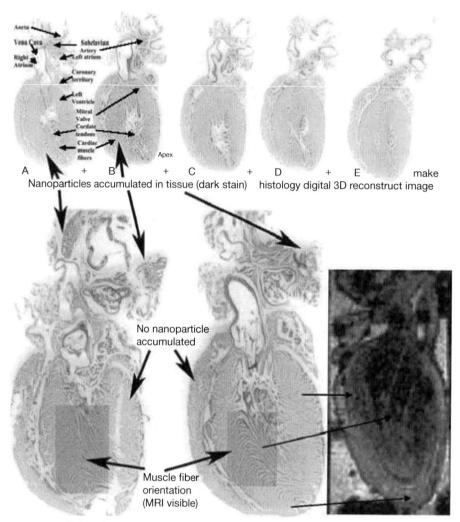

Figure 31.4 Herbal and drug testing of heart muscles and heart structures by *ex vivo* MRI and corresponding *ex vivo* histopathology to observe cytomorphic changes in cardiac structures. *Reproduced from Sharma, R., 2011. Antibodies in nanomedicine and bioimaging. In: Pathak, Y., Benita, S. (Ed.), Antibody Mediated (mAB) Drug Delivery Systems (DDS): Concepts, Technology and Applications. John Willey and Sons, New York (Chapter 17), with permission.*

thinning, and cardiac muscle strengthening, in the following sections based on imaging strategy for CHD (Berman et al., 2006; Sharma and Singh, 2010).

Three main goals to be accomplished to keep the heart healthy are
- opening the blood vessels
- strengthening the heart muscle
- controlling free radical damage – consumption of antioxidants.

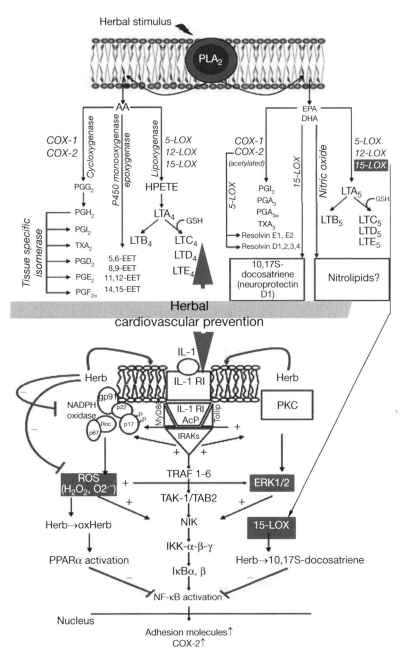

Figure 31.5 Metabolic reactions in COX, IL-1 signaling pathways and lipooxygenases. FA, fatty acid(s); PGH$_2$, prostaglandin H$_2$; PGI$_2$, prostacyclin; TXA$_2$, thromboxane A$_2$; PGD$_2$, prostaglandin D$_2$; PGE$_2$, prostaglandin E$_2$; PGF$_{2\alpha}$, prostaglandin F$_{2\alpha}$; HPETE, hydroperoxy eicosatetraenoic acids; EET, epoxyeicosatrienoic acids; LT, leukotrienes; PGI$_3$, prostaglandin I$_3$; PGA$_3$, prostaglandin A$_3$; TXA$_3$, thromboxane A$_3$; PGF$_{3\alpha}$, prostaglandin F$_{3\alpha}$; GSH, glutathione; PLA$_2$, phospholipases A$_2$. *Modified from Massaro, M., Scofitti, E., Carluccio, M.A., Caterina, R.D., 2008. Basic mechanisms behind the effects of n-3 fatty acids on cardiovascular disease. Prostaglandins, Leukotrienes, and Essential Fatty Acids 79 (3–5), 109–115.*

3.5 Biomarkers in Evaluation of Herbs

Herbal testing is a standard procedure using different biomarkers, as shown in schematics in Figure 31.1, to evaluate herbal response to improve cardiac recovery. The following reports are extracted from original sources in both preclinical and clinical herbal trials for readers (Sharma and Singh, 2004; Wei et al., 2004; Young, 2006).

3.5.1 Antimyocardial infarction protection of vascular epithelial heart tissue in patients

The observation includes counting clinical symptoms before and after treatment, for the changes inmyocardial TIB, ET, cGRP, NO, and SOD and MDA.

TIB is done with Holter inspection. Before and after medication, venous blood is drawn for determining plasma RT, NO, density of serum SOD and MDA, and changes in TIBN. With regard to the treatment of blood shortage to the heart, it is important to effectively improve myocardial blood shortage and, to the greatest possible extent, to restore oxygen resupply and protect vascular epithelial cells from vascular oxygen shortage and oxygen resupply damage.

- Vascular ET is a strong and lasting polyprotoplasm that shrinks vascular byczenol®. Its primary biological effects are multifunctional such as shrinking vascular plain muscle, stimulating breeding of cells, inhibiting release of renal hormone, strengthening depotassium adrenaline and vascular nervous hormone II, refining vascular amino acid inhibition hormone, matter revolving, self-secretion, and side-secretion. In fact, it plays an important role in the biological and pathological process of cardiac and cerebral vascular diseases such as those of reversal of damage, generation of blood vessels, and formation of thrombosis. However, from the biological standpoint, vascular epithelial tissue is also the most vulnerable functional interface. It can be affected by various pathological situations, and produces morphological and biochemical changes. Damage to vascular epithelial tissue is the main mechanism for increasing ET release. Its excessive release can lead to coronary artery convulsion, myocardial blood shortage, and even necrosis. Thus, reducing ET is an important means of protecting the health of the myocardium.
- cGRP is a byczenol polyprotoplasm that dilates blood vessels. It leads to dropping of blood pressure and strong diastolic capillary function. It is able to prevent tissues of the heart, brain, and kidney from damage of blood shortage and reconcentration. It protects the myocardium from shortage of blood and damage, and enhances systole and myocardial discharge capacity of the myocardium (reduced flare up of heart rhythm, ET-1) to strengthen vascular resistance and breeding of muscle cells.
- NO has the capability of dilating blood vessels, reducing blood pressure, and inhibiting platelet adherence and polymerization. It has the most significant function of safeguarding the regular cardiac mechanism of maintaining myocardial blood flow. It is

able to resist the vascular systole effect of ET. It is an internal myocardial protective substance. Two different biological effects take part in the adjustment of cardiac vascular function and the flare-up process of coronary disease. Therefore, protecting vascular epithelial tissue from being damaged; effectively inhibiting secretion of ET-1; improving release of NO; adjusting the plasma density balance of both in order to improve the supply of blood and oxygen to myocardium: these are the important ways of treating CHD.

- Reduction in plasma ET density and the obvious rise in plasma NO indicate the positive adjustment function on internal vascular active substance and metabolism of cardiac protective substance. In myocardial blood shortage, the herbal mixture provides good protection and restoration in vascular epithelial tissue damage or antimyocardial blood shortage as it has protective effects on vascular epithelial tissue.
- Myocardial blood shortage of CHD and damage of blood shortage refilling, increase lipoperoxide reaction to cause an oxygen–unrestrained base in vascular epithelial tissue. Antioxidation or superoxide anion scavenger herbal actions are the protective functions in vascular epithelial tissue damage and myocardial blood shortage.
- To enhance blood circulation, improve later developments related to blood, resist fibrosolvent thrombosis of hemolysis, dilate coronary arteries, prevent spasms of minor arteries, and increase blood flow capacity of coronary arteries indicated by the rise in SOD activity and reduced MDA density in conjunction with lipoperoxide removal as internal and external antioxidant.

3.5.2 CHD, angina pectoris, change of ET-1, and decalcification

Gene-related protoplasm (cGRP) of pre- and posttreatment: antihypertrophic cardiomyopathy in patients is standard for symptomatic diagnosis of CAD:

- Angina pectoris in $A \rightarrow D$ grades. Herbal treatment restricts or reverts the events of angina pectoris for a longer time with the disappearance of the symptoms.
- Sex, age, disease course, angina pectoris types, and degree of seriousness of angina pectoris.
- Irregular heart rhythm and diabetic complications are comparable ($p > 0.05$).
- Clinical symptoms, physical manifestation, heart rate and blood pressure, lab tests of blood, urine and stool, liver and renal function, electrocardiogram for ST section. Tall T wave and suppressed ST section appear after herbal treatment.
- Reduced ET-1 and rise in cGRP comparison (pg ml^{-1} X±S) of two groups after treatment.
- ET is a strong and lasting polyprotoplasm with biological effects: shrinking vascular plain muscle; stimulating breeding of cells; inhibiting release of renal hormone; strengthening depotassium adrenaline and vascular nervous hormone II; and refining vascular amino acid inhibition hormone. It has an inhibitory effect on cardial mechanism.

- cGRP is a byczenol polyprotoplasm with biological effects: dilating blood vessels; dropping of blood pressure and thus a strong diastole function on capillaries; preventing the heart, brain, liver, and kidney from damage of blood shortage and reconcentration; protecting the myocardium from shortage of blood and enhancing myocardium systole and cardial discharge capacity. As a result, flare-up of heart rhythm can be prevented or reduced; cGRP strengthens the vascular resistance and prevents the myocardium from damage. Herbal mixture raises the plasma cGRP level.

3.5.3 CHF: Experimental rat model

Symptoms:

- Palpitation, tightness of chest, coughing, pain in the front of the chest, shortness of breath, paroxysmal breathing difficulty at night, fatigue and weakness, upper body pain and discomfort, sweating, night sweating, cold phobia and reduced urination.
- Physical manifestation: heart rate and heart rhythm, blood pressure, breathing, lip cyanosis, expanded cervical vein, wheezing lungs, stagnant thorax water, abdominal distension, enlarged liver, edema of lower limbs, head, and face dropsy.
- Improved cardial function index: heartbeat volume (SV), CO, CI, cardial EF, and LVEDV.
- Higher content of MDA, ANP-SOD, SOD, GSH-Px, and ANP after herbal treatment.
- Improved systolic capacity of cardial muscle by measuring LVSP, left ventricle maximum systole speed rate $(+dp/dt)$, and left ventricle minimum systole speed rate $(-dp/dt)$.
- With regard to animal experiment, pathological slice of animal model's heart shows hypertrophy of left ventricle myocardial cells; muscular tissue breaks; and inflammation by histology-MR microscopy.

4. CARDIOPROTECTIVE HERBAL ACTIVE COMPONENTS IN HUMAN USE APPROVED BY CDC AND REGULATED BY FDA

The herbs are rich in different metabolites playing a possible role in active intermediary metabolism and these are needed in the body in a minimum amount daily, the so-called recommended daily allowances (RDAs), through diets or herbal supplements (Table 31.3). Saponoin glycosides, antioxidents, flavonoids, and oligomeric proanthocyanidin fractions are major players along with other ingredients. Readers are referred to section 5.5 for details (Sharma and Singh, 2010). A number of herbal active ingredients are listed in Table 31.1 and some of them have been identified to be abundant in herbs, as shown in Table 31.2.

5. PHARMACEUTICAL APPROACH OF HERBICEUTICAL FORMULA WITH ANTIARRHYTHMIC PROPERTIES

5.1 Carrier of Different Herbiceutical Components

The said herbal mixture in water, saline, starch, sugar, gel, lipids, waxes, glycerol, solvents, oils, liquids, proteins, glycols, electrolyte solutions, alcohols, fillers, binders, emulsifiers, preservatives, buffers, colorants, emollients, sweeteners, surfactants, additives, and solvents may be used in a solid, liquid, powder, paste, gel, or tablet form; or as a foam, pack, aerosol, solvent, diluents, capsule, pill, liposome, syrup, solution, suppository, emulsion, suspension, or biodelivery agent. The herbiceutical mixture may be delivered as an oral, injectable, or external administration for treating cancer of the skin, breast, breast, colon, kidney, bone, blood, lymph, stomach, gastrointestinal tract, ovary, prostate, liver, lung, head and neck, adrenal gland, brain, bronchial tract, hypothalamus, parathyroid, thyroid, pancreas, pituitary gland, sinus, endometrium, and bile duct; and leukemia, AIDS, astrocytoma, glioma, and lymphoma.

Controversial status: Several bioactive compounds, such as $CoQ_{2,4,6}$, and CoQ_{10}, and herbs, such as knotwood rhizome, elecampane root, Turkey rhubarb, are less understood and their antiarrhythmic properties remain controversial. Recently, the safe use of herbiceutical and nutraceutical supplementation formulas was reviewed by the author, focusing on the preclinical and clinical evidence and the role of regulatory federal governments in approving bioactive foods, herbs, and the use of herbiceuticals (Haller et al., 2002; Sharma and Singh, 2010).

5.2 What Remains to be Solved in the Cardioprotection by Herbiceuticals?

The major issues that remain unsolved are the herbiceutical side effects, dosage and mechanisms, follow-up consequences, and mandatory guidelines for usage. The diet and lifestyle guidelines for prevention of coronary artery disease (CAD) have been evidenced as a major interest during the last few decades. Recommendations of the American Heart Association have been reformulated for better understanding based on new scientific evidence after the publication of guidelines in 2007 (Warnes et al., 2008). However, none of these guidelines emphasize the role of the diet in patients with acute myocardial infarction (AMI) and stroke. Patients presenting with AMI are highly motivated to follow the advice of the cardiologist because of their serious AMI condition. AMI is associated with hyperglycemia, hyperinsulinemia, hypertriglyceridemia, free radical stress, rise in free fatty acid, and proinflammatory cytokines, leading to endothelial dysfunction. An acute generation of proinflammatory milieu is in evidence among AMI patients, which is known to cause disruption of atheroma plaques, resulting in reinfarction and death. The synergy of these mechanisms in chronic disease is not clear enough to decide the intervention by herbiceuticals such as walnuts, ginko, and vegetables (Almario et al., 2001; Din et al., 2004; Jump, 2002; Kris-Etheron et al., 2003; Lopez-garcia et al., 2004; Khan et al., 2002). Most American experts very diligently prescribe cardioprotective dietary patterns including grains, vegetables, fruits, nuts, seeds and legumes, fat, and oils based on limited research studies. Most of the time, the side effects of newly introduced products in the market are not documented, for example, there is no recommendation for refined starches in the prevention of endothelial dysfunction (Hjerkinn et al., 2005; Khan et al., 2002). There is no guideline for the type of fatty acid rich oil and the type of nuts for omega-3 fat and monounsaturated fatty acid (MUFA) content in supplemented processed cardioprotective foods. While foods and beverages with added sugars and refined starches as well as excess of omega-6, total and saturated fat and trans-fatty acids, may be proinflammatory, increased intake of omega-3 fatty acid and MUFA may not be cardioprotective against the surge of TNF-alpha, IL-6, IL-18, and adhesion molecules such as VCAM-1 (vascular cell adhesion molecule-1) and IVAM-1 (intravascular cell adhesion molecule-1) caused by high glycemic, rapidly absorbed proinflammatory foods (De Caterina et al., 2000; Harris et al., 2007; Hu and Willett, 2002). These foods are known to initiate a proinflammatory milieu in the body that is similar to that of AMI, causing a further increase in complications among these patients (Haller et al., 2002). Keeping these facts in mind, it is necessary to identify concrete evidence of cardioprotective mechanisms in animals and from clinical trials under controlled conditions with thorough investigations, careful nutritional formula design, and analysis of success rate versus fallacies of earlier clinical experiences in favor of herbiceuticals in public use.

5.3 Animal Studies

A large volume of literature is available on the inhibitory effects of herbiceuticals on cardiovascular disease (CVD) cell growth based on observations of cultured CVD cell proliferation, enhanced apoptosis, antioxidant action, and so on. Attempts are still on in the direction of morphological, cytomorphic, and histopathologic evidence for herbiceutical-induced lipid inhibition and thrombosis by using 3D localized molecular imaging techniques. Previous studies on micro-MRI and immunostaining suggested reduced apoptosis in experimental models – rats, mice, rabbits, pigs, and dogs (Harris et al., 2007). The major benefits were reduced oxidative stress, slowed apoptosis, reduced proliferation, small plaque size, less necrosis, and poor atherosclerosis growth in treated groups (Coombes et al., 2000). The mechanisms of these herbiceuticals are still not established and it remains to be investigated with more scientifically diet-controlled experimental methods (Oudit et al., 2004; Racasan et al., 2004; Wang et al., 2005; Zhou et al., 2003). Moreover, the beneficial effects of herbiceuticals in experimental animals were reviewed and two-third of the literature reports on herbiceuticals are documented on experimental animal CVD studies as either reviews or animal bench experiments on CVD prevention without confirmation. The clinical evidence of CVD prevention with herbiceuticals is poorly reported or is still based on the biochemical mechanisms of nutrients in diets reported over several decades. Some mechanisms of herbiceutical action are reported to be immune modulatory, apoptosis inducing, free radical removing, cell proliferation inhibiting, and necrosis inhibiting. New

Ayurvedic (Indian traditional medicine) concepts are also emerging as powerful herbiceuticals in CVD prevention (Zampolli et al., 2006). The growing literature on the mechanism of herbiceutical action in the CVD supports the extended benefits of herbiceuticals, but it needs more investigations as described in the following section on new literature evidence (El-Badry et al., 2007; Esterhuyse et al., 2005; Zahid et al., 2005).

5.4 Clinical Trials

Singh et al. (1992a,b,c) used 400 g day^{-1} of fruits, vegetables, and legumes in conjunction with mustard oil to decrease the risk of hypertension, diabetes, and CAD in the 1990s, similar to DART, DART II, and GISSI (Samuel et al., 2008). This diet was reexamined by DASH investigators and subsequently by other groups to observe the reduced risk of hypertension in the USA (Nilsen et al., 2001; Singh et al., 1992a,b,c). In further randomized, controlled intervention trials, Singh et al. (2002) and Sharma and Singh (2010), administered 400 g day^{-1} of fruits, vegetables, and nuts (almonds and walnuts) and another 400 g day^{-1} of whole grains including legumes in conjunction with 25–50 g day^{-1} of mustard oil (ALA 2.9 g day^{-1}) in patients with high risk of vascular disease, which showed significant benefits (Almario et al., 2001; Obarzanek et al., 2001; Singh et al., 2008). Other workers also found a beneficial effect of fruit, vegetables, nuts, and ℵ-3 fatty acid (EPA + DHA 1.8 g day^{-1})-rich foods in patients at risk of CAD (Singh et al., 1992a,b,c, 2008). A randomized, double-blind placebo-controlled trial on 300 patients after MI supplemented with EPA + DHA 3.4–3.5 g day^{-1} or corn oil showed no change. Increased intake of MUFA and ℵ-3 fatty acids has been suggested to be protective against diabetes and metabolic syndrome, whereas increased consumption of trans-fatty acids, saturated fat, and refined starches can predispose to CVD. India has been through a rapid economic development causing increased consumption of salt, tobacco, fat, sugar, and energy in the past four decades. There has been an increase in per capita income, gross domestic product, food production, and automobile production in the last four decades (Singh et al., 1992a,b,c, 2008).

The period from 1970 to 2008 has witnessed a marked shift toward a nutraceutical-rich diet and lifestyle, particularly in the urban population in India. New bioactive factors have come to light regarding cardiovascular mechanisms likely affected by nutrients; (1) iodine induces T3 and nitric oxide decreases SVR by dilation of the arterioles protein kinase akt pathway via smooth muscle relaxation through nuclear transcription mechanisms (Singh et al., 1992a,b,c); (2) fish consumption >300 g week^{-1} reduces nonfatal coronary syndrome (CARDIO 2000 study) (Sampath and Ntambi, 2004); (3) transcription of the positively regulated genes (alpha-myosin heavy chain (MHC) and calcium ATPase, SERCA2) downregulate the expression of negatively regulated genes (beta-MHC and phospholamban) to increase cardiac contractile performance. It may be possible to repair cardiac contractility and improve ejection time with nutraceutical protection (LVET) (Kim et al., 1999; Sampath and Ntambi, 2004); (4) improved cardiac output, reduced cardiac preload (low rennin state and decreased erythropoietin secretion), increased vascular resistance, bradycardia, slightly depressed myocardial contractility, and some increase in LV mass (Leaf et al., 2003); (5) IF channel, L-type and T-type calcium channel, potassium channel, and the ryanodine channel contribute to pacemaker functions and heart rate (De Caterina et al., 2003); (6) dyslipidemia due to total cholesterol (TC) and low-density lipoproteins (LDL) cholesterol, triglycerides, very low-density lipoproteins (VLDL), intermediate-density lipoproteins, apoprotein A-1, and apoprotein B are observed as well (Connor et al., 1993; Zampelas et al., 1994); (7) cholesteryl ester transfer protein and hepatic lipase, increased levels of high-density lipoproteins (HDL); (8) endothelial dysfunction, increased arterial stiffness, increased vascular resistance, and hypercoagulability with CAD (Abeywardena and Head, 2001).

However, it is not known whether bioactive food affects cardiovascular morbidity or mortality. It might be beneficial to use bioactive food or herbiceuticals as supplements simultaneously with cardioprotective drug therapy. Recently available noninvasive imaging methods such as Doppler echocardiography, carotid intima-media thickness, pulsed tissue Doppler imaging, cardiac MRI, and radionuclide ventriculography to evaluate the preejection/ejection ratio in systolic dysfunction may be more useful to establish the beneficial effects of herbiceuticals. Overall, trials evaluating cardiovascular mortality and mortality have yielded conflicting results (Hooper et al., 2006).

5.5 Biochemical Basis of Herbiceuticals in Cardiac Prevention

Natural vegetables, herbs, plants, and wild foods are complex in structural composition. The biochemical basis of the individual sources of these foods has not been explored because of their complex nature. Some of the evidence is in favor of the active food principles as herbiceuticals to show cardioprotective or preventive supplements. Some of the herbiceuticals are in the phase of clinical trial or already available as food supplements.

Complementary and alternative medicine (CAM) is emerging as a safe practice in the prevention of chronic coronary and heart diseases because of the high risk of mortality and long-term morbidity associated with surgical procedures of CAD and the severe side effects of chemotherapy. Herbal medicines have shown reduced myocyte cell necrosis in cultured cells. Vitamins, minerals, and dietary fat play a role in cardioprevention and control. The mechanisms of herbiceutical action can be discussed broadly in the following categories based on the active metabolites present in herbiceuticals.

1. Niacin-bound chromium is reported to enhance myocardial protection in ischemia-reperfusion injury (Thirunavukkarasu et al., 2006).
2. The mechanism of the antithrombotic effect was introduced by dietary diacylglycerol in atherogenic mice (Roche and Gibney, 2000).
3. The protective effect of potassium against hypertensive cardiac dysfunction was associated with reactive oxygen species reduction (Matsui et al., 2006).

4. The atherogenic process is reduced by regulation of coenzyme Q10 biosynthesis and breakdown.

5. The n-3 fatty acids reduce the risk of CVD. The evidence was explained and the mechanisms were explored (Dallner et al., 2003; Matsui et al., 2006).

6. The Mediterranean diet and optimal diets play a role in prevention of CHD.

7. Alpha-tocopherol therapy was evidenced to reduce oxidative stress and atherosclerosis (Harris et al., 2002).

8. Genetic deficiency of inducible nitric oxide synthase reduces atherosclerosis and lowers plasma lipid peroxides in apolipoprotein E-knockout mice.

9. Glutathione is the liver's most abundant protective constituent of antioxidant glutathione reductase enzyme. Glutathione functions as a substrate for the two key detoxification processes in the liver: (1) transforming toxins into water-soluble forms; (2) neutralizing and 'conjugating' with toxins for elimination through the gut or the kidneys. If either of these processes is impaired for any reason, toxins will accumulate in the body and lead to disease. The best nutrition with liver CVD focuses on improving the body's glutathione reserves (Calder, 2004).

10. The Soy isoflavone Haelan951 (genistein and genistin) and garlic allicin were reported to have some role as a cardioprotective in humans (Santo et al., 2010). Beta-glycoside conjugate, genistin, is abundant in fermented soybeans and soybean products such as soymilk and tofu. The beta-glycosyl bond of genistin is cleaved to produce genistein by microbes during fermentation to yield miso and natto. Soy sauce has high isoflavone but low miso and natto content.

How much of soy isoflavone is needed in the diet? 1.5–4.1 mg per person miso isoflavone and 6.3–8.3 mg per person natto, respectively (Santo et al., 2010).

11. Green tea has always been considered by the Chinese and Japanese as a potent medicine for the maintenance of health, as being endowed with the power to prolong life (Basu and Lucas, 2007).

12. CVD has been reported to be associated with vascular endothelial growth factor (Gurley et al., 2008).

13. Some herbal plants act as cardioprotective medicines. The herbal extracts are known to reduce the circulating markers of inflammation, including CRP, interleukine-6 (IL-6), tumor necrosis factor-α (TNF-α), and serum amyloid A (SAA).

14. Combination of garlic, ginko biloba, and herbs with resveratrol inhibited nearly 92% of age-related gene changes in the heart (Gurley et al., 2008).

5.6 Lipid Metabolism and Fatty Acid Modifiers as the Basis of CVD and the Role of Herbiceuticals

Lipid metabolism has been established as a major factor in cardiovascular protection by supplementing omega fatty acids as described with recent developments for interested readers (Sharma and Singh, 2010). The possible reversal of increased TC, increased

LDL cholesterol, apolipoprotein B, and decreased HDL concentrations in cardiovascular patients on bioactive foods and herbiceuticals is controversial (Slavin, 2008). In several trials, TC levels, HDL, LDL-cholesterol, triglycerides, apolipoprotein A and B, and lipoprotein A were not significantly improved with nutraceutical or vitamin–mineral treatment (Slavin, 2008). A trend was noted in favor of nutraceutical therapy with reduced TC level >240 mg dl^{-1} and LDL > 155 mg dl^{-1} TC levels (significant only for >240 mg dl^{-1}), and body mass index >25 kg m^{-2} was associated with better improvements (Chagan et al., 2005).

Control of lipid metabolism and cholesterol desaturation in the blood has been cited as a major factor in CVD. Herbiceuticals have been reported as inhibitors of cholesterol synthesis and enhancers of HDL lipoproteins in the body. Two major mechanisms play significant roles in cholesterol saturation and lipoprotein synthesis. First, the HMG CoA synthase enzyme controls the mevalonate to HMG CoA formation that is subsequently used in cholesterol formation while the cholesterol oxidase enzyme oxidizes cholesterol to desaturate it. Second, cholesterol esterification by LCAT and ACAT enzymes and subsequently apoprotein binding controls the lipoprotein formation (Okuyama et al., 2007a). Mainly HDL plays a significant role in scavenging cholesterol from blood, as shown in Figure 31.5. LDL transport is controlled by LDL receptors in the cells. LDL lipoproteins get metabolized by lipo-oxygenase pathways, as shown in Figure 31.5. The anti-inflammatory effects and antithrombogenic effects of omega-3 fatty acids are eicosanoid-dependent processes. More intake of EPA and DHA fatty acids increases these fatty acids in tissue, and cellular and circulating lipids, along with a simultaneous reduction in omega-6 fatty acids. EPA acts as a substrate for both cyclooxygenase (COX) and 5-lipoxygenase (5-LOX) enzymes to make derivatives from arachidonic acid (α, β) such as leucotriene B5 (LTB5), which is only about 10% as potent as LTB4 as a chemotactic agent and in promoting lysosomal enzyme release. The omega-3 fatty acids also result in reduced formation of thomboxane-2 (TxA2) and prostacyclin I2 (PGI2), as AA is a TxA2 and PGI2 precursor inhibiting platelet aggregation (a less thrombogenic state), as shown in Figure 31.5.

5.7 The Unsaturated Omega-3 and Omega-6 Fatty Acids Display Major Beneficial Effects

The established beneficial effects are as follows: (1) Lipid lowering in blood; (2) antiarrhythmic effect in CHD; (3) antithrombotic effects; (4) antiatherosclerotic and anti-inflammatory effects; (5) improved endothelial function; and (6) lowering blood pressure. From the biochemical standpoint, the beneficial effect of β-3 fatty acids on blood lipids is by the stimulation of the gene expression of lipoprotein lipase (LPL) enzyme in human adipose tissue with an increase in the LPL mRNA. It results in post-heparin LPL activity, in conjunction with the lowering effect of these fatty acids on the triglyceride levels, postprandial lipidemia, and the levels of the highly atherogenic, small and dense LDL particles (Khan et al., 2002). These fatty acids increase the expression of genes encoding enzymes critical to hepatic and skeletal muscle fatty acid β-oxidation while repressing genes encoding glycolytic, lipogenic, and cholesterolgenic enzymes. This twofold action results in a decrease in lipid synthesis and a subsequent increase in lipid oxidation favorable for nutraceutical intervention. Despite the fact that the exact mode of action of β-3 fatty acids is not fully understood, it is speculated that N-3 fatty acids interact with three nuclear receptors – hepatic nuclear factor (HNF)-4α, liver X receptors (LXR) α and β, and peroxisome proliferator-activated receptors (PPARs) α, β, and γ and by regulating the transcription factor sterol regulatory element binding proteins (SREBPs) 1 and 2 (Jump, 2002). β-3 fatty acids also decrease excitability and the cytosolic calcium fluctuations of ventricular myocytes via inhibition of Na^+ and L-type Ca^{2+} channels. The mechanisms of action of omega-3 and omega-6 fatty acids are known but mechanisms of β-3 fatty acids have not been fully elucidated.

6. TREATMENT RECOMMENDATIONS FOR HERBICEUTICALS IN CARDIOVASCULAR PREVENTION

6.1 Who Needs the Alternative Approaches of Herbiceuticals in CVD?

Children below 18 years probably do not need herbiceuticals. Adults over 20–40 years need herbiceuticals in monitoring of CVD. Persons over 60 years of age need a CVD/CHD watch and herbiceuticals as mandatory daily dietary supplements in practice. These senior persons may show the following major symptoms of cardiovascular disorders and CVD development (Mozaffarian et al., 2004).

- Poor cytokines, inflammatory proteins gradually lead to apoptosis and loss of immunity.
- Arteries and veins (and other tissues) become less elastic, as evidenced by the skin. Blood pressure may rise, as arteries lose their elasticity. (The amino acid taurine, found in fish, softens arteries and veins, as well as other connective tissue.)
- Inflammation and cholesterol-filled growths (plaques) in our blood vessels reduce their rates of flow. The loss of elasticity causes the heart to pump with less power and force.
- Insulin levels begin to rise as old cells become less responsive to insulin, and the pancreas increases its output to compensate. This eventually leads to Type II diabetes and pancreatic CVD in which old cells no longer respond to insulin and end up with heavy cardiovascular damage and CVD.
- Kidneys lose reserve capacity, gradually fail to perform normal function and develop CVD.
- Reduced cell-mediated immunity and humoral immunity lead to immune deficiency and cardiovascular disorders.

6.2 Present State of Art on Herbiceutical Medicine in Cardiovascular Prevention

The FDA requires appropriate scientific evidence regarding safety of nutraceutical use as a daily prescription. However, new recommendations have suggested that the daily diet must contain 6.25 g of soy protein per serving, microcompound allicin (a small component of garlic) ad libitum amount, and ecosapentanoic acid/docosahexanoic acid as polyunsaturated fatty acids (PUFAs) from fish or fish oils. The complementary medicine and alternative medicine approach is emerging as a regulated tool to prescribe the norms of herbiceuticals as daily supplements in CVD and other diseases (Lane et al., 2008).

6.3 Insurance and Prescription

National and federal agencies such as NCI and FDA need evidence and established data in large trials to approve herbiceuticals in clinical practice. In the absence of such evidence and such a database, nutraceutical practice remains at the doorstep as nonprescription self-prescription available over the counter. As a result, insurance companies shy away from accepting herbiceuticals as prescription medicines.

6.4 Government Policy: Criteria for Suggested Use of Herbiceuticals in Cardiovascular Prevention

Awareness regarding CAM is increasing rapidly among the common public in developed countries (Lane et al., 2008). Government agencies are actively participating in the safe delivery of bioactive foods and dogwatch for any side effect. Several government reports have shown positive support for the introduction of new functional foods and herbiceuticals in CVD/CHD prevention, such as guava, dietary fibers, soy, phytoesterogens, herbs, and cruciferous vegetables (Singh et al., 1992a,b,c). Both bioactive food and herbiceuticals in diets were suggested as preventive measures in CVD. The main causative factors of CVD were free radicals, vitamin C, D, and E deficiency, selenium deficiency, and loss of cellular immunity in patients on a daily diet (Anon, 1999). Recently, the National Heart and Lung Institute suggested alternative ways of CVD prevention with the main focus on life style, prevention and control care measures, eating habits, avoidance of hazardous contaminants and consumption of antioxidants, garlic, and vitamins (NIH statement, 2006). Most of the bioactive foods are available over the counter, and herbiceuticals are marketed under supervision and dogwatch; some of them are listed in Table 31.3.

6.5 Bioactive Foods and Herbiceuticals in CVD/CHD: A Survey

During 2002–2010, the major focus was on more evidence-based use of omega-3 fatty acids combined with multivitamin–multimineral and isolated bioactive components from plants and functional foods in various CVD types. In the last 4 years, maximum efforts were devoted to reviews and compilation of evidenced experimental effects of vegetarianism on reducing CVD progress and identification of associations of active food components in diets in reduced lipids, myocardial necrosis, and apoptosis. However, NHLI is of the view that sequential events during the nutraceutical-treated cell growth or arrest of CVD are controversial (Heinrich et al., 2005). The use of fish oils in elderly patients was revisited if there was any relation to arrhythmia and contractility. The literature during years 2002–2010 provided important information for the following: (1) direct link of vitamins and minerals in CVD prevention; (2). new bioactive food components with new mechanisms of lipid lowering; (3) more controlled trials and regulated studies under federal support; (4) new awareness about unpopular foods and common shelf food supplements in CVD prevention; and (5) new federal and statuary guidelines on recommended allowances for nutraceuticals and their marketing. The following information is grouped based on the literature on herbiceuticals and herbiceuticals in CVD management with the focus on controlled randomized trials in experimental CVDs and clinical CVD subjects. The description is divided into three sections.

I. Bioactive foods and herbiceuticals in cardiovascular prevention during years 2000–2008:

Herbiceuticals and local foods were suggested as they were readily available and their use could be an alternative pharmacotherapy to prevent CVDs (Chagan et al., 2002; Heinrich et al., 2005; Wildman, 2001). Less-known bioactive foods containing ephedra and caffeine were reported to improve electrocardiographic and hemodynamic effects (Wildman, 2001). A clear cardioprotective role for vitamin E and antioxidant supplements was reviewed in the prevention of CVDs (Borochov-Neori et al., 2008; Eastwood, 1999; Maxwell, 2000; McBride et al., 2004; Pham and Plakogiannis, 2005; Tran, 2001).

Homocysteine, taurine, vitamins, and omega-3 fatty acids were reinvestigated and their value confirmed in cardiovascular prevention (Carlsson, 2006; Erdmann et al., 2008; Marchioli et al., 2002; McCarty, 2004; Simopoulos, 2003).

Mechanism of cardiovascular prevention by herbiceuticals: cholesterol-rich dietary fats enhance the risk of CHD while omega-3/omega-6 fatty acids reduce the risk of CVDs and play a cardioprotective role in primary, secondary, and late-onset diseases (Okuyama et al., 2007a,b). Interestingly, excessive linoleic acid is manifested as 'linoleic acid syndrome' in CHD (Okuyama et al., 2007c,d). Conjugated linoleic acid was reported to be protective against cardiac hypertrophy (Malinowski and Metka, 2007). Omega-3 fatty acids mainly lower the blood lipids.

II. The possible reasons of cardioprotection by omega-3 fatty acids in bioactive foods were the following:
- Lipid lowering (reduction of fasting triglycerides, attenuation of postprandial triglyceride response)
- Antiarrhythmic effects
- Antithrombotic and other effects on the haemostatic systems (i.e., reduced platelet reactivity, slightly longer bleeding times, reduced plasma viscosity)
- Inhibition of atherosclerosis and inflammation via inhibition of smooth muscle cell proliferation, altered eicosanoid synthesis, reduced expression of cell adhesion

Table 31.3 The Table Represents the FDA Approved Herbiceuticals with Recommended Quantity and Sources of Herbiceuticals on Shelf in Super Markets

Herbiceuticals	Quantity needed	Common American sources
Vitamin D	400 IU a day (2000 IU)	Walmart's 'OneSource' multivitamins
Multivitamin-minerals As	1 pill daily	Centrum silver A–Z with minerals
Natural vitamin E (4 tocopherols + 4 tocotrienols)	Two 400 IU capsules a week (800 mg)	GNC natural vitamin E
Selenium	200 mcg a day	Walmart's 'OneSource' multivitamins
Aspirin or ibuprofen[a]	Baby aspirin a day	Nonprescription counter
Chocolate (best if fat-free)?	Three servings	Home-made, Food emporium
Green tea?	Three servings	Home-made, Food emporium
Lycopene	Cooked tomato sauces	Domino's Pizza
Fish (tuna, salmon, mackerel)[b] or EHA + DHA	Two servings a week	Fresh phytosterols at Publix
Soy 'meat,' cheese, milk, mozzarella, sausage, burgers, broccoli, cabbage, cauliflower	Ad libitum	Publix, at the edge of the produce section
Sulfhydrals	Ad libitum	Piccadilly's tastes pretty good
Blueberries	A few tablespoons a day	Publix' frozen foods (N. side, S. aisle)
Strawberries	Four or five large a day	Publix' frozen foods (N. side, S. aisle)
Old-fashioned oatmeal	One ounce?	Publix, all supermarkets
Legumes (beans)	Two servings a week	Publix, all supermarkets
Low-fat blueberry yogurt	Two or three times a week	Publix, all supermarkets
Yellow vegetables	Ad libitum	Publix (Piccadilly's tastes pretty good).
Purple grape juice, or red wine	A glass a day	Publix, for Welsh's grape juice
Turmeric roots	Two capsules daily	GNC natural body products
Herbs	Two pills daily	St John Warts natural source
Garlic, soy products	Ad libitum	Walmart's 'OneSource' ampoules

Source: Sharma (2009).

[a] Aspirin and ibuprofen primarily act as anti inflammation. (Other agents such as fish also have anti-inflammatory properties.)

[b] Tuna and mackerel contain mercury, dioxin, and PCBs; salmon fish is safe. Winn Dixie farm-raised salmon. Canned salmon provides omega-3 fatty acids and, taurine, which are vital to the nervous and cardiovascular systems.

molecules and suppression of inflammatory cytokines production (IL's, TNF-α) and mitogens

- Improvement of the endothelial function (through enhancement of nitric oxide – dependent and nitric oxide independent vasodilatation)
- Improvement in blood pressure.

III. CVD/CHD in the human body and herbiceutical protection (Table 31.3):

Fish oil supplementation dominates the scenario of lipid lowering in CVDs (Malinowski and Metka, 2007). New candidates such as cinnamon, ginko biloba, and bioactive peptides have been introduced to the list of herbiceuticals with cardioprotective properties (Alibin et al., 2008; Baker et al., 2008; Erdmann et al., 2008). In a recent detailed report, the authors have validated that Guggul (*Commiphora mukul*), a herb rich in guggusterones, lowers both cholesterol (30% in 3 months) and triglycerides. It maintains LDL levels (35% lowering in 3 months) and improves HDL level (20% in 12 weeks) to maintain a higher HDL/LDL ratio. It keeps the blood flow smooth and maintains thin blood with continuous detoxification and reduced platelet aggregation. It relaxes the muscles and keeps muscle strain low. Additionally, it has properties of rejuvenation and blood purification. Other unique properties are immunomodulation and lipid lowering. The presence of guggulsterones in Guggul increases the body's metabolic rate, improves thyroid function and heat production (Nohr et al., 2009; Szapary et al., 2003). Today it is believed that bioactive foods are digested by natural enzymes and their digested metabolite products target many cardiovascular-related intracellular metabolic abnormalities, both focal (targeted cure) and whole body in origin (whole individual or global cure) while its counterparts, artificial synthesized pharmaceutical drugs either inhibit or elevate only one biochemical reaction with the assumption of a complete cure. In this single-step cure approach, several naturally active enzymes, cofactors, and assembly proteins lose their conformation and functionality (bioactive behavior), leading to several side effects. These are less in the case of bioactive foods or herbiceuticals because of their wider acceptance in the body, but side effects are very often caused by pharmaceutical drugs and minimizing these side effects remains a challenge. Several negative results advocate further investigations (Nohr et al., 2009; Szapary et al., 2003).

6.6 Challenges, Hypes, Hopes, and Futuristic Role of Herbiceuticals in Cardioprotection

Most of the success of herbiceuticals is based on self-prescription and individual experiences. It is too early to legitimize the miraculous benefits of herbiceuticals unless controlled clinical trials support the evidence for the preventive therapeutic efficacy of nutraceuticals. A major challenge is the early detection of CVD and timely effective treatment. In spite of all the tools available, CVD is a major health hazard. The majority of available data on nutraceutical benefits in CVD come from epidemiological health and population statistics. The reduced CVD incidence due to herbiceuticals seems overhyped but greater successes are anticipated with the advancements in food science. However, CVD remains a major threat because of high mortality compounded with the incomplete success of chemotherapy and surgery intervention. In future, bioengineered herbiceuticals will play a significant role in CVD prevention as alternative therapeutics.

Bioactive foods with rich herbiceuticals are growing in number as healthy food products introduced by companies and investigations give high hopes of CVD prevention with herbiceuticals. The primary focus still remains on dyslipidemia and lipid lowering by fish oils and bioactive foods. Governments and globalization will certainly support the health risks and clinical trials on new bioactive foods and herbiceuticals. Herbiceuticals are becoming popular as they are harmless and natural food constituents. They are still food supplements and the past 5 years have demonstrated an enormous change in the perception of herbiceuticals as CVD preventive and therapeutic supplements in CVDs of different organs. Chinese herbal medicine is making advances in introducing herbs such as hawthorn, and cassa italica herbal combinatorial medicine on priority within medical ethics to claim the success of herbs in arresting cardiovascular injury (An and Yang, 2006; El-Menyar et al., 2006; Gao et al., 2010; Jia et al., 2001; Tam et al., 2009). It is believed that the future trend in CAD treatment will be a mixture of complementary approaches such as medical treatment (vasodilators + antiplatelet agents) → herbal supplements (Chinese or Arjun herbs) → dietary (L-carnitine, magnesium) → body physique (exercise, chelation therapy, acupuncture) → Mind (esteem build up) → life style change (nonsmoking/nonalcoholic spirit).

7. CONCLUSION

In this chapter, herbs are reviewed for possible use as antihypertensive, antiarrhythmic, and cardioprotective supplements. The pharmacological action and biochemical mechanisms of herbs are highlighted with examples of their possible antihypertensive, antiarrhythmic, and cardioprotective effects on heart tissue and their cardioprotective action. A possible antihypertensive, antiarrhythmic, and cardioprotective composition is proposed for making an effective cardioprotective herbal formula. The focus of this chapter is the review and comparison of the antihypertensive, antiarrhythmic, and cardioprotective strengths of different herbs in the light of current knowledge. The toxic effects of herbal overintake are highlighted to show their side effects. Finally, the aim is to draw the attention of regulatory government bodies to the increasingly negligent use of herbs among the general population having no knowledge of the side effects of the herbs they are using so that the government or health authorities can remain vigilant in informing the public and insurers before it is too late.

ACKNOWLEDGMENTS

The author acknowledges the permission to do advanced level internship at Heart and Vascular Surgery Center, Tallahassee Memorial Hospital, Mikusukee Road, Tallahassee, Florida for Cardiovascular Technology

Research program under Drs. Julian Hurt, Murrah, Al Saint, and Khairullah. The author also acknowledges the opportunity of engineering and biotechnology internship under the supervision of Dr. Ching J. Chen at FAMU-FSU College of Engineering, Tallahassee, Florida.

REFERENCES

Abeywardena, M.Y., Head, R.J., 2001. Long chain n-3 polyunsaturated fatty acids and blood vessel function. Cardiovascular Research 52, 361–371.

Alibin, C.P., Kopilas, M.A., Anderson, H.D., 2008. Suppression of cardiac myocyte hypertrophy by conjugated linoleic acid: role of peroxisome proliferator-activated receptors alpha and gamma. Journal of Biological Chemistry 283 (16), 10707–10715.

Almario, R.U., Vonghavaravat, V., Wong, R., Kasim-Karakas, S.E., 2001. Effect of walnut consumption on plasma fatty acids and lipoproteins in combined hyperlipidemia. American Journal of Clinical Nutrition 74, 72–79.

An, W., Yang, J., 2006. Protective effects of Ping-Lv-Mixture (PLM), a medicinal formula on arrhythmias induced by myocardial ischemia-reperfusion. Journal of Ethnopharmacology 108 (1), 90–95.

Anon, 1999. MRC/BHF Heart Protection Study of cholesterol-lowering therapy and of antioxidant vitamin supplementation in a wide range of patients at increased risk of coronary heart disease death: early safety and efficacy experience. European Heart Journal 20 (10), 725–741.

Baker, W.L., Gutierrez-Williams, G., White, C.M., Kluger, J., Coleman, C.I., 2008. Effect of cinnamon on glucose control and lipid parameters. Diabetes Care 31 (1), 41–43.

Basu, A., Lucas, E.A., 2007. Mechanisms and effects of green tea on cardiovascular health. Nutrition Reviews 65 (8), 361–375.

Berman, D.S., Hachamovitch, R., Shaw, L.J., et al., 2006. Roles of nuclear cardiology, cardiac computed tomography, and cardiac magnetic resonance. Journal of Nuclear Medicine 47 (7), 1107–1118.

Borochov-Neori, H., Judeinstein, S., Greenberg, A., et al., 2008. Phenolic antioxidants and antiatherogenic effects of Marula (*Sclerocarrya birrea* subsp. caffra) fruit juice in healthy humans. Journal of Agricultural and Food Chemistry 56 (21), 9884–9891.

Calder, P.C., 2004. n-3 Fatty acids and cardiovascular disease: evidence explained and mechanisms explored. Clinical Science (London, England) 107 (1), 1–11.

Carlsson, C.M., 2006. Homocysteine lowering with folic acid and vitamin B supplements: effects on cardiovascular disease in older adults. Drugs & Aging 23 (6), 491–502.

Chagan, L., Bernstein, D., Cheng, J.W., et al., 2005. Use of biological based therapy in patients with cardiovascular diseases in a university hospital in New York City. BMC Complementary and Alternative Medicine 5, 4.

Chagan, L., Ioselovich, A., Asherova, L., Cheng, J.W., 2002. Use of alternative pharmacotherapy in management of cardiovascular diseases. The American Journal of Managed Care 8 (3), 270–285.

Connor, W.E., De Franchesco, C.A., Connor, S.L., 1993. n-3 Fatty acids from fish oil: effects on plasma lipoproteins and hypertriglyceridemic patients. Annals of the New York Academy of Sciences 683, 16–34.

Coombes, J.S., Powers, S.K., Hamilton, K.L., et al., 2000. Improved cardiac performance after ischemia in aged rats supplemented with vitamin E and alpha-lipoic acid. American Journal of Physiology – Regulatory, Integrative and Comparative Physiology 279 (6), R2149–R2155.

Dallner, G., Brismar, K., Chojnacki, T., Swiezewska, E., 2003. Regulation of coenzyme Q biosynthesis and breakdown. Biofactors 18 (1–4), 11–22.

De Caterina, R., Liao, J.K., Libby, P., 2000. Fatty acid modulation of endothelial activation. American Journal of Clinical Nutrition 71, 213S–223S.

De Caterina, R., Madonna, R., Zucchi, R., La Rovere, M.T., 2003. Antiarrhythmic effects of omega-3 fatty acids: from epidemiology to bedside. American Heart Journal 146, 420–430.

Din, J.N., Newby, D.E., Flapan, A.D., 2004. Omega 3 fatty acids and cardiovascular disease – fishing for a natural treatment. BMJ 328, 30–35.

Eastwood, M.A., 1999. Interaction of dietary antioxidants *in vivo*: how fruit and vegetables prevent disease? QJM 92 (9), 527–530.

El-Badry, A.M., Moritz, W., Contaldo, C., Tian, Y., Graf, R., Clavien, P.A., 2007. Prevention of reperfusion injury and microcirculatory failure in macrosteatotic mouse liver by omega-3 fatty acids. Hepatology 45 (4), 855–863.

El-Menyar, A.A., Helmy, A.H., Mubarak, N.M., Arafa, S.E., 2006. Acute myocardial infarction with patent epicardial coronary vessels following Cassia italica ingestion. Cardiovascular Toxicology 6 (2), 81–84.

Erdmann, K., Cheung, B.W., Schröder, H., 2008. The possible roles of food-derived bioactive peptides in reducing the risk of cardiovascular disease. The Journal of Nutritional Biochemistry 19 (10), 643–654.

Esterhuyse, A.J., Toit, E.D., Rooyen, J.V., 2005. Dietary red palm oil supplementation protects against the consequences of global ischemia in the isolated perfused rat heart. Asia Pacific Journal of Clinical Nutrition 14 (4), 340–347.

Gao, Z.Y., Zhang, J.C., Xu, H., et al., 2010. Analysis of relationships among syndrome, therapeutic treatment, and Chinese herbal medicine in patients with coronary artery. Zhong Xi Yi Jie He Xue Bao 8 (3), 238–243.

Gurley, B.J., Swain, A., Hubbard, M.A., et al., 2008. Clinical assessment of CYP2D6-mediated herb–drug interactions in humans: effects of milk thistle, black cohosh, goldenseal, kava kava, St. John's wort, and Echinacea. Molecular Nutrition & Food Research 52 (7), 755–763.

Haller, C.A., Anderson, I.B., Kim, S.Y., Blanc, P.D., 2002. An evaluation of selected herbal reference texts and comparison to published reports of adverse herbal events. Adverse Drug Reactions and Toxicological Reviews 21 (3), 143–150.

Harris, A., Devaraj, S., Jilal, I., 2002. Oxidative stress, alpha-tocopherol therapy, and atherosclerosis. Current Atherosclerosis Reports 4 (5), 373–380.

Harris, W.S., Reid, K.J., Sands, S.A., Spertus, J.A., 2007. Blood omega-3 and trans fatty acids in middle aged acute coronary syndrome patients. The American Journal of Cardiology 99, 154–158.

Heinrich, M., Leonti, M., Nebel, S., Peschel, W., 2005. Local food – nutraceuticals: an example of a multidisciplinary research project on local knowledge. Journal of Physiology and Pharmacology 56 (S1), 5–22.

Hjerkinn, E.M., Seljeflot, I., Ellingsen, I., et al., 2005. Influence of long-term intervention with dietary counseling, long-chain *n*-3 fatty acid supplements, or both on circulating markers of endothelial activation in men with long-standing hyperlipidemia. American Journal of Clinical Nutrition 81, 583–589.

Hooper, L., Thompson, R.L., Harrison, R.A., et al., 2006. Risks and benefits of omega 3 fats for mortality, cardiovascular disease, and cancer: systematic review. BMJ 332, 752–755.

Hu, F.B., Willett, W.C., 2002. Optimal diets for prevention of coronary heart disease. Journal of the American Medical Association 288 (20), 2569–2578.

Jia, Y., Sun, X., Jia, M., Cui, Z., Li, C., 2001. One hundred and seven middle-aged and senile cases of coronary heart disease with ventricular premature beat treated by qing xin an shen fang. Journal of Traditional Chinese Medicine 21 (4), 247–251.

Jump, D.B., 2002. Dietary polyunsaturated fatty acids and regulation of gene transcription. Current Opinion in Lipidology 13, 155–164.

Khan, S., Minihane, A.M., Talmud, P.J., et al., 2002. Dietary long-chain *n*-3 PUFA's increase LPL gene expression in adipose tissue of subjects with an atherogenic lipoprotein phenotype. Journal of Lipid Research 43, 979–985.

Kim, H.J., Takahashi, M., Ezaki, O., 1999. Fish oil feeding decreases mature sterol regulatory element-binding protein 1 [SREBP-1] by downregulation of SREBP-1c mRNA in mouse liver. A possible mechanism for downregulation of lipogenic enzyme mRNAs. Journal of Biological Chemistry 274, 25892–25898.

Kris-Etheron, P.M., Harris, W.S., Appel, L.J., 2003. Fish consumption, fish oil, omega-3 fatty acids and cardiovascular disease. Arteriosclerosis, Thrombosis, and Vascular Biology 23, e20–e31.

Lane, J.S., Magno, C.P., Lane, K.T., Chan, T., Hoyt, D.B., Greenfield, S., 2008. Nutrition impacts the prevalence of peripheral arterial disease in the United States. Journal of Vascular Surgery 48 (4), 897–904.

Leaf, A., Kang, J.X., Xiao, Y.F., Billman, G.E., 2003. Clinical prevention of sudden cardiac death by *n*-3 polyunsaturated fatty acid mechanism of prevention arrhythmias by *n*-3 fish oils. Circulation 107, 2646–2652.

Lopez-Garcia, E., Schulze, M.B., Manson, J.E., et al., 2004. Consumption of (*n*-3) fatty acids is related to plasma biomarkers of inflammation and endothelial activation in women. Journal of Nutrition 134, 1806–1811.

Malinowski, J.M., Metka, K., 2007. Elevation of low-density lipoprotein cholesterol concentration with over-the-counter fish oil supplementation. The Annals of Pharmacotherapy 41 (7), 1296–1300.

Marchioli, R., Barzi, F., Bomba, E., et al., 2002. Early protection against sudden death by *n*-3 polyunsaturated fatty acids after myocardial infarction: time-course analysis of the results of the Gruppo Italiano per lo Studio della Sopravvivenza nell'Infarto Miocardico (GISSI)-Prevenzione. Circulation 105 (16), 1897–1903.

Massaro, M., Scofitti, E., Carluccio, M.A., Caterina, R.D., 2008. Basic mechanisms behind the effects of *n*-3 fatty acids on cardiovascular disease. Prostaglandins, Leukotrienes, and Essential Fatty Acids 79 (3–5), 109–115.

Matsui, H., Shimosawa, T., Uetake, Y., et al., 2006. Protective effect of potassium against the hypertensive cardiac dysfunction: association with reactive oxygen species reduction. Hypertension 48 (2), 225–231.

Maxwell, S.R., 2000. Coronary artery disease-free radical damage, antioxidant protection and the role of homocysteine. Basic Research in Cardiology 95 (1), I65–I71.

McBride, B.F., Karapanos, A.K., Krudysz, A., Kluger, J., Coleman, C.I., White, C.M., 2004. Electrocardiographic and hemodynamic effects of a multicomponent dietary supplement containing ephedra and caffeine: a randomized controlled trial. Journal of the American Medical Association 291 (2), 216–221.

McCarty, M.F., 2004. A taurine-supplemented vegan diet may blunt the contribution of neutrophil activation to acute coronary events. Medical Hypotheses 63 (3), 419–425.

Mozaffarian, D., Psaty, B.M., Rimm, E.B., et al., 2004. Fish intake and risk of incident of atrial fibrillation. Circulation 110, 368–373.

Nilsen, D.W., Albrektsen, G., Landmark, K., Moen, S., Aarsland, T., Woie, L., 2001. Effects of a high dose concentrate of *n*-3 fatty acids or corn oil introduced after an acute myocardial infraction on serum triglycerides and HDL cholesterol. American Journal of Clinical Nutrition 57, 193–200.

Nohr, L.A., Rasmussen, L.B., Straand, J., 2009. Resin from the mukul myrrh tree, guggul, can it be used for treating hypercholesterolemia? A randomized, controlled study. Complementary Therapies in Medicine 1 (1), 16–22.

Obarzanek, E., Sacks, F.M., Vollmer, W.M., et al., 2001. Effects on blood lipids of a blood pressure-lowering diet: the Dietary Approaches to Stop Hypertension (DASH) Trial. American Journal of Clinical Nutrition 74, 80–89.

Okuyama, H., Ichikawa, Y., Sun, Y., Hamazaki, T., Lands, W.E., 2007a. The cholesterol hypothesis - its basis and its faults. World Review of Nutrition and Dietetics 96, 1–17.

Okuyama, H., Ichikawa, Y., Sun, Y., Hamazaki, T., Lands, W.E., 2007b. New directions of lipid nutrition for the primary and secondary prevention of coronary heart disease and other late-onset diseases. World Review of Nutrition and Dietetics 96, 151–158.

Okuyama, H., Ichikawa, Y., Sun, Y., Hamazaki, T., Lands, W.E., 2007c. Mechanisms by which dietary fats affect coronary heart disease mortality. World Review of Nutrition and Dietetics 96, 119–141.

Okuyama, H., Ichikawa, Y., Sun, Y., Hamazaki, T., Lands, W.E., 2007d. Omega3 fatty acids effectively prevent coronary heart disease and other late onset diseases – the excessive linoleic acid syndrome. World Review of Nutrition and Dietetics 96, 83–103.

Oudit, G.Y., Trivieri, M.G., Khaper, N., et al., 2004. Taurine supplementation reduces oxidative stress and improves cardiovascular function in an iron-overload murine model. Circulation 109 (15), 1877–1885.

Pham, D.Q., Plakogiannis, R., 2005. Vitamin E supplementation in cardiovascular disease and cancer prevention: part 1. The Annals of Pharmacotherapy 39 (11), 1870–1878.

Racasan, S., Braam, B., Van der Giezen, D.M., et al., 2004. Perinatal L-arginine and antioxidant supplements reduce adult blood pressure in spontaneously hypertensive rats. Hypertension 44 (1), 83–88.

Roche, H.M., Gibney, M.J., 2000. Effect of long-chain *n*-3 polyunsaturated fatty acids on fasting and post-prandial triacylglycerol metabolism. American Journal of Clinical Nutrition 71 (1), 232S–237S.

Sampath, H., Ntambi, J.M., 2004. Polyunsaturated fatty acid regulation of gene expression. Nutrition Reviews 62, 333–339.

Samuel, S.M., Thirunavukkarasu, M., Penumathsa, S.V., Paul, D., Maulik, N., 2008. Akt/FOXO3a/SIRT1-mediated cardioprotection by *n*-tyrosol against ischemic stress in rat *in vivo* model of myocardial infarction: switching gears toward survival and longevity. Journal of Agricultural and Food Chemistry 56 (20), 9692–9698.

Santo, A.S., Santo, A.M., Browne, R.W., et al., 2010. Postprandial lipemia detects the effect of soy protein on cardiovascular disease risk compared with the fasting lipid profile. Lipids 45 (12), 1127–1138.

Sharma, R., 2011. Antibodies in nanomedicine and bioimaging. In: Pathak, Y., Benita, S. (Eds.), Antibody Mediated (mAB) Drug Delivery Systems (DDS): Concepts, Technology and Applications. John Willey and Sons, New York (Chapter 17).

Sharma, R., Singh, R.B., 2004. Human coronary artery lesions: magnetic resonance imaging, NMR spectroscopy, histopathology and oxidative stress markers. World Heart Journal 1 (2), 179–184.

Sharma, R., Singh, R.B., 2010. Bioactive foods and nutraceutical supplementation criteria in cardiovascular protection. The Open Nutraceuticals Journal 3, 141–153.

Sheu, S.J., Shen, C.G., 2004. Herbal Pharmaceutical Composition for Prophylaxis and/or Treatment of Cardiovascular Diseases and the Method of Preparing the Same. US Patent US2004/0234627.

Simopoulos, A.P., 2003. Importance of the ratio of omega-6/omega-3 essential fatty acids: evolutionary aspects. World Review of Nutrition and Dietetics 92, 1–22.

Singh, R.B., DeMeester, F., Mechirova, V., Pella, D., Otsuka, K., 2008. Fatty acids in the causation and therapy of metabolic syndrome. In: Watson, R.R., DeMesster, F. (Eds.), Wild Type Foods in Health Promotion and Disease Prevention. Humana Press, Totowa, NJ, pp. 263–284.

Singh, R.B., Dubnov, G., Niaz, M.A., et al., 2002. Effect of an Indo-Mediterranean diet on progression of coronary disease in high risk patients: a randomized single blind trial. Lancet 360, 1455–1461.

Singh, R.B., Rastogi, S.S., Ghosh, S., Singh, R., Niaz, M.A., 1992a. Effects of guava intake on serum total and high density lipoprotein cholesterol levels and on systemic blood pressure. The American Journal of Cardiology 70, 1287–1291.

Singh, R.B., Rastogi, S.S., Niaz, M.A., Ghosh, S., Singh, R., Gupta, S., 1992b. Effect of fat modified and fruits and vegetable enriched diets on blood lipids in the Indian diet heart study. The American Journal of Cardiology 69, 869–874.

Singh, R.B., Sharma, V.K., Gupta, R.K., 1992c. Nutritional modulators of lipoprotein metabolism in patients with risk factors for coronary heart disease. Journal of the American College of Nutrition 11, 391–398.

Slavin, J.L., 2008. Position of the American Dietetic Association: health implications of dietary fiber. Journal of the American Dietetic Association 108 (10), 1716–1731.

Szapary, P.O., Wolfe, M.L., Bloedon, L.T., et al., 2003. Guggulipid for the treatment of hypercholesterolemia: a randomized controlled trial. Journal of the American Medical Association 290 (6), 765–772. Available at http://www.ayurvediccure.com/guggul.htm.

Tam, W.Y., Chook, P., Qiao, M., et al., 2009. The efficacy and tolerability of adjunctive alternative herbal medicine (*Salvia miltiorrhiza* and *Pueraria lobata*) on vascular function and structure in coronary patients. Journal of Alternative and Complementary Medicine 15 (4), 415–421.

Thirunavukkarasu, M., Penumathsa, S.V., Juhasz, B., et al., 2006. Niacinbound chromium enhances myocardial protection from ischemiareperfusion injury. American Journal of Physiology – Heart and Circulatory Physiology 291 (2), H820–H826.

Tran, T.L., 2001. Antioxidant supplements to prevent heart disease. Real hope or empty hype? Postgraduate Medicine 109 (1), 109–114.

Wang, Q., Simonyi, A., Li, W., et al., 2005. Dietary grape supplement ameliorates cerebral ischemia-induced neuronal death in gerbils. Molecular Nutrition & Food Research 49 (5), 443–451.

Warnes, C.A., Williams, R.G., Bashore, T.M., et al., 2008. ACC/AHA 2008 Guidelines for the management of adults with congenital heart disease. Journal of the American College of Cardiology 52, 143–263.

Wei, F., Li, D., Luo, C., Yue, H., Chen, Q., Huang, Z., 2004. Pharmaceutical Composition for the Treatment of Cardiovascular and Cerebrovascular Diseases. US Patent 7438935.

Wei, Q.Y., Ma, J.P., Cai, Y.J., Yang, L., Liu, Z.L., 2005. Cytotoxic and apoptotic activities of diarylheptanoids and gingerol-related compounds from the rhizome of *Chinese ginger*. Journal of Ethnopharmacology 102 (2), 177–184.

Wildman, R.E.C., 2001. Classifying nutraceuticals. In: Wildman, R.E.C. (Ed.), Handbook of Nutraceuticals and Functional Foods. CRC Series in Modern Nutrition, pp. 13–30.

Young, J., 2006. Composition of Natural Herb Extract for Treating Cardiovascular Disease and Its Method of Preparation Thereof. US Patent 0083798.

Zahid, A.M., Hussain, M.E., Fahim, M., 2005. Antiatherosclerotic effects of dietary supplementations of garlic and turmeric: restoration of endothelial function in rats. Life Sciences 77 (8), 837–857.

Zampelas, A., Peel, A.S., Gould, B.J., Wright, J., Williams, C.M., 1994. Polyunsaturated fatty acids of the *n*-6 and *n*-3 series: effects on postprandial lipid and apolipoprotein levels in healthy men. European Journal of Clinical Nutrition 48, 842–848.

Zampolli, A., Bysted, A., Leth, T., Mortensen, A., De Caterina, R., Falk, E., 2006. Contrasting effect of fish oil supplementation on the development of atherosclerosis in murine models. Atherosclerosis 184 (1), 78–85.

Zhou, J., Møller, J., Ritskes-Hoitinga, M., Larsen, M.L., Austin, R.C., Falk, E., 2003. Effects of vitamin supplementation and hyperhomocysteinemia on atherosclerosis in apoE-deficient mice. Atherosclerosis 168 (2), 255–262.

CHAPTER 32

Fish Proteins in Coronary Artery Disease Prevention: Amino Acid–Fatty Acid Concept

R. Sharma*, J. Katz[†,‡]
*Florida State University, Tallahassee, FL, USA
[†]Dr. Katz Cardiology Center, New York, NY, USA
[‡]Columbia University, New York, NY, USA

1. INTRODUCTION

A daily diet that includes fish, one of the best sources of dietary protein, has been routine since the origin of the human race (Brown, 1990). Till the latter half of the nineteenth century, the very low incidence of cardiovascular heart disease among Eskimos in Greenland, and the tribals in Australia and Japan remained an unsolved puzzle. In the last half-century, cholesterol was identified as responsible for heart disease, and lipoproteins as the main risk factors for heart attacks and atherosclerosis (Côté et al., 2004; Kristensen et al., 2001; Singh et al., 2010; O'Dea 1988, 1991). At present, the omega-3 fatty acids in fish oil are a controversial choice in cardiovascular disease prevention while statins show serious side effects (Albert et al., 2010). Several omega fatty acid CVD prevention trials in Asia, Europe, and the West have documented mixed views on the benefits of omega fatty acid therapy. Fish protein supplementation is emerging as a better source of dietary protein than other protein sources in cardioprotection (Bergeron and Jacques, 1989; Bergeron et al., 1992a,b). American Heart Association (AHA), NECP ATP III has evidenced significantly the prospects of lipid lowering by dietary means. Marine fish protein can also benefit the heart (NCEP Report, 2001). Recent studies provide little or no direct evidence that fish proteins and amino acids taurine and methionine can prolong life, or prevent or delay CAD events (Yamori et al., 2009). Today, it is an open question. Authors propose the 'one amino acid-one fatty acid concept' that amino acid (in fish protein) may be an alternative approach to keep high HDL or low (LDL) or (LDL+TG+C) lipids.

In light of these recommendations, the possibility of using fish proteins as an emerging option in cardioprotective food is explored; most other diets and foods remain, at large, unidentified, without a scientific basis for their action (Alne et al., 2009; Andersen et al., 2004; Andreassen et al., 2009; Bower et al., 2010; Capilla et al., 2004; Cleveland et al., 2010; Fernandes, 2002; Heine-Broring et al., 2010; Jordal et al., 2006; Krauss et al., 2000; Krawczenko et al., 2005; Mikalsen et al., 2005; Murashita et al., 2009; Nalbone

Bioactive Food as Dietary Interventions for Cardiovascular Disease
http://dx.doi.org/10.1016/B978-0-12-396485-4.00029-3

© 2013 Elsevier Inc.
All rights reserved.

et al., 1988; Owen et al., 2000; Sales, 2009; Sharma et al., 2010; Siddiqui et al., 2008; Sidhu, 2003; Sinnatamby et al., 2008; Undeland et al., 2004; van Rooyen et al., 2008; von Schalburg et al., 2008; Xiao et al., 2011; Zhang et al., 1999; Zheng et al., 2005; Zhong et al., 2003). Fish proteins in food practice and their major mechanistic action in controlling lipids are quite unknown (Singh et al., 2010). This chapter describes the methods and the benefits of consumption of proteins in commonly used fish in central India. Fish are an excellent source of protein. About 100 g of cooked fish provides 18–20 g of protein (or one-third of RDA) containing abundant essential amino acids. The protein content in most of the fish is constant, and does not vary with season. The author reported variation in fish proteins based on fish feed and month of breeding in different seasons (Shriniwas et al., 2008).

This chapter presents an introduction to fish food as a source of proteins beneficial in cardiac protection, the protein and amino acid composition of fish foods, the new 'one amino acid–one fatty acid' concept (one amino acid+one fatty acid can lower lipid+stabilize heart), intervention trials, and a futuristic approach to fish food as an option in CHD.

2. FISH PROTEINS AND AMINO ACIDS

The essential amino acid compositions of fish given in Tables 32.1–32.3 indicate an abundance of lysine, methionine, threonine, and low collagen. It enhances the digestibility

Table 32.1 Apparent Crude Protein and Amino Acid Availabilities (%) from Various Fish in Cardioprotection to Meet FAO/WHO Daily Recommended Values[a]

Amino acid	Atlantic salmon	Coho salmon	Cherry salmon	Channel catfish	Rainbow trout	Herring menhaden
Alanine	6.52	6.08	6.35	6.31	6.57	
Arginine	6.61	5.99	6.23	6.67	6.41	9.13
Aspartate	9.92	9.96	9.93	9.74	9.94	8.54
Cystein	0.80	0.95	1.23	1.34	0.86	0.80
Glutamine	14.31	15.25	15.39	14.39	14.22	
Glycine	7.41	7.31	7.62	8.14	7.76	
Histidine	3.02	2.99	2.39	2.17	2.96	
Isoleucine	4.41	3.70	3.96	4.29	4.34	8.93
Leucine	7.72	7.49	7.54	7.40	7.59	9.06
Lysine	9.28	8.64	8.81	8.51	8.49	8.41
Methionine	1.83	3.53	3.14	2.92	2.88	
Phenylalanine	4.36	4.14	4.63	4.14	4.38	8.92
Proline	4.64	4.76	4.33	6.02	4.89	
Serine	4.61	4.67	4.48	4.89	4.66	
Threonine	4.95	5.11	4.63	4.41	4.76	8.51
Tryptophan	0.93	1.40	0.83	0.78	0.93	7.27
Tyrosine	3.50	3.44	3.58	3.28	3.38	
Valine	5.09	4.32	4.85	5.15	5.09	8.97

[a] FAO/WHO daily recommended values for an 80 kg man/60 kg woman are: Isoleu 800/600; Leu 1120/840; Lys 960/720; Meth/Cys 1040/780; Phenylala/Tyr 1120/840; Thr 560/420; Tryp 280/210; Val 800/600.

Table 32.2 Energy and Fat Contents in Different Fish

Fish (84 g/3 oz)	Calories	Total fat[a] (g/%DV)	Saturated fat[a] (g/%DV)	Protein (g)
Cod	100	1/2	0/0	20
Halibut	110	2/3	0/0	23
Mackerel	210	13/20	1.5/8	21
Salmon[1]	160	7/11	1/5	22
Salmon[2]	130	4/6	1/5	22
Salmon[3]	180	9/14	1.5/8	23
Salmon[4]	200	12	3	21
Tuna	320	24/30	1.2/6	21

Serving size: 3 Oz skinless cooked fish portion.
Source: US FDA data source for daily 2000 calorie diet.
[a] Nutrient value/% daily value of nutrient.

Table 32.3 Nutritive Profiles of Fish (in 100 g Whole Flesh) in Cardioprotection

Fish (100 g)	Calories (kcal)	protein (g)	Fat (g)	Ca (mg)	Iron (mg)	Vit A IU	Vit D IU	EPA (mg)	DHA (mg)
Salmon/ Sake	167	20.7	8.4	14	0.9	200	1300	492	820
Tuna/ Maguro	322	21.4	24.6	11	1	100	720	1290	2880
Tuna red meat	133	28.3	1.4	5.0	2.0	20	210	27	115
Sardine/ Iwashi	213	19.2	13.8	70.0	1.7	60	390	1390	1140
Bonito/ Katsuo	129	25.8	2.0	10.0	1.9	17.0	400	78	310
Mackerel/ Saba	230	19.8	16.5	22.0	1.5	100	440	1210	1780
Cod/tara	70.0	15.7	0.4	42.0	0.6	100	–	37	72

coefficient to near 100, and a fish intake of 100 g/day supplies around 25% of RDA of the adult male. A less known fact is that fish protein consumption decreases the atherogenic risk of vascular diseases. Even less known is the result of one study showing that a sole fish diet increased blood HDL lipoprotein relative to other proteins such as soy or milk (Beauchesne-Rondeau et al., 2003). Nonprotein nitrogen compounds are common in fish, mostly in the sarcoplasm, which includes free amino acids, peptides, amines, amine oxides, guanidine compounds, quaternary ammonium molecules, nucleotides, and urea (Ackman, 1995). Creatine is the main component in fish protein. Creatine plays an important role in fish muscle metabolism in its phosphorylated form. Endogenous proteases yield some free amino acids such as glycine, taurine, and histidine (>1%) in the red muscles of tuna fish. Proper cooking of mahi-mahi, mackerel, skipjack, and tuna fish is important as improper cooking only converts histidine to histamine. Histamine is not affected by heat and becomes a hazard to consumers because of 'scombroid poisoning' (Arino et al., 2003; Food and Drug Administration, 1989; Haard, 1995) (Figure 32.1).

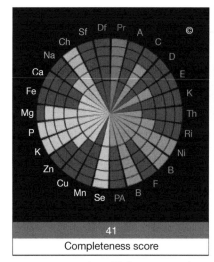
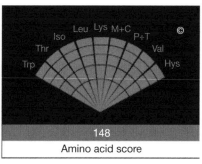

Figure 32.1 Nutrition value of fish protein is shown as micronutrients amino acid composition. Notice the scores of nutrition value 41 for micronutrients and 148 for amino acids.

Salmon fish is an oily fish, high in protein, omega-3 fatty acids, and vitamin D. It is abundant in the Atlantic and Pacific oceans, farm-raised roe and raw sashimi in origin. Salmon fish contains dioxanes, polychlorinated biphenyl compounds. Salmon flesh is red in color, but the natural color is white because of the presence of astaxanthin or canthaxantin carotinoid antioxidant pigments. (Food Standards Agency, 2004; Mozaffarian, 2006).

Sardines are an excellent low calorie, low carbohydrate fish food. Small, silver-colored fish, also known as pilchard, they can be a healthy snack or a regular meal due to the various nutrients in them. Pilchards are oily fish, very rich in omega-3 fatty acids; they have no carbohydrates and are rich sources of fish protein, vitamins A, B, C, D, and E, and various minerals such as iron, calcium, selenium, magnesium, phosphorous, and potassium. Sardines contain the coenzyme Q10, which is an antioxidant and promotes heart health. Oily sardine fish contains omega-3 fatty acids, which play a vital role in regulating blood cholesterol levels to promote heart health. Fish intake helps to lower bad cholesterol and maintain good cholesterol levels. The improved ratio between good and bad cholesterol helps to sustain good heart health. It also reduces the risk of stroke and cardiovascular disease. Vitamin B12, also found in high concentrations in the fish, helps to protect the walls of the arteries. It promotes cardiovascular health.[1]

Tuna is an excellent source of protein, and while some vitamin and mineral losses occur during canned tuna processing, the protein nutritive values are not dramatically changed. Tuna is an excellent source of the omega-3 fatty acids EPA and DHA,

---

[1] http://www.buyomegaprotein.com/benefits.aspx.

protein, potassium, selenium, and vitamin B12. Every 100 g of fish food contains: carbohydrates, 0.00 g; dietary fiber, 0.0 g; fat, 0.95 g; protein, 23.38 g; vitamin A, 60 IU; thiamine (vitamin B_1), 0.434 mg; riboflavin (vitamin B_2), 0.047 mg; niacin (vitamin B_3), 9.800 mg; pantothenic acid (B_5), 0.750 mg; vitamin B_6, 0.900 mg; folate (Vitamin B_9), 2 µg; vitamin B_{12}, 0.52 µg; vitamin C, 1.0 mg; vitamin E, 0.50 mg; vitamin K, 0.1 µg; calcium, 16 mg; iron, 0.73 mg; magnesium, 50 mg; phosphorus, 191 mg; potassium, 444 mg; sodium, 37 mg; zinc, 0.52 mg; and manganese, 0.015 mg.

Cod, hake, flounder, and sole contain <100 kcal per 100 g fish flesh, while mackerel, herring, and salmon contain 250 kcal in 100 g flesh. Lean type fish have 40–60 mg cholesterol per 100 g muscle. Salmon, tuna, mackerel, and sardine fish also have plenty of omega-3 fatty acids, which is considered to be beneficial in cardiac prevention. Major beneficial effects of fish eating are long life expectancy, antiarrhythmic, antithrombosis, lowering triglycerides and VLDL cholesterol and antihypertensive action.

3. FISH PROTEINS IN CARDIAC PREVENTION

Fat intake is not culprit at all. We analyze this issue based on recent studies. The Harvard School of Public Health showed that total fat intake bore no significant relation to the risk of CAD, but fish intake in the diet reduces the risk. Other studies suggested high omega fatty acid intake with adverse effect or stimulating fibrillation and reducing platelet aggregation or antithrombotic effect (Aarsetov et al., 2008; Harris, 2007; Kowey et al., 2010; Pratt et al., 2010; Saravanan et al., 2010). Investigators clearly advocated that claims of fish omega fatty acids in cardioprotection are fishy and not conclusive (Albert et al., 2010). In fact, several studies over the last four decades have suggested that a diet that includes fish is rich in proteins with the potential to reduce the risk of CAD (ADA report, 2003a,b; Bernstein et al., 2010; Das, 2000; De Lao et al., 2009; Mozaffarian, 2008). Saturated fats in other animal meats and foods appear to carry more risk than fish, refined carbohydrates, other food classes representing the bulk of recommended *daily calories*.[2] Fish diet is rich in unsaturated fatty acids (mono- and polyunsaturated fatty acids) and good proteins (45–80%). However, fish foods contain mercury, arsenic etc. as contaminants and appear to have adverse effects. Several other epidemiological studies (Gordon et al., 1981) have shown no evidence that man who eat less fat live longer or have fewer myocardial infarctions (MI). Epidemiological evidence suggests that fish-eating populations on a low carbohydrate diet for 6 months had low fat and low risk of heart disease (Westman et al., 2002). Other groups have reported that fish protein was better than other cardioprotective dietary and omega-3 options (Bergeron and Jacques, 1989; Bergeron et al., 1992a,b). Fish muscle protein characteristics in different seasons, including casein content and W-6/W-3 contents, were shown to be correlated with improved blood pressure and fewer episodes of

---

[2] http://www.13.waisays.com/protein.htm.

heart complications after dietary fish intake. In this context, our question was whether fish proteins have cardioprotective effects. Recently, a study reported the protein content of *Heteropneustes fossilis* (BLOCH) fish to evaluate its nutritive value and the impact it has on the fish-eating community in Nagpur (Shriniwas et al., 2008). In Western world and Southeast Asia, fish eating concept is emerging as affluent style of cardiac protection. We propose that fish protein content analysis can highlight the additional potential of eating fish, rich in omega fatty acids, fish oils, and protein values, in cardiac protection. Authors reported a short cross sectional study on patients with cardiac heart disease (arrhythmia, early myocardial infraction sign, high blood pressure) having treatment of betablocker and diuretics for last known 3–6 months. Patients were monitored and intervened with W-3/W-6 EPA/DHA rich oils or with fish eating for at least 100 g/100 kg weight/day in last 1–3 months. Cross sectional routine BP, Heart indicators, dietary intake of fish proteins, and oil content was calculated. To further calculate the fish protein content, electrophoretic mobility indices were screened in the *H. fossilis*. The casein content, oil content, and heart indicators were correlated to establish the effect of fish protein and oil content as effective measures of cardiac protection. Intervention of fish eating and withdrawal of chemotherapy improved the serum lipid profile (HDL-3), BP, EKG. After 3 months, the fish-rich diet intervention showed a further improvement in BP, lipid profile (HDL-3), and EKG finding. However, during the next 3 months, the intervention effect was slower. The *H. fossilis* protein content analysis suggested several proteins on electrophoresis bands with possibility of other protein candidates in cardioprotection. Casein protein was distinct candidate. During seasonal protein patterns, male fish protein suggested April–June and female Dec–Jan period as high protein yield cardioprotective diet (Shriniwas et al., 2008).

Cardioprotection by fish eating is a dilemma despite known fish infection, environmental hazards. The authors believe that fish proteins supplement essential amino acids (taurine, methionine, cysteine, glycine, threonine, leucine) to enhance the excitation–contraction coupling rate in sarcolemma (Ca^{++} and troponin mediated actin–tropomyosine binding) across T-tubule and SR-junction. Fish breeding industries have a significant role to play in providing infection-free, protein-rich fish food throughout the year by measures of spawning in different seasons, especially in the resting phase of fish. The combined use of liver oil and proteins has proven to be the best known nonchemotherapeutic measure for cardiac protection. Our growing understanding of fish eating intervention with slow withdrawal of betablockers/diuretics has become routine clinical practice. In this report, the major points are as follows: (1) W-3/W-6 fatty acid-rich oils with fish casein protein provide enhanced cardiac protection, perhaps due to a casein sparing effect and reduce free radicals sufficiently to retard further progress of cardiac injury; (2) fish breeding with spawning in the rest phase shows an impact on the quality of fish value; (3) cardiac protection is multifactorial and is enhanced by the combined effects of the fish liver oil, omega fatty acids, and amino acids present in fish proteins. Fish high quality proteins with fish liver oils serve best cardiac protection.

Fish meat or muscle has good protein quality. Salmon, halibut, tuna are major fish foods. Casein, taurine are major fish proteins. In following sections, we focus on fish protein contents and their role in hypertension and heart disease.

Essential hypertension is associated with higher lipoperoxidation and imbalanced antioxidant status (means oxidative stress) with increased RBC enzymes (Yuan et al., 2002). The mechanisms are not well established yet, but some experimental studies have established the modulation of HDL and reverse cholesterol transport, lipoprotein lipase activity in the liver, and the action of actinopectin, ACE inhibitory peptides on heart (De Lao et al., 2009; Hersberger and Von Eckardstein, 2005; Jung et al., 2008; Siddiqui et al., 2004). Blocking of AHR2 and ARNT1 gene expression was reported as cardioprotective (Antkiewicz et al., 2006).

3.1 One Amino Acid-One Fatty Acid Concept

One amino acid in fish protein may be alternative approach to keep high HDL, low (LDL+TG+C) lipids for cardioprotection. Author reported the benefits of casein protein in hypercholesterolemic hamsters. In gallstone-bearing hamsters with high plasma cholesterol, casein (250 g/kg wt) showed cholesterol lowering after 4 weeks. Cholesterol lowering effect against cholesterol saturation and cholelithiasis in hamsters was shown by using cytochrome P450 and cholesterol 7α Hydroxylase biomarker proteins. In casein-fed animals, plasma lipids including total cholesterol, phospholipids, lipoproteins, and biliary lipids were brought down in a time-dependent manner (Sharma et al., 2010). The following studies present evidence supporting the cardioprotective effect of casein:

1. Researchers from Algeria compared fish protein consumption to casein in an animal model of hypertension. The fish protein-rich diet lowered blood pressure and plasma total cholesterol to a higher degree compared with casein, leading the researchers to conclude that fish protein attenuated the development of hypertension (Yahia et al., 2003a). Casein intake changed the tissue antioxidant status in rats (Yahia et al., 2003b).

2. Dietary cod fish consumption, rich in casein, influenced muscle physiology by the insulin-induced activation of glutamate transfer protein and translocation characteristics in fish muscle (Tremblay et al., 2003).

3. Bergeron and Jacques (1989) reported the influence of fish proteins and compared to casein and soy protein for their effect on serum and liver lipids, and serum lipoprotein cholesterol levels in the rabbits. The investigators established the mechanism of cardioprotection by fish protein at the molecular level as modulation of HDL and lipoprotein lipase activity. Casein effect was closer with fish protein benefits in cardioprotection and regulation of plasma lipids (Bergeron et al., 1992a; Jacques et al., 1995; Santos et al., 1996). Furthermore, interaction between fish proteins and lipids was responsible in regulation of serum and lipids in liver that gives benefit

of cardioprotection (Bergeron et al., 1991). Fish protein actually showed effect in proportion of its incremental amounts in diet or factorial manner (Bergeron et al., 1992b). In the following section, the individual amino acids are discussed for their value in cardiac prevention.

3.1.1 Taurine in fish proteins

Taurine (T) was first noted as beneficial for stroke and cardiovascular diseases (CVD) prevention in genetic rat models, stroke-prone spontaneously hypertensive rats (SHRSP) (Yamori, 1984). The preventive mechanisms of T were ascribed to sympathetic modulation for reducing blood pressure (BP) and anti–inflammatory action. Recent epidemiological surveys revealed that taurine was effective in experimental arterio–lipidosis prone SHRSP selectively bred rats with higher reactive hypercholesterolemia. In fact, sulfur containing amino acids taurine and methionine showed an attenuated effect on severe hypertension and stroke as a result of activation of 7α hydroxylase to accelerate cholesterol excretion into bile acids. Rats quickly developed arterial fat deposition and fatty liver, which was attenuated by dietary Taurine supplementation. In fact, investigators suggested the role of rate limiting enzyme cholesterol 7α hydroxylase to bile synthesis to decrease cholesterol and inverse correlation between mRNA levels and enzyme gene CYP7A1 as contributor to increased serum triglycerides.

3.1.2 Methionine, cysteine, and cystine in fish protein

Sulfur-containing amino acids are abundant in fish muscle. Their role in lowering lipid has not been established, but these amino acids play a role in the sarcoplasm in muscle cells and in contractility (Ackman, 1995; Arino et al., 2003). Amino acid requirements in different age groups are specific as amino acid contents of fish foods stated below. In general, the amino acid requirement pattern is clear; typically, methionine and cystine are most scarce in our daily food. The National Institute of Nutrition (ICMR) monitored the following requirements and suggested fish foods as shown in Tables 32.4 and 32.5 (NNMB report, 2007; FAO/WHO report).

For adults, methionine and cystine always are most scarce (100%). Even if only minimal amounts of amino acids are consumed, in 81% of foods, methionine and cystine are again the most scarce; in 19%, tryptophan is scarce.

For school children, again methionine and cystine are most scarce in all foods except grains. In 47% of grains, methionine and cystine are the scarcest, but in 53%, lysine is, depending on the applied amino acid requirements. However, nobody eats grains like bread and cornflakes *only*, again making methionine and cystine the scarcest amino acids in diets comprising lots of grains.

For younger children, protein requirements match food protein contents better, leveling relative availability; in 57%, methionine and cystine are the scarcest; in 25%, phenylalanine and tyrosine; in 13%, tryptophan; and in 5% of foods, isoleucine is the scarcest, depending

Table 32.4 Other Potential Fish/Nonfish Foods Available in India with Their Protein Nutritive Values in Cardiac Prevention

Fish foods	Energy (kcal)	Protein (g)	Carbohydrates (g)	Fat (g)	Ca (mg)	P (mg)	Fe (mg)
Bhetki (fresh)	79	14.9	3.0	0.8			
Crab (muscle)	59	8.9	3.3	1.1			
Crab (small)	169	11.2	9.1	9.8			
Hilsa	273	21.8	2.9	19.4	180	280	2.1
Katla	111	19.5	2.9	2.4	530	235	0.9
Mackerel	93	19.9	0.5	2.7	429	305	4.5
Pomfrets black	111	20.3	1.5	2.6	286	306	2.3
Pomfrets white	87	17.0	1.8	1.3	200	290	0.9
Surumai	92	19.9	NIL	1.4	92	161	2.0
Lobster	90	20.5	NIL	0.9			
Prawn	89	19.1	0.8	1.0			
Rohu	97	16.6	4.4	1.4			
Sardine	101	21.0	NIL	1.9	90	360	2.5
Shrimp (small, dried)	349	68.1	NIL	8.5			

Source: Nutritive Value of Indian Foods: National Institute of Nutrition (ICMR).

Table 32.5 Requirement of Total Amino Acids Available from Fish Foods in Different Age Groups

Fish	Lysine	TRP	Valine	Phenylala	Tyrosine	Leucine	Isoleu	Threonine	Meth/cys
Herring	389	**47**	269	<u>167</u>	<u>149</u>	389	231	231	*100*
Cod	482	**56**	256	<u>198</u>	<u>167</u>	396	<u>233</u>	228	*100*
Saith	488	**45**	295	<u>186</u>	<u>162</u>	417	271	243	*100*
Mackerel	398	62	278	<u>193</u>	<u>147</u>	414	251	223	*100*
Tuna	491	67	316	<u>233</u>	<u>216</u>	482	<u>269</u>	262	*100*
Trout	487	58	301	<u>222</u>	<u>164</u>	429	258	260	*100*
Salmon	408	**53**	281	<u>164</u>	<u>145</u>	358	234	224	*100*
Brown shrimp	412	**43**	202	<u>180</u>	<u>133</u>	402	<u>204</u>	173	*100*
Mussel	363	**56**	284	<u>191</u>	<u>191</u>	353	<u>219</u>	214	*100*

Source: US FDA data source for daily 2000 calorie diet.
Requirements as % Daily Values (%DV) are Shown in bold for Adults, in italic for Schoolchildren, and in underline in Adolescents Fed on Fish Food.

on the applied amino acid requirements. But, again, methionine and cystine are the scarcest amino acids.

3.1.3 Guanidine, histidine, creatine, glycine

Creatine is considered as an essential amino acid to keep the creatine kinase enzyme CK-MB and other isozymes working in cardiac muscle contraction, and it is also recommended for athletic activity (Food and Drug Administration, 1989; Haard, 1995). The mechanism of guanidine ME10092 is not known in cardiac prevention, but its analogue CARIPORIDE is thought to provide cardiac prevention by sodium–hydrogen exchange inhibition in mitochondria (Oliver et al., 2004). Histidine is converted to histamine in cooked fish but gives constipation problems (Arino et al., 2003; Food and Drug Administration, 1989). Glycine is basically a novel anti-inflammatory, immunomodulatory cytoprotective agent and believed beneficial in cardiac prevention (Haard, 1995).

3.1.4 Squalene in fish

Squalene is bioactive isoprenoid substance present in shark liver oil. It is explored to neutralize the harmful effects of free radicals and improve membrane stabilizing properties. Squalene has been proven to be a safe dietary supplement without any side effects (Farvin et al., 2006; Thankappan, 2003).

3.2 Interventional Studies

Fish proteins showed similarity in casein for short-term metabolic effects of dietary interventions on various risk factors of CAD. Casein was given as supplements in the form of beta casein A1 and A2, and the effect on plasma lipoproteins was observed. The major effect was seen on HDL and triglycerides (Chin-Dusting et al., 2006; Nilausen and Meinertz, 1999; Venn et al., 2006). Studies provide little or no direct evidence that fish proteins and amino acids taurine and methionine can prolong life or prevent or delay CAD events (Yamori et al., 2009). These studies also suffer from a major design flaw that has only recently been recognized in cardiovascular medicine: metabolic or biochemical measures can provide mechanistic insights and are essential building blocks in therapeutic development, but they cannot reliably predict the effect of proposed interventions on clinical events. Authors describe metabolic and biochemical insight on fish protein composition and muscle physiological influence on heart physiology.

Cardiovascular Diseases and Alimentary Comparison Study, CARDIAC, trial was designed to study biological markers of hypertension and CVD mortality from the diet (Yamashita and Konagaya, 1990). The CARDIAC (CVD and Alimentary Comparison)–WHO-coordinated multi-center epidemiological survey on diets and CVD risks in 61 populations showed that twenty-four-hour urinary (24 h) taurine excretion was inversely related with significant coronary heart disease mortality Yamori, 1989. Higher 24U-T excreters had significantly lower body mass index, systolic and diastolic BP, total cholesterol (T-Cho), and atherogenic index (AI: T-Cho/high density lipoprotein-cholesterol) than lower T excreters. T effects on CVD risks were intensified in individuals whose 24U-T and –magnesium (M) excretions were higher. Furthermore, higher Na excreters with higher heart rates, whose BP was significantly higher than that of individuals with lower heart rates, were divided into two groups by the mean of 24U-T, high and low T excreters.

Since the former showed significantly lower BP than the latter, T may beneficially affect salt-sensitive BP rise. In other study on 61 populations including Guiyang, China and St. John's, Newfoundland, Canada where in which the means of both 24U-T and -M were high and low, respectively. The former and the latter had low and high CVD risks, respectively (Yamori et al., 2006). Australian aborigines living in the coastal areas in Victoria eat T- and M-rich bush and mainly sea foods, and were free from CVD, till 200 years ago. Such a diet pattern indicated that T- and/or M-containing seafood, vegetables, fruits, nuts, milk, etc., was similar to the food of prehistoric hunters and gatherers, and should be good for CVD prevention. Now same population had highest CVD risks in those areas. In recent study, preventive effects of T good for health and longevity were first noted experimentally and later were proven epidemiologically in humans (Yamori et al., 2006, 2009).

EXPEDITION study was an important, large, drug intervention study that tested the hypothesis that targeting an ischemia/reperfusion injury mechanism can result in a reduction in the incidence of MI after coronary bypass (CABG). The results of EXPEDITION revealed (1) compelling evidence that the incidence of intraoperative myocardial necrosis in patients undergoing CABG occurs more frequently than previously appreciated; (2) a reduction in the primary endpoint of all-cause death or nonfatal MI was achieved with cariporide (a guanidine analogue); and (3) the reduction in the primary endpoint was due almost exclusively to a reduction in nonfatal MI; however, this benefit was offset by a higher incidence of CVEs and mortality in patients receiving cariporide (Mentzer et al., 2008). It needs further research on other alternative amino acid or analogue with better outcome.

3.3 Nutrient Composition of Fish and Environment

There is some knowledge available to address whether fish protein composition can affect appetite or quality of life. High quality fish meal is a complete source of amino acids. It contains high levels of lysine and methionine, essential trace elements. Due to the high nutritional value of dietary fish, research on alternative sources of protein, such as unsaturated fatty acid-rich oils, legumes, meat by-product, brewery by-products with high nutritive value, or available essential amino acids, is continuing. The protein quality of fish is evaluated by freshness of flesh by volatile nitrogen content, intact proteins.

Methods of assessing quality fall into three catagories: (1) Inspection; (2) chemical analysis; and (3) biological evaluation. Chemical tests of protein quality include tests for acid-corrected pepsin-digestible protein (AOAC and Torry methods), protein extraction methods by electrophoresis and SDS-PAGE, multienzyme digestible proteins, total volatile basic nitrogen, lysine, sulfhydryl groups, and disulphide bonds. Biological tests are multienzyme and Torry pepsin solubility tests. Protein data in fish after PAGE electrophoresis is shown in Table 32.6. In a collaborative study, electrophoresis SDS-PAGE on Excel 15% homogeneous gels was easy and cheap; the silver staining method

Table 32.6 Protein Content of Different Fish are Shown by Using Urea Immunoelectrophoresis and SDS-PAGE Methods

Fish species (common name)	Protein content (mg/g flesh)	
	Urea IEF	SDS-PAGE
Oncorhynchus gorbuscha (pink salmon)	182.4	215.6
Oncorhynchus keta (chum salmon)	125.8	135.2
Oncorhynchus mykiss (rainbow trout)	170.5	153.2
Salmo trutta (sea trout)	170.3	170.3
Salmo salar (Atlantic salmon)	208.1	167.1
Hippoglossus hippoglossus (halibut)	124.8	136.9
Reinhardtius hippoglossoides (Greenland halibut)	171.2	155.6
Thunnus alalunga (albacore)	185.9	197.3
Thunnus albacores (yellow fin tuna)	148.8	173.9
Katsuwonis pelamis (skipjack tuna)	139.6	179.6

Source: Etienne, M., Jérôme, M., Fleurence, J., et al., 2000. Identification of fish species after cooking by SDS-PAGE and urea IEF: a collaborative study. Journal of Agricultural and Food Chemistry 48(7), 2653–2658.

was a better option than the urea immuno–electrophoresis (IEF) method for the identification of fish species and for distinguishing the different proteins in salmon, halibut, and tuna fish food extracts (Etienne et al., 2000). Species differentiation was easy in different fish family by spot analysis as shown in Figure 32.2. For details of the technique, readers are referred to read original paper (Etienne et al., 2000).

Biogenic amines (cadaverine, putrescine, histamine, tyramine) are used to assess fish food quality (Chen et al., 2007) as shown in Table 32.7. Thiamine content was used as indicator of high quality as function of thermal processing conditions in canned salmon fish industry (Quitral et al., 2006). The temperature and the food processing method used are two major factors that change fish protein, especially the composition of methionine, cysteine, and taurine in fish food (Lipka and Ganowiak, 1993) (Table 32.8).

Temperature around the year in different months plays a significant role in fish breeding and fish growth. The fish protein content, amino acid composition, and growth hormone action are dependent on the dietary composition of a fish meal and its quality. In a recent study, Shriniwas et al., 2008 reported the effect of temperature on the fish liver proteins identifiable in *H. fossalis* and *Catla catla,* as shown in Figure 32.3, and on the protein contents on PAGE-electrophoresis in catala fish (a common human fish food in Nagpur, Central India). Investigators established better SDS–PAGE electrophoresis method (see Appendix 1).

4. EFFECT OF FISH DIETARY PROTEINS ON CORONARY ARTERY DISEASE

In a randomized, single-blind, controlled intervention trial, Singh et al. (2010), an Indo-Mediterranean dietary 24-week trial on 59 patients with high blood pressure, and a

M M M R₁₂ C₄ R₁₃ R₄ R₅ R₆ C₂ R₆ M C₃ R₄ C₃ R₄ C₃ R₂ C₃ R₂ C₁ R₁ M

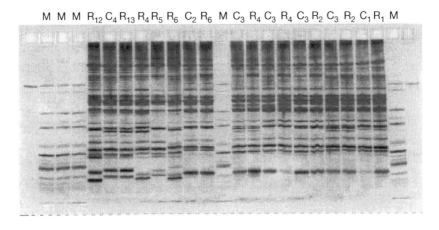

M   M M   C₄ C₁₂ R₂₁ R₁₂ R₁₀ M C₄ R₁₃ R₁₈ R₁₅ R₁₃ R₁₄ R₁₁ R₁₅ M

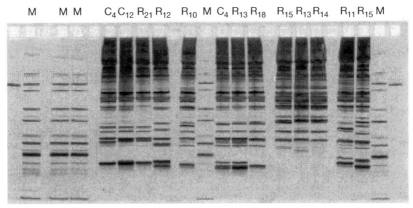

Figure 32.2 SDS-PAGE. Extracts of raw (references R1–R21) and cooked (samples C1–C10) fish muscle were run on Excel gel homogeneous 15% M) p*l* calibration proteins. The cathode is at the top of the gel. *Reproduced from Etienne, M., Jérôme, M., Fleurence, J., et al., 2000. Identification of fish species after cooking by SDS-PAGE and urea IEF: a collaborative study. Journal of Agricultural and Food Chemistry 48(7), 2653–2658, with permission.*

subsequent preliminary study by Shriniwas et al. (2008), both demonstrated the effects of fish supplementation on blood pressures and blood lipids, and nitric oxide in patients with hypertension and dyslipidemia. Epidemiological studies and intervention trials indicated that fish intake can decrease cardiovascular events in patients with high risk of coronary

Table 32.7 Biogenic Amine Content in Fish Meals

Fish	Histamine mg/100 g[a]	Putrescine mg/100 g[a]	Cadaverine mg/100 g[a]	Tyramine mg/100 g[a]
Sardine	5.1	33.2	41.6	4.9
Tuna	17.9	95.7	159.0	36.6

[a] Expressed as a concentration of the dry matter.

Table 32.8 Public Online Resources on Fish Diet and Proteins for Cardiovascular Protection

http://www.fao.org/docrep/003/w7499e/w7499e13.htm
http://linkinghub.elsevier.com/retrieve/pii/S0045653504010173
http://www.pulsus.com/CARDIOL/home.htm
www.banglajol.info/index.php/JARD/article/viewPDFInterstitial/762/800
http://linkinghub.elsevier.com/retrieve/pii/S1050464801903742
http://linkinghub.elsevier.com/retrieve/pii/S1050464807000186
http://www.blackwell-synergy.com/doi/abs/10.1111/j.1365-2761.2006.00722.x
http://ohioline.osu.edu/sc172/sc172_17.html
http://aem.asm.org/cgi/content/abstract/74/11/3551
http://findarticles.com/p/articles/mi_m0887/is_6_20/ai_75818427

artery disease (CAD). It was evidence that total or whole fish intake can also decrease blood pressures and blood lipids. The beneficial effects of fish intake may be due to long chain w-3 (EPA and DHA) fatty acids and amino acids in the fish proteins. Investigators examined the effects of mild fish intake on cardiovascular risk factors, in patients with hypertension and dyslipidemia. The effects of Indian fish (30 g/day) and the AHA-step 1 diet were compared for a period of 24 weeks in patients with mild hypertension (140/90–160/110 mmHg) and dyslipidemia. All patients with known hypertension, with low HDL (<40 mg/dl) or high triglycerides (>150 mg/dl) or hypercholesterolemia (T-C > 200 mg/dl), were randomly divided into a fish intake group (Gr A, $n=30$) and a control group (Gr B, $n=29$) by the dietitian for computer-generated data after

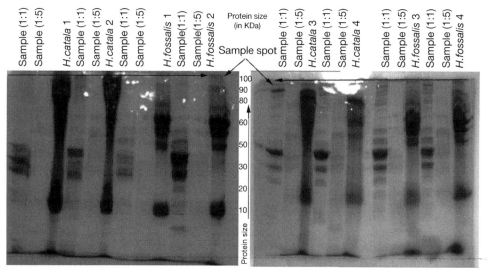

Figure 32.3 SDS-PAGE electrophoresis is shown for two fish species *H. fossilis* (a) and *C. catla* (b) muscle proteins.

an observation period of 1 week. Mean age (57.1 ± 9.5 vs. 58.5 ± 8.7 years), body mass index (25.2 ± 2.5 vs. 24.6 ± 2.6 kg/m^2), and waist circumferences (89.8 ± 8.8 vs. 90.8 ± 6.8 cm) were comparable at entry to the study. Mean systolic (155.6 ± 11.5 vs. 153.7 ± 13.4 mmHg) and diastolic (100.4 ± 8.8 vs. 101.0 ± 7.2 mmHg) blood pressures in fish intake group and control groups were comparable, at entry to the study. However, after 24 weeks, there was a significant fall in both mean systolic (146.3 ± 9.5 vs. 152.5 ± 12.0 mmHg, $P < 0.03$) and diastolic (92.4 ± 9.8 vs. 98.6 ± 7.6 mmHg, $P < 0.05$) blood pressures in the intervention group compared to the control group, respectively. Mean concentrations of blood glucose (126.8 ± 35.1 vs. 120.5 ± 31.8 mg/dl) were comparable at entry to the study. Plasma levels of antioxidant vitamins E (20.5 ± 3.2 vs. 21.5 ± 3.3 pmol/l), and C (19.2 ± 3.3 vs. 19.6 ± 3.4 pmol/l) were comparable at the entry to the study. After 24 weeks, plasma levels of vitamin E (28.6 ± 3.8 vs. 21.6 ± 3.1 pmol/l) and C (25.4 ± 4.0 vs. 19.2 ± 3.4 pmol/l) showed a significant increase, and TBARS and MDA (0.88 ± 0.26 vs. 1.52 ± 0.31 pm/dl) showed a significant ($P < 0.02$) decrease in the fish intake group compared to the control group, respectively. HDL-C and triglycerides showed no significant differences before entry to the study. However, after 24 weeks of treatment with fish, HDL-C (40.5 ± 7.2 vs. 35.2 ± 8.5 mg/dl, $P < 0.01$) showed a significant increase. T-C/HDL-C ratio (4.6 ± 1.0 vs. 5.6 ± 1.1 mg/dl, $P < 0.05$) and LDL cholesterol (120 ± 12 vs. 132 ± 15 mg/dl, $P < 0.04$) showed a significant decrease, while T–C and TG showed a nonsignificant decline in the intervention group compared to the control group. Serum concentrations of nitrite, which is an indicator of nitric oxide, were comparable at baseline (0.57 ± 0.12 vs. 0.63 ± 0.16 μmol/l). After 24 weeks, there was a significant increase in nitrite levels in the intervention group compared to the control group (0.93 ± 0.21 vs. 0.71 ± 0.13 μmol/l), respectively. Increase in nitrite is an indicator of nitric oxide, which is known to decrease endothelial function and blood pressure. The investigators indicated that even a low fish intake can decrease blood pressure, modulate oxidative stress, and increase the HDL-C, T-C/HDL-C ratio and nitric oxide in patients with high risk of CAD.

4.1 Indian Fish Proteins in Lipid Lowering: One Amino Acid-One Fatty Acid Concept

Although the benefits of specific lipid-lowering drugs are unquestioned, the relation between these drug effects and the potential of the diet to improve outcomes is unclear. Fish diet is emerging as cardioprotective food. Fish protein, amino acid, and omega–3/6 eicosapentanoic/docosahexanoic fatty acid (EPA/DHA)–rich fish oils are considered to reduce total blood fat LDL (Bad) cholesterol, and simultaneously raise the HDL (Good) cholesterol. Eating 30 g of fish (muscles) every day reduces the chances of coronary heart disease by >70%. Fish proteins, along with their omega-3/omega-6 (EPA/DHA) polyunsaturated fatty acid content, protect the heart by keeping the HDL3 ratio high and rapidly converting cholesterol to its products by cholesterol oxidase. Shriniwas et al. (2008)

analyzed diets with fish protein contents, omega-3/omega-6 (EPA/DHA) contents, and essential amino acid composition, and correlated diets with their lipid lowering effect. The idea was that fish muscle proteins and essential amino acid compositions provide better cardiac protection along with omega-3/omega-6 fatty acids against sudden death from cardiovascular diseases. The investigators proposed the possibility of 'one amino acid-one fatty acid concept' that fish proteins and amino acids may be an alternative approach to maintaining high HDL and low (LDL+TG+C) lipids, and preventing the formation of blood clots to avoid the build up of plaque in the coronary and cardiovascular arteries, especially in patients showing sensitivity to omega fatty acids. In preliminary experiments, different fish proteins, oil compositions, and amino acids were analyzed and compared. Borderline hypertensive patients with a cardiac problem (high BP with risk of heart attack) were advised to take 30 g of fish in the diet every day [to keep up the recommended omega-3/omega-6 (EPA/DHA) content] over 6 months. After follow-up, fish oil content, fish protein content, fish amino acid contents were correlated with heart indicators to establish the effect of fish protein and oil content on cardiovascular diseases. Simultaneously, the biochemical analysis of less known Indian fish protein content and protein composition were analyzed by electrophoretic mobility. In the following section, fish protein compositions, omega fatty acids, and their benefits in cardiovascular prevention are discussed.

The source of Indian fish is important in fish protein quality to decrease hypertension (see Table 32.9). The amino acid composition and fish protein content, and the omega-3/omega-6 (EPA/DHA) contents in fish differ (see Table 32.10). The progressive increase in lipids leads to coronary heart disease and hyperlipidemia, the two being the main causes of death in most fast growing urban cities. Several previous studies report that fish protein, fish amino acid content were determinants to lower the blood lipids with possibility of cardiac prevention if taken in specific quantity not exceeding fat energy 10% intake. The protein content of fish *H. fossilis* and *C. catla* suggested specific proteins of size 35, 41, 67, and 94 kDa as SDS-PAGE electrophoretic bands (see Figure 32.3). The fish grown during December and January months possibly served as better cardiac protector fish food and served as high yield cardioprotective proteins. On an average, fish intake brings down BP by −8/2.5 mmHg systolic/diastolic pressure. However, strong belief is in favor of fish proteins playing significant role in Okinawa community. Fish proteins and omega-3/omega-6 (EPA/DHA) appear to be effective measures to keep fat energy intake below 10% and prevent coronary heart disease and stroke by maintaining normal levels of hypertension, BP, and hypercholesterolemia. The main player in lipid lowering is HDL-3 molecule composed of Apolipoprotein E2 and apo-A moieties bound with major cholesterol esters. Its main component LP-A apolipoprotein has been established as cholesterol scavenger to keep low total lipid content (LDL+TG+free cholesterol). However, the link between HDL-3 synthesis and effect of fish protein intake is not established. An alternate possibility appears of

Table 32.9 Fish Protein and Energy Contents

Indian fish	Protein g%	Energy cal/g	BP (mmHg)–Sys/Dia
Hilsa	21.8	273	−10/2.5
Rohu	16.6	97	−6/2
Catla	19.5	111	−9.5/3
Sardine	21.0	101	−5/3
Surmai	19.9	92	−
Mackerel	18.9	93	−10/2.5
Black Pomfret	20.3	111	−
White Pomfret	17.3	87	−

Source: Shariniwas, B.D., 2011. Ph.D dissertation submitted to Nagpur University, Nagpur, India.

Table 32.10 Omega-3/6 Fatty Acid Content of Popular Fish and EAA (%) in Fish Protein

Fish	Omega-3/6 PUFA	Amino acid	mg/g
Sardine	0.98–1.70	Lysine	8.8
Trout	0.98–0.84	Tryptophan	1.0
Anchovy	1.4	Histidine	2.0
Herring	1.2–1.8	Phenylalanine	3.9
Catfish	0.3–0.4	Leucine	8.4
Crab	0.35	Isoleucine	6.0
Lobster	0.07–0.41	Threonine	4.6
Mackerel	0.34–1.57	Methionine/cystine	4.0
		Valine	6.0

Source: Shariniwas, B.D., 2011. Ph.D dissertation submitted to Nagpur University, Nagpur, India.

specific amino acid for specific fatty acid during synthesis of HDL-3 and Lp-A protein synthesis. If it is true, it amounts to support the fish diet intake and its effect on BP and lipid lowering. Fish proteins are effective diet components in lipid lowering. The amino acid–fatty acid combination may be an effective tool to synthesize the HDL-3 protein–lipid composition in favor of keeping cholesterol ester-rich Apo-protein moieties in HDL molecules as scavengers of cholesterol.

Different fish have different protein composition and its nutrition value. Temperature and fish feed also play important roles in fish protein quality and muscle growth over months. The other fact can be attributed to calcium-mediated tropomyosin–actin activity in muscle contraction at low temperatures in the December and January months. However, much remains unknown about fish muscle and its protein composition differing during fish growth in different months of the year. Also, it has not been established if fish eaten in different months of the year provides different levels of cardioprotection.

Table 32.9: Fish protein and energy contents Table 32.10: Omega-3/6 fatty acid content of popular fish and essential amino acids (mg/g) in fish proteins.

5. EFFECT OF FISH PROTEINS ON ATHEROSCLEROSIS

Randomized, controlled trials have been conducted to know the effects of fish dietary interventions alone as a strategy to arrest the progression of CAD as shown in Table 32.9. The Lifestyle Heart Trial randomly allocated 48 patients to either a diet very low in fat (10% of daily energy intake) and intensive lifestyle intervention (exercise, stress management, smoking cessation, group counseling) or to usual care. After 1 year, the experimental group showed more favorable changes in angina frequency and angiographic stenosis. After 5 years, the experimental group still had more favorable changes in low coronary stenoses and fewer cardiac events (unpublished data).

In the St. Thomas' Atherosclerosis Regression Study (STARS), 90 men were randomized to one of three arms: usual care; a low-fat, low-cholesterol diet, high in omega-6 and omega-3 fatty acids and in fiber (similar to AHA diet recommendations); or this diet plus cholestyramine. Patients in the fish diet-only group had significant improvements in several angiographic variables and fewer cardiac events or interventions compared with the usual-care group. Fish intake (two meals containing fish meat weekly) may offer some promise in the secondary prevention of CAD. Fish is a functional food which is rich in n-3 fatty acids, coenzyme Q10, and selenium, which are protective against CAD.

6. PREVENTION OF CAD: FISH DIET

There is a strong necessity for fish dietary research to eschew the type of data that would no longer be accepted to recommend a drug for prevention or treatment of CAD. In contrast to drugs, the basic fish diet will not change in the future in view of its firm biological basis, ability to reduce one or more risk factors for CAD with better clinical outcomes, or the epidemiological data favoring the safety and feasibility of continuing with a fish diet over a lifetime. Advanced understanding of trial methods can overturn many an erroneous principle or public policy. 'Does a program of dietary advice that can be followed by a typical person lead to fewer cardiovascular events?' sounds effectiveness or pragmatic type to answer the public-policy question.

7. CONCLUSION

This is appropriate time to apply to fish protein diet research. It is believed that indications or claims made regarding weight loss or health improvement via a fish diet – whether made by authors, the government, or other associations – must be supported by three types of evidence: (1) proof that the diet provides essential nutrients in actual patients; (2) proof from efficacy studies; and (3) proof from randomized, controlled trials with clinical events as endpoints.

APPENDIX 1 NEW METHOD DEVELOPED: SDS-PAGE ELECTROPHORESIS

The muscle was homogenized in lyses buffer separately containing 50 mM Tris–HCL, pH 7.5, 50 mM MgCl$_2$, 1 mM EDTA, 1% Triton X-100 and 1 mM PMSF (Phenyl methyl sulfonyl fluoride) as protease inhibitor. The homogenized tissues were centrifuged and supernatants were taken as a protein sample. These protein samples were stored at $-20\degree$ C and used for gel electrophoresis.

Chemicals
1. Acrylamide stock solution (30%)
   Acrylamide 29.2 g.
   Bis Acrylamide 0.8 gm.
   Double distilled water (DDW) upto 100 ml.
   (Stored in refrigerator in the dark)
2. Running gel buffer (1.5M, Tris–HCl, pH 8.8):
   Tris 18.17 g
   D.D.W. upto 100 ml
3. Stacking Gel buffer (0.05M, Tris–HCl, pH 6.8):
   Tris 1.5 g
   D.D.W. upto 25 ml
4. 10% SDS:
   SDS 10 g
   D.D.W. upto 100 ml
5. 10% APS (Ammonium per sulfate):
   APS0.1 g
   D.D.W. upto 10 ml
6. Treatment buffer (pH 6.8)
   Tris 2.5 ml (pH 6.8)
   SDS 4.0 ml
   Glycerol 2.0 ml
   β-Mercaptoethanol 1.0 ml
   D.D.W. upto 10 ml
   Bromophenol blue (pinch)
7. Tank buffer
   Tris 3.0 g
   Glycine 14.4 g
   SDS 10.0 ml
   D.D.W. upto 1000 ml
8. Stain stalk (1% Coomassie brilliant blue R$_{250}$):
   Coomassie brilliant blue 2 g
   D.D.W. upto 200 ml

9. Working stain:

Stain stock 12.5 ml

Methanol 50 ml

Glacial acetic acid (GAA) 10 ml

D.D.W. upto 100 ml

10. Destaining solution (50% Methanol, 10% acetic acid):

Methanol 500 ml

GAA 100 ml

D.D.W. upto 1000 ml

11. Preparation of separating gel (15%):

30% Acrylamide (stock) 10 ml

Tris (pH 8.8) 5.0 ml

D.D.W. 4.6 ml

Ammonium per sulfate 200 μl

SDS 200 μl

TEMED 8.0 μl

12. Preparation of staking gel

30% Acrylamide (stock) 1.0 ml

Stacking gel buffer (pH 6.8) 750 ml

D.D.W. 4.1 ml

Ammonium per sulfate 60 μl

SDS 60 μl

TEMED 6 μl

Procedure: The 15% sodium dodecyl sulfate-polyacrylamide gel electrophoresis (SDS-PAGE) was prepared on a vertical gel (16×14 cm) system (Bangalore Genei, India) in between two glass plates using a 1-mm spacer up to the desired level. Stacking gel was poured in the vacant space. The comb of 1-mm well was inserted in the stacking gel. After solidification of the gel, the comb was taken out.

Meanwhile, the protein sample was added with an equal volume of sample buffer (0.1M Tris–HCL, pH 6.8;10% glycerol; 1% SDS, 0.02% bromophenol blue), treated with 1% β-mercaptoethanol and denatured at 98°C for 3 min. The gel plates were attached to the electrophoretic chamber. The upper and lower tanks of the chamber were filled with tank buffer. Nearly 50 μl of sample was taken and mixed with 50 μl of treatment buffer and denatured. Then 30 μl of sample was loaded in each well with a micropipette. A lane containing molecular weight marker (Bangalore Genei, India) was included in a well and 50 mA current was supplied to electrophoretic chamber. After running the samples, the gel was then stained with Coomassie Brilliant Blue R-$_{250}$ (SRL, India) and destained.

REFERENCES

Ackman, R.G., 1995. Composition and nutritive value of fish and shellfish. In: Ruiter, A. (Ed.), Fish and Fishery Products: Composition, Nutritive Properties and Stability. CAB International, Willingford, pp. 117–156.

Albert, C., London, B., Anderson, M., Nattel, S., 2010. Omega 3 oil: a fishy protection in heart. Nature Medicine 16 (11).

Alne, H., Thomassen, M.S., Takle, H., et al., 2009. Increased survival by feeding tetradecylthioacetic acid during a natural outbreak of heart and skeletal muscle inflammation in S0 Atlantic salmon, *Salmo salar* L. Journal of Fish Diseases 32 (11), 953–961.

American Dietetic Association; Dietitians of Canada, 2003a. Position of the American Dietetic Association and Dietitians of Canada: vegetarian diets. Canadian Journal of Dietetic Practice and Research 64 (2), 62–81.

American Dietetic Association, Dietitians of Canada, 2003b. Position of the American Dietetic Association and Dietitians of Canada: vegetarian diets. Journal of the American Dietetic Association 103 (6), 748–765.

Andersen, Ø., Østbye, T.K., Gabestad, I., Nielsen, C., Bardal, T., Galloway, T.F., 2004. Molecular characterization of a PDZ-LIM protein in Atlantic salmon (*Salmo salar*): a fish ortholog of the alpha-actinin-associated LIM-protein (ALP). Journal of Muscle Research and Cell Motility 25 (1), 61–68.

Andreassen, R., Lunner, S., Høyheim, B., 2009. Characterization of full-length sequenced cDNA inserts (FLIcs) from Atlantic salmon (*Salmo salar*). BMC Genomics 10, 502.

Antkiewicz, D.S., Peterson, R.E., Heideman, W., 2006. Blocking expression of AHR2 and ARNT1 in zebrafish larvae protects against cardiac toxicity of 2,3,7,8-tetrachlorodibenzo-p-dioxin. Toxicological Sciences 94 (1), 175–182.

Arino, A., Beltran, J.A., Roncales, P., 2003. Dietary importance of fish and shellfish. In: Caballero, B., Trugo, L., Finglas, P. (Eds.), Encyclopedia of Food Sciences and Nutrition. second ed. Elsevier Science Ltd., Oxford, pp. 2471–2478.

Arsetoy, H., Ponitz, V., Nilsen, O.B., et al., 2008. Low levels of cellular omega-3 increase the risk of ventricular fibrillation during the acute ischaemic phase of a myocardial infarction. Resuscitation 78 (3), 258–264.

Beauchesne-Rondeau, E., Gascon, A., Bergeron, J., Jacques, H., 2003. Plasma lipids and lipoproteins in hypercholesterolemic men fed a lipid-lowering diet containing lean beef, lean fish, or poultry. American Journal of Clinical Nutrition 77 (3), 587–593.

Bergeron, N., Deshaies, Y., Jacques, H., 1992b. Factorial experiment to determine influence of fish protein and fish oil on serum and liver lipids in rabbits. Nutrition 8 (5), 354–358.

Bergeron, N., Deshaies, Y., Jacques, H., 1992a. Dietary fish protein modulates high density lipoprotein cholesterol and lipoprotein lipase activity in rabbits. Journal of Nutrition 122 (8), 1731–1737.

Bergeron, N., Deshaies, Y., Lavigne, C., Jacques, H., 1991. Interaction between dietary proteins and lipids in the regulation of serum and liver lipids in the rabbit. Effect of fish protein. Lipids 26 (9), 759–764.

Bergeron, N., Jacques, H., 1989. Influence of fish protein as compared to casein and soy protein on serum and liver lipids, and serum lipoprotein cholesterol levels in the rabbit. Atherosclerosis 78, 113–121.

Bernstein, A.M., Sun, Q., Hu, F.B., Stampfer, M.J., Manson, J.E., Willett, W.C., 2010. Major dietary protein sources and risk of coronary heart disease in women. Circulation 122 (9), 876–883.

Bower, N.I., Johnston, I.A., 2010. Discovery and characterization of nutritionally regulated genes associated with muscle growth in Atlantic salmon. Physiological Genomics 42A (2), 114–130.

Brahmam, S.N.V., 2007. National nutrition Monitoring Bureau in India-An overview. Indian Journal of Community Medicine 32 (1), 1–9.

Brown, W.V., 1990. Dietary recommendations to prevent coronary heart disease. Annals of the New York Academy of Sciences 598, 376–388.

Capilla, E., Díaz, M., Albalat, A., et al., 2004. Functional characterization of an insulin-responsive glucose transporter (GLUT4) from fish adipose tissue. American Journal of Physiology, Endocrinology and Metabolism 287 (2), E348–E357.

Chen, Y.C., Tou, J.C., Jaczynski, J., 2007. Amino acid, fatty acid, and mineral profiles of materials recovered from rainbow trout (*Oncorhynchus mykiss*) processing by-products using isoelectric solubilization/precipitation. Journal of Food Science 72 (9), C527–C535.

Chin-Dusting, J., Shennan, J., Jones, E., Williams, C., Kingwell, B., Dart, A., 2006. Effect of dietary supplementation with beta-casein A1 or A2 on markers of disease development in individuals at high risk of cardiovascular disease. British Journal of Nutrition 95 (1), 136–144.

Cleveland, B.M., Evenhuis, J.P., 2010. Molecular characterization of atrogin-1/F-box protein-32 (FBXO32) and F-box protein-25 (FBXO25) in rainbow trout (Oncorhynchus mykiss): expression across tissues in response to feed deprivation. Comparative Biochemistry and Physiology. Part B, Biochemistry and Molecular Biology 157 (3), 248–257.

Côté, S., Dodin, S., Blanchet, C., et al., 2004. Very high concentrations of n-3 fatty acids in peri- and post-menopausal Inuit women from Greenland. International Journal of Circumpolar Health 63 (Suppl 2), 298–301.

Das, U.N., 2000. Beneficial effect(s) of *n*-3 fatty acids in cardiovascular diseases: but, why and how? Prostaglandins, Leukotrienes, and Essential Fatty Acids 63 (6), 351–362.

De Lao, F., Panarese, S., Gallerani, R., Ceci, L.R., 2009. Angiotensin converting enzyme (ACE) inhibitory peptides: production and implementation of functional food. Current Pharmaceutical Design 15 (31), 3622–3643.

Etienne, M., Jérôme, M., Fleurence, J., et al., 2000. Identification of fish species after cooking by SDS–PAGE and urea IEF: a collaborative study. Journal of Agricultural and Food Chemistry 48 (7), 2653–2658.

Farvin, K.H.S., Anandan, R., Kumar, H.S., et al., 2006. Cardioprotective effect of squalene on lipid profile in isoprenaline-induced myocardial infarction in rats. Journal of Medicinal Food 9 (4), 531–536.

Fernandes, J., 2002. Nutrition and health-recommendations of the Health Council of the Netherlands regarding energy, proteins, fats and carbohydrates. Nederlands Tijdschrift voor Geneeskunde 146 (47), 2226–2229.

Food and Drug Administration, 1989. The Fish List, FDA Guide to Acceptable Market Names for Food Fish sold in Interstate Commerce 1988. US Government Printing Office, Washington, DC pp. 30–34.

Gordon, T., Kagan, A., Garcia- palmieri, M., et al., 1981. Diet and its relation to coronary heart disease and death in three populations. Circulation 63, 500–515.

Haard, N.F., 1995. Composition and nutritive value of fish proteins and other nitrogen compounds. In: Ruiter, A. (Ed.), Fish and Fishery Products: Composition, Nutritive Properties and Stability. ACB International, Wallingford, pp. 77–115.

Harris, W.S., 2007. Omega-3 fatty acids and cardiovascular disease: a case for omega-3 index as a new risk factor. Pharmacological Research 55 (3), 217–223.

Heine-Bröring, R.C., Brouwer, I.A., Proença, R.V., et al., 2010. Intake of fish and marine *n*-3 fatty acids in relation to coronary calcification: the Rotterdam Study. American Journal of Clinical Nutrition 91 (5), 1317–1323.

Hersberger, M., von Eckardstein, A., 2005. Modulation of high-density lipoprotein cholesterol metabolism and reverse cholesterol transport. Handbook of Experimental Pharmacology 170, 537–561.

Jacques, H., Gascon, A., Bergeron, N., et al., 1995. Role of dietary fish protein in the regulation of plasma lipids. Canadian Journal of Cardiology 11 (Suppl G), 63G–71G.

Jordal, A.E., Hordvik, I., Pelsers, M., Bernlohr, D.A., Torstensen, B.E., 2006. FABP3 and FABP10 in Atlantic salmon (*Salmo salar* L.) – general effects of dietary fatty acid composition and life cycle variations. Comparative Biochemistry and Physiology. Part B, Biochemistry and Molecular Biology 145 (2), 147–158.

Jung, U.J., Torrejon, C., Tighe, A.P., Deckelbaum, R.J., 2008. n-3 Fatty acids and cardiovascular disease: mechanisms underlying beneficial effects. American Journal of Clinical Nutrition 87 (6), 2003S–2009S.

Kowey, P.R., Reiffel, J.A., Ellenbogen, K.A., et al., 2010a. Efficacy and safety of prescription omega-3 fatty acids for the prevention of recurrent symptomatic atrial fibrillation: a randomized controlled trial. Journal of American Medical Association 304 (21), 2363–2372.

Krauss, R.M., Eckel, R.H., Howard, B., et al., 2000. AHA Dietary Guidelines: revision 2000: a statement for healthcare professionals from the Nutrition Committee of the American Heart Association. Circulation 102 (18), 2284–2299.

Krawczenko, A., Ciszak, L., Malicka-Blaszkiewicz, M., 2005. Carp liver DNase – isolation, further characterization and interaction with endogenous actin. Comparative Biochemistry and Physiology. Part B, Biochemistry and Molecular Biology 140 (1), 141–151.

Kristensen, S.D., Iversen, A.M., Schmidt, E.B., 2001. n-3 polyunsaturated fatty acids and coronary thrombosis. Lipids 36 (Suppl), S79–S82.

Lipka, E., Ganowiak, Z., 1993. Nutritional value of protein subjected to technologic processing. Changes in content of biologically active amino acids – methionine, cysteine and taurine under the influence of sterilization. Roczniki Państwowego Zakładu Higieny 44 (2–3), 151–158.

Mikalsen, A.B., Sindre, H., Torgersen, J., Rimstad, E., 2005. Protective effects of a DNA vaccine expressing the infectious salmon anemia virus hemagglutinin-esterase in Atlantic salmon. Vaccine 23 (41), 4895–4905.

Mozaffarian, D., 2006. Fish intake, contaminants and human health evaluating the risks and the benefits. Journal of the American Medical Association 296 (15), 1885–1899.

Mozaffarian, D., 2008. Fish and n-3 fatty acids for the prevention of fatal coronary heart disease and sudden cardiac death. American Journal of Clinical Nutrition 87 (6), 1991S–1996S.

Murashita, K., Kurokawa, T., Ebbesson, L.O., Stefansson, S.O., Rønnestad, I., 2009. Characterization, tissue distribution, and regulation of agouti-related protein (AgRP), cocaine- and amphetamine-regulated transcript (CART) and neuropeptide Y (NPY) in Atlantic salmon (Salmo salar). General and Comparative Endocrinology 162 (2), 160–171.

Nalbone, G., Termine, E., Léonardi, J., et al., 1988. Effect of dietary salmon oil feeding on rat heart lipid status. Journal of Nutrition 118 (7), 809–817.

NCEP REPORT, 2001. Executive summary of the third report of the National Cholesterol Education Program (NCEP) Expert Panel on Detection, Evaluation, and Treatment of High Blood Cholesterol in Adults (Adult Treatment Panel III). Journal of the American Medical Association 285, 2486–2497.

Nilausen, K., Meinertz, H., 1999. Lipoprotein(a) and dietary proteins: casein lowers lipoprotein(a) concentrations as compared with soy protein. American Journal of Clinical Nutrition 69 (3), 419–425.

O'Dea, K., 1988. The hunter gatherer lifestyle of Australian aborigines: implications for health. In: McLean, A.J., Wahlqvist, M.L. (Eds.), Current Problems in Nutrition, Pharmacology and Toxicology. John Libbey & Co Ltd., London, pp. 27–36.

O'Dea, K., 1991. Cardiovascular disease risk factors in Australian aborigines. Clinical and Experimental Pharmacology and Physiology 18 (2), 85–88.

Oliver, D.W., Dormehl, I.C., Wikberg, J.E., Louw, W.K., Dambrova, M., et al., 2004. In vivo measurements of the cerebral perfusion and cardiovascular effects of the novel guanidine ME10092 in the non-human primate, Papio ursinus. Life Sciences 75 (17), 2057–2064.

Owen, R.W., Giacosa, A., Hull, W.E., et al., 2000. Olive-oil consumption and health: the possible role of antioxidants. The Lancet Oncology 1, 107–112.

Pratt, C.M., Reiffel, J.A., Ellenbogen, K.A., et al., 2010. Efficacy and Safety of prescription omega-3 ethyl esters for the prevention of recurrent symptomatic atrial fibrillation: a prospective study. American Heart Journal 158 (2), 163–169.e1–3.

Quitral, V., Romero, N., Avila, L., Marín, M.E., Nuñez, H., Simpson, R., 2006. Thiamine retention as a function of thermal processing conditions: canned salmon. Archivos Latinoamericanos de Nutricion 56 (1), 69–76.

Sales, J., 2009. Prediction of digestible energy content across feed ingredients and fish species by linear regression. Fish Physiology and Biochemistry 35 (4), 551–565.

Saravanan, P., Bridgewater, B., West, A.L., et al., 2010. Omega-3 fatty acid supplementation does not reduce risk of arial fibrillation after coronary artery bypass aurgery: a randomized double-blind, placebo-controlled clinical trial.Circulation: Arrhythmia and Electrophuysiology 3 (1), 46–53.

Sharma, R., Singh, R.B., Moffatt, R.J., Katz, J., 2010. Dietary fat intake: promotion of disease in carotid artery disease: lipid lowering versus side effects of statins. In: Meester, F.D., Zibadi, S., Watson, R.R. (Eds.), Modern Dietary Fat Intakes in Disease Promotion, Nutrition and Health. Springer Science+Business Media, New York, pp. 151–185.

Sharma, R., Tandon, R., 2010. Comparison of cholesterol lowering diets: apple, casein cytochrome p450 protein and cholesterol 7α hydroxylase activities in hamsters. http://dx.doi.org/10.1038/npre.2010. 4205.1 Available from Nature Proceedings.

Shriniwas, B.D., Sharma, R., Sharma, A., Baile, V.V., Chen, C.J., Raghukumar, V., 2008. Particles as protein markers: nanoscale microscopy towards picoscale. Nanotechnology Research Journal 2 (3), 25–32.

Siddiqui, R.A., Harvey, K.A., Zaloga, G.P., 2008. Modulation of enzyme activities by n-polyunsaturated fatty acids to support cardiovascular health. The Journal of Nutritional Biochemistry 19 (7), 417–437.

Siddiqui, R.A., Shaikh, S.R., Sech, L.A., Yount, H.R., Stillwell, W., Zaloga, G.P., 2004. Omega 3-fatty acids: health benefits and cellular mechanisms of action. Mini Reviews in Medicinal Chemistry 4 (8), 859–871.

Sidhu, K.S., 2003. Health benefits and potential risks related to consumption of fish or fish oil. Regulatory Toxicology and Pharmacology 38 (3), 336–344.

Singh, R.B., de Meester, F., Wilczynska, A., 2010. The tsim tsoum approaches for prevention of cardiovascular disease. Cardiology Research and Practice 2010, 824938. 10.4061/2010/824938.

Sinnatamby, R.N., Dempson, J.B., Power, M., 2008. A comparison of muscle- and scale-derived delta13C and delta15N across three life-history stages of Atlantic salmon, *Salmo salar*. Rapid Communications in Mass Spectrometry 22 (18), 2773–2778.

Food Standards Agency, 2004. What's an oily fish? 2004-06-24. http://www.food.gov.uk/news/newsarchive/2004/jun/oilyfishdefinition.

Thankappan, T.K., 2003. Isolation of squalene from shark liver oil. In: Surendran, P.K., Mathew, P.T., Nirmala, T., Narayan, N., Jose, J., Boopendranath, M.R., Lakshmanan, P.T., Nair, P.G.V. (Eds.), Seafood Safety. Society of Fisheries Technologists, Cochin, pp. 173–175.

Tremblay, F., Lavigne, C., Jacques, H., Marette, A., 2003. Dietary cod protein restores insulin-induced activation of phosphatidylinosol 3-kinase/Akt and GLUT4 translocation to the T-tubules in skeletal muscle of high-fat-fed obese rats. Diabetes 52, 29–37.

Undeland, I., Ellegard, L., Sandberg, A.S., 2004. Fish and cardiovascular health. Scandinavian Journal of Food and Nutrition 48 (3), 119–130.

van Rooyen, J., Esterhuyse, A.J., Engelbrecht, A.M., du Toit, E.F., 2008. Health benefits of a natural carotenoid rich oil: a proposed mechanism of protection against ischaemia/reperfusion injury. Asia Pacific Journal of Clinical Nutrition 17 (Suppl 1), 316–319.

Venn, B.J., Skeaff, C.M., Brown, R., Mann, J.I., Green, T.J., 2006. A comparison of the effects of A1 and A2 beta-casein protein variants on blood cholesterol concentrations in New Zealand adults. Atherosclerosis 188 (1), 175–178.

von Schalburg, K.R., Yazawa, R., de Boer, J., et al., 2008. Isolation, characterization and comparison of Atlantic and Chinook salmon growth hormone 1 and 2. BMC Genomics 9, 522.

Westman, E.C., Yancy, W.S., Edman, J.S., et al., 2002. Effect of 6-month adherence to a very low carbohydrate diet program. American Journal of Medicine 113, 30–36.

Xiao, X., Qin, Q., Chen, X., 2011. Molecular characterization of a toll-like receptor 22 homologue in large yellow croaker (*Pseudosciaena crocea*) and promoter activity analysis of its 5′-flanking sequence. Fish and Shellfish Immunology 30 (1), 224–233.

Yahia, D.A., Madani, S., Savelli, J.L., Prost, J., Bouchenak, M., Balleville, J., 2003a. Dietary fish protein lowers the blood pressure and alters tissue polyunsaturated fatty acid composition in spontaneously hypertensive rats. Nutrition 19, 342–346.

Yahia, D.A., Madanni, S., Prost, E., Prost, J., Bouchenak, M., Belleville, J., 2003b. Tissue antioxidant status differs in spontaneously hypertensive rats fed fish protein or casein. Journal of Nutrition 133, 479–482.

Yamashita, M., Konagaya, S., 1990. Purification and characterization of cathepsin L from the white muscle of chum salmon, *Oncorhynchus keta*. Comparative Biochemistry and Physiology B 96 (2), 247–252.

Yamori, Y., 1984. The stroke-prone spontaneously hypertensive rat: contribution to risk factor analysis and prevention of hypertensive diseases. In: de Jong, W. (Ed.), Handbook of Hypertension. Elsevier, Amsterdam, pp. 240–255.

Yamori, Y., 1989. Hypertension and biological dietary markers in urine and blood: a progress report from the CARDIAC study group. In: Yamori, Y., Strasser, T. (Eds.), New Horizons in Preventing Cardiovascular Diseases. Elsevier, Amsterdam, pp. 111–126.

Yamori, Y., Liu, L., Mizushima, S., Ikeda, K., Nara, Y., CARDIAC Study Group, 2006. Male cardiovascular mortality and dietary markers in 25 population samples of 16 countries. Journal of Hypertension 24, 1499–1505.

Yamori, Y., Liu, L., Mori, M., et al., 2009. Taurine as the nutritional factor for the longevity of the Japanese revealed by a world-wise epidemiological survey. Advances in Experimental Medicine and Biology 643, 13–25.

Yuan, Y.V., Kitta, D.D., Godin, D.V., 2002. Heart and red blood cell antioxidant status and plasma lipids in the spontaneously hypertensive and normotensive wistar Kyoto rats. Canadian Journal of Physiology and Pharmacology 74, 290–297.

Zhang, J., Sasaki, S., Amano, K., Kesteloot, H., 1999. Fish consumption and mortality from all causes, ischemic heart disease, and stroke: an ecological study. Preventive Medicine 28 (5), 520–529.

Zheng, X., Tocher, D.R., Dickson, C.A., Bell, J.G., Teale, A.J., 2005. Highly unsaturated fatty acid synthesis in vertebrates: new insights with the cloning and characterization of a delta 6 desaturase of Atlantic salmon. Lipids 40 (1), 13–24.

Zhong, Z., Wheeler, M.D., Li, X., et al., 2003. L-Glycine: a novel antiinflammatory, immunomodulatory, and cytoprotective agent. Current Opinion in Clinical Nutrition and Metabolic Care 6 (2), 229–240.

CHAPTER 33

Herbs Used in Traditional Chinese Medicine in Treatment of Heart Diseases

W. Cai, J. Chen
Shanghai Rundo Biotech Japan Co., Ltd., Kobe, Hyogo, Japan

ABBREVIATIONS

CVD Cardiovascular disease
I/R Ischemia and reperfusion
ROS Reactive oxygen species
TCM Traditional Chinese medicine

1. INTRODUCTION

Cardiovascular disease (CVD) is one of the top menaces of human lives and quality of life and constitutes a major public concern in industrialized nations and developing nations like China. While modern medicine remains the most important method in treating these disorders, numerous patients are looking for alternative methods for a cure for various reasons, such as unsatisfying treatment results, unwanted side effects of modern medication, or even for economic reasons. For example, dan shen, wu wei zi, and he shou wu are used as cardiotonics; hong hua, dan gui, and ge geng are used to treat arrhythmia; huang qin, ye ju hua, and ku shen are used to lower blood pressure. To introduce generally the Chinese herbs used in treatment of CVDs, we had summarized the information about dozens of such herbs and had organized the information briefly and concisely (Table 33.1).

Traditional Chinese medicine (TCM) usually approaches a patient in a holistic way. And the remedies actually prescribed for patients usually consist of different kinds of herbs in each remedy. Nevertheless, to make it easier to understand and to study these herbs, in this chapter, we chose to introduce these herbs one by one individually and even introduce the main components in molecular level.

In TCM, a unique theory is used to guide the diagnosis and treatment. Some of the most basic conception in TCM includes yin and yang, wu xing, and so on (Williams, 2003). Yin and yang describe the contrary forces that interconnected and interdependent in human body as well as in the natural world. Another unique conception wu xing is used for describing interactions and relationships between phenomena. These concepts

Bioactive Food as Dietary Interventions for Cardiovascular Disease
http://dx.doi.org/10.1016/B978-0-12-396485-4.00030-X

© 2013 Elsevier Inc.
All rights reserved.

are difficult to understand, but one can benefit from Chinese herb medicines, even without understanding these concepts at first.

2. TCM HERBS

2.1 bing pian

1. Name in simplified Chinese: 冰片.
2. Pinyin of name: bing pian.
3. Botany description: resin of *Dryobalanops aromatica* Gaertn.f., family Dipterocarpaceae, or chemically synthesized from camphor and turpentine oil.
4. Effective components: DL-Borneol.
5. Effects: analgesia, inhibit the growth of bacteria, and anti-inflammation.
6. Research: Li et al. (2008) investigated the antithrombotic and antiplatelet activities of borneol on thrombosis *in vivo* and on platelet aggregation *ex vivo* and reported that borneol had concentration-dependent inhibitory effects on arteriovenous shunt and venous thrombosis but no effect on adenosine diphosphate (ADP) and arachidonic acid-induced platelet aggregation. Meanwhile, borneol prolonged the coagulation parameters for prothrombin time (PT) and thrombin time (TT) but did not show any fibrinolytic activity. It suggested that the antithrombotic activity of borneol and its action in combined formula for preventing CVDs might be due to anticoagulant activity rather than antiplatelet activity.

2.2 chi shao

1. Name in simplified Chinese: 赤芍.
2. Pinyin of name: chi shao.
3. Botany description: dried root of *Paeonia lactiflora* Pall and plants of the same genus such as *Paeonia obovata* Maxim and *Paeonia veitchii* Lynch (State Pharmacopoeia Board, 2005).
4. Effective components: paeoniflorin, albiflorin, hydroxy-paeoniflorin, benzoylpaeoniflorin, and paeonin.
5. Effects: calcium channel blocker, dilate coronal arteries, improve cardiac output, inhibit platelet aggregation, and enhance thrombolysis.
6. Research: Li et al. (2011) reported that total glucosides of peony (TGP) may attenuate the development of atherosclerotic disease. The beneficial effects are associated with its efficacy of lowering blood lipids and inhibiting the expression of inflammatory cytokines. In another report, paeonol, paeoniflorin, benzoylpaeoniflorin, and benzoyloxypaeoniflorin were found to be the major common active constituents, and they would collectively contribute to improving blood circulation through their inhibitory effects on both platelet aggregation and blood coagulation (Koo et al., 2010).

Table 33.1 Summary of Herbs Used in Traditional Chinese Medicine in Treatment of Heart Diseases

Name in simplified Chinese	Name in Chinese pinyin	Description	Effective components	Effects	Side effects and cautions
冰片	bing pian	Resin of *Dryobalanops aromatica* Gaertn.f., family Dipterocarpaceae, or chemically synthesized from camphor and turpentine oil	DL–Borneol	Analgesia Inhibit the growth of bacteria Anti-inflammation	Generally not used alone but together with some herb components to make suxiao jiuxin pills, suhexiang pills, huatuo zaizao pills (Ren, 2002)
赤芍	chi shao	Dried root of *Paeonia lactiflora* pall and plants of the same genus such as *Paeonia obovata* Maxim and *Paeonia veitchii* Lynch (State Pharmacopoeia Board, 2005)	Paeoniflorin, albiflorin, hydroxy-paeoniflorin, benzoylpaeoniflorin, paeonin	Calcium channel blocker, dilate coronal arteries, and improve cardiac output; inhibit platelet aggregation, enhance thrombolysis	
臭梧桐	chou wu ton	Leaf of *Clerodendron trichotomum* Thunb	Clerodolone, clerodone, clerostorol	Sedative Analgesia Dilate blood vessels and lowering blood pressure Anti-inflammation	May cause nausea and vomiting
川芎	chuan qiong	Root and stem of *Ligusticum chuanxiong* Hort	Tetramethylpyrazine, ferulic acid, chuanxingol, chrysophanol, volatile oil, and alkylbenzenes	Dilate coronal vessels Enhance endurance to oxygen-deficient condition Lowering blood pressure Inhibit aggregation of platelets Antithrombotic	May cause rash

Continued

Table 33.1 Summary of Herbs Used in Traditional Chinese Medicine in Treatment of Heart Diseases—cont'd

Name in simplified Chinese	Name in Chinese pinyin	Description	Effective components	Effects	Side effects and cautions
刺五加	ci wu jia	Root and root stem of *Acanthopanax senticosus* (Rupr. Et Maxim.) Harmes (Eleuther. *Ococus senticosus* (Rupr. Et Maxim.))	Eleutheroside A, β, eleutheroside B, syrigin Bl, eleutheroside B1, C, D, F, G	May dilate blood vessels and improve cerebral blood circulation	
丹参	dan shen	Root of *Salvia miltiorrhiza* Bge	Tanshinone I, II A, II B, isotanshinone I, IA, cryptotanshinone, isocryptotanshinone, methyltanshinone, and hydroxyltanshinone	Protect damaged myocardial cell Dilate limbic vessels Reduce blood viscosity Sedative Analgesia Anti-inflammation Inhibit bacteria growth	
当归	dang gui	Root of *Angelica sinensis* (Oliv) Diels	Ligustilide, n–butylidenephthalide, n–valerophenone–O–carboxylic acid, Δ2.4dihydrophthalic anhydride, and sesquiterpenes	Inhibit excitability of central nervous system, Inhibit the contraction of heart	
党参	dang shen	Root of *Codonopsis pilosula* (French.) Nannf or plants of the same family	The main components are Lobetyolin A, saponin, polysaccharides, inulin and in details they are Scutellarein glucoside, friedelin, taraxeryl acetate, α-spinasterol and its glucopyranoside, stigmastenol and its glucopyranoside, spinesterone, atractylenolide	Ameliorate memory, sedative, enhance cardio output, increase blood supply to brain, lower limbs, and viscera. Enhance endurance to oxygen-deficient condition and radiation. Inhibit the	Over dosage (>60 g/per each dose) may lead to discomfort at precordial region and arrhythmia, both can be retrieved by stopping taking it

丁公藤	ding gong teng	Vine stem of erycibe	III, atractylenolide II, syringaldehyde, syringin, vanillic acid,5-hydroxy-2-pyridinemethanol, α-furancarboxylic acid, *n*-hexyl-β-D-glucopyranoside,ethyl-α-D-fructofuranoside (Wang, 1954) 2β-Hydroxy-6β-acetoxynortropane, 2β, 6β-dihydroxynortropane, scopoletin, scopolin, caffeic acid, chlorogenic acid	adhesion and aggregation of platelets Lowering blood pressure, analgesia, anti-inflammation, anti-histamine	
杜仲	du zhong	Bark of *Eucommia ulmoides* Oliv	Lignans, iridoids, phenylpropanoids, flavoids, and triterpenes	Reduce blood pressure Inhibit Prevent atherosclerosis Promote growth of osteoblast Enhance immunity Inhibit absorption of glucose in intestine Enhance sensitivity of insulin	
莪术	e shu	Root stem of *Curcuma zedoaria* Rosc, *Curcuma kwangsiensis* S, G. Lee, et C.F. Liang and Curcuma Wenyujin Y, H, Chen et C, Ling	Volatile oil: curzerenone, epicurzerenone, curzenene, curdione, and curcumol	Improve femoral artery blood flow, useful in treating thromboangiitis obliterans	
福寿草	fu shou cao	Whole body of *Adonis amurensis* Reg. Et Radde	The components of the root of Fu shou cao include cardiac glycosides, noncardiac	Cynarin has quick digitalis effect. The total glycosides are effective	May induce nausea, vomiting, and arrhythmia

Continued

Table 33.1 Summary of Herbs Used in Traditional Chinese Medicine in Treatment of Heart Diseases—cont'd

Name in simplified Chinese	Name in Chinese pinyin	Description	Effective components	Effects	Side effects and cautions
			glycosides and coumarins. The cardiac glycosides include cymarin, cymarol, corchoroside A, convallatoxin, K-strophanthin-β, somalin, etc. From the noncardiac glycosides, the following are isolated: lineolone, isolineolone, adonilide, fukujusone, fukujusonorone, 12-o-Nico-tinoylisolineolone, 12-o-Ben-zoylisolineolone, etc. Also isolated are coumarins including umbelliferone, scopoletin	in treating acute heart failure and the infusion is effective in treating chronic heart failure. Fu shou cao affect quickly, has less storage effect and is less toxic, has quick and long-lasting diuretic effect and has sedative effect which digitalis lacks	
			In the overground part of the grass body, there are glycosides and noncardiac glycosides: isoramanone, nicotinoylisoramanone, digitoxigenin, linelone, pergularin, stro-pbanthidin, adonilide, fukujusone, benzoylisolinelone, nicotinoylieolone, fukujusonorone, and coumarins such as umbelliferone, scopoletin		

附子	fu zi	Lateral root of *Aconitum carmichaelii* Debx	Aconitine, mesaconitine, and hypaconitine	Cardiotonic Raise blood pressure Sedative, analgesia Immunoenhance	0.2 mg of aconitine is toxic and 3–4 mg of it is lethal to human. Do not use it to treat patients with atrioventricular block. Raw material of fu zi is toxic and decoction with licorice, dried ginger, or ingestion with honey greatly reduced toxicity of Fuzi, without destroying much of the cardiotonic effects
葛根	ge gen	Root of *Pueraria lobata* (Willd.) Ohwi	Glycosides and flavonoids such as puerarin-7-xyloside, 4',6'-O-diacetylpuerarin, puerarin, daidzin, daidzein	Protect myocardial tissue from shock-reinfusion damage Dilate coronal arteries and peripheral arteries Antiarrhythmic Reduce blood lipids and sugar levels	
钩藤	gou teng	Stem and leaf of *Uncaria rhynchophylla* (Miq.) Jacks. and plants of the same genus	Rhynchophylline, isorhynchophylline, corynoxeine, isocorynoxeine, corynantheine, dihydrocorynantheine, hirsuteine, rhynchophine	Sedative Dilate blood vessels and lowering blood pressure Inhibit platelet aggregation and thrombosis Relieve dyspnea Improve digestion	
汉防己	han fang ji	Mass root of *Stephania tetrandra* S. Moore	Alkaloids: tetrandrine, demethyltetrandrine, fangchinoline, cyclanoline,	Sedative Antiarrhythmic	

Continued

Table 33.1 Summary of Herbs Used in Traditional Chinese Medicine in Treatment of Heart Diseases—cont'd

Name in simplified Chinese	Name in Chinese pinyin	Description	Effective components	Effects	Side effects and cautions
			dimethyltetrandrine, and berbamine	Protect cardiac tissue from ischemia Lowering blood pressure	
红花	hong hua	Corolla of *Carthamus tinctorius* L. and the upper chapiter and the upper part of the stilet of *Crocus sativus* L	Components consist mainly of flavones and fatty acids. Among the flavones, safflor yellow is the most important component. The following flavones are also found in hong hua: kaempferol, quercertin, myricetin, apigenin, and luteoline. The fatty acids of hong hua include palmitic acid, myristic acid, lauric acid, dipalmitin, oleic acid, and linoleic acid	Lowering blood pressure by reduce peripheral resistance Improve peripheral microcirculation Inhibit aggregation of platelets and enhance hydrolysis of fibrin Anti-inflammation Analgesia	Avoid treating women in pregnancy and patients suffering hemorrhage diseases and ulceration
黄芪	huang qi	Root of *Astragalus membranaceus* (Fisch.) Bunge or *A. membranaceus* (Fisch.) Bge. Var. mongholicus (Bge.)Haiao	Flavoids: calycosin, astragaloside I, V, III; astragalus polysacharinand A, B, C, D, volatile oils, amino acids	Improve immunity, cardiotonic, lowering blood pressure, diuretic, anti-inflammation	Dilation of blood vessels in the head may lead to headache
黄芩	huang qin	Root of *Scutellaria baicalensis* Georgi	Flavonoids: baicalin, baicalein, wogonoside, wogonin, neobaicalein, 7-methoxybaicalein, 7-methoxynorwogonin, oroxylin A, skullcapflavone I, II	Lowering blood pressure Lowering serum lipids Anti-inflammation Anti-hypersensitivity	

Continued

降香	jiang xiang	Root and core of the stem of *Dalbergia odorifera* T. Chen	Contains various flavoids: formononetin, bowdichione, liquiritigenin, medicarpin, 9-O-methyl-nissolin, melilotocarpanC, D, odoricarpinobtustyrene, volatile oils: β-bisalolene, *trans*–β–farnesene, *trans*– nerolidol	Inhibit thrombosis in rat, inhibit mitosis of cancer cells	
决明子	jue ming zi	Seed of *Cassia tora* Linn	Emodin, chrysophanol, physcion, obtusin, obtusifolin, and glycosides	Lowering blood pressure and blood lipid level	
苦参	ku shen	Root of *Sophora flavescens* Ait	Include various flavonoids and alkaloids. The alkaloids include matrine, oxymatrine, dihydroxy matrine, cytisine, methylcytisine, anagyrine, bap-iifoline. And the alkaloids include kuraridin, kurarinone, norkurarinone, kuraridinol, kurarinol, neokurarinol, norkurarinol, isokurarinol. Ku shen also contains isoflavonoids like formononetin	Ku shen can relieve myocardial ischemia and has functions such as diuretic, vermicide, cough-suppressing, calming panting-calming and phlegm-dispelling; sedative, immunoinhibitive, bile secretion enhancement, hepatoprotective and anti-inflammation	Taking Ku shen orally may cause acid reflux, stomachache, nausea, constipation, and loss of appetite
莱菔子	lai fu zi	Seed of *Raphanus sativus* L	The main components classify into volatile oils (45%) and fatty acids. The volatile oils are methyl-mercaptan, α, β-hexenal, and β, γ-Hexenol; the fatty acids are erucic acid, glycerol sinapate	Lowering blood pressure Inhibit bacterial growth Inhibit inflammation Bind with exotoxin to prevent intoxication	

Table 33.1 Summary of Herbs Used in Traditional Chinese Medicine in Treatment of Heart Diseases—cont'd

Name in simplified Chinese	Name in Chinese pinyin	Description	Effective components	Effects	Side effects and cautions
铃兰	ling lan	Root or the whole plant of Convallaria Keiskei	Convallatoxin, convallatoxol, convalloside, deglucosheirotoxin, keioside, rhodeasapogenin, isorhodea sapogenin	Has digitalis-like effect. The infusion is prone to hydrolysis and make it unstable. Has significant diuretic effect and has better effect in treating edema. Has sedative effect	It has milder side effect and is less toxic than digitalis. Anorexia, nausea, vomit or dizziness, headache, palpitation occurred in some patients
鹿蹄草	lu ti cao	Whole plant body of *Pyrola rotundifolia* L. subsp. Chinesis H. Andres, *Pyrola decorata* H. Andres or *Pyrola rotundifolia* L	Arbutin, methyl hydroquinone, homoarbutin, isohomoarbutin, chimaphillin, monotropein, volatile oil, and tanin	Cardiotonic and antibacterial effects	
罗布麻	Luo bu ma	Leaf and root of *Apocynum venetum* L	Neoisorutin, rutin, quercetin, isoquercitrin, hyperin, fumaric acid, succinic acid	Cardiotonic Dilate blood vessels and lowering blood pressure Relieve dyspnea and remove phlegm Lowering serum lipids Inhibit platelet aggregation and thrombosis Enhance immunity	
麦门冬	mai men dong	Mass root of *Ophiopogon japonicus* (Thunb.) Ker-Gawl and *Liriope spicata* Lour	Contains steroidal saponins, of which the aglycone parts are ruscogenin, β–sitosterol, stigmasterol, β–sitosterol, β–	Enhance endurance to oxygen-deficient condition Regulate blood sugar	–

		Source	Components	Functions	Notes
毛冬青	mao dong qing	Root and leaf of *Ilex pubescens* Hook. Et Am	D-glucoside. It also contains methylophiopogonanone A, B; ophiopogonanone A, methylophiopogonone A, B; ophiopogonone A, B; isoophiopogonone A; desmethylisoophiopogonone B; 6-aldehydoisoophiopogonone A, B; and terpenoids such as calciombornyl sulfate and terpenoid glycoside	Inhibit bacteria growth	
青皮	qing pi	Immature fruit proper or the cover of the immature fruit of *Citrus reticulata* Blanco and plants of the same genus	Contains volatile oil: lemonene, cital, and flavoids: hesperidin, neohesperidin, and synephrine	Improve blood flow to coronal arteries Improve metabolism and reduce oxygen consumption of cardiac muscles Inhibit aggregation of platelets Reduce blood pressure Anti-inflammation Inhibit bacteria growth Raise blood pressure in rescue of shock, relieve asthma, and remove phlegm	Toxicity very low
三七	san qi	Root of *Panax notoginseng* (Burk.) F.H. Chen	Notoginsenosides and flavone glycosides. The total glycosides amount to 8–12% and the glycosides are	Antiarrhythmic Anti-inflammatory Cardio-protective	

Continued

Table 33.1 Summary of Herbs Used in Traditional Chinese Medicine in Treatment of Heart Diseases—cont'd

Name in simplified Chinese	Name in Chinese pinyin	Description	Effective components	Effects	Side effects and cautions
			ginsenoside Rb1, Rb2, Rc, Rd, Re, Rf, Rg1, Rg2, Rh, among them, ginsenoside Rb1, Rbg are the most common ones. The aglycones are panoxadiol and panaxatriol. Different from ren sheng, san qi lacks oleanolic acid	Reduce blood cholesterol levels	
苏合香	su he xiang	Resin of *Liquidambar orientalis* Mill	*Liquidambar orientalis* Mill consists of resin (36%) and oil-like liquid. The resin mainly contains of olease and oleanolic acid. The oil-like liquid consists styrene, ethyl cinnamate, phenypropyl cinnamate, vanillin, and free cinnamic acid	Inhibit the adhesion and aggregation of platelets Increase blood flow to coronal arteries Relieve itch Accelerate wound healing	—
万年青	wan nian qing	Root or the whole plant of *Rohdea japonica* Roth	Its main effective components are cardiac glycosides including rhodexin A, B, C, and D and rhodenin, bipindogenin-D-allopyranoside, bipindogenin-D-xy-lopyranosyl, D-allopyranoside, digitoxigenin, periplogenin,	Have digitalis-like effect and can inhibit atrioventricular block. It stimulates smooth muscle of bladder and uterus. It is also an emetic	Over dose of it may lead to premature cardio contraction and complete block of cardio conduction

五味子	wu wei zi	Mature fruit of *Schisandra chinensis* (Turez.) Baill. and *Schisandra sphenanthera* Rehd. Et Wils	rhodeasapogenin, isorhodeasapogenin, 22-epirhodeasapogenin, convallamarogenin, D-glucopyranoside, sitosterol, and octadecenoic acid Lignans: schizandrin A, B, C, schizandrol A, B and volatile oils, fatty acids	Cardiotonic, enhance excitability of central nervous system, protect hepatocytes, antiulceration. Induce contraction of ovary	Avoid treating women in pregnancy
细辛	xi xin	Whole plant body of *Asarum heterotropoides* Fr. Schmidt var. mandshuricum (Maxim.) kitag. and *Asarum sieboldii* Miq	Volatile oil: methyl eugenol, borneol, pinene, safrole, elemicin, asarone, limonene, and isobutyldodecatetraenamine	Anesthetic, sedative, analgesia, anti-inflammation, increase coronary artery blood flow	
夏枯草	xia ku cao	Whole plant body of *Prunella vulgaris* L	In the whole plant, the main components are ursolic acid, oleanolic acid, glycoside of oleanolic acid, rutin, hyperoside, caffeic acid, vitamins C and D, carotene, tannin, alkaloids, camphor, fenchone (Liu et al., 2003)	Anti-inflammation Lowering blood pressure Inhibit bacterial growth Lowering blood sugar level in animal model of diabetes	
羊角拗	yang jiao niu	Root, stem, leaf or seed of *Strophanthus divaricatus* (Lour.) Hook. Et Arm	Cardiac glycosides: most plentiful in the seeds and consists of diavricoside, divostroside, coudoside, D-strophanthin-I, II	Has digitalis-like effect, it has weaker and longer cardiotonic effect comparing with strophanthin K. Increase smooth muscle	Side effect such as gastric intestinal reactions rarely occurred. When total dosage exceeds 1.5 mg, arrhythmia may occur

Continued

Table 33.1 Summary of Herbs Used in Traditional Chinese Medicine in Treatment of Heart Diseases—cont'd

Name in simplified Chinese	Name in Chinese pinyin	Description	Effective components	Effects	Side effects and cautions
				tone. Also have sedative, antiarrhythmic and diuretic effects	which is correlated with the extent of myocardial damage but not the accumulated dosage. Intoxication dosage may lead to coronary artery contraction, so it must be used carefully in patients suffering coronary artery disorders
野菊花	ye ju hua	Capitate of *Chrysanthemum indicum* L	Flavoids: acacetin, luteolin, apigenin, eupatilin, tricin, tetrahydroxy-dimethoxyflavone, apigenin-glucopyranoside, luteolin-glucopyranoside, linarin; and sesquiterpenoids: cumambrin-A, yejuhualactone	Lowering blood pressure, Improve coronary circulation, Antioxidation, Inhibit bacterial growth	
益母草	yi mu cao	Whole plant of *Leonurus heterophyllus* Sweet	Alkaloids such as leonurine, betonicine, stachydrine, rutin, and fumaric acid	Induce contraction of ovary, Cardiotonic, increase coronal blood flow, Improve tolerance to myocardial ischemia, Relieve angina	Avoid treating women in pregnancy

| 银杏叶 | yin xing ye | Leaf of *Ginkgo biloba* L | Flavonoids such as ginkgetin, isoginkgetin, bibobetin, quercetin, kaempferd, rhamnetin, ginkgolide A, B, C, bilobalide, and rutin | Inhibit platelet aggregation Antithrombotic Diuretic Sedative Dilate coronal and cerebral vessels Protect central nervous system in oxygen-deficient condition by clearing free radicals Lowering blood viscosity Inhibit aggregation of platelets Antithrombotic | |
| 淫羊藿 | yin yang huo | Whole plant of *Epimedium grandiflorum* Morr. or *Epimedium sagittatum* (s. et z.) Maxim. or *Epiomedium brevicornum* Maxim | Flavonoids: icariin, noricariin; it also contains volatile oil, stererol, fatty acids, and alkaloids | Experiment in mice indicated it may act on hypothalamus–pituitary–adrenal axis to improve sexual ability Increase cardio cerebral blood flow Enhance calcify of bone Antiaging Antivirus Reduce peripheral resistance and increase coronal arteries blood flow Reduce blood pressure | Do not use it to treat patients with hypersexual disorder |

Continued

Table 33.1 Summary of Herbs Used in Traditional Chinese Medicine in Treatment of Heart Diseases—cont'd

Name in simplified Chinese	Name in Chinese pinyin	Description	Effective components	Effects	Side effects and cautions
郁金	yu jin	yu jin is the tuber on the rhizome of *Curcuma wenyujin* Y.H. chen et C. Ling, *Curcuma Longa* L, *C. kwangsiensis* S.G. Lee et C.F. Liang and *Curcuma phacocaulis* Val	The tuber contains 6.1% of volatile oil, which consists of L. Curcumene, canphene, camphor, and sesquiterpenes	Antiarrhythmic, lowering serum cholesterol, lipid proteins, and triglyceride; reduce blood viscosity, red blood cell aggregation index, and improve red blood cell deformation index. It also resists ADP induced platelet aggregation	
玉米须	yu mi xu	Ear of maize	Cryptoxanthin, pantothenic acid, inositol, sitosterol, stigmasterol, vitamins C and K, malic acid, citric acid, oxalic acid, tartaric acid and fatty acids, volatile oils, resin	Diuretic effect Lowering blood pressure	

Note: The information are ranked in an alphabet order of the 'Names in Chinese pinyin,' a system which is often used to spell Chinese names.

2.3 chou wu tong

1. Name in simplified Chinese: 臭梧桐.
2. Pinyin of name: chou wu tong.
3. Botany description: leaf of *Clerodendron trichotomum* Thunb.
4. Effective components: clerodolone, clerodone, and clerostorol.
5. Effects: sedative, analgesia, dilate blood vessels and lowering blood pressure, and anti-inflammation.
6. Research: Lu et al. (1994) reported intravenous administration of the extract of *C. trichotomum* Thunb elicited renal vasodilation and increased urine flow and urinary sodium excretion and acute oral administration of the extract reduced blood pressure of spontaneously hypertensive rats but not of normotensive control rats. Chronic daily administration for 6 weeks prevented the increase of blood pressure in spontaneously hypertensive rats.
7. Side effects and cautions: may cause nausea and vomiting.

2.4 chuan qiong

1. Name in simplified Chinese: 川芎.
2. Pinyin of name: chuan qiong.
3. Botany description: root and stem of *Ligusticum chuanxiong* Hort.
4. Effective components: tetramethylpyrazine, ferulic acid, chuanxingol, chrysophanol, volatile oil, and alkylbenzenes.
5. Effects: dilate coronal vessels, enhance endurance to oxygen-deficient condition, lowering blood pressure, inhibit aggregation of platelets, antithrombotic.
6. Research: *L. chuanxiong* Hort. (Umbelliferae) is often prescribed together with nitric oxide (NO) donors for treating coronary heart diseases such as angina in China, Chan et al. (2009) examined the interaction between the *L. chuanxiong* major active constituent butylidenephthalide (BDPH) and the NO donor sodium nitroprusside (SNP) in vasorelaxation of rat isolated aorta and demonstrated the synergistic relaxation between BDPH and SNP.

2.5 ci wu jia

1. Name in simplified Chinese: 刺五加.
2. Pinyin of name: ci wu jia.
3. Botany description: root and root stem of *A. senticosus* (Rupr. Et Maxim.) Harmes (Eleuther. *Ococus senticosus* (Rupr. Et Maxim.)).
4. Effective components: eleutheroside A, β, eleutheroside B, syrigin Bl, eleutheroside B1, C, D, F, and G.
5. Effects: may dilate blood vessels and improve cerebral blood circulation.

6. Research: In traditional Chinese medicine, *A. senticosus* (Rupr.et Maxim.) Harms is used in a variety of diseases in traditional Chinese system of medicine including hypertension, ischemic heart disease, and hepatitis. *A. senticosus* Harms aqueous extracts (ASE) attenuated the morphological injury of liver induced by tert-butyl hydroperoxide and increased the activity of antioxidant enzymes and the ratio of GSH/GSSG (GSH is the abbreviation for glutamylcysteinlyglycine and GSSG is the abbreviation for glutathione-S-S-glutathione) in serum and liver homogenates and elevated the gene expression of NF-E2-related factor-2 (Nrf2). Protein expression results showed that Nrf2 and the antioxidant enzymes were all increased significantly by medium and high doses of ASE. The results indicated that ASE protects against oxidative stress possibly via the induction of Nrf2 and related antioxidant enzymes (Wang et al., 2010).

2.6 dan shen

1. Name in simplified Chinese: 丹参.
2. Pinyin of name: dan shen.
3. Botany description: root of *Salvia miltiorrhiza* Bge.
4. Effective components: tanshinone I, II A, II B, isotanshinone I, IA, cryptotanshinone, isocryptotanshinone, methyltanshinone, and hydroxyltanshinone.
5. Effects: protect damaged myocardial cell, dilate limbic vessels, reduce blood viscosity, sedative, analgesia, anti-inflammation, and inhibit bacteria growth.
6. Research: ischemia and reperfusion (I/R) exerts multiple insults in microcirculation, frequently accompanied by endothelial cell injury, enhanced adhesion of leukocytes, macromolecular efflux, production of oxygen free radicals, and mast cell degranulation and results in injury of organs. *S. miltiorrhiza* root has long been used in Asian countries for clinical treatment of various microcirculatory disturbance-related diseases. For example, NADPH oxidase and platelet aggregation are inhibited by tanshinone IIA and tanshinone IIB, respectively, and the mast cell degranulation is blunted by cryptotanshinone and 15,16-dihydrotanshinone I (Han et al., 2008).
7. Side effects and cautions: Danshen can affect hemostasis in several ways, including inhibition of platelet aggregation, interference with the extrinsic blood coagulation, antithrombin III–like activity, and promotion of fibrinolytic activity. Single-dose and steady-state studies in rats indicated that danshen increased the absorption rate constants, area under curves, maximum concentrations, and elimination half-lives, but decreased the clearances and apparent volume of distribution of both R- and S-warfarin. Consequently, the anticoagulant response to warfarin was exaggerated. Three cases have previously been published reporting gross overanticoagulation and bleeding complications when patients receiving chronic warfarin therapy also took danshen. In conclusion, because of both pharmacokinetic and pharmacodynamic interactions, danshen should be avoided in patients taking warfarin (Chan, 2001).

2.7 dang gui

1. Name in simplified Chinese: 当归.
2. Pinyin of name: dang gui.
3. Botany description: root of *Angelica sinensis* (Oliv) Diels.
4. Effective components: ligustilide, butylidene phihalide, ferulic acid, and volatile oil which contains sesquiterpene A, B, carvacrol, and angelicone.
5. Effects: inhibit excitability of central nervous system and inhibit the constriction of heart.
6. Research: the importance of stress-activated protein/mitogen-activated protein kinase (SAP/MAPK) pathway signaling (involving c-Jun-*N*-terminal kinase (JNK), extracellular signal-regulated kinase (ERK), and p38 kinase) in normal cellular proliferation, differentiation, and programmed cell death has led to significant recent advances in people's understanding of the role of SAP/MAPK signaling in inflammatory disorders such as arthritis and CVD, cancer, and pulmonary and neurodegenerative diseases (Malemud, 2007). Su et al. (2011) showed that ligustilide, the most abundant ingredient of *A. sinensis* (Oliv) Diels, exhibits anti-inflammatory activities by blocking the activation of MAPKs/IKK and the downstream transcription factors AP-1 and NF-kappaB, which may result from ligustilide's downregulation of iROS production.

2.8 dang shen

1. Name in simplified Chinese: 党参.
2. Pinyin of name: dang shen.
3. Botany description: root of *Codonopsis pilosula* (French.) Nannf or plants of the same family.
4. Effective components: the main components are Lobetyolin A, saponin, polysaccharides, and inulin, and in details, they are Scutellarein glucoside, friedelin, taraxeryl acetate, α-spinasterol and its glucopyranoside, stigmastenol and its glucopyranoside, spinesterone, atractylenolide, atractylenolide α, syringaldehyde, syringin, vanillic acid, hydroxy-pyridinemethanol, α-furancarboxylic acid, *n*-hexyl-β-D-glucopyranoside, and ethyl-α-D-fructofuranoside (Wang, 1954).
5. Effects: ameliorate memory, sedative, enhance cardio output, and increase blood supply to brain, lower limbs, and viscera. Enhance endurance to oxygen-deficient condition and radiation. Inhibit the adhesion and aggregation of platelets.
6. Research: in a report by Ng et al. (2004), the roots of Panax quinquefolium, *Panax notoginseng*, *Glehnia littoralis*, *C. pilosula*, and *Pseudostellaria heterophylla* were extracted with an aqueous extraction method and also with an organic extraction method. The aqueous extracts of *G. littoralis* and *C. pilosula* were the most potent in inhibiting erythrocyte hemolysis. The aqueous extracts of Panax quinquefolium and

P. notoginseng had lower potencies, while the aqueous extract of *P. heterophylla* and the organic extract of Panax quinquefolium were only weakly active. The organic extracts of *G. littoralis*, *Panax heterophylla*, and Panax quinquefolium were potent in inhibiting lipid peroxidation, while the organic extracts of *C. pilosula* and *P. notoginseng* had weaker potencies.

7. Side effects and cautions: overdosage (>60 g per each dose) may lead to discomfort at precordial region and arrhythmia, and both can be retrieved by stopping taking it.

2.9 ding gong teng

1. Name in simplified Chinese: 丁公藤.
2. Pinyin of name: ding gong teng.
3. Botany description: vine stem of *Erycibe obtusifolia* Benth.
4. Effective components: 2β-hydroxy-6β-acetoxynortropane, 2β,6β-dihydroxynortropane, scopoletin, scopolin, caffeic acid, and chlorogenic acid.
5. Effects: lowering blood pressure, analgesia, anti-inflammation, and antihistamine.
6. Research: Pan et al. (2011) reported that scopoletin, the main bioactive constituent of *E. obtusifolia* Benth stems, exerted antiarthritic activity *in vivo* partly by preventing synovial angiogenesis as well as antiangiogenic activity in chick chorioallantoic membrane model. Their findings suggest that scopoletin is a candidate of angiogenesis inhibitors, and it functions by interrupting the autophosphorylation of vascular endothelial growth factor (VEGF) receptor 2 (VEGFR2) and the downstream signaling pathways.

2.10 du zhong

1. Name in simplified Chinese: 杜仲.
2. Pinyin of name: du zhong.
3. Botany description: bark of *Eucommia ulmoides* Oliv.
4. Effective components: lignans, iridoids, phenylpropanoids, flavoids, and triterpenes.
5. Effects: lowering blood pressure, inhibit atherosclerosis, promote growth of osteoblast, enhance immunity, inhibit absorption of glucose in intestine, and enhance sensitivity of insulin.
6. Research: Fujikawa et al. (2010) used a metabolic syndrome-like rat model, produced by feeding a 35% high-fat diet (HFD), to examine potential antiobesity and antimetabolic syndrome effects and mechanisms of chronic administration of Eucommia leaf as an extract or green leaf powder. Eighty rats were studied for 3 months in ten groups. Both forms of Eucommia leaves minimized increases in body weight and visceral fat in a dose-dependent fashion. Increases in plasma levels of triacylglycerol and nonesterified fatty acid and insulin resistance secondary to HFD were lessened by both forms of Eucommia leaf. Concomitantly, an increase in plasma adiponectin levels and suppression of plasma resistin and tumor necrosis factor (TNF)-α levels were confirmed. Real-time PCR studies showed that both forms of Eucommia leaf enhanced metabolic function

across several organs, including diminishing ATP production (white adipose tissue), accelerating β-oxidation (liver), and increasing the use of ketone bodies/glucose (skeletal muscle), all of which may exert antiobesity effects under HFD conditions. These findings suggest that chronic administration of either form of Eucommia leaves stimulates the metabolic function in rats across several organs. The antiobesity and antimetabolic syndrome activity in this rat model may be maintained through secretion and regulation of adipocytokines that depend on the accumulation of visceral fat to improve insulin resistance or hyperlipemia.

2.11 e shu

1. Name in simplified Chinese: 莪术.
2. Pinyin of name: e shu.
3. Botany description: root stem of *Curcuma zedoaria* Rosc, *Curcuma kwangsiensis* S, G. Lee, et C.F. Liang and Curcuma Wenyujin Y, H, Chen et C, Ling.
4. Effective components: volatile oil: curzerenone, epicurzerenone, curzenene, curdione, and curcumol.
5. Effects: improve peripheral blood circulation and inhibit atherosclerosis.
6. Research: Chen et al. (2011) reported that essential oil of *C. zedoaria* presented anti-angiogenic activity *in vitro* and *in vivo* by downregulating MMPs.

2.12 fu shou cao

1. Name in simplified Chinese: 福寿草.
2. Pinyin of name: fu shou cao.
3. Botany description: whole body of *Adonis amurensis* Reg. Et Radde.
4. Effective components: the components of the root of Fu shou cao include cardiac glycosides, noncardiac glycosides, and coumarins. The cardiac glycosides consist of cymarin, cymarol, corchoroside A, convallatoxin, K-strophanthin-b, somalin, etc. The noncardiac glycosides consist of lineolone, isolineolone, adonilide, fukujusone, fukujusonorone, 12-*o*-Nico-tinoylisolineolone, 12-*o*-Ben-zoylisolineolone, etc. The coumarins include umbelliferone and scopoletin. In the overground part of the grass body, there are glycosides and noncardiac glycosides: isoramanone, nicoti-noylisoramanone, digitoxigenin, linelone, pergularin, stro-pbanthidin, adonilide, fukujusone, benzoylisolinelone, nicotinoylieolone, fukujusonorone, and coumarins such as umbelliferone and scopoletin.
5. Effects: cymarin has quick digitalis effect. The total glycosides are effective in treating acute heart failure, and the infusion is effective in treating chronic heart failure. Fu shou cao has quick and long-lasting diuretic effect, and nevertheless has less storage effect, is less toxic, and has sedative effect which digitalis lacks.
6. Side effects and cautions: may induce nausea, vomiting, and arrhythmia.

2.13 fu zi

1. Name in simplified Chinese: 附子.
2. Pinyin of name: fu zi.
3. Botany description: lateral root of *Aconitum carmichaelii* Debx.
4. Effective components: aconitine, mesaconitine, and hypaconitine.
5. Effects: cardiotonic, raise blood pressure, sedative, analgesia, and immunoenhancement.
6. Research: Huang et al. (2010) reported that polysaccharide extracted from fu zi has cholesterol-lowering effect in hypercholesteremic rats.
7. Side effects and cautions: 0.2 mg of aconitine is toxic and 3–4 mg of it is lethal to human. Do not use it to treat patients with atrioventricular block. Raw material of fu zi is toxic and decoction with licorice, dried ginger, or ingestion with honey greatly reduced toxicity of Fuzi, without destroying much of the cardiotonic effects.

2.14 ge gen

1. Name in simplified Chinese: 葛根.
2. Pinyin of name: ge gen.
3. Botany description: root of *Pueraria lobata* (Willd.) Ohwi.
4. Effective components: glycosides and flavonoids such as puerarin-7-xyloside, 4′,6′-O-diacetylpuerarin, puerarin, daidzin, and daidzein.
5. Effects: antioxidative.
6. Research: in a diabetic rat model, where diabetes and the accompanying oxidative stress were induced by intraperitoneal administration of streptozotocin, 500 mg kg^{-1} of the root extract which contains $10.42 \pm 0.15\%$ puerarin as the main constituent and smaller amounts of the related isoflavonoids 3′-hydroxypuerarin, 3′-methoxypuerarin, 6″-xylosylpuerarin, daidzin, genistin, daidzein, and genistein was administrated orally. The level of malondialdehyde (MDA) in plasma, used as a marker of oxidative damage to lipids, was reduced to the same level as in healthy control animals. No obvious signs of toxicity were observed by administration of 10× the treatment dose (Bebrevska et al., 2009).

2.15 gou teng

1. Name in simplified Chinese: 钩藤.
2. Pinyin of name: gou teng.
3. Botany description: stem and leaf of *Uncaria rhynchophylla* (Miq.) Jacks. and plants of the same genus.
4. Effective components: rhynchophylline, isorhynchophylline, corynoxeine, isocorynoxeine, corynantheine, dihydrocorynantheine, hirsuteine, and rhynchophine.
5. Effects: sedative, dilate blood vessels and lowering blood pressure, inhibit platelet aggregation and thrombosis, relieve dyspnea, improve digestion, isorhynchophylline as one important constituent extracted from *U. rhynchophylla* (Miq.) Jacks.

6. Research: as one important constituent extracted from a TCM, *U. rhynchophylla* (Miq.) Jacks, isorhynchophylline has been used to treat hypertension, epilepsy, head-ache, and other illnesses. Gan et al. reported that they used ouabain and calcium chloride to establish *in vivo* experimental arrhythmic models in guinea pigs and rats and the whole-cell patch-lamp technique to establish *in vitro* model and their results suggested that isorhynchophylline could inhibit the onset of cardiac arrhythmias in-duced by ouabain and shorten the arrhythmias time. Their results also showed that isorhynchophylline could significantly decrease action potential duration (APD) and inhibit calcium currents in isolated guinea pig and rat cardiomyocytes in a dose-dependent manner. In summary, isorhynchophylline played a remarkably preventive role in cardiac arrhythmias through the inhibition of calcium currents in rats and guinea pigs (Gan et al., 2011).

2.16 han fang ji

1. Name in simplified Chinese: 汉防己.
2. Pinyin of name: han fang ji.
3. Botany description: mass root of *Stephania tetrandra* S. Moore.
4. Effective components: alkaloids: tetrandrine, demethyltetrandrine, fangchinoline, cyclanoline, dimethyltetrandrine, and berbamine.
5. Effects: sedative, antiarrhythmic, protect cardiac tissue from ischemia, and lowering blood pressure.
6. Research: pretreatment with tetrandrine protects the myocardial tissue from injuries caused by isoproterenol. It counteracted the appearance of myocardial necrotic lesions and ischemic electrocardiographic modifications, such as ST segment alterations, prevented the appearance of the plasma cardiac necrosis markers c-troponin I and myoglobin, lowered MDA levels, and prolonged partial thromboplastin time. The protective effects of tetrandrine can be attributed to its antioxidant action in lowering peroxide levels and its ability to counteract coagulating activity. Tetrandrine seems to offer full protection against myocardial infarction experimentally induced by the noninvasive treatment of rabbits with isoprotenerol (Pinelli et al., 2010).

2.17 hong hua

1. Name in simplified Chinese: 红花.
2. Pinyin of name: hong hua.
3. Botany description: corolla of *Carthamus tinctorius* L. and the chapiter and the upper part of the stilet of *Crocus sativus* L.
4. Effective components: components consist mainly of flavones and fatty acids. Among the flavones, safflor yellow is the most important component. The following flavones are also found in hong hua: kaempferol, quercertin, myricetin, apigenin, and

luteoline. The fatty acids of hong hua include palmitic acid, myristic acid, lauric acid, dipalmitin, oleic acid, and linoleic acid.

5. Effects: lowering blood pressure by reduce peripheral resistance, improve peripheral microcirculation, inhibit aggregation of platelets, and enhance hydrolysis of fibrin, anti-inflammation, analgesia.

6. Research: Han et al. (2009) investigated the antimyocardial ischemia effects of a purified extract of *C. tinctorius* (ECT) both *in vivo* and *in vitro*. An animal model of myocardial ischemia injury was induced by left anterior descending coronary artery occlusion in adult rats. Pretreatment with ECT (100, 200, 400, and 600 mg kg^{-1} body wt.) could protect the heart from ischemia injury by limiting infarct size and improving cardiac function. In the *in vitro* experiment, neonatal rat ventricular myocytes were incubated to test the direct cytoprotective effect of ECT against H_2O_2 exposure. Pretreatment with 100–400 μg ml^{-1} ECT prior to H_2O_2 exposure significantly increased cell viability as revealed by 3-(4,5-dimethylthiazol-2-yl)-2, 5-diphenyl tetrazolium bromide (MTT) assay.

2.18 huang qi

1. Name in simplified Chinese: 黄芪.
2. Pinyin of name: huang qi.
3. Botany description: root of *Astragalus membranaceus* (Fisch.) Bunge or *A. membranaceus* (Fisch.) Bge. var. mongholicus (Bge.) Haiao.
4. Effective components: flavoids: calycosin, astragaloside I, V, III; astragalus polysacharinand A, B, C, D, volatile oils, amino acids.
5. Effects: improve immunity, cardiotonic, lowering blood pressure, diuretic anti-inflammation.
6. Research: *A. membranaceus* extract (AME) is a widely used herbal product for the treatment of CVDs in China. In a study to evaluate the cardiac protective effects of AME and to probe the underlying molecular mechanism related to angiogenesis, AME with 75 μg ml^{-1} significantly increased proliferation, migration, and tube formation on human umbilical vein endothelial cells (HUVECs). Moreover, *in vivo* experiments on rats with ligation of left anterior descending artery were performed to study the cardiac protective and angiogenic effect of AME (50 and 100 mg kg^{-1} i.g . for 3, 7, and 14 days). The results showed that AME inhibited cardiac fibrosis, reduced infarct size, and increased capillary and arteriole densities. Meanwhile, Western blot was used to determine protein levels of VEGF, p-AKT, p-GSK3beta, and p-mTOR. AME significantly elevated protein expression of VEGF and increased phosphorylation of AKT, GSK3beta, and mTOR. In conclusion, AME exerted cardiac protective and angiogenic effects in the ischemic injured heart. The activation of AKT/GSK3beta and AKT/mTOR pathways and elevated expression of VEGF may contribute to the promoted neovascularization by AME (Zhang et al., 2011).

Another study investigated the effect of Astragalus on hemodynamic changes in Adriamycin (ADR)-injured rat hearts and its underlying molecular mechanism. Sprague–Dawley rats were divided into four groups: control, ADR only, ADR + low dose of Astragalus, and ADR + high dose of Astragalus. Rats were injected intraperitoneally with six equal doses of ADR (cumulative dose, 12 mg kg^{-1}) over a period of 2 weeks. Treatment of Astragalus began 1 day before the onset of ADR injection and was given orally once a day for 50 days (3.3 or 10 g kg^{-1} day^{-1}). Five weeks after the final injection of ADR, rats treated with ADR only showed a significant inhibition of cardiac diastolic function accompanied by the presence of ascites, a remarkable reduction in body weight and heart weight as well as survival rate compared to the controls. Moreover, SERCA2a mRNA and protein expressions in hearts were obviously downregulated by ADR. However, this impaired cardiac function was significantly improved in both doses of Astragalus feeding groups. The amount of ascites was also reduced in a similar extent in these two groups. Only the high-dose treatment of Astragalus significantly attenuated the changes of SERCA2a expression in injured hearts and improved survival. These results indicated that Astragalus could improve cardiac function of ADR-injured rat hearts, which was partly mediated by upregulation of SERCA2a expression (Su et al., 2009).

7. Side effects and cautions: dilation of blood vessels in the head may lead to headache.

2.19 huang qin

1. Name in simplified Chinese: 黄芩.
2. Pinyin of name: huang qin.
3. Botany description: root of *Scutellaria baicalensis* Georgi.
4. Effective components: flavonoids: baicalin, baicalein, wogonoside, wogonin, neobaicalein, 7-methoxybaicalein, 7-methoxynorwogonin, oroxylin A, and skullcapflavone I, II.
5. Effects: lowering blood pressure, lowering serum lipids, anti-inflammation, antihypersensitivity, and antioxidants (Wang et al., 2007).
6. Research: Shao et al. (2002) studied the antioxidative effects of baicalein, in a chick cardiomyocyte model of reactive oxygen species (ROS) generation during hypoxia, simulated ischemia–reperfusion, or mitochondrial complex III inhibition with antimycin A. They found baicalein attenuated oxidant stress during all conditions studied and acted within minutes of treatment. It was concluded that baicalein can scavenge ROS generation in cardiomyocytes and that it protects against cell death in an ischemia–reperfusion model. In addition to the direct radical scavenging mechanism, *S. baicalensis* extract and its constituents may exert antioxidant effects via indirect mechanisms. Shieh et al. (2000) showed that although wogonin does not possess direct radical scavenging activities, it can significantly inhibit enzyme xanthine oxidase activity.

2.20 jiang xiang

1. Name in simplified Chinese: 降香.
2. Pinyin of name: jiang xiang.
3. Botany description: root and core of the stem of *Dalbergia odorifera* T. Chen.
4. Effective components: contains various flavoids: formononetin, bowdichione, liquiritigenin, medicarpin, 9-*O*-methyl-nissolin, melilotocarpan C, D, odoricarpinobtustyrene, volatile oils: β-bisalolene, *trans*-β-farnesene, and *trans*-nerolidol.
5. Effects: inhibit thrombosis in rat, inhibit mitosis of cancer cells.
6. Research: Wu et al. (2010a) evaluated the vasorelaxation effects of formononetin, an isoflavone/phytoestrogen on rat isolated aorta. Formononetin increased endothelial NO synthase (eNOS), but not inducible NO synthase, activity with an upregulation of eNOS mRNA and p-eNOS (Ser1177) protein expression. The results suggest that formononetin caused vascular relaxation via endothelium/NO-dependent mechanism. Isoflavones (formononetin, daidezein) reduce arterial stiffness. In a clinical trial in overweight men and postmenopausal women, isoflavones reduced blood pressure and central arterial stiffness, a predictor of cardiovascular events (Nestel et al., 2007).

2.21 jue ming zi

1. Name in simplified Chinese: 决明子.
2. Pinyin of name: jue ming zi.
3. Botany description: seed of *Cassia tora* Linn.
4. Effective components: emodin, chrysophanol, physcion, obtusin, obtusifolin, and glycosides.
5. Effects: lowering blood pressure and blood lipid level.
6. Research: In a study of the effect of emodin on cultured vascular smooth muscle cells (VSMCs) proliferation induced by angiotensin II (Ang II) and the expression of proto-oncogene c-myc. It was found that emodin inhibited VSMCs proliferation induced by Ang II. Inhibition of the expression of c-myc might be correlated with the inhibitory effects (Wang et al., 2008). Hyun et al. (2009) screened the bioactivity of seeds from raw and roasted *C. tora* via angiotensin-converting enzyme (ACE) inhibitory assays. They found that both of the MeOH extracts from the raw and roasted *C. tora* exhibited significant inhibitory properties against ACE.

2.22 ku shen

1. Name in simplified Chinese: 苦参.
2. Pinyin of name: ku shen.
3. Botany description: root of *Sophora flavescens* Ait.

4. Effective components: include various flavonoids and alkaloids. The alkaloids consist of matrine, oxymatrine, dihydroxy matrine, cytisine, methylcytisine, anagyrine, and bap–iifoline. And the alkaloids consist of kuraridin, kurarinone, norkurarinone, kuraridinol, kurarinol, neokurarinol, norkurarinol, and isokurarinol. Ku shen also contains isoflavonoids like formononetin.

5. Effects: ku shen can relieve myocardial ischemia and has functions such as diuretic, vermicide, cough suppressing, panting calming, and phlegm dispelling; sedative, immunoinhibitive, bile secretion enhancement, hepatoprotective, and anti-inflammation.

6. Research: in a study, rats with acute myocardial infarction (AMI) induced by ligation of left anterior descending branch were randomly assigned to receive oxymatrine 50 and 25 $mg\,kg^{-1}$ intragastrically, and model group which were further compared with sham–operated group and positive group treated with captopril. The effects of 4-week therapy with oxymatrine starting 24 h after infarction had been investigated based on (1) hemodynamics, (2) tissue weights, (3) biochemical indicator (hydroxyproline contents in left ventricle), and (4) TGF-beta1, TGF-beta1 receptor (TbetaR(1)), Smad3, Smad4, Smad7, Col1, and Col3 expression by semiquantitative reverse transcription PCR. Treatment with oxymatrine significantly ameliorated hemodynamics, inhibited the expression of TbetaR(1) mRNA and Smad3 mRNA, and reduced the left ventricle weight/body weight. The results of this research indicated that oxymatrine might protect against myocardial fibrosis and the mechanism may be involved in modulating TGF-beta1–Smads signal pathway (Shen et al., 2011).

    In another study designed to evaluate the antiarrhythmic effects as well as the electrophysiological properties of oxymatrine. The antiarrhythmic activity of oxymatrine was observed in a rat model of arrhythmia induced by coronary ligation. APD, L–type calcium current (I_{Ca-L}), transient outward potassium current (I_{to}), and inward rectifier potassium current (I_{K1}) in rat ventricular myocytes were recorded by utilizing the whole-cell patch–clamp technique. The results showed that administration of oxymatrine significantly delayed the onset of ventricular arrhythmia, decreased the duration of ventricular arrhythmia, and reduced the arrhythmia score of arrhythmic rats. The beneficial effects of oxymatrine may be related to the shortening of APD through reduction of I_{Ca-L}, enhancement of I_{to}, and inhibition of I_{K1} (Cao et al., 2010).

7. Side effects and cautions: taking ku shen orally may cause acid reflux, stomachache, nausea, constipation, and loss of appetite.

2.23 lai fu zi

1. Name in simplified Chinese: 萊菔子.
2. Pinyin of name: lai fu zi.
3. Botany description: seed of *Paphanus sativus* L.

4. Effective components: the main components classify into volatile oils (45%) and fatty acids. The volatile oils are methyl–mercaptan, α, β–hexenal, and β, γ–hexenol; the fatty acids are erucic acid and glycerol sinapate.

5. Effects: lowering blood pressure, inhibit bacterial growth, inhibit inflammation, and bind with exotoxin to prevent intoxication.

6. Research: the abnormal growth of VSMC is a prominent feature of vascular disease, including atherosclerosis, restenosis after angioplasty. Suh et al. (2006) reported the antiproliferative activity of *Raphanus sativus* crude extract on mouse aortic smooth muscle cell proliferation and the related mechanisms. The viability of VSMC decreased with treatment with *R. sativus* crude extract and total isothiocyanates (ITC) including 4-(methylthio)-3-butenyl isothiocyanate (MTBITC), allyl isothiocyanate (AITC), benzyl isothiocyanate (BITC), and phenethyl isothiocyanate (PEITC), isolated from *n*-hexane extracts of *R. sativus*. Treatment of *R. sativus* crude extract may inhibit the DNA synthesis of cultured VSMC and induce apoptosis. These inhibitory effects were associated with G1 cell cycle arrest and downregulation of cyclins and CDKs and upregulation of the CDK inhibitor p21 expression. Ghayur and Gilani (2006) studied the hypotensive, cardiomodulatory, and endothelium-dependent vasodilator actions of *R. sativus* (radish) seed crude extract to provide scientific basis for its traditional use in hypertension. *In vivo* blood pressure was monitored in anesthetized normotensive rats. The results suggested cardiovascular inhibitory effects of the plant are mediated through activation of muscarinic receptors thus possibly justifying the use of *R. sativus* seed in hypertension.

2.24 ling lan

1. Name in simplified Chinese: 铃兰.
2. Pinyin of name: ling lan.
3. Botany description: root or the whole plant of Convallaria Keiskei.
4. Effective components: convallatoxin, convallatoxol, convalloside, deglucosheirotoxin, keioside, rhodeasapogenin, and isorhodea sapogenin.
5. Effects: has digitalis–like effect. Its infusion is prone to hydrolysis and thus is unstable, has significant diuretic effect, has better effect in treating edema, and has sedative effect.
6. Research: the positive inotropic effect of the aqueous extract of Convallaria keiskei (ACK) and the possible mechanisms responsible for this effect were investigated in beating rabbit atria. The results suggest that the ACK-induced positive inotropic effect in beating rabbit atria may, at least in part, be due to the digitalis-like activity of convallatoxin (Choi et al., 2006).

The effects of ouabain and other cardiotonic steroids were examined to investigate whether changes in Na, K-adenosine triphosphatase (ATPase) activity modified the actions of palytoxin (PTX) in rabbit aortic vascular smooth muscle. The results suggest that the specific sugar moiety of cardiac glycosides is important for the inhibitory effect exerted by these compounds on the PTX-induced responses and that the inhibition is not related to the activity of the Na, K-ATPase (Ozaki et al., 1984).

7. Side effects and cautions: it has milder side effect and is less toxic than digitalis. Anorexia, nausea, vomit or dizziness, headache, and palpitation occurred in some patients.

2.25 lu ti cao

1. Name in simplified Chinese: 鹿蹄草.
2. Pinyin of name: lu ti cao.
3. Botany description: whole plant body of *Pyrola rotundifolia* L. subsp. Chinesis H. Andres, *Pyrola decorata* H. Andres, or *Pyrola rotundifolia* L.
4. Effective components: arbutin, methyl hydroquinone, homoarbutin, isohomoarbutin, chimaphillin, monotropein, volatile oil, and tanin.
5. Effects: cardiotonic and antibacterial effects.
6. Research: Lu et al. (2010) investigated the protective effect of total flavonoid of Herba Pyrolae (TFHP) on acute myocardial ischemic injury induced by isoproterenol in rats and the primary mechanisms. They established acute myocardial ischemic models by i.s. of isoproterenol. ECG of the rats was recorded, activities of creatine phosphokinase (CK), lactate dehydrogenase (LDH), and the superoxide dismutase (SOD), and the levels of MDA, NO, and free fatty acid (FFA) in rat serum were determined, heart index was measured, and histopathological changes of myocardium were observed. In comparison with model group, TFHP raised the height of T wave, reduced CK, LDH activities and FFA levels in serum, decreased heart index, and relieved myocardial ischemic injury. The primary study of its mechanism showed that TFHP decreased MDA level, increased SOD activity and NO levels in the rat serum. In summary, TFHP has protective effect on acute myocardial ischemic injury possibly via antioxidation and increasing the release and production of NO.

2.26 luo bu ma

1. Name in simplified Chinese: 罗布麻.
2. Pinyin of name: luo bu ma.
3. Botany description: leaf and root of *Apocynum venetum* L.
4. Effective components: neoisorutin, rutin, quercetin, isoquercitrin, hyperin, fumaric acid, succinic acid.
5. Effects: cardiotonic, dilate blood vessels and lowering blood pressure, relieve dyspnea and remove phlegm, lowering serum lipids, inhibit platelet aggregation and thrombosis, and enhance immunity.

6. Research: the leaves of *A. venetum* L. (AV), a native Chinese plant, have been used as folk medicine in China and Japan. This study evaluated the content of the active antioxidant component and antioxidant activities of AV, and its two alternative species, *Poacynum pictum* (Schrenk) Baill. (PP) and *Poacynum hendersonii* (Hook.f.) Woodson (PH). The total phenolic and total flavonoid contents were determined. In addition, the quantitative analysis of two major flavonoid compounds (hyperoside and isoquercitrin) was carried out by HPLC. The antioxidant activities were investigated by the 1,1-diphenyl-2-picrylhydrazyl (DPPH) radical scavenging activity method, the reducing power test, and the chelating ability of ferrous ions. The highest total phenolic and flavonoid contents were observed in the AV methanolic extract, followed by the PP and PH methanolic extracts. HPLC analysis indicated that isoquercitrin was one of the major components in all three species; however, hyperoside was only detected in AV at high levels. All the antioxidant assays we performed demonstrated that the AV extract was markedly superior to those of the other two species (Liang et al., 2010).

2.27 mai men dong

1. Name in simplified Chinese: 麦门冬.
2. Pinyin of name: mai men dong.
3. Botany description: mass root of *Ophiopogon japonicus* (Thunb.) Ker-Gawl and *Liriope spicata* Lour.
4. Effective components: contains steroidal saponins, of which the aglycone parts are ruscogenin, β-sitosterol, stigmasterol, and β-sitosterol-β-D-glucoside. It also contains methylophiopogonanone A, B; ophiopogonanone A, methylophiopogonone A, B; ophiopogonone A, B; isoophiopogonone A; desmethylisoophiopogonone B; 6-aldehydoisoophiopogonone A, B; and terpenoids such as calciombornyl sulfate and terpenoid glycoside.
5. Effects: enhance endurance to oxygen-deficient condition, regulate blood sugar, inhibit bacteria growth, antithrombosis.
6. Research: the *in vivo* inhibitory effects of the ethanol extract of Radix *O. japonicus* (ROJ-ext) on venous thrombosis were studied in mouse and rat models, and *in vitro* endothelial cell-protective and antiadhesive activities were observed in ECV304 cells injured by sodium dithionite and HL-60 adhesion to ECV304 cells injured by TNF-α. The *in vivo* results showed that ROJ-ext significantly inhibited venous thrombosis induced by tight ligation of the inferior vena cava for 6 h in mice and for 24 h in rats by once oral administration at doses of 12.5 and 25 mg kg^{-1}. Meanwhile, ROJ-ext had no obvious effect on some coagulation parameters, which was different from warfarin, which remarkably prolonged activated partial thromboplastin time (APTT), TT, and PT in rats at the same time. Histological analysis under light microscope and scanning electron microscope (SEM) of inferior vena cava

indicated that ROJ-ext could protect endothelial cells from anoxic injury and alleviate inflammatory changes in the vein wall. On the other hand, the *in vitro* studies approved that ROJ-ext significantly enhanced viability of ECV304 cells injured by sodium dithionite at the concentrations of 0.1, 1.0, and 10 $\mu g\,ml^{-1}$ when given before and after the anoxic induction. Meanwhile, ROJ-ext remarkably inhibited adhesion of HL-60 cells to ECV304 cells injured by rh TNF-α at above concentrations in a dose-dependent manner. The results showed that ethanol extract of Radix *O. japonicus* (ROJ-ext) inhibited venous thrombosis, which linked with its endothelial cell-protective and antiadhesive activities (Kou et al., 2005).

2.28 mao dong qing

1. Name in simplified Chinese: 毛冬青.
2. Pinyin of name: mao dong qing.
3. Botany description: root and leaf of *Ilex pubescens* Hook. Et Am.
4. Effective components: most of the components are triterpenoids and saponins such as ilexsaponin A1, ilexsaponinB1, ilexsaponin B2, ilexsaponin O, etc., and the other components are flavones and polyphenols.
5. Effects: improve blood flow to coronal arteries, improve metabolism and reduce oxygen consumption of cardiac muscles, inhibit aggregation of platelets, reduce blood pressure, anti-inflammation, and inhibit bacteria growth.
6. Research: ilexonin A (IA), purified from the Chinese herbal medicine Maodongqing (*I. pubescens* Hook, et Arn), has been commonly used in China to treat thrombotic disorders. Li et al. found von Willebrand factor (vWF) binding and vWF-mediated platelet activation and aggregation occurring under high shear rate were inhibited by IA. They suggested that IA may be a unique antithrombotic drug inhibiting the vWF-GP Ibalpha interaction and may thus facilitate drug design targeting arterial thrombosis (Li et al., 2004).

2.29 san qi

1. Name in simplified Chinese: 三七.
2. Pinyin of name: san qi.
3. Botany description: root of *P. notoginseng* (Burk.) F.H. Chen.
4. Effective components: notoginsenosides and flavone glycosides. The total glycosides amount to 8–12% and the glycosides are ginsenoside Rb1, Rb2, Rc, Rd, Re, Rf, Rg1, Rg2, Rh, among them, ginsenoside Rb1, Rbg are the most common ones. The aglycones are panoxadiol and panaxatriol. Different from ren sheng, san qi lacks oleanolic acid.

5. Effects: antiarrhythmic, anti-inflammatory, cardioprotective, and reduce blood cholesterol levels.

6. Research: *P. notoginseng* saponins (PNS) was reported to have antiatherosclerotic effects. In a study exploring the molecular mechanisms responsible for the antiatherosclerotic effects of PNS and the inflammatory response, rats were administered liquid paraffin (i.p.), zymosan A (20 mg kg^{-1}, i.p., once every 3 days) or zymosan A and PNS (100 mg kg^{-1}, i.p., once daily), respectively. In the study, typical pathological changes associated with atherosclerosis in rats following induction by zymosan A were alleviated by PNS treatment. In the PNS-treated group, there was a marked reduction in total serum cholesterol, triglycerides, and blood viscosity. In addition, PNS treatment significantly decreased the gene expression of some inflammatory factors, such as integrins, interleukin (IL)-18, IL-1beta, and matrix metalloproteinases 2 and 9. The expression of NF-kappaB/p65 was attenuated, whereas the expression of IkappaBalpha was significantly increased, after treatment with PNS. In conclusion, it appears that PNS exerts its therapeutic effects on atherosclerosis through an anti-inflammatory action and regulation of the blood lipid profile and that an NF-kappaB signaling pathway is involved (Zhang et al., 2008). Trilinolein is a triacylglycerol purified from a commonly used TCM *P. notoginseng*. Trilinolein has been reported to provide a number of beneficial effects including reducing thrombogenicity and arrhythmias and increasing erythrocyte deformability. Additionally, trilinolein has been reported to be an antioxidant, which can counteract free radical damage associated with atherogenesis, and myocardial damage seen with ischaemia and reperfusion. These pharmacologic effects may explain the perceived benefits derived from treating circulatory disorders with the herb over the centuries (Chan et al., 2002).

2.30 wan nian qing

1. Name in simplified Chinese: 万年青.
2. Pinyin of name: wan nian qing.
3. Botany description: root or the whole plant of *Rohdea japonica* Roth, Ornithogalum caudatum Ait.
4. Effective components: its main effective components are cardiac glycosides including rhodexin A, B, C, and D and rhodenin, bipindogenin-D-allopyranoside, bipindogenin-D-xy-lopyranosyl, D-allopyranoside, digitoxigenin, periplogenin, rhodeasapogenin, isorhodeasapogenin, 22-epirhodeasapogenin, convallamarogenin, D-glucopyranoside, sitosterol, and octadecenoic acid.
5. Effects: have digitalis-like effect and can inhibit atrioventricular block. It stimulates smooth muscle of bladder and uterus. It is also an emetic.
6. Research: Iida (1955) examined the effect of rhodexin on isolated hearts of guinea pigs and observed digitalis-like effect of rhodexin.

7. Side effects and cautions: overdose of it may lead to premature cardio contraction and complete block of cardio conduction.

2.31 wu wei zi

1. Name in simplified Chinese: 五味子.
2. Pinyin of name: wu wei zi.
3. Botany description: mature fruit of *Schisandra chinensis* (Turez.) Baill. and *Schisandra sphenanthera* Rehd. Et Wils.
4. Effective components: lignans: schizandrin A, B, C, schizandrol A, B and volatile oils, fatty acids.
5. Effects: cardiotonic, enhance excitability of central nervous system, protect hepatocytes, antiulceration, and induce constriction of ovary.
6. Side effects and cautions: avoid treating women in pregnancy.

2.32 xi xin

1. Name in simplified Chinese: 细辛.
2. Pinyin of name: xi xin.
3. Botany description: whole plant body of *Asarum heterotropoides* Fr. Schmidt var. mandshuricum (Maxim.) kitag. and *Asarum sieboldii* Miq.
4. Effective components: volatile oil: methyl eugenol, borneol, pinene, safrole, elemicin, asarone, limonene, and isobutyldodecatetraenamine.
5. Effects: anesthetic, sedative, analgesia, anti-inflammation, and increase coronary artery blood flow.
6. Research: the radix of *A. sieboldii* Miq. (AR) has been used to treat pain and inflammation in Korea. A study was conducted to gain insights into the mechanism of actions regarding antinociceptive and anti-inflammatory activities of AR. Administration of methanol extract of AR caused dramatic antinociceptive effects based on acetic acid writhing and tail-flick assay. When naloxone (Nx) was pretreated, AR extract failed to exert such antinociceptive effect in the tail-flick assays. These results suggest that AR extract has opioid-like activity. It also exerted significant anti-inflammatory effects in the rat paw edema assay. AR extract caused inhibition in the bradykinin (BK)/histamine-mediated ileum contractions of guinea pig. Taken together, these results provide evidence that the methanol extract of AR exerts antinociceptive and anti-inflammatory effects by activating opioid receptor as well as by inhibiting bradykinin and histamine-mediated actions (Kim et al., 2003).

2.33 xia ku cao

1. Name in simplified Chinese: 夏枯草.
2. Pinyin of name: xia ku cao.

3. Botany description: whole plant body of *Prunella vulgaris* L.
4. Effective components: in the whole plant, the main components are ursolic acid, oleanolic acid, glycoside of oleanolic acid, rutin, hyperoside, caffeic acid, vitamins C and D, carotene, tannin, alkaloids, camphor, and fenchone.
5. Effects: anti-inflammation, lowering blood pressure, inhibit bacterial growth, lowering blood sugar level in animal model of diabetes.
6. Research: *P. vulgaris* L. (PV, Labiatae) is known as a self-heal herb. The different extracts of dried spikes were studied for the best antioxidant active compounds. The 60% ethanol extract (P-60) showed strong antioxidant activity based on the results of 2,2′-azino-di(3-ethylbenzthiazoline-6-sulfonic acid) (ABTS +), 2,2-diphenyl-1-picrylhydrazyl (DPPH), and ferric reducing antioxidant power (FRAP) assay methods. High performance liquid chromatography (HPLC) and LC/MS analysis showed that the main active compounds in P-60 were phenols, such as caffeic acid, rosmarinic acid, rutin, and quercetin. Total phenols were highly correlated with the antioxidant activity ($R^2 = 0.9988$ in ABTS +, 0.6284 in DPPH, and 0.9673 FRAP tests). P-60 could inhibit significantly the tumor growth in C57BL/6 mice (Feng et al., 2010).

    The purported effects of 'circulation-improving' herbs used in TCM show striking similarities with the vascular actions of NO produced by the eNOS. Xia et al. studied the effect on eNOS gene expression of 15 Chinese herbs with potential effects on the vasculature and identified *P. vulgaris* L. (PVL) (flowering spike) as a potent eNOS-upregulating agent. In EA.hy 926 cells, a cell line derived from HUVEC, an aqueous extract of PVL increased eNOS promoter activity, eNOS mRNA and protein expressions, as well as NO production in concentration- and time-dependent manners (Xia et al., 2010).

2.34 yang jiao niu

1. Name in simplified Chinese: 羊角拗.
2. Pinyin of name: yang jiao niu.
3. Botany description: root, stem, leaf, or seed of *Strophanthus divaricatus* (Lour.) Hook. Et Arn.
4. Effective components: cardiac glycosides: most plentiful in the seeds and consists of diavricoside, divostroside, coudoside, and D-strophanthin-I, II.
5. Effects: has digitalis-like effect and has weaker and longer cardiotonic effect comparing with strophanthin K. Increase smooth muscle tone. Also have sedative, antiarrhythmic, and diuretic effects.
6. Side effects and cautions: side effect such as gastric-intestinal reactions rarely occurred. When total dosage exceeds 1.5 mg, arrhythmia may occur which is correlated with the extent of myocardial damage but not the accumulated dosage. Intoxication dosage

may lead to coronary artery contraction, so it must be used carefully in patients suffering coronary artery disorders.

2.35 ye ju hua

1. Name in simplified Chinese: 野菊花.
2. Pinyin of name: ye ju hua.
3. Botany description: capitate of *Chrysanthemum indicum* L.
4. Effective components: flavoids: acacetin, luteolin, apigenin, eupatilin, tricin, tetrahydroxy-dimethoxyflavone, apigenin-glucopyranoside, luteolin-glucopyranoside, linarin; and sesquiterpenoids: cumambrin-A, yejuhualactone.
5. Effects: lowering blood pressure, improve coronary circulation, antioxidation, and inhibit bacterial growth.
6. Research: Wu et al. explored the effects and mechanism of *C. indicum* on experimental ventricular remodeling induced by isoprenaline (ISO) and L-thyroxine (L-Thy) and their results suggested *C. indicum* can significantly attenuate the experimental ventricular remodeling; the mechanism may be related with restricting the activity of the sympathetic nervous system and decreasing the levels of Ang II, aldosterone, and TNF-α (Wu et al., 2010a,b).

2.36 yi mu cao

1. Name in simplified Chinese: 益母草.
2. Pinyin of name: yi mu cao.
3. Botany description: whole plant of *Leonurus heterophyllus* Sweet.
4. Effective components: alkaloids such as leonurine, betonicine, stachydrine, rutin, and fumaric acid.
5. Effects: induce contraction of ovary, cardiotonic, increase coronal blood flow, improve tolerance to myocardial ischemia, relieve angina, inhibit platelet aggregation, antithrombotic, diuretic, sedative.
6. Research: stachydrine is a major constituent of Chinese herb *L. heterophyllus* Sweet, which is used in clinics to promote blood circulation and dispel blood stasis. To investigate the role of stachydrine in HUVECs injury induced by anoxia–reoxygenation, Yin et al. (2010) divided the cultured HUVECs randomly into control group, anoxia–reoxygenation (A/R) group and four A/R + stachydrine groups. HUVECs in the control group were exposed to normoxia for 5 h, while in all A/R groups, HUVECs underwent 3 h anoxia followed by 2 h reoxygenation, and HUVECs in the four A/R + stachydrine groups were treated with 10^{-8}, 10^{-7}, 10^{-6}, and 10^{-5} M (final concentration) of stachydrine, respectively. After anoxia–reoxygenation, tissue factor (TF) was overexpressed, cell viability and the concentrations of SOD, glutathione peroxidase (GSH-PX), and NO were declined, while

LDH, MDA, and endothelin-a (ET-1) were overproduced ($p < 0.05$–0.001 vs. the control group). However, in stachydrine-treated groups, TF expression was inhibited at both mRNA and protein levels, while the declined cell viability and SOD, GSH-PX, NO, as well as the enhanced LDH, MDA, and ET-1 levels occurred during anoxia–reoxygenation were ameliorated and reversed effectively ($p < 0.05$–0.01 vs. A/R group). Consequently, the results indicate that TF plays an important role in the development of anoxia–reoxygenation injury of HUVECs, stachydrine ameliorates HUVECs injury induced by anoxia–reoxygenation, and its putative mechanisms are related to inhibition of TF expression.

7. Side effects and cautions: avoid treating women in pregnancy.

2.37 yin xing ye

1. Name in simplified Chinese: 银杏叶.
2. Pinyin of name: yin xing ye.
3. Botany description: leaf of *Ginkgo biloba* L.
4. Effective components: flavonoids such as ginkgetin, isoginkgetin, bibobetin, quercetin, kaempferd, rhamnetin, ginkgolide A, B, C, bilobalide, and rutin.
5. Effects: dilate coronal and cerebral vessels, protect central nervous system in oxygen-deficient condition by clearing free radicals, lowering blood viscosity, inhibit aggregation of platelets, antithrombotic.
6. Research: results from clinical trials demonstrate that extract of *Ginkgo biloba* may be useful in preventing and treating CVD, particularly ischemic cardiac syndrome. Since many patients with CVD are already taking anticoagulants and antiplatelet drugs, self-medication with extract of *Ginkgo biloba* is not recommended without the advice of their physician (Mahady, 2002).

2.38 yu mi xu

1. Name in simplified Chinese: 玉米须.
2. Pinyin of name: yu mi xu.
3. Botany description: ear of maize.
4. Effective components: cryptoxanthin, pantothenic acid, inositol, sitosterol, stigmasterol, vitamins C and K, malic acid, citric acid, oxalic acid, tartaric acid and fatty acids, volatile oils, resin.
5. Effects: diuretic effect, lowering blood pressure.
6. Research: consumption of flavonoid-rich foods and beverages is thought to reduce the risk of CVDs. Whereas the biological activities of flavonoids have been characterized *in vitro*, there are no clear experimental data demonstrating that chronic dietary intake and intestinal absorption of flavonoids actually protects the heart against ischemia–reperfusion injury. We tested whether long-term consumption of specific flavonoids (anthocyanins, ACNs) included in normal food could render the heart of

rats more resistant to myocardial infarction. Maize kernels that differed specifically in their accumulation of ACNs were used to prepare rodent food in which ACNs were either present or absent. Male Wistar rats were fed the ACN-rich or the ACN-free diet for a period of 8 weeks. ACNs were significantly absorbed and detected in the blood and urine of only rats fed the ACN-rich diet. In Langendorff preparations, the hearts of rats fed the ACN-rich diet were more resistant to regional I/R insult. Moreover, on an *in vivo* model of coronary occlusion and reperfusion, infarct size was reduced in rats that ate the ACN-rich diet than in those that consumed the ACN-free diet ($p < .01$). Cardioprotection was associated with increased myocardial glutathione levels, suggesting that dietary ACNs might modulate cardiac antioxidant defenses. Our findings suggest important potential health benefits of foods rich in ACNs and emphasize the need to develop ACN-rich functional foods with protective activities for promoting human health (Toufektsian et al., 2008).

3. DISCUSSION

This chapter summarized the TCM herbs used in the treatment of CVDs. In the past decades, plenty of researches and studies on these herbs were done, and most of the results were published in Chinese, to help non-Chinese speakers to retrieve the relative information further by themselves, we have included the names of the herbs in original simplified Chinese characters, as well as pinyin, which is the official system to transcribe Chinese characters, and to teach Mandarin Chinese in mainland China, Hong Kong, Taiwan, Malaysia, and Singapore. It is also often used to spell Chinese names in foreign publications and used as an input method to enter Chinese characters into computers.

The information on the effective components of the TCM herbs is included for two considerations. One is to introduce the results in the field of phytochemistry of the TCM herbs; another is to help the reader to retrieve the original TCM herbs from the chemical names of the effective components, since lots of academic publications only indicate the chemical names of the effective components without mention the name of the original herbs in which the components exist.

Although TCM herbs have been using in medical practice for hundreds or even thousands of years, they are still very active in the modern pharmaceutical market, especially the East Asian market. In China, TCM herbs are frequently used in treating ischemic heart diseases, congestive heart failure, arrhythmias, and hypertension.

In the past decades, TCM herbs have been studied phytochemically, biochemically, cell biologically, and currently even molecular biologically; for example, the intracellular signal transduction induced by TCM herbs is intensively studied in laboratories around the world. Nevertheless, TCM takes a holistic approach in understanding human being. While exploring the herbs and action of the herbs on human being chemically, cell biologically, and molecular biologically, we need to think holistically as well.

REFERENCES

Bebrevska, L., Foubert, K., Hermans, N., et al., 2009. In vivo antioxidative activity of a quantified Pueraria lobata root extract. Journal of Ethnopharmacology 127 (1), 112–117.

Cao, Y.G., Jing, S., et al., 2010. Antiarrhythmic effects and ionic mechanisms of oxymatrine from *Sophora flavescens*. Phytotherapy Research 24 (12), 1844–1849.

Chan, T.Y., 2001. Interaction between warfarin and danshen (Salvia miltiorrhiza). Annal of Pharmacotherapy 35 (4), 501–504.

Chan, S.S., Jones, R.L., et al., 2009. Synergistic interaction between the *Ligusticum chuanxiong* constituent butylidenephthalide and the nitric oxide donor sodium nitroprusside in relaxing rat isolated aorta. Journal of Ethnopharmacology 122 (2), 308–312.

Chan, P., Thomas, G.N., et al., 2002. Protective effects of trilinolein extracted from *Panax notoginseng* against cardiovascular disease. Acta Pharmacologica Sinica 23 (12), 1157–1162.

Chen, W., Lu, Y., et al., 2011. Anti-angiogenesis effect of essential oil from *Curcuma zedoaria in vitro* and *in vivo*. Journal of Ethnopharmacology 133 (1), 220–226.

Choi, D.H., Kang, D.G., et al., 2006. The positive inotropic effect of the aqueous extract of Convallaria keiskei in beating rabbit atria. Life Sciences 79 (12), 1178–1185.

Feng, L., Jia, X., et al., 2010. Antioxidant activities of total phenols of *Prunella vulgaris* L. in vitro and in tumor-bearing mice. Molecules 15 (12), 9145–9156.

Fujikawa, T., Hirata, T., Wada, A., et al., 2010. Chronic administration of Eucommia leaf stimulates metabolic function of rats across several organs. British Journal of Nutrition 104 (12), 1868–1877.

Gan, R., Dong, G., Yu, J., Wang, X., Fu, S., Yang, S., 2011. Protective effects of isorhynchophylline on cardiac arrhythmias in rats and guinea pigs. Planta Medica 77 (13), 1477–1481.

Ghayur, M.N., Gilani, A.H., 2006. Radish seed extract mediates its cardiovascular inhibitory effects via muscarinic receptor activation. Fundamental and Clinical Pharmacology 20 (1), 57–63.

Han, J.Y., Fan, J.Y., et al., 2008. Ameliorating effects of compounds derived from *Salvia miltiorrhiza* root extract on microcirculatory disturbance and target organ injury by ischemia and reperfusion. Pharmacology and Therapeutics 117 (2), 280–295.

Han, S.Y., Li, H.X., et al., 2009. Protective effects of purified safflower extract on myocardial ischemia *in vivo* and *in vitro*. Phytomedicine 16 (8), 694–702.

Huang, X., Tang, J., Zhou, Q., Lu, H., Wu, Y., Wu, W., 2010. Polysaccharide from fuzi (FPS) prevents hypercholesterolemia in rats. Lipids in Health and Disease 9, 9.

Hyun, S.K., Lee, H., et al., 2009. Inhibitory activities of *Cassia tora* and its anthraquinone constituents on angiotensin-converting enzyme. Phytotherapy Research 23 (2), 178–184.

Iida, M., 1955. Effect of rhodexin on isolated heart of guinea-pig. Japanese Journal of Pharmacology 4, 145–154.

Kim, S.J., Gao, Z.C., et al., 2003. Mechanism of anti-nociceptive effects of *Asarum sieboldii* Miq. radix: Potential role of bradykinin, histamine and opioid receptor-mediated pathways. Journal of Ethnopharmacology 88 (1), 5–9.

Koo, Y.K., Kim, J.M., et al., 2010. Platelet anti-aggregatory and blood anti-coagulant effects of compounds isolated from *Paeonia lactiflora* and *Paeonia suffruticosa*. Pharmazie 65 (8), 624–628.

Kou, J., Yu, B., et al., 2005. Inhibitory effects of ethanol extract from Radix *Ophiopogon japonicus* on venous thrombosis linked with its endothelium-protective and anti-adhesive activities. Vascular Pharmacology 43 (3), 157–163.

Li, J., Chen, C.X., Shen, Y.H., 2011. Effects of total glucosides from paeony (Paeonia lactiflora Pall) roots on experimental atherosclerosis in rats. Journal of Ethnopharmacology 135 (2), 469–475.

Li, M., Wu, W.K., et al., 2004. Specific inhibiting effects of Ilexonin A on von Willebrand factor-dependent platelet aggregation under high shear rate. Chinese Medical Journal 117 (2), 241–246.

Li, Y.H., Sun, X.P., Zhang, Y.Q., Wang, N.S., 2008. The antithrombotic effect of borneol related to its anticoagulant property. The American Journal of Chinese Medicine 36 (4), 719–727.

Liang, T., Yue, W., et al., 2010. Comparison of the phenolic content and antioxidant activities of *Apocynum venetum* L. (Luo–Bu–Ma) and two of its alternative species. International Journal of Molecular Sciences 11 (11), 4452–4464.

Liu, Y., Song, S.J., Xu, S.X., 2003. Advances in the study on the chemical constituents and biological activities of *Prunella vulgaris* L. Journal of Shenyang Pharmaceutical University. 20, 55–59.

Lu, P.P., Liu, J.T., et al., 2010. Protective effect of total flavonoid of Herba Pyrolae on acute myocardial ischemic injury induced by isoproterenol in rats. Zhong Yao Cai 33 (1), 73–76.

Lu, G.W., Miura, K., Yukimura, T., Yamamoto, K., 1994. Effects of extract from Clerodendron trichotomum on blood pressure and renal function in rats and dogs. Journal of Ethnopharmacology 42 (2), 77–82.

Mahady, G.B., 2002. Ginkgo biloba for the prevention and treatment of cardiovascular disease: a review of the literature. Journal of Cardiovascular Nursing 16 (4), 21–32.

Malemud, C.J., 2007. Inhibitors of stress-activated protein/mitogen–activated protein kinase pathways. Current Opinions of Pharmacology 7 (3), 339–343.

Nestel, P., Fujii, A., et al., 2007. An isoflavone metabolite reduces arterial stiffness and blood pressure in overweight men and postmenopausal women. Atherosclerosis 192 (1), 184–189.

Ng, T.B., Liu, F., et al., 2004. The antioxidant effects of aqueous and organic extracts of Panax quinquefolium, Panax notoginseng, Codonopsis pilosula, Pseudostellaria heterophylla and Glehnia littoralis. Journal of Ethnopharmacology 93 (2–3), 285–288.

Ozaki, H., Nagase, H., et al., 1984. Involvement of the sugar moiety in the inhibitory action of the cardiac glycosides on the palytoxin-induced responses in vascular smooth muscles. Journal of Pharmacology and Experimental Therapeutics 231 (1), 153–158.

Pan, R., Dai, Y., et al., 2011. Inhibition of vascular endothelial growth factor-induced angiogenesis by scopoletin through interrupting the autophosphorylation of VEGF receptor 2 and its downstream signaling pathways. Vascular Pharmacology 54 (1–2), 18–28.

Pinelli, A., Trivulzio, S., et al., 2010. Pretreatment with tetrandrine has protective effects against isoproterenol-induced myocardial infarction in rabbits. In Vivo 24 (3), 265–270.

Ren, D.Q., 2002. Clinical-Oriented Traditional Chinese Medicine (Chinese). People's Medical Publication House, Beijing.

Shao, Z.H., Vanden, H.T., et al., 2002. Baicalein attenuates oxidant stress in cardiomyocytes. American Journal of Physiology. Heart and Circulatory Physiology 282 (3), H999–H1006.

Shen, X.C., Yang, Y.P., et al., 2011. Protective effect of oxymatrine on myocardial fibrosis induced by acute myocardial infarction in rats involved in TGF-beta(1)-Smads signal pathway. Journal of Asian Natural Products Research 13 (3), 215–224.

Shieh, D.E., Liu, L.T., et al., 2000. Antioxidant and free radical scavenging effects of baicalein, baicalin and wogonin. Anticancer Research 20 (5A), 2861–2865.

State Pharmacopoeia Board, 2005. People's Republic of China Pharmacopoeia. Chemical Industry Press, Beijing.

Su, Y.W., Chiou, W.F., Chao, S.H., Lee, M.H., Chen, C.C., Tsai, Y.C., 2011. Ligustilide prevents LPS-induced iNOS expression in RAW 264.7 macrophages by preventing ROS production and down-regulating the MAPK, NF-kappaB and AP-1 signaling pathways. International Immunopharmacology 11 (9), 1166–1172.

Su, D., Li, H.Y., et al., 2009. Astragalus improved cardiac function of adriamycin-injured rat hearts by upregulation of SERCA2a expression. The American Journal of Chinese Medicine 37 (3), 519–529.

Suh, S.J., Moon, S.K., et al., 2006. Raphanus sativus and its isothiocyanates inhibit vascular smooth muscle cells proliferation and induce G(1) cell cycle arrest. International Immunopharmacology 6 (5), 854–861.

Toufektsian, M.C., de Lorgeril, M., et al., 2008. Chronic dietary intake of plant-derived anthocyanins protects the rat heart against ischemia–reperfusion injury. Journal of Nutrition 138 (4), 747–752.

Wang, J.M., 1954. Pharmacology of Traditional Chinese Medicine (Chinese). People's Medical Publication House, Beijing.

Wang, X., Hai, C.X., et al., 2010. The protective effects of Acanthopanax senticosus Harms aqueous extracts against oxidative stress: role of Nrf2 and antioxidant enzymes. Journal of Ethnopharmacology 127 (2), 424–432.

Wang, S., Liu, Y., et al., 2008. Inhibitory effects of emodin on the proliferation of cultured rat vascular smooth muscle cell-induced by angiotensin II. Phytotherapy Research 22 (2), 247–251.

Wang, C.Z., Mehendale, S.R., et al., 2007. Commonly used antioxidant botanicals: active constituents and their potential role in cardiovascular illness. The American Journal of Chinese Medicine 35 (4), 543–558.

Williams, T., 2003. The Complete Illustrated Guide to Chinese Medicine, a Comprehensive System for Health and Fitness. Element Books Limited, London.

Wu, Q., Chen, C.X., et al., 2010a. Effect of *Chrysanthemum indicum* on ventricular remodeling in rats. Zhong Yao Cai 33 (7), 1112–1115.

Wu, J.H., Li, Q., et al., 2010b. Formononetin, an isoflavone, relaxes rat isolated aorta through endothelium-dependent and endothelium-independent pathways. The Journal of Nutritional Biochemistry 21 (7), 613–620.

Xia, N., Bollinger, L., et al., 2010. *Prunella vulgaris* L. upregulates eNOS expression in human endothelial cells. The American Journal of Chinese Medicine 38 (3), 599–611.

Yin, J., Zhang, Z.W., et al., 2010. Stachydrine, a major constituent of the Chinese herb *Leonurus heterophyllus* Sweet, ameliorates human umbilical vein endothelial cells injury induced by anoxia-reoxygenation. The American Journal of Chinese Medicine 38 (1), 157–171.

Zhang, L., Yang, Y., et al., 2011. *Astragalus membranaceus* extract promotes neovascularisation by VEGF pathway in rat model of ischemic injury. Pharmazie 66 (2), 144–150.

Zhang, Y.G., Zhang, H.G., et al., 2008. *Panax notoginseng* saponins attenuate atherosclerosis in rats by regulating the blood lipid profile and an anti-inflammatory action. Clinical and Experimental Pharmacology and Physiology 35 (10), 1238–1244.

CHAPTER 34

Protective Effect of Garlic (*Allium sativum* L.) Against Atherosclerosis

M.S. Baliga*, A.R. Shivashankara*, P.L. Palatty*, J.J. Dsouza*, R. Arora[†]
*Father Muller Medical College, Kankanady, Mangalore, Karnataka, India
[†]Institute of Nuclear Medicine and Allied Sciences, Brig, Delhi, India

ABBREVIATIONS

ADP Adenosine diphosphate
CAD Coronary artery disease
CVD Cardiovascular diseases
HDL High-density lipoprotein
IFN-γ Interferon gamma
IL-1 Interleukin 1
IL-6 Interleukin 6
LDL Low-density lipoprotein
L-NAME *L*-NG-Nitroarginine methyl ester
MCP-1 Monocyte chemoattractant protein 1
PKC Protein kinase C
RNS Reactive nitrogen species
ROS Reactive oxygen species
SdLDL Small dense LDL
TNF-α Tumor necrosis factor alpha
VCAM-1 Vascular cell adhesion molecule 1

1. INTRODUCTION

Cardiovascular diseases (CVD) are the world's leading cause of death and atherosclerosis, commonly referred to as a hardening or furring of the arteries. Atherosclerosis is a condition affecting arterial blood vessels in which the artery wall thickens as the result of a build-up of fatty materials such as cholesterol. In humans, atherogenesis typically occurs over a period of many years, usually many decades, and has severe clinical consequences such as myocardial infarction, stroke, cerebral ischemia, angina pectoris, renal artery stenosis, intermittent claudication, and gangrene. The condition arises either due to a chronic inflammatory response in the walls of the arteries, in large part due to the accumulation of macrophage or white blood cells, and is promoted by low-density

Bioactive Food as Dietary Interventions for Cardiovascular Disease
http://dx.doi.org/10.1016/B978-0-12-396485-4.00031-1

© 2013 Elsevier Inc.
All rights reserved.

lipoproteins (LDL), which lead to the formation of multiple plaques within the arteries (Libby, 2008).

2. ETIOPATHOGENESIS OF ATHEROSCLEROSIS

Atherosclerosis is a multifocal, smoldering immunoinflammatory disease of medium and large arteries, fuelled by lipids, and superimposed by thrombosis. Important risk factors contributing to the process of atherogenesis are hypercholesterolemia, high levels of LDL, low levels of high-density lipoprotein (HDL), diabetes mellitus, hypertension, high fat diet, smoking, obesity, sedentary life style with decreased physical activity, and family history of coronary heart diseases (Figure 34.1) (Libby, 2008).

The process of atherogenesis is complex and the oxidized LDL and advanced glycation end products initiate the process. Surplus plasma LDL cholesterol accumulates in the arterial linings and initiates the free radical-induced oxidation of LDL. This leads to the formation of small dense LDL particles and causes functional alteration. Concomitantly, increase in the expression of atherogenic signal molecules, adhesion molecules (such as vascular cell adhesion molecule 1, VCAM-1), chemoattractants (such as monocyte chemoattractant protein 1, MCP-1), and a host of growth factors and cytokines (macrophage colony-stimulating factor; CD40 ligand (CD154); interferon gamma, IFN-γ, tumor necrosis factor alpha, TNF-α, interleukin 1, IL-1; and interleukin 6, IL-6) occurs (Libby, 2008).

These signaling molecules facilitate the adhesion of monocytes and T-lymphocytes to the arterial endothelium and their penetration into the intima. Monocytes undergo transformation to macrophages and ultimately form the lipid-rich foam cells that are

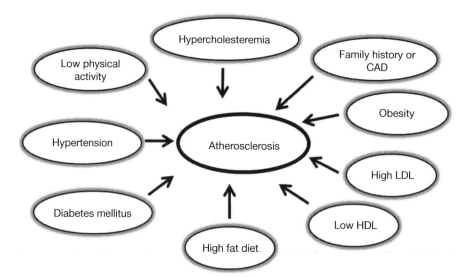

Figure 34.1 Risk factors associated with atherosclerosis.

characteristic of the fatty streak, the first morphologically recognizable precursor of the atherosclerotic plaque. The same-signal molecules are also responsible for the growth and the eventual destabilization of the plaque, as they are able to promote plaque rupture and the thrombogenic nature of the plaque content itself through the increased expression of molecules such as tissue factor (Libby, 2008).

3. PREVENTION OF ATHEROSCLEROSIS

Conventionally, atherogenesis can be prevented or retarded through changes in lifestyle and by regular consumption of medications. In early stages, practice of regular exercise, abstinence from smoking and excess alcohol consumption, and dietary modification are suggested. Of these, dietary modification is known to play a major role as studies have shown that reduction in consumption of fat, cholesterol, sucrose, trans-fat-rich diet, and increase in the consumption of polyunsaturated fatty acids (especially omega-3 fatty acids) and dietary fibers can have beneficial effects (Libby, 2008). When lifestyle changes fail or the levels of serum cholesterol are in excess, the use of medications, especially the hypolipidemic drugs affecting the lipoprotein and cholesterol metabolism, is recommended (Libby, 2008). However, although useful, the regular use of hypolipidemic drugs is associated with untoward effects and may necessitate additional prophylaxis for the ensuing side effects. The various hypolipidemic drugs available, their actions, and side effects are represented in Table 34.1.

Table 34.1 The Different Class of Hypolipidemic Drugs Used, Their Mode of Action, and the Associated Side Effects

Class of hypolipidemic drugs	Mode of action	Side effects
HMG-co A reductase inhibitors (lovastatin, simvastatin)	Inhibit rate-limiting step in cholesterol synthesis (HMG CoA reductase)	Headache, sleep disturbances, muscle tenderness
Fibric acid derivatives (gemfihozil, clofibrate)	Increased lipoprotein lipase activity. Inhibit release of fatty acids from adipose store	Loose motions, skin rash, impotence, eosinophilia, myopathy
Bile acid-binding resin (cholestyramine, cholestipol)	Increases LDL receptors on hepatocytes. Reduces absorption of bile acids and other fats. Increases cholesterol conversion to bile acids	Vitamin A, D, E, K unabsorbed
Nicotinic acid	Inhibits VLDL formation Reduces lipolysis in adipose tissue	Flushing, dyspepsia hyperpigmentation

Source: Libby, P., 2008. The pathogenesis, prevention, and treatment of atherosclerosis. In: Fauci, A.S., Braunwald, E., Kasper, D.L., Hauser, S.L., Longo, D.L., Jameson, J.L., Loscalzo, J. (Eds.), Harrison's Principles of Internal Medicine, 17th ed., vol. II. McGraw Hill, New York, pp. 1501–1509.

4. PLANTS IN THE PREVENTION OF ATHEROSCLEROSIS

Preclinical studies suggest certain dietary agents like *Allium sativum* and *Allium cepa*, and medicinal plants like *Terminalia chebula*, *Terminalia arjuna*, *Ocimum sanctum*, *Emblica officinalis*, and *Asparagus racemosus* possess cardioprotective properties. Scientific studies carried out in the past two decades have shown that the dietary as well as medicinal plant *Allium sativum* Linn, commonly known as garlic, is a well-studied and extensively investigated plant for its cardioprotective and antiatherosclerotic effects. In the following sections, the various observations and mechanisms contributing toward the prevention of atherosclerosis by garlic are addressed.

5. ALLIUM SATIVUM

Allium sativum Linn, commonly known as garlic, belongs to the onion family Alliaceae. Since antiquity, garlic is one of the most important medicinal and culinary plants and finds mention in the various traditional and folk systems of medicine. The bulb of the plant is the most commonly used part and is divided into numerous fleshy sections called cloves. The cloves have a characteristic pungent, spicy flavor that mellows and sweetens considerably with cooking. The leaves and flowers (bulbils) on the head (spathe) are also of dietary use and are less mild in flavor than the bulbs (Amagase et al., 2001). Depending on the needs, garlic is used in different forms such as raw, aged, tablet, and powdered. Additionally, oil is also extracted from the cloves and marketed (Banerjee and Maulik, 2002).

6. BIOACTIVE COMPOUNDS IN GARLIC

Phytochemical studies carried out in the past have shown that garlic is rich in sulfur-containing compounds. However, their composition and ratio alters with the type of processing and length of aging. Studies have shown that the raw garlic is rich in allicin (allyl 2-propenethiosulfinate or diallyl thiosulfinate), allylmethyl thiosulfonate, 1-propenyl allylthiosulfonate, and γ-glutamyl γ−S-alkyl-L-cysteine and adenosine. Allicin is the principal bioactive compound and is produced by the action of allinase on alliin (S-allyl cysteine sulphoxide) when garlic is chopped or crushed. The enzyme allinase responsible for converting alliin (S-allyl cysteine sulphoxide) to allicin is heat-sensitive and because of this, heat-treated garlic contains alliin. However, in the aged garlic, due to the process of aging, there is a considerable loss of allicin content and increased activity of S-allylcysteine, allixin, and N-alpha-(1-deoxy-D-fructos-1-yl)-L-arginine (Fru-Arg), and selenium. On the contrary, the major ingredients of garlic oil are diallyl disulfide, diallyl trisulfide, diallyl tetrasulfide, allylmethyl tetrasulfide, and dimethyl trisulfide. Oil-macerated garlic oil contains the vinyl-dithiins and ajoenes (Amagase et al., 2001; Banerjee and Maulik, 2002). The proximate and phytochemical compositions of garlic are enlisted in Tables 34.2, 34.3, and 34.4, and structures of the important phytochemicals are depicted in Figure 34.2.

Table 34.2 Chemical Compounds Found in Garlic Bulb

Chemical compounds	Amount (ppm)
1,2-Dimercaptocyclopentane	2.4
1,2-Epithiopropane	0.1–1.66
1,3-Dithiane	0.08–3
1-Hexanol	0.23
2-Methyl-benzaldehyde	0.1
2-Propen-1-ol	0.1–21
2-Vinyl-4H-1,3-dithiin	2–29
2,5-Dimethyl-tetrahydrothioptene	0.6
3,5-Diethyl-1,2,4-trithiolane	0.15–43
3-Methyl-2-cyclopenthene-1-thione	0.16–1.6
3-Vinyl-4H-1,2-dithiin	0.34–10.65
4-Methyl-5-vinylthiazole	0.75
Allicin	1500–27 800
Alliin	5000–10 000
Allyl-propyl-disulfide	36–216
Beta-carotene	0.17
Caffeic acid	20
Diallyl-disulfide	16–613
Diallyl-sulfide	2–99
Diallyl-trisulfide	10–1061
Dimethyl-difuran	5–30
Dimethyl-disulfide	0.6–2.5
Dimethyl trisulfide	0.8–19
Ferulic acid	27
Methyl-allyl-disulfide	6–104
Methyl-allyl-sulfide	0.5–4.6
Methyl-allyl-trisulfide	6–279
Methyl-propyl-disulfide	0.03–0.66
Nicotinic acid	4.8
p-Coumaric acid	58
Protodegalactotigonin	10
Protoeruboside B	100
Quercetin	200
Riboflavin	0.5–3
S-(2-Carboxy-propyl)-glutathione	92.5
S-Allo-mercapto-cysteine	2
S-Allyl-cysteine	10
Scordine	250
Scordinine-A	39 000
Scordinine-B	800
Trans-1-propenyl-methyl-disulfide	0.9
trans-Ajoene	268
Scordinine-A-3	333
Scordinine-A-2	250–8000
Sativoside-B-1	30
Scordinine-A-1	67–30 000

Source: Ejaz, S., Woong, L.C., Ejaz, A., 2003. Extract of garlic *Allium sativum* L. in cancer chemoprevention. Experimental Oncology 25, 93–97.

Table 34.3 Chemical Compounds Found in Garlic Counterparts

Compound	Amount (ppm)		
	Leaf	Shoot	Flower
Ascorbic acid	390–2868	420–1883	440–3793
Ash	10 000–74 000	7000–31 000	6000–52 000
Calcium	580–4265	120–538	250–2155
Carbohydrates	95 000–699 000	201 000–901 000	94 000–810 000
Fat	5000–37 000	3000–13 000	2000–17 000
Fiber	18 000–132 000	17 000–76 000	8000–69 000
Iron	6–44	17–76	9–78
Niacin	6–44	5–22	4–34
Phosphorus	460–3382	520–2332	460–3966
Potassium	3260–23 971	2730–12 242	
Protein	26 000–191 000	12 000–54 000	14 000–121 000
Riboflavin	1.4–10.3	0.6–2.7	0.6–5.2
Sodium	40–294		
Thiamin	1.1–8.1	1.4–6.3	1.1–9.5
Water	864 000	777 000	884 000

Source: Ejaz, S., Woong, L.C., Ejaz, A., 2003. Extract of garlic *Allium sativum* L. in cancer chemoprevention. Experimental Oncology 25, 93–97.

7. PROTECTIVE EFFECT OF GARLIC AGAINST ATHEROSCLEROSIS

7.1 Garlic Ameliorates Dyslipidemia

Hyperlipidemia is the major risk factor for atherosclerosis and several preclinical studies by different investigators have conclusively shown that garlic possesses antihyperlipidemic effects and can reduce atheromatous lesions (Figure 34.3). The term "atherogenic dyslipidemia" denotes a combination of elevated triglycerides and small-dense LDL particles, and low levels of HDL cholesterol. LDL, very low-density lipoprotein (VLDL) remnants, chylomicron remnants, small dense LDL (sdLDL), Lp(a), and oxidized LDL are pro-atherogenic and HDLs are antiatherogenic (Libby, 2008). An increase in serum triglycerides leads to increased triglyceride component of VLDL.

Table 34.4 Chemical Compounds Found in Garlic Root

Compound	Amount (ppm)
Desgalactotigonin	400
Gitonin	300
Sativoside-R-1	500
Sativoside-R-2	300

Source: Ejaz, S., Woong, L.C., Ejaz, A., 2003. Extract of garlic *Allium sativum* L. in cancer chemoprevention. Experimental Oncology 25, 93–97.

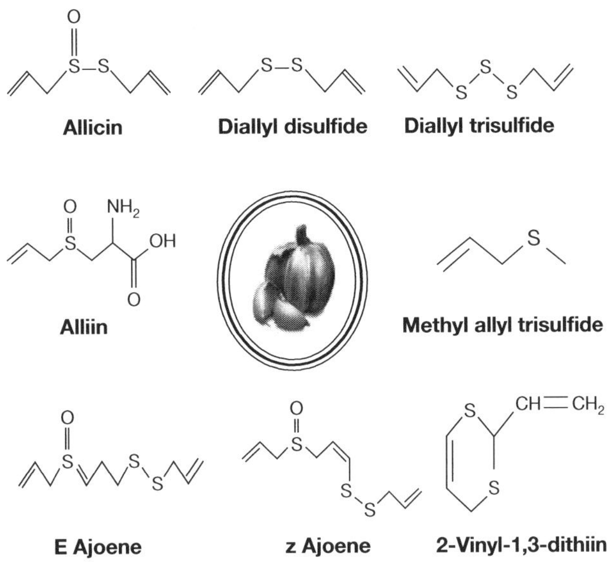

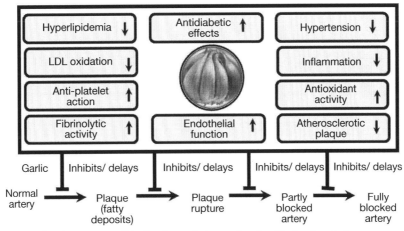

Allicin   **Diallyl disulfide**   **Diallyl trisulfide**

Alliin   **Methyl allyl trisulfide**

E Ajoene   **z Ajoene**   **2-Vinyl-1,3-dithiin**

Figure 34.2 Important phytochemicals of garlic.

When a triglyceride from VLDL is exchanged for a cholesterol ester in LDL by the action of cholesterol transfer protein, the VLDL becomes enriched in cholesterol ester and LDL becomes enriched in triglyceride. Enzymatic hydrolysis of triglyceride in LDL results in a smaller, denser LDL particle. Small-dense LDL particles promote atherogenesis by rapid infiltration into the arterial wall, and have longer residence time and higher affinity to the extracellular matrix and increased susceptibility for oxidation (Libby, 2008).

Hyperlipidemia ↓	Antidiabetic effects ↑	Hypertension ↓
LDL oxidation ↓		Inflammation ↓
Anti-platelet action ↑		Antioxidant activity ↑
Fibrinolytic activity ↑	Endothelial function ↑	Atherosclerotic plaque ↓

Garlic   Inhibits/ delays   Inhibits/ delays   Inhibits/ delays   Inhibits/ delays

Normal artery → Plaque (fatty deposits) → Plaque rupture → Partly blocked artery → Fully blocked artery

Figure 34.3 Mechanisms responsible for the antiatherosclerotic effects of garlic (*arrows up* = increase; *arrows down* = decrease).

Studies have shown that garlic reduces the plasma levels of total cholesterol, triglycerides, and LDL cholesterol, and increases the levels of HDL cholesterol in plasma (Banerjee and Maulik, 2002; Gorinstein et al., 2007; Orekhov and Grunwald, 1997). Additionally, garlic also rectifies the altered levels of LDL cholesterol and helps to achieve a balance between the good cholesterol (HDL) and bad cholesterol (LDL) (Banerjee and Maulik, 2002).

Multiple studies have shown that garlic possesses protective effects against high fat or high cholesterol diet-induced hyperlipidemia in laboratory animals. Seminal studies by Gorinstein et al. (2006a, b, 2007) have shown that oral administration (500 mg kg^{-1} b. wt.) of raw or boiled garlic to rats for 28–30 days caused a marked decrease in the levels of plasma lipids, decreased the levels of total cholesterol, LDL cholesterol, triglycerides, and liver cholesterol. Studies have also shown that administering raw garlic daily for 4 weeks (2 g kg^{-1} b.wt.) to hyperlipidemic guinea pigs (achieved by feeding cholesterol for 4 weeks before giving garlic) caused a significant decrease in serum cholesterol, triglyceride, LDL cholesterol, and atherogenic index (Choudhary, 2008). Oral administration of the aqueous extract of garlic (1% solution kg^{-1} b.wt.) for 30 consecutive days to diabetic rabbits is also shown to reduce the serum cholesterol level (Mahesar et al., 2010). Studies have also shown that raw garlic was better than boiled garlic in reducing serum cholesterol and triglycerides (Thomson et al., 2006).

In addition to animal studies, clinical trials performed with hyperlipidemic individuals have shown that garlic possesses antihyperlipidemic effects. Garlic, when administered in the form of enteric-coated garlic powder tablets (Kojuri et al., 2007), as garsin tablets (Afkhami-Ardekani et al., 2006), raw garlic (Parastouei et al., 2006), aged garlic extract (Yeh and Liu, 2001), and allicor, a long-active garlic (Sobenin et al., 2005), is reported to reduce serum cholesterol, triglycerides, and LDL cholesterol, and to increase the levels of HDL cholesterol when administered for a prolonged period.

Mechanistic studies have shown that garlic mediates its antihyperlipidemic effects by multiple mechanisms. *In vitro* studies with cultured rat hepatocytes have shown that the water-extractable fraction, methanol-extractable fraction, and petroleum ether-extractable fraction of fresh garlic and kyolic, the liquid form of aged garlic extract, inhibit cholesterol synthesis (Gorinstein et al., 2007; Yeh and Liu, 2001). The garlic phytochemicals S-ethyl cysteine, S-propyl cysteine, γ-glutamyl-S-methylcysteine, γ-glutamyl S-allylcysteine, γ-glutamyl-S-propylcysteine, diallyl sulfide, diallyl disulfide, diallyl trisulfide, dipropyl sulfide, and dipropyl trisulfide were also effective in inhibiting cholesterol synthesis (Gorinstein et al., 2007; Yeh and Liu, 2001). Studies indicate that the cholesterol synthesis inhibition by garlic was possibly due to its effect on sterol 4 alpha-methyl oxidase (Singh et al., 2006).

Studies have also shown that garlic affects the lipogenic enzymes glucose 6-phosphate dehydrogenase, malate dehydrogenase, and HMG CoA reductase (Gebhardt, 1993; Sendl et al., 1992), and also prevents/inhibits intracellular accumulation of lipids in tissues

(Orekhov and Grunwald, 1997). Additionally, garlic is also shown to decrease the levels of free and esterified cholesterol in arterial cells by decreasing the activities of acyl CoA: cholesterol acyl transferase, an enzyme involved in the intracellular esterification of cholesterol, and concomitantly stimulating the activity of cholesterol ester hydrolase, an enzyme responsible for degrading cholesteryl esters in the atherosclerotic cells (Orekhov and Grunwald, 1997).

7.2 Garlic Enhances Antioxidant Activity and Prevents/Inhibits LDL Oxidation

Oxidative stress refers to a condition resulting from excessive generation of reactive nitrogen species (RNS) and reactive oxygen species (ROS), and decreased antioxidants. It is implicated in the etiopathogenesis of many diseases. Antioxidant molecules provide protection against the detrimental effects of ROS or RNS. Oxidative modification of proteins and lipids in plasma LDL leads to abnormal LDL that is not recognized by the liver LDL receptors, and so is not cleared by the liver. The modified LDL is taken up by macrophage scavenging receptors. Oxidized LDL entering the macrophages triggers recruitment of macrophages in the atherogenesis process, infiltration of macrophages in blood vessel endothelium. This process further triggers inflammatory responses to the formation of foam cells rich in oxidized LDL, thereby causing formation of an atherosclerotic plaque (Libby, 2008). Antioxidants, which make LDL less susceptible to oxidation, are likely to be considered antiatherogenic. Multiple studies have shown that both water-soluble and lipid-soluble organosulfuric compounds, notably allixin and the trace element selenium present in raw and aged garlic, possess antioxidant properties, and that they prevent the oxidative damage to the LDL and the ensuing atherogenic events (Borek, 2001).

Investigative studies have shown that the hexane extract had the highest antioxidant activity, followed by water extracts, bulb pressings, and commercial products, indicating that the nonpolar molecules are highly effective (Leelarungrayub et al., 2006). With regard to phytochemicals, studies have shown that alliin scavenged superoxide, allicin suppressed the formation of superoxide by the xanthine oxidase system, and alliin, allylcysteine and allyl disulfide scavenged hydroxyl radicals (Chung, 2006).

Aged garlic extract is shown to have more potent antioxidant action than raw garlic (Gorinstein et al., 2007; Orekhov and Grunwald, 1997). Comparative studies aimed at understanding the antioxidant efficacy have shown that the aged garlic was better than the raw garlic. The aged garlic extract as well as its phytochemicals *S*-allylcysteine (SAC) and *S*-allylmercaptocysteine decreased the t-butyl hydroperoxide-induced lipid peroxidation in a liver microsome fraction, while the raw and heat-treated raw garlic extract produced an oxidant effect (Imai et al., 1994). The antioxidant compounds from aged garlic extract like *S*-allyl cysteine, *S*-methyl cysteine, *N*-fructosyl arginine, and *N*-fructosyl glutamate exhibited potent free radical scavenging effects in various assays (Imai et al., 1994).

Additionally, *in vitro* studies with human LDL have shown that both aged garlic extract and its diethyl ether extracts were effective in preventing oxidant-induced damage. The aged garlic extract was observed to be more effective than the diethyl ether extract in inhibiting the production of superoxide. Diethyl ether extract was effective in reducing the copper and 15-lipooxygenase-mediated lipid peroxidation on isolated LDL. Aged garlic extract also reduced the LDL oxidation by chelating cupric ions and inhibited the formation of lipid peroxides (Dillon et al., 2003).

Animal studies have also shown that administering garlic to high cholesterol-fed rats (25 mg kg^{-1} b.wt.) of lyophilized garlic powder extract obtained from raw and boiled garlic) for over a period of 30 days increases the plasma total antioxidant activity (Gorinstein et al., 2007). Administering 1 ml of garlic juice (100 g kg^{-1} b.wt.) daily to alloxan-induced diabetic rats for 4 weeks is also reported to enhance the antioxidant activity (El-Demerdash et al., 2005). Studies have also shown that the administration of pure allicin (9 mg kg^{-1} b.wt.) significantly inhibited both native LDL and oxidized LDL degradation in the isolated mouse macrophages of mice developing atherogenesis (Gonen et al., 2006).

7.3 Garlic Has Antiplatelet Action

Platelet aggregation and clot formation is an important stage in the atherogenesis process. Initially, platelets are activated by binding to collagen at the site of the vessel wall injury to form thromboxane A2 and release adenosine diphosphate (ADP), which activates other platelets flowing in the vicinity of the injury. Thrombin, formed from the coagulation cascade, is the most potent activator of platelets and initiates activation by interacting with its receptors on the platelet membrane, triggering signal transduction by phosphoinositide and other pathways. Upon activation, platelets change shape and in the presence of fibrinogen aggregate to form the platelet plug of the thrombus. Further, a more stable thrombus is formed by a fibrin mesh binding to the platelet aggregate. Endothelial cells in the vessel walls synthesize thromboxane A2 (activator/inducer of platelet aggregation), and prostacyclin PGI2 (inhibitor of platelet aggregation) from arachidonic acid, by the cyclooxygenase pathway (Libby, 2008).

Antiplatelet drugs act by inhibiting the key processes or motionecules which induce platelet aggregation. Inhibitors of COX-1 (e.g., Aspirin), ADP receptor (e.g., Clopidogrel), or glycoprotein GPIIb-IIIa (e.g., Abciximab) that bind to fibrinogen are used as antiplatelet drugs (Libby, 2008). Among the most studied indices of antithrombotic effects of garlic, the reduction of platelet aggregation is important. *In vitro* studies have shown that raw garlic, garlic oil, and garlic extracts inhibit platelet aggregation. However, studies are not able to clearly demonstrate whether the effects are due to the inhibition of cyclooxygenase, the key enzyme of thromboxane synthesis, but suggest that the effect of garlic may be on the platelet activation phase. Adenosine present in garlic might increase adenosine 3′,5′-monophosphate (cyclic AMP) levels, which might decrease the thromboxane synthesis and action (Srivastava, 1984).

Garlic suppresses thromboxane production and also inhibits collagen-, ADP-, and epinephrine-induced platelet aggregation (Bordia et al., 1998). Garlic inhibits the activity of phospholipase A2, the enzyme releasing arachidonate from membrane phospholipids, and this concomitantly inhibits the synthesis of thromboxanes (Makheja et al., 1979). The antiplatelet effects of garlic are thought to be caused by allicin, SAC, adenosine, methyl allyltrisulfide, diallyl disulfide, and diallyl trisulfide (Bordia et al., 1998).

Among the different forms of garlic, raw garlic is supposed to be more effective than boiled in inhibiting platelet aggregation (Ali et al., 1999; Makheja et al., 1979). *In vitro* studies by Cavagnaro et al. (2007) have shown that raw garlic extract was effective in inhibiting the aggregatory activity of human platelets while similar results were not observable with the cooked garlic extract. Aged garlic is also shown to reduce platelet adhesion to collagen-coated surfaces, fibrinogen, and Von Willebrand factor (Ali et al., 1999). Garlic also inhibits platelet aggregation induced by the ADP pathway and to a lesser extent by epinephrine but is ineffective when induced by adenosine diphosphate, collagen, A23187, epinephrine, and arachidonic acid (Hiyasat et al., 2009).

Experimental studies with laboratory animals have validated the *in vitro* observations for garlic's inhibitory effects on platelet aggregation. Administering rabbits with an aqueous extract of garlic (500 mg kg^{-1}) is shown to inhibit thromboxane synthesis and protect them against thrombocytopenia caused by collagen or arachidonic acid (Ali et al., 1990). Garlic also inhibited the thrombin-induced platelet synthesis of thromboxane B-2 in rats. The effect was both dose- and time-dependent and maximum inhibition was observed between 0.5 and 6 h at 25 and 100 mg kg^{-1} garlic (Thomson et al., 2000).

Human studies with both healthy volunteers and patients with coronary artery disease (CAD) have also shown that raw garlic, garlic oil, dried garlic powder, fried garlic, and ethyl acetate extract possess platelet inhibitory effects (Bordia et al., 1998). In a randomized, placebo-controlled, double-blind crossover study, garlic has been shown to increase the threshold concentrations for ADP, collagen, and epinephrine to induce platelet aggregation (Bordia et al., 1998; Steiner and Li, 2001). In another double-blind, randomized, placebo-controlled study, administering 800 mg dried garlic powder for 4 weeks reduced the ratio of circulating platelet aggregates and spontaneous platelet aggregation (Kiesewetter et al., 1993a). Additionally, administering 800 mg of dried garlic powder daily for 6 weeks to patients with arterial occlusive disease reduced plasma cholesterol, plasma viscosity, and spontaneous platelet aggregation (Kiesewetter et al., 1993b).

7.4 Garlic Has Fibrinolytic Activity

Garlic is also reported to possess fibrinolytic properties and to dissolve fibrin clots. The coagulation system is normally in a state of dynamic equilibrium in which fibrin clots are constantly laid down and dissolved. Fibrin is present in large quantities in the form of mural thrombus on the intact wall of the plaque or within the layers of the fibrous cap and distributed throughout the plaque. Fibrinolysis, the process of dissolving the fibrin clots, is catalyzed by the serine protease plasmin. Plasmin exists as an inactive precursor plasminogen, which is activated by tissue plasminogen activator (Libby, 2008).

Animal studies have shown that feeding garlic juice (raw garlic 250 mg day^{-1}) for 13 weeks to rabbits on a high cholesterol diet enhanced fibrinolytic activity (Bordia et al., 1998; Gorinstein et al., 2007). Studies have also shown that garlic oil (with 2 g twice daily treatment after 3 months) increases fibrinolytic activity (Bordia et al., 1998). Garlic is shown to increase plasminogen activator activity (Gorinstein et al., 2007).

7.5 Garlic Has Antihyperglycemic and Antidiabetic Effect

Diabetes is one of the major risk factors for atherosclerosis and the prolonged exposure to hyperglycemia is regarded to be the major factor for diabetes-induced atherosclerosis. At the cellular level, hyperglycemia alters vascular tissue and accelerates the process of atherosclerosis. Prolonged exposure to hyperglycemia leads to the glycosylation of both proteins and lipoproteins by a nonenzymatic pathway known as Maillard reaction, thereby resulting in the formation of different classes of heterogeneous sugar–protein adducts collectively called advanced glycation end products (AGE). These glycated proteins interact with receptors present on cells relevant to the atherosclerotic process, including monocyte-derived macrophages, endothelial cells, and smooth muscle cells (Libby, 2008). The interaction of glycosylated proteins with their receptors results in the induction of oxidative stress, proinflammatory responses, and activation of Protein kinase C (PKC) activation with subsequent enhanced expression of growth factors. Glycosylation of apo-B in LDL is increased in correlation with glucose levels, and glycosylation of ApoB results in a significant impairment of LDL receptor-mediated uptake, decreasing the clearance of LDL (Libby, 2008).

With regard to garlic's antidiabetic effects, observations have been mixed and contradictory, especially in humans. Studies suggest garlic possesses hypoglycemic effects in subjects with normal blood glucose levels but similar effects were not seen in diabetic patients (Banerjee and Maulik, 2002; Orekhov and Grunwald, 1997). However, it is quite possible that the hypoglycemic effect of garlic in the normal individuals may contribute to the initiation and progression of atherosclerosis and needs to be validated.

Preclinical studies have shown that garlic was effective in reducing the blood glucose levels in diabetic rats, rabbits, and mice (Banerjee and Maulik, 2002; Orekhov and Grunwald, 1997). Administering a garlic-containing diet (12.5%) to alloxan-induced diabetic rats for 15 days is shown to reduce fasting blood glucose (Jelodar et al., 2005). Recently, Mahesar et al. (2010) have also observed that administering the aqueous extract of garlic (1% solution kg^{-1} b.wt.) to diabetic rabbits for 30 consecutive days decreased the blood glucose level.

Oral or intraperitoneal administration of 500 mg kg^{-1} raw garlic for four consecutive weeks reduced hyperglycemia in diabetic rats. However, similar effects were not seen when the boiled garlic extract was fed, suggesting that the heat-labile molecules contribute to the effects (Thomson et al., 2006). The phytochemical alliin also reduced hyperglycemia in diabetic rats with effects being equal to that of insulin and glibenclamide (Augusti and Sheela, 1996; Banerjee and Maulik, 2002). Mechanistic studies suggest that garlic acts as an insulin secretagogue probably through increased secretion of insulin from the pancreas or by releasing it from the bound insulin (Banerjee and Maulik, 2002).

With respect to humans, the antihyperglycemic effects of garlic have been inconclusive (Banerjee and Maulik, 2002; Orekhov and Grunwald, 1997). Studies by Afkhami-Ardekani et al. (2006) have shown that administering garsin tablets (300 mg of effective extract of garlic) three times a day for 4 weeks did not reduce the blood glucose levels. However, studies by Sobenin et al. (2008) have shown that administering garlic powder tablet allicor to type 2 diabetes mellitus patients for 4 weeks decreased fasting blood glucose and serum fructosamine and decreased the levels of glycation of proteins and accumulation of advanced glycation end products.

7.6 Garlic Improves Endothelial Function of Arteries and Reduces Atherosclerotic Plaque Volume

Various studies with both raw and aged garlic extract have shown to be able to restore endothelial function of arteries to normal in both preclinical and human studies. Preclinical studies with laboratory rats have shown that raw garlic was effective in preventing monocrotaline-induced vasoconstrictory responses on the coronary arteries (Banerjee and Maulik, 2002; Gorinstein et al., 2007; Orekhov and Grun wald, 1997). Clinical trials have also shown that administering aged garlic extract improves the impaired endothelial function in men with CAD by decreasing aortic stiffness, increasing elasticity of the aorta, preventing oxidative injury to endothelial cells, and restoring endothelial cell functions (Banerjee and Maulik, 2002; Gorinstein et al., 2007; Orekhov and Grunwald, 1997).

In a randomized, placebo-controlled, cross-over design with 2 weeks garlic treatment and washout period in men suffering from CAD, coadministration of garlic improved the brachial artery flow-mediated endothelium-dependent dilation, especially in men with lower baseline flow-mediated endothelium-dependent dilation. Additionally, the markers of oxidant stress (plasma-oxidized LDL and peroxides), systemic inflammation (plasma C-reactive protein and IL-6), and VCAM-1 did not change significantly during the study. These data suggest that short-term treatment with aged garlic extract may improve impaired endothelial function in men with CAD treated with aspirin and a statin. Additionally, in a randomized, double-blind, placebo-controlled clinical trial, continuous intake of high-dose garlic powder reduced the increase in arteriosclerotic plaque volume by 5–18% in 48 months (Koscielny et al., 1999).

7.7 Garlic Has Anti-inflammatory Action

Inflammation plays an important role in both the initiation of atherosclerosis and development of atherothrombotic events. The migration and proliferation of leukocytes/monocytes into the endothelium is an early event in atherogenesis. Rassoul et al. (2006) evaluated *in vitro* the influence of water-soluble garlic extract on the cytokine-induced expression of endothelial leukocyte adhesion molecules such as intercellular adhesion molecule-1 (ICAM-1, CD54) and vascular cell adhesion molecule-1 (VCAM-1, CD106). Results of the study suggested that garlic components act to suppress VCAM-1 and ICAM-1 expression in primary human coronary artery endothelial cell with a consequent decrease in monocyte adherence. These effects provide a complementary explanation for the antiatherogenic properties of garlic. Garlic is also shown to inhibit the cyclooxygenase pathway responsible for synthesis of inflammation-mediating molecules (Gorinstein et al., 2007). Garlic powder extracts (GPE) and single garlic metabolites modulated lipopolysaccharide (LPS)-induced cytokine levels in human whole blood. GPE-altered cytokine levels in human blood sample supernatants reduced nuclear factor (NF-κB) activity in human cells exposed to these samples. Pretreatment with GPE (100 mg l^{-1}) reduced LPS-induced production of proinflammatory cytokines IL-1β and TNF-α (Keiss et al. 2003). The garlic metabolite diallyl disulfide (1–100 μmol l^{-1}) also significantly reduced IL-β and TNF-α (Keiss et al. 2003).

7.8 Garlic Has Antihypertensive Action

Hypertension is not only a well-established cardiovascular risk factor but also increases the risk of atherosclerosis. There is increasing evidence that hypertension, like hyperlipidemia, induces oxidative stress in the arterial wall. It has even been suggested that superoxide anions might trigger the development of hypertension in some models, presumably by inactivating endothelium-derived nitric oxide and thus mitigating this important vasodilator mechanism. In varying degrees, abnormalities of volume regulation, enhanced vasoconstriction, and remodeling of the arterial wall (decreasing lumen diameter and increasing resistance) contribute to the development of hypertension, these processes triggering the atherosclerosis process (Libby, 2008).

Studies with experimental animals have shown that garlic and its components possess hypotensive effects and this is partly due to its vasodilatory property (Orekhov and Grunwald, 1997). Additionally, gamma-glutamyl cysteines, the compounds present in garlic, are also known to inhibit angiotensin-converting enzyme (Gorinstein et al., 2007). Additionally, studies have also shown that garlic reduced the *L*-NG-nitroarginine methyl ester (*L*-NAME) induced BP in rats, indicating that the garlic phytochemicals possess stimulatory effects on the activity of nitric oxide synthase, an enzyme responsible for the synthesis of nitric oxide, a known vasodilator (Al-Qattan, 2006).

Human studies have also shown that administering the dried garlic preparation of Kwai (600–900 mg) daily for at least 4 weeks decreased the systolic blood pressure by 10 mmHg and diastolic pressure by 7 mmHg (Gorinstein et al., 2007). Administering a higher dose of 2400 mg Kwai powder containing 1.3% allicin to patients with persistent severe hypertension was also observed to be effective in reducing diastolic blood pressure by 16 mmHg (Gorinstein et al., 2007). Allicor, the long-acting garlic tablet, at doses of 600 mg day^{-1} or 2400 mg day^{-1} for 8 weeks is also reported to be effective in decreasing both systolic and diastolic blood pressure (Sobenin et al., 2009). Together, all these observations indicate the usefulness of garlic in the prevention of hypertension.

8. CONCLUSIONS

Garlic has been used for many millennia as a cure for a wide variety of different conditions including CVD. Scientific studies have shown that the organosulfur compounds present in garlic are responsible for the observed myriad cardioprotective effects. Multiple studies have confirmed that garlic possesses lipid-lowering, anticoagulant, antioxidant properties to correct the impaired endothelial function. However, certain observations that garlic is devoid of lipid-lowering effects need to be considered and merit detailed investigation. It is quite probable that the contradictory observations may be due to the differences in garlic preparations, variations in the ratio of the active constituents and their bioavailability, inadequate randomization, selection of inappropriate subjects, and differences in the duration of study. The pharmacological activity of garlic is due to the presence of various organosulfuric compounds and the final ratio of these compounds in garlic is determined by a number of factors, including the geographic origin, the maturity of the rhizomes at the time of harvest, and the method by which the extracts are prepared. As there is considerable variation in the chemical composition among various samples of garlic, it is imperative that a quality control be established for the presence of active phytochemicals in the required levels. Due to its abundance, low cost, and safety in consumption, garlic remains a species with tremendous potential and countless possibilities for further investigation.

ACKNOWLEDGMENT

The authors dedicate this chapter to Dr. Ashalatha Rao, Professor and Founder Head of Department of Biochemistry, Father Muller Medical College, Mangalore, India, for her seminal studies on the molecular mechanisms of various diseases and oxidative stress markers. The authors are grateful to Rev. Fr. Patrick Rodrigus (Director), Rev. Fr. Denis D'Sa (Administrator), and Dr. Jaya Prakash Alva (Dean) of Father Muller Medical College for providing the necessary facilities and support.

REFERENCES

Afkhami-Ardekan, M., Kamali-Ardekani, A.R., Shojaoddiny-Ardekani, A., 2006. Effects of garlic on serum lipids and blood glucose of type 2 diabetic patients. International Journal of Diabetes in Developing Countries 26, 86–88.

Ali, M., Thomson, M., Alnaqeeb, M.A., et al., 1990. Antithrombotic activity of garlic: its inhibition of the synthesis of thromboxane-B2 during infusion of arachidonic and collagen in rabbits. Prostaglandins Leukotrienes and Essential Fatty Acids 41, 95–99.

Ali, M., Bordia, T., Mustafa, T., 1999. Effect of raw versus boiled aqueous extract of garlic and onion on platelet aggregation. Prostaglandins Leukotrienes and Essential Fatty Acids 60, 43–47.

Al-Qattan, K.K., 2006. Nitric oxide mediates the blood-pressure lowering effect of garlic in the rat two-kidney, one-clip model of hypertension. The Journal of Nutrition 136, 774S–776S.

Amagase, H., Petesch, B.L., Matsuura, H., Kasuga, S., Itakura, Y., 2001. Intake of garlic and its bioactive components. The Journal of Nutrition 131, 955S–962S.

Augusti, K.T., Sheela, C.G., 1996. Antiperoxide effect of S-allyl cysteine sulfoxide, an insulin secretagogue, in diabetic rats. Experientia 52, 115–120.

Banerjee, S.K., Maulik, S.K., 2002. Effect of garlic on cardiovascular disorders: a review. Nutrition Journal 1, 4–14.

Bordia, A., Verma, S.K., Srivastava, K.C., 1998. Effect of garlic extract (*Allium sativum*) on blood lipids, blood sugar, fibrinogen and fibrinolytic activity in patients with coronary artery disease. Prostaglandins Leukotrienes and Essential Fatty Acids 58, 257–263.

Borek, C., 2001. Recent advances on the nutritional effects associated with the use of garlic as a supplement: antioxidant health effects of aged garlic extract. The Journal of Nutrition 131, 1010S–1015S.

Cavagnaro, P.F., Camargo, A., Galmarini, C.R., Simon, P.W., 2007. Effect of cooking on garlic (*Allium sativum* L.) antiplatelet activity and thiosulfinates content. Journal of Agricultural and Food Chemistry 55, 1280–1288.

Choudhary, R., 2008. Benificial effect of *Allium sativum* and *Allium tuberosum* on experimental hyperlipidemia and atherosclerosis. Pakistan Journal of Physiology 4, 7–9.

Chung, L.Y., 2006. The antioxidant properties of garlic compounds: allyl cysteine, alliin, allicin and allyl disulfide. Journal of Medicinal Food 9, 205–213.

Dillon, S.A., Burmi, R.S., Lowe, G.M., Billington, D., Rahaman, K., 2003. Antioxidant properties of aged garlic extract: an *in vitro* study incorporating human low-density lipoprotein. Life Sciences 72, 1583–1594.

Ejaz, S., Woong, L.C., Ejaz, A., 2003. Extract of garlic *Allium sativum* L. in cancer chemoprevention. Experimental Oncology 25, 93–97.

El-Demerdash, F.M., Yousef, M.I., Abou El-Naga, N.I., 2005. Biochemical study on the hypoglycemic effects of onion and garlic in alloxan-induced diabetic rats. Food and Chemical Toxicology 43, 57–63.

Gebhardt, R., 1993. Multiple inhibitory effects of garlic extracts on cholesterol biosynthesis in hepatocytes. Lipids 28, 613.

Gonen, A., Harats, D., Rabinkov, A., et al., 2006. The antiatherogenic effect of allicin: possible mode of action. Pathobiology 72, 325–334.

Gorinstein, S., Leontowicz, M., Leontowicz, H., et al., 2006a. Supplementation of garlic lowers lipids and increases antioxidant capacity in plasma of rats. Nutrition Research 26, 362–368.

Gorinstein, S., Leontowicz, M., Drzewiecki, J., et al., 2006b. Raw and boiled garlic enhances plasma antioxidant activity and improves plasma lipid metabolism in cholesterol-fed rats. Life Sciences 9, 205–213.

Gorinstein, S., Zenon, J., Namiesnik, J., et al., 2007. The atherosclerotic heart disease and protecting properties of garlic: contemporary data. Molecular Nutrition & Food Research 51, 1365–1381.

Hiyasat, B., Sabha, D., Grötzinger, K., et al., 2009. Antiplatelet activity of *Allium ursinum* and *Allium sativum*. Pharmacology 83, 197–204.

Imai, J., Ide, N., Nagae, S., et al., 1994. Antioxidants and free radical scavenging effects of aged garlic extract and its constituents. Planta Medica 60, 417–420.

Jelodar, G.A., Maleki, M., Motadayen, M.H., Sirus, S., 2005. Effect of fenugreek, onion and garlic on blood glucose and histopathology of pancreas of alloxan-induced diabetic rats. Indian Journal of Medical Sciences 59, 64–69.

Keiss, H.P., Dirsch, V.M., Hartung, T., et al., 2003. Garlic (Allium sativum L.) modulates cytokine expression in lipopolysaccharide-activated human blood thereby inhibiting NF-kappaB activity. The Journal of Nutrition 133(7), 2171–2175.

Kiesewetter, H., Jung, E., Jung, E.M., 1993a. Effect of garlic coated tablets in peripheral arterial occlusive disease. The Clinical Investigator 71, 383–386.

Kiesewetter, H., Jung, E., Jung, E.M., 1993b. Effect of garlic on platelet aggregation in patients with increased risk of juvenile ischaemic attack. European Journal of Clinical Pharmacology 43, 333–336.

Kojuri, J., Vosoughi, A.R., Akram, M., 2007. Effects of *Anethum graveolens* and garlic on lipid profile in hyperlipidemic patients. Lipids in Health and Disease 6, 5–9.

Koscielny, J., Klussendirf, D., Latza, R., et al., 1999. The antiatherosclerotic effect of *Allium sativum*. Atherosclerosis 144, 237–249.

Leelarungrayub, N., Rattanapanone, V., Chanarat, N., Gebicki, J.M., 2006. Quantitative evaluation of the antioxidant properties of garlic and shallot preparations. Nutrition 22, 266–274.

Libby, P., 2008. The pathogenesis, prevention and treatment of atherosclerosis. In: Fauci, A.S., Braunwald, E., Kasper, D.L., Hauser, S.L., Longo, D.L., Jameson, J.L., Loscalzo, J. (Eds.), 17th Edition Harrison's Principles of Internal MedicineII, McGraw Hill, New York, pp. 1501–1509.

Mahesar, H., Bhutto, M.A., Khand, A.A., Narejo, N.T., 2010. Garlic used as an alternative medicine to control diabetic mellitus in alloxan-induced male rabbits. Pakistan Journal of Physiology 6, 39–41.

Makheja, A.N., Vanderhoek, J.Y., Bailey, J.M., 1979. Inhibition of platelet aggregation and thromboxane synthesis by onion and garlic. Lancet 1, 781.

Orekhov, A.N., Grunwald, J., 1997. Effects of garlic on atherosclerosis. Nutrition 13, 655–663.

Parastouei, K., Ravanshad, Sh., Mostaphavi, H., Setoudehmaram, E., 2006. Effects of garlic tablet on blood sugar, plasma lipids and blood pressure in type 2 diabetes patients with hyperlipidemia. Journal of Medicinal Plants 5, 48–54.

Rassoul, F., Salvetter, J., Reissig, D., Schneider, W., Thiery, J., Richter, V., 2006. The influence of garlic (Allium sativum) extract on interleukin 1alpha-induced expression of endothelial intercellular adhesion molecule-1 and vascular cell adhesion molecule-1. Phytomedicine 13, 230–235.

Sendl, A., Schliack, M., Loser, R., Stanislaus, F., Wagner, H., 1992. Inhibition of cholesterol synthesis *in vitro* by extracts and isolated compounds prepared from garlic and wild garlic. Atherosclerosis 94, 79.

Singh, D.K., Todd, D., Porte, T.D., 2006. Inhibition of sterol 4alpha-methyl oxidase is the principal mechanism by which garlic decreases cholesterol biosynthesis. The Journal of Nutrition 136, 759S–764S.

Sobenin, I.A., Pryanishnikov, V.V., Kunnova, L.M., Rabinovich, E.A., Orekhov, A.N., 2005. Allicor efficacy in lowering the risk of ischemic heart disease in primary prophylaxis. Terapevticheski Arkhiv 77, 9–13.

Sobenin, S.A., Nedosugova, L.V., Filatova, L.V., Balabolkin, M.I., Gorchakova, T.V., Orekhov, A.N., 2008. Metabolic effects of time-released garlic powder tablets in type 2 diabetes mellitus: the results of double-blinded placebo-controlled study. Acta Diabetologica 45, 1–6.

Sobenin, I.A., Andrianova, I.V., Forchenkov, I.V., Gorchakova, I.V., Orekhov, A.N., 2009. Time-released garlic powder tablets lower systolic and diastolic blood pressure in men with mild and moderate arterial hypertension. Hypertension Research 32, 433–437.

Srivastava, K.C., 1984. Effects of aqueous extracts of onion, garlic, and ginger on platelet aggregation and metabolism of arachidonic acid in the blood vascular system: *in vitro* study. Prostaglandins, Leukotrienes and Medicine 13, 227–235.

Steiner, M., Li, W., 2001. Aged garlic extract, a modulator of cardiovascular risk factors: a dose finding study on the effects of AGE on platelet functions. The Journal of Nutrition 131, 980S–984S.

Thomson, M., Mustafa, M., Ali, M., 2000. Thromboxane-B2 levels in serum of rabbits receiving a single intravenous dose of aqueous extract of garlic and onion. Prostaglandins, Leukotrienes, and Essential Fatty Acids 63, 217–221.

Thomson, M., Al-Qattan, K.K., Bordia, T., Ali, M., 2006. Including garlic in the diet may help lower blood glucose, cholesterol, and triglycerides. The Journal of Nutrition 136, 800S–802S.

Yeh, Y.Y., Liu, L., 2001. Cholesterol-lowering effect of garlic extracts and organosulfur compounds: human and animal studies. The Journal of Nutrition 131, 989S–993S.

CHAPTER 35

Potential of Soy Phytochemicals in Cardiomyocyte Regeneration and Risk Reduction of Coronary Heart Disease

J.M. Wu, G.R. Tummuri, T.-C. Hsieh
New York Medical College, Valhalla, NY, USA

ABBREVIATIONS

AC–MS An experimental approach in which affinity chromatography is coupled with mass spectrometry
ApoB Apo-lipoprotein B
CDKs Cyclin-dependent kinases
CHD Coronary heart disease
CHF Chronic heart failure
ChiP–Seq An experimental approach involving chromatin immunoprecipitation followed by sequencing of immunoprecipitated genes
CRP C-reactive protein
E2F A transcription factor involved in cell cycle control
FGF1/p38i FGF1/p38 MAP kinase inhibitor
HDL high-density lipoprotein
IP–MS An experimental approach in which immunoprecipitation is combined with mass spectrometry to identify specific genes
LDL low-density lipoprotein
MAPK mitogen-activated protein kinase
NOS nitric oxide synthase
PCNA Proliferating cell nuclear antigen
SMC Smooth muscle cells
VCAM-1 Vascular cell adhesion molecule-1

1. INTRODUCTION AND OVERVIEW

Coronary heart disease (CHD) is the leading cause of death worldwide and results from reduction in the blood supply owing to narrowing of coronary arteries secondary to atherosclerotic pathology (Wu et al., 2001); inadequate coronary circulation induces death of cardiomyocytes and the bulk of heart muscle and surrounding tissue leading to functional deterioration (Goldspink et al., 2003). Restoration of function and integrity to the damaged heart remains challenging, as the ability of the injured adult heart is restricted by the limited proliferative potential of cardiomyocytes.

Bioactive Food as Dietary Interventions for Cardiovascular Disease
http://dx.doi.org/10.1016/B978-0-12-396485-4.00032-3

© 2013 Elsevier Inc.
All rights reserved.

The adult myocardium is considered incapable of regenerating itself after ischemic or other forms of injury; growth is limited to hypertrophy of remaining viable cardiomyocytes. Recurring cardiac injury may result in formation of scarred tissues and impaired functions, which may manifest as arrhythmias, loss of compliance, and other complications, contributing significantly to morbidity and mortality. Thus, prevention of cardiomyocyte death is urgently needed to reduce the social and medical burdens of cardiac disorders (Chien et al., 2008). Equally important are strategies to reactivate cardiomyocyte regeneration to replace injured or dysfunctional cells in order to reduce the incidence of heart failure (Goldspink et al., 2003).

Epidemiological studies have shown that consumption of soy-containing diets has an inverse association with CHD risks and may act by preventing or retarding the development of CHD (Hanson et al., 2006; Mink et al., 2007; Steinberg, 2007; Xiao, 2008). Soy contains naturally occurring plant phytochemicals, for example, isoflavones such as genistein, daidzein, and glycitein. Cardiovascular benefits of dietary isoflavones have been reported (Wenzel et al., 2008). Intake of soy isoflavones reduces total and low-density lipoprotein (LDL) cholesterol along with other CHD risk factors, for example, prevention of LDL oxidation; oxidized LDL is atherogenic and leads to the narrowing of coronary arteries (Wu et al., 2001). Dietary intake of ≥ 25 g day^{-1} of soy protein in women resulted in mean reduction of 1.9 and 0.9 mm Hg in systolic and diastolic blood pressures, respectively, when compared with women with soy intake <2.5 g day^{-1} (Yang et al., 2005). These results suggest that isoflavones and other bioactive ingredients in soy may act as cardioprotective agents by slowing or prolonging the events that culminate in heart failure, marked by the death of incumbent cardiomyocytes.

Cardiomyocytes become terminally differentiated shortly after birth. Therefore, the regeneration of the cardiomyocytes affording the replacement of dead or dysfunctional cells and reinvigorating the activity of a weakened heart is an important strategy to reduce the incidence of heart failure. Scientific literature shows that soy isoflavones can fulfill the key aspects required for cardiomyocyte replication and progression in the new niche of the regenerating heart. Engel and Keating show that the cardiomyocytes can resume proliferation by inhibiting the p38 mitogen-activated protein kinase (MAPK), which acts as a negative regulator of cardiomyocyte replication (Engel et al., 2005). Isoflavone genistein has been shown to enhance the activity of enzyme telomerase, which is important in cell and tissue regeneration (Chau et al., 2007).

This chapter will summarize CHD pathogenesis and evidence supporting the potential of soy phytochemicals as cardioprotective agents and their role in the control and restoration of cardiomyocyte regeneration. Demonstrating and understanding how soy phytochemicals play a potential role in cardiomyocyte regeneration may lead to development of new strategies and future directions for managing these lethal diseases.

2. PATHOGENESIS OF CHD

The primary underlying cause of CHD is atherosclerosis, a generic term used to describe thickening or loss of elasticity of arterial walls due to formation of fibrous fatty plaques, which comprises smooth muscle cells (SMC), macrophages, lipoproteins, and cellular waste products. An earliest visible lesion of atherosclerosis is fatty streak, attributed to the accumulation of lipid-laden foam cells in the intimal layer of the arterial wall (Ross and Glomset, 1976b; Wu et al., 2001).

The pathogenesis of atherosclerosis is rooted in the response-to-injury hypothesis (Ross and Glomset, 1976a,b). The formation of atherosclerotic plaques follows a sequence of events depicted in Figure 35.1, consisting of

(1) *Chronic endothelial injury.* Damage to the endothelium is a pivotal event in the initiation of CHD. Many endothelium–damaging factors have been identified; elevation in cholesterol and hypertension are among ones most extensively studied. Endothelial damage is accompanied by numerous responses, such as increased permeability of lipoproteins and expression of adhesion molecules, adherence of monocytes/macrophages and leukocytes, and release of cytokines, vasoactive agents, and growth factors.

(2) *Inflamed endothelium facilitates recruitment of leukocytes/monocytes and adhesion of platelets.* Damage to the endothelium produces mediators that facilitate the recruitment and adhesion of leukocytes, mediated by selectin molecules, including P-selectin and E-selectin, and adhesion molecules such as integrins, selectins, and immunoglobulins on endothelial cells and vascular cell adhesion molecule-1 (VCAM-1) on leukocytes (Haverslag et al., 2008). Over time, these damage-elicited responses culminate in the establishment of an inflammatory state marked by migration of SMC into the intima and their proliferation to form an intermediate lesion; the asymptomatic foam cell lesions are called 'fatty streaks' (Ross, 1999; Wu et al., 2001).

(3) *Extravasation of lipoproteins and oxidative modification.* Following entry into subendothelial space through leaky, defective endothelium, the lipoprotein particles acquire proinflammatory, cytotoxic, and atherogenic properties, in coordination with their oxidative modification by nitric oxide produced by nitric oxide synthase (NOS; Glass and Witztum, 2001) and by 15-lipoxygenase (Rankin et al., 1991) from macrophages. In addition, phospholipase A2 in LDL releases reactive intermediates, which modify lysine residues in the adjacent apo-lipoprotein B (ApoB), thereby inhibiting the binding of LDL to its cognate receptor, while promoting LDL recognition by macrophage scavenger receptors (Steinbrecher et al., 1987).

(4) *Migration and proliferation of SMC to intima.* Convergent, activated platelets, macrophages, and vascular endothelial cells release cytokines that cause proliferation and migration of SMC to the intima (Wu et al., 2001).

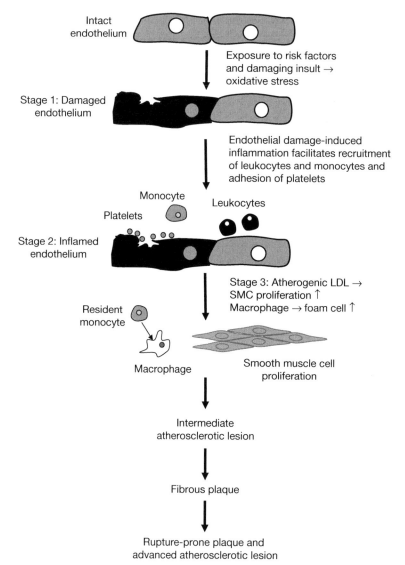

Figure 35.1 Injury to the endothelium is the cornerstone to the hypothesis, which is due to several factors like hyperlipidemia, infectious agents, and stress. The injured endothelium becomes leaky, permeable, and express adhesion molecules like intercellular adhesion molecule and VCAM. The inflammation of endothelium results in recruitment of inflammatory cells like monocytes that adhere to endothelium with adhesion molecules and migrate to subendothelium. The oxidized LDL particles are taken by monocyte-derived macrophages and results in initial fatty streak formation, which transforms into fatty fibrous plaque, which is a mixture of inflammatory, smooth muscle cells, and debris. The rupture of fibrous plaque results in thrombus formation with severe complications of CHD.

(5) *Establishment of fibrous plaques and rupture-prone advanced atherosclerotic lesions.* The atheroma is further modified by the accumulation of collagen and proteoglycans synthesized by SMC, ultimately converting the fatty streak into mature fibrous lesions (Ross, 1999; Wu et al., 2001), marked by connective tissue-rich fibrous cap, and a central core endowed with lipid-laden cells and fatty debris. Moreover, during progression of atherosclerotic lesions, death of the endothelial cells, macrophages, and SMC occur by apoptosis, promoting the disintegration of foam cells and loss of SMC and destabilizing the lipid-rich core to form the fibrous cap (Schaar et al., 2004). Importantly, the fibrous cap is fragile and rupture-prone and is the most common cause of coronary artery thrombosis, which far exceeds lumen narrowing by atherosclerotic plaque as the clinical contribution and manifestations of the atherosclerotic arterial disease. Notably, plaque rupture accounts for 76% of all fatal heart attacks caused by coronary thrombosis, which is responsible for the majority of acute ischemic syndromes – unstable angina, acute myocardial infarction, and sudden death (Falk, 2004, 2006). Factors capable of triggering the rupture of plaques include strenuous physical activity, severe emotional trauma, exposure to cocaine, and marijuana (Willich et al., 1993).

3. CARDIOMYOCYTE REGENERATION

3.1 Injury and Repair

Ischemic heart diseases are among the leading causes of death. Following injury, the natural compensatory processes of the damaged heart are limited to hypertrophy of the remaining cardiomyocytes and replacement of necrotic regions with fibrotic scar tissue. The cardiac function is lost at the site of injury. Cardiac scarring and loss of contractile tissue cause arrhythmias, dilation, and heart failure and contribute significantly to morbidity and mortality (Rosamond et al., 2008). The underlying cause of CHD is due to loss of cardiomyocytes accompanied by functional derangements in contraction and relaxation (Pasumarthi and Field, 2002). The capacity of the heart to regenerate functional myocardium is limited or absent; since as noted, the cardiomyocytes *in vivo* lose the ability to proliferate and exit cell cycle shortly after birth (Pasumarthi and Field, 2002).

3.2 Compromised Ability to Undergo Cell Division in Mammalian Cardiomyocytes

In mammals, heart growth is based on increase in cell size (hypertrophy) in response to increase in cardiac load. It is estimated that only 0.01% of adult cardiomyocytes in the human heart are capable of cell division following myocardial infarction (Borchardt and Braun, 2007). The transition from proliferation to hypertrophy is characterized by maturation of contractile apparatus and occurs without the completion of cytokinesis. However, it was observed in 1977 that a limited percentage of adult mammalian cardiomyocytes can traverse all phases of mitotic cycle. The molecular and cellular mechanisms that contribute to the exit of mammalian cardiomyocytes from cell cycle in concert with the arrest of proliferation have not been definitively elucidated.

3.3 Cell Cycle Control

The switch in the growth potential of cardiomyocytes from a proliferative cell phenotype to a hypertrophy phenotype occurs at different stages of development in different species. In mice, it occurs at or shortly after birth, whereas in rats, it occurs between 3 and 4 days postnatally. It is estimated that in 85% of adult rats, cardiomyocytes nuclei are arrested in G_0/G_1 phases of cell cycle with the remaining nuclei being blocked in G_2/M phase. In humans, cardiomyocytes essentially no longer possess the capacity for cell division after 7 months of age (Li et al., 1996).

A correlation has been demonstrated to exist between the proliferative capacity of cardiomyocytes and expression of cell cycle regulatory molecules. Positive regulators like cyclins, cyclin-dependent kinases, and majority of a transcription factor involved in cell cycle control (E2F) are mostly downregulated in adult cardiomyocytes (Brooks et al., 1997). The negative regulators of cell cycle progression like p21, p27, and E2F are robustly expressed in cell cycle-arrested cardiomyocytes. Partial reactivation of the cell cycle occurs in adult myocytes during growth by hypertrophy; a significant proportion of cells progresses through the G_1/S transition and undergoes replication but becomes arrested in G_2/M phase (Poolman and Brooks, 1998). Injury of cardiomyocytes is accompanied by downregulation of cell cycle inhibitors like p21 and p27 and upregulation of cell cycle perpetuating factors like proliferating cell nuclear antigen (PCNA) and cyclin-dependent kinase (CDK)-1: cyclin complexes. Induction of DNA synthesis after injury results in endoreplication or polynucleation; thus, the detection of mitotic figures and expressed cell cycle genes may not be a definitive proof for cardiomyocyte cell division. In end-stage heart failure in humans, the expressions of p21 and p27 are downregulated and p57 is upregulated and, despite reverting to the fetal pattern of expression of CDK inhibitors, cardiomyocyte hypertrophy but not proliferation is observed (Brodsky et al., 1991).

4. SOY PHYTOCHEMICALS AND CARDIOPROTECTION

Phytochemicals are present naturally in plants including soy and soy products, which are widely consumed by humans as whole soybeans, tofu, tempeh, and soy milk. Among the most extensively studied soy phytochemicals are isoflavones, which are mainly derived from soy and soy-based foods in the human diet (Hanson et al., 2006; Xiao, 2008). The principal soy isoflavones are daidzein, genistein, and glycitein and their glycoside conjugates including 7-O-glucosides, 6-O-acetyl, and 6-O-malonyl-7-O-glucosides. After ingestion of isoflavone-rich foods, the isoflavone glycosides undergo deglycosylation (Gee et al., 1998) by enzymes located in the small intestinal brush border (lactose phlorizin hydrolase) and in enterocytes (cytosolic β-glucosidases), releasing aglycones daidzein and genistein, which are further converted to other metabolites including equol or are conjugated with glucuronic acid and sulfate by hepatic enzymes. Isoflavones are predominantly conjugated with glucuronides and to a lesser extent with sulfates (Coward et al., 1996). These conjugates are more readily transported in the blood and excreted in bile or urine than parent aglycone. The absorption of isoflavones by gastrointestinal mucosa may partly depend on their relative hydrophobicity and hydrophilicity. The most readily absorbed isoflavones are aglycones. Limited studies have shown that the time to attain peak plasma concentrations after ingesting aglycones is 4–7 h, whereas it is 8–11 h when the glycoside conjugates are ingested. This shift indicates that the rate-limiting step for absorption is initial hydrolysis of sugar moiety (Setchell et al., 2001). Ingestion of 50 mg of isoflavones per day in human adults yields plasma concentrations ranging from 50 to 800 ng ml^{-1}. Soy food processing appears to influence isoflavone bioavailability. The urinary isoflavone excretion was similar in 17 males consuming either 112 g of fermented soy tempeh or 125 g of unfermented soybean pieces for 9 days each. Urinary recovery of daidzein and genistein was higher when the subjects consumed fermented tempeh diet (9.7+0.6 and 1.9+0.1%) than when they consumed unfermented soy diet (5.7+0.6 and 1.3+0.1%), suggesting that isoflavone aglycones in fermented foods are more bioavailable (Hutchins et al., 1995). The metabolism of isoflavones is variable among individuals and influenced by components of the diet.

4.1 Evidence of Cardioprotection by Soy Consumption

4.1.1 Epidemiological studies

Several countries including the United States have approved the intake of soy protein as a measure to reduce the levels of cholesterol. Of note, the mean daily intake of soy protein is 30 g in Japan, 20 g in Korea, 7 g in Hong Kong, 8 g in China, and less than 1 g in the United States. The first study was conducted as early as 1967 by Hodges and coworkers, which showed that the intake of 100 g day^{-1} of isolated soy protein may reduce the mean cholesterol levels by >2.5 mmol l^{-1} in hypercholesterolemic men (Hodges et al., 1967). Several additional human studies were conducted in the ensuing years between 1977 and 1994. In a meta-analysis of 38 controlled studies with 30 involving hypercholesterolemic subjects, it was observed that the mean intake of 47 g day^{-1} of soy protein resulted in significant reduction in total cholesterol by 9.3%, LDL cholesterol by 12.9%, and triglycerides by 10.5% without affecting the high–density lipoprotein (HDL) levels (Anderson et al., 1995). The daily intake of 25 g of soy protein and 101 mg of aglycone isoflavones repressed the levels of LDL cholesterol and ApoB levels by 11% and 8% and lowered the systolic and diastolic blood pressures by 9.9% and 6.8% in hypertensive women (Welty et al., 2007).

The effect of soy protein with varying levels of isoflavones on lipids has been studied in young men. Thirty-five males who consumed milk protein isolate, low-isoflavone soy protein isolate, and high-isoflavone soy protein isolate were analyzed. Total, LDL, HDL, triacylglycerols, apoB, and C-reactive protein were measured in serum. The ratios of total to HDL cholesterol, LDL to HDL cholesterol, and apoB were significantly lower in the group consuming both soy protein isoflavone diets than milk protein. These results demonstrate that regardless of the isoflavone content, serum lipids were reduced in a direction beneficial for cardiovascular disease risk in healthy young men (McVeigh et al., 2006). Thorp and coworkers have examined the effect of soy protein, isoflavones, and equol in the hypocholesterolemic effects of soy foods. Results of their studies show that consumption of 24 g of soy protein per day had no significant effect on plasma LDL cholesterol regardless of its equol-producing status (Thorp et al., 2008).

A study to investigate the effect of soy on *in vivo* biomarkers of lipid peroxidation and resistance of LDL to oxidation has been studied in 24 subjects. F(2)-isoprostane, a biomarker of *in vivo* lipid peroxidation, and resistance of LDL to copper in induced oxidation were measured. The 8-Epi-prostaglandin F2-α was lower after high-isoflavone treatment than after low-isoflavone treatment (326 ± 32 and 405 ± 50 ng l^{-1}, respectively). Lag time for copper-induced LDL oxidation was also longer (48 ± 2.4 and 44 ± 1.9 min, respectively). This suggests that isoflavones reduce lipid peroxidation *in vivo* and increased the resistance of LDL to oxidation (Wiseman et al., 2000).

4.1.2 Animal studies

Several studies using animal models provide evidence for a role of soy in the prevention of atherosclerosis and subsequent CHD. A 2-month study was conducted in 20 rabbits with diets containing 1% cholesterol and 27% casein or 27% soy protein isolate. Results showed that soy protein, in comparison with casein, decreased lipid peroxides, cholesterol, and triglyceride content of atherogenic lipoproteins (VLDL, LDL) (Damasceno et al., 2001). To test whether genistein affects atherosclerosis, rabbits challenged a hypercholesterolemic diet for periods of 4 months were continuously exposed to the same diet for an additional 4.5 months, with and without dietary supplementation of genistein. Dietary fortification with genistein was found to suppress progression of atherogenesis, marked by stabilization of the lesions (Lee et al., 2004). The antiatherosclerotic effects of isoflavones have also been studied in rhesus monkeys, comparing a diet that contained soy protein devoid of isoflavones (by extraction, SPI−) with a diet fortified with isoflavone-containing soy protein (SPI+), and additionally a casein-containing diet. Animals fed the three diets were evaluated regarding the prevalence of coronary artery disease. The results showed atherosclerotic lesions in 73% of casein-fed, 64% of (SPI−)-exposed, and 45% of (SPI+)-fed groups, respectively. Moreover, the average plaque area of 0.02 mm was least in the group given the (SPI+) diet, compared with 0.06 mm in (SPI−) group and 0.13 mm in casein-fed group, clearly showing that soy isoflavones are antiatherosclerotic (Anthony et al., 1998). Addition of soy genistein in diets to hypertensive rats restores aortic endothelial NOS levels, alleviates hypertension, and improves aortic wall thickness. Genistein for 6 weeks lowered blood pressure and the blood pressure-lowering effect of genistein was still significant at 6 weeks after genistein withdrawal from the diet (Si and Liu, 2008).

4.1.3 In vitro *studies*

Several studies indicate that soy phytoestrogens have cardioprotective properties in human cell lines. Human aortic endothelial cells and human umbilical vein endothelial cells when treated with soy genistein and other soy phytochemicals show enhanced NOS and elevated nitric oxide synthesis and improved vascular function (Chung et al., 2008; Si and Liu, 2008).

4.2 Cardioprotective Properties and Mechanisms

According to US Food and Drug Administration and American Heart Association, daily consumption of above 25 g of soy protein reduces the risk of heart disease (Sacks et al., 2006). Several risk factors of heart diseases like hyperlipidemia, atherosclerotic plaque formation, blood pressure, and lipid peroxidation have been shown to respond positively to intake of soy products. Research studies suggest that the high consumption of soy foods may be one of the reasons possibly explaining the low risk of CHD in Asian populations (Zhang et al., 2003).

Several mechanisms have been proposed by which soy protein or isoflavones alleviate the risk factors of CHD. These include lowering of blood cholesterol levels and atherosclerosis-related events by (1) increased excretion of bile acids that in turn shift cholesterol to bile acid synthesis, and increase the LDL receptor expression (Potter, 1995); (2) altering regulation of plasma insulin, glucagon, and thyroid hormone concentrations (Forsythe, 1990); (3) preventing the development of atherosclerosis and subsequent CHD, through inhibition of platelet-derived growth factor, suppression of SMC proliferation, and modulation of platelet activity and function (Helmeste and Tang, 1995); (4) suppression of the oxidation of LDL (Hwang et al., 2000), thereby decreasing the formation of atherosclerotic plaques and cardiovascular disease; and (5) modulating other risk factors of heart disease like blood pressure, arterial compliance, and vascular reactivity (Figure 35.2).

When soy was consumed >25 g per day, systolic blood pressure and diastolic blood pressure was observed to be 1.9 and 0.9 mm Hg lower in women whose intake of soy protein is <2.5 g day^{-1} (Yang et al., 2005). Antihypertensive potential of soy milk was studied in 40 men and women with mild to moderate hypertension who consumed 500 ml of soy milk and cow milk. Systolic blood pressure was lowered by 18.4+10.7 mm Hg compared with 1.4+7.2 mm Hg in cow milk group. Diastolic blood pressure was lowered by 15.9+9.8 mm Hg compared with 3.7+5.0 mm Hg in cow milk group (Rivas et al., 2002). Arterial compliance, considered one of the important risk factor for pathogenesis of hypertension and arterial elasticity, has shown 26% improvement when 45 mg of soy

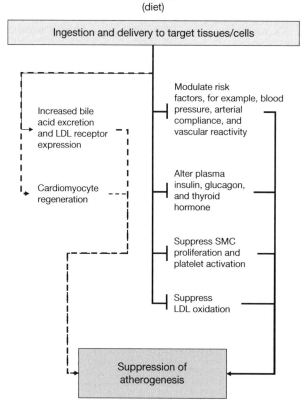

Figure 35.2 Multiple proposed mechanisms by which soy consumed in the diet act to suppress atherogenesis.

genistein was taken for 10 weeks in perimenopausal and menopausal women (Honore et al., 1997).

5. ROLE OF SOY ISOFLAVONES IN CONTROL OF CARDIOMYOCYTE PROLIFERATION, CELL CYCLE REENTRY, AND REGENERATION

Impairment of the circulatory vasculature leading to chronic heart failure (CHF) is a significant contributor to morbidity and mortality of CHD (Aranda et al., 2009). Formidable challenges and obstacles remain in the restoration of function to the damaged heart resulting from CHF. Even with surgical advances, improved use of mechanical assistance devices, availability and timely administration of drugs, and organ transplantation, a high percentage of CHF patients die within years of initial diagnosis. Currently available therapies for CHF are insufficiently specific and may have untoward side effects. Thus, alternative, preferably, diet-based agents with CHF preventative and/or therapeutic potentials are urgently needed. A better understanding of the beneficial effects of identified agents is also imperative.

The devastating effects of heart failure are in part attributed to the destruction of heart muscle cells known as cardiomyocytes, which constitute the bulk of the ventricle wall. Cardiomyocytes play an integral role in normal and pathophysiological growth responses in the cardiovascular system and are considered terminally differentiated shortly after formation of the heart. Cardiomyocytes are known to adapt to the stress of intermittent increased hemodynamic load by undergoing hypertrophy; however, when sustained, excessive workload increases are placed on the heart, such as in conditions of induced and essential hypertension and myocardial infarction, pathological hypertrophy might ensue that ultimately leads to the demise of cardiomyocytes, and heart failure.

The long-held scientific view that cardiomyocytes are restricted from entry into cell replication and mitosis in mammals, that is, totally devoid of regeneration capabilities, has been a limiting factor in the development of strategies and drugs to combat CHF and related myocardial pathologies. Moreover, impaired progenitor cell activity contributes to age-dependent endothelial cell dysfunction (Goldspink et al., 2003). Accordingly, prevention of cardiomyocyte cell death and discovery of ways to reactivate their silenced regeneration state, for example, by inducing the reentry into cell cycling, are both considered novel approaches since they are expected to enlarge the pool of living cells as well as afford the replacement of dead or dysfunctional cells, thereby preserving and restoring the pumping activity of weakened heart and potentially reducing the incidence of CHF. The same considerations should apply to discovering ways of bolstering progenitor cell activity in age-related decline in endothelial cell function.

Cardiomyocytes withdraw from the cell cycle in the early neonatal period, rendering the adult heart incapable to regenerate after injury. Engel and coworkers have reported the establishment of a cell-free system that enables investigation of the control of cell cycle reentry and to specifically address whether nuclei from terminally differentiated cardiomyocytes can be stimulated to reenter S phase (Engel et al., 1999). Incubation of cardiomyocyte nuclei with nuclei and cytoplasmic extract of synchronized H9c2 muscle cells or cardiac nonmyocytes, combined with assays of DNA synthesis based on biotinylated-dUTP incorporation and PCNA expression and localization, showed that nuclei and cytoplasmic extract from S-phase H9c2 cells but not from H9c2 myotubes induced DNA synthesis in 92% of neonatal cardiomyocyte nuclei. These results demonstrate that postmitotic ventricular myocyte nuclei are responsive to stimuli derived from S-phase cells and can thus bypass the cell cycle block (Engel et al., 1999).

5.1 Inhibition of p38 MAPK

Further studies revealed that control of the cell cycle of cardiomyocytes involves the p38 MAPK gene family, which comprises four genes encoding the p38 MAPK isoforms, respectively, p38α, p38β, p38δ, and p38γ. The p38α and p38β are present ubiquitously in adult tissues, while p38δ is expressed mainly in lung, kidney, and pancreas and p38γ mainly occurs in skeletal muscle (Li et al., 1996). The p38 pathway has an implicated role in the heart, particularly in cardiac gene regulation, myocyte hypertrophy, inflammatory response, cardiomyocyte proliferation, and cell death. The activities of the p38 MAPK controls both cell cycle entry and G_2/M phase transition by inhibiting transcription of cyclin D1 and CD25 phosphatase activity. Engel and coworkers showed that one mechanism controlling the proliferation and cell cycle regulation in mammalian cardiomyocytes involves negative regulation of p38 activity (Engel, 2005; Engel et al., 2005). Thus, inhibition of p38 has been shown to induce mitosis and cytokinesis in neonatal cardiomyocyte cultures. Further, the effect of p38 inhibition on cardiomyocyte cell cycle is enhanced significantly by costimulation with growth factors such as fibroblast growth factor and interleukin (Engel, 2005). In recent study, the FGF1/p38 MAP kinase inhibitor (FGF1/p38i) treatment in 8- to 10-week-old rats after acute myocardial infarction increases cardiomyocyte mitosis. The FGF1/p38i treatment showed the best outcome regarding preservation of cardiac structure and function. It improves the capillary density >40% at 3 months after injury. Cardiac function as analyzed by echocardiography after 4 weeks of FGF1/p38i showed signs of improvement. Specifically, FGF1/p38i improved the percentage of left ventricular fractional shortening at day 1 and 3 months, but p38i alone improved percentage of left ventricular fractional shortening only at day 1. It preserved the wall thickness and improved cardiac function and reduced the volume of scar (Engel et al., 2006). Huang and coworkers showed that in human prostate cancer cell lines, soy phytochemical genistein inhibited the p38 MAPK activation by inhibiting transforming growth factor-β and lowering the matrix metalloprotein-2 activity, which plays a role in destroying extracellular matrix proteins required for cell invasion and prostate cancer cell metastasis. Further, genistein has been reported to inhibit the p38 MAPK-dependent leukotriene synthesis by eosinophil in asthma patients, in a concentration-dependent manner with significant inhibition at 100 nm and higher (Kalhan et al., 2008).

Taken together, the above studies indicate that p38 MAPK is a key negative regulator of the cardiomyocyte proliferation and play a role in cardiomyocyte cell cycle exit. Soy phytochemical genistein, which inhibits the p38 pathway in human prostate cancer cell lines and eosinophils, can be tested in cardiomyocytes on whether it can circumvent the restrictive potential of the cardiomyocytes by inhibiting the negative regulator of its proliferation.

5.2 Induction of Telomerase Activity

Telomerase is an enzyme that adds specific DNA sequence repeats (TTAGGG) to the end of DNA of eukaryotic chromosomes. It has reverse transcriptase activity that is responsible for the extension of telomeric DNA. The telomerase complex is composed of telomerase reverse transcriptase (TERT), telomerase RNA (TERC), telomerase associated protein 1, and chaperone proteins (p23 and HSP 90) (Cong et al., 2002). Because telomerase is expressed in germ line cells and cancer cell lines but not expressed in normal somatic cells, it is thought to contribute to the progressive loss of telomeres with each cell division. Studies by Leri and coworkers suggest that telomere shortening and telomerase dysfunction may contribute to some of the pathologies associated with human aging, including the aging heart and demise of cardiomyocytes (Leri et al., 2003). Telomerase ablation affects cardiomyocyte size, number, proliferative potential, and death, as evidenced by experiments comparing cardiac function using G2 and G5 (second- and fifth-generation) telomerase knockout mice (Terc−/−) in comparison with wild-type (WT) mice. When cardiomyocyte proliferation was measured by bromodeoxyuridine (Brdu) and Ki67 staining, it was shown that cardiomyocyte replication was reduced in G2 and G5 Terc−/− mice hearts. Cell growth impairment was twofold higher in G5 mice and death by apoptosis was 67% and 39% higher in G5-mice compared with WT and G2-mice. Functional abnormalities like severe left ventricular failure and diastolic wall stress were observed in G5 Terc−/− mice, but not in G2 Terc−/−, suggesting that the dysfunctional features were associated with critical telomere shortening in G5 Terc−/− cardiomyocytes rather than telomerase deficiency. Taken as a whole, these studies support the notion that the impaired cardiomyocyte regeneration coupled with cardiomyocyte death as a consequence of telomerase deficiency and telomere shortening may lead to establishment of pathological conditions, and further suggest that telomere shortening with increasing age in human heart could be a biological determinant of heart failure in the elderly (Leri et al., 2003). Additional studies by Hidemasa and coworkers showed that cardioprotection is associated with TERT of telomerase. Specifically, prevention or disruption of the downregulation of TERT is accompanied by a delay in timing of cardiac cell cycle exit and appearance of the postmitotic phenotype, suggesting that TERT protects cardiomyocytes from undergoing apoptosis.

Soy phytochemical genistein has been shown to stimulate as well as inhibit the telomerase activity. Studies by Banerjee and coworkers showed that at physiological doses, genistein acts to enhance the telomerase activity and in turn the proliferation of human prostate cancer cell lines (Chau et al., 2007). Moreover, the positive stimulatory effect of genistein on telomerase is mediated by activation of STAT3 via stimulation of binding of STAT3 to the promoter elements of telomerase, specifically targeting the hTERT component that contains the reverse transcriptase (Chau et al., 2007). Thus, it may be suggested that restoration of telomerase in cardiomyocytes, in concert with exposure to soy phytochemicals, such as genistein at physiologically relevant concentrations, may confer protection on the heart by promoting and facilitating regeneration of cardiomyocytes.

6. CONCLUSION AND FUTURE STUDIES

In conclusion, the seemingly timeless biological adage that the majority of human cells, once reached specialization status, are permanently banned from cell division or acquisition of a different phenotype is, in recent years, rapidly being transformed on two fronts: first, through the discovery of endowed innate stem cells, damaged differentiated cells can now be recreated, replaced, and expanded; second, the apparent irrevocable dormant, locked-down state of specialized cells can be cued to reenter the precise and dynamically regulated process of cycling, proliferation, and division. These features underlying tissue/cell regeneration have been realized and accepted in cardiovascular and heart research, thus offering increasingly larger windows of hope that disease of the heart, involving an organ regarded absolutely refractory to regeneration, may no longer be considered the most common birth defect in humans but rather is open to therapeutic intervention, rejuvenation, and healing.

Soy phytochemicals fulfill at least several key aspects required for cardiomyocyte replication and progression in the new niche of the regenerating heart (Figure 35.3). *First*, the elegant studies of Engel and Keating pioneered the thesis that the restrictive ability of cardiomyocytes to undergo proliferation and hence regeneration may be readily reversed by inhibiting an enzyme known as p38 MAP kinase, which normally suppresses cardiomyocyte replication (Engel, 2005; Engel et al., 1999, 2006). Genistein, an extensively studied soy phytochemical, has been reported to inhibit p38 MAPK (Huang et al., 2005). *Second*, improvements in both cardiomyocyte proliferation and heart function are

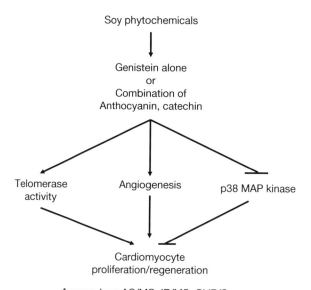

Figure 35.3 Soy phytochemicals are hypothesized to induce cardiomyocyte regeneration by (i) activating telomerase, (ii) inhibiting p38 MAP kinase, and (iii) inducing angiogenesis. Collectively, they relieve the proliferation restriction imposed on cardiomyocytes, by promoting and facilitating their recommitment to cell growth and regeneration. We propose to use AC–MS, IP–MS, and ChiP–Seq, to study soy phytochemical-induced cardiomyocyte regeneration.

predicated on cardiomyocyte replication occurring in concomitance with angiogenesis to ensure supply of nutrients and oxygen; soy phytochemicals have demonstrated ability to induce angiogenesis (Banerjee et al., 2008). *Third*, the soy phytochemical genistein has been shown to enhance telomerase activity (Chau et al., 2007), a key enzyme in cell and tissue regeneration.

Future studies should be focused on testing several aspects of the above, specifically, whether telomerase in cardiomyocytes can be activated by genistein and other phytochemicals present in soy, and as corroboration, whether control of telomerase is more effective with grouped soy-derived phytochemicals, and moreover, whether replicative restriction in cardiomyocytes can be lifted by genistein and other soy phytochemicals, and whether control of cell replication will respond better to grouped soy phytochemicals, compared with single soy phytochemicals. Additionally, the ability of soy phytochemicals to regulate cardiomyocyte regeneration in animal studies must also be considered. One might envisage proposing experimental approaches integrating an experimental approach in which affinity chromatography is coupled with mass spectrometry (AC–MS), an experimental approach in which immunoprecipitation is combined with mass spectrometry to identify specific genes (IP–MS), an experimental approach involving chromatin immunoprecipitation followed by sequencing of immunoprecipitated genes (ChiP–Seq), and MA-Sig analysis, with the overall objective of discovering and identifying triggers and activators/coregulators that differentiate progenitor cells into cardiomyocytes (Figure 35.3). A better understanding of whether and how soy phytochemicals mediate cardiomyocyte regeneration may lead to diet-based CHD prevention and management strategies.

ACKNOWLEDGMENTS

Studies in this chapter were supported in part by the Intramural Sponsored Research Program of New York Medical College and by Phillip Morris USA Inc. and Phillip Morris International (to J. M. W.).

REFERENCES

Anderson, J.W., Johnstone, B.M., Cook-Newell, M.E., 1995. Meta-analysis of the effects of soy protein intake on serum lipids. The New England Journal of Medicine 333, 276–282.

Anthony, M.S., Clarkson, T.B., Williams, J.K., 1998. Effects of soy isoflavones on atherosclerosis: potential mechanisms. The American Journal of Clinical Nutrition 68, 1390S–1393S.

Aranda Jr., J.M., Johnson, J.W., Conti, J.B., 2009. Current trends in heart failure readmission rates: analysis of Medicare data. Clinical Cardiology 32, 47–52.

Banerjee, S., Li, Y., Wang, Z., Sarkar, F.H., 2008. Multi-targeted therapy of cancer by genistein. Cancer Letters 269, 226–242.

Borchardt, T., Braun, T., 2007. Cardiovascular regeneration in non-mammalian model systems: what are the differences between newts and man? Thrombosis and Haemostasis 98, 311–318.

Brodsky, V., Chernyaev, A.L., Vasilyeva, I.A., 1991. Variability of the cardiomyocyte ploidy in normal human hearts. Virchows Archiv. B, Cell Pathology Including Molecular Pathology 61, 289–294.

Brooks, G., Poolman, R.A., McGill, C.J., Li, J.M., 1997. Expression and activities of cyclins and cyclin-dependent kinases in developing rat ventricular myocytes. Journal of Molecular and Cellular Cardiology 29, 2261–2271.

Chau, M.N., El Touny, L.H., Jagadeesh, S., Banerjee, P.P., 2007. Physiologically achievable concentrations of genistein enhance telomerase activity in prostate cancer cells via the activation of STAT3. Carcinogenesis 28, 2282–2290.

Chien, K.R., Domian, I.J., Parker, K.K., 2008. Cardiogenesis and the complex biology of regenerative cardiovascular medicine. Science 322, 1494–1497.

Chung, J.E., Kim, S.Y., Jo, H.H., et al., 2008. Antioxidant effects of equol on bovine aortic endothelial cells. Biochemical and Biophysical Research Communications 375, 420–424.

Cong, Y.S., Wright, W.E., Shay, J.W., 2002. Human telomerase and its regulation. Microbiology and Molecular Biology Reviews 66, 407–425 Table of contents.

Coward, L., Kirk, M., Albin, N., Barnes, S., 1996. Analysis of plasma isoflavones by reversed-phase HPLC-multiple reaction ion monitoring-mass spectrometry. Clinica Chimica Acta 247, 121–142.

Damasceno, N.R., Gidlund, M.A., Goto, H., Dias, C.T., Okawabata, F.S., Abdalla, D.S., 2001. Casein and soy protein isolate in experimental atherosclerosis: influence on hyperlipidemia and lipoprotein oxidation. Annals of Nutrition and Metabolism 45, 38–46.

Engel, F.B., 2005. Cardiomyocyte proliferation: a platform for mammalian cardiac repair. Cell Cycle 4, 1360–1363.

Engel, F.B., Hauck, L., Cardoso, M.C., Leonhardt, H., Dietz, R., von Harsdorf, R., 1999. A mammalian myocardial cell-free system to study cell cycle reentry in terminally differentiated cardiomyocytes. Circulation Research 85, 294–301.

Engel, F.B., Hsieh, P.C., Lee, R.T., Keating, M.T., 2006. FGF1/p38 MAP kinase inhibitor therapy induces cardiomyocyte mitosis, reduces scarring, and rescues function after myocardial infarction. Proceedings of the National Academy of Sciences of the United States of America 103, 15546–15551.

Engel, F.B., Schebesta, M., Duong, M.T., et al., 2005. p38 MAP kinase inhibition enables proliferation of adult mammalian cardiomyocytes. Genes & Development 19, 1175–1187.

Falk, E., 2004. Widespread targets for friendly fire in acute coronary syndromes. Circulation 110, 4–6.

Falk, E., 2006. Pathogenesis of atherosclerosis. Journal of the American College of Cardiology 47, C7–C12.

Forsythe 3rd., W.A., 1990. Dietary proteins, cholesterol and thyroxine: a proposed mechanism. Journal of Nutritional Science and Vitaminology 36 (supplement 2), S101–S104.

Gee, J.M., Dupont, M.S., Rhodes, M.J., Johnson, I.T., 1998. Quercetin glucosides interact with the intestinal glucose transport pathway. Free Radical Biology & Medicine 25, 19–25.

Glass, C.K., Witztum, J.L., 2001. Atherosclerosis. The road ahead. Cell 104, 503–516.

Goldspink, D.F., Burniston, J.G., Tan, L.B., 2003. Cardiomyocyte death and the ageing and failing heart. Experimental Physiology 88, 447–458.

Hanson, L.N., Engelman, H.M., Alekel, D.L., Schalinske, K.L., Kohut, M.L., Reddy, M.B., 2006. Effects of soy isoflavones and phytate on homocysteine, C-reactive protein, and iron status in postmenopausal women. The American Journal of Clinical Nutrition 84, 774–780.

Haverslag, R., Pasterkamp, G., Hoefer, I.E., 2008. Targeting adhesion molecules in cardiovascular disorders. Cardiovascular & Hematological Disorders Drug Targets 8, 252–260.

Helmeste, D.M., Tang, S.W., 1995. Tyrosine kinase inhibitors regulate serotonin uptake in platelets. European Journal of Pharmacology 280, R5–R7.

Hodges, R.E., Krehl, W.A., Stone, D.B., Lopez, A., 1967. Dietary carbohydrates and low cholesterol diets: effects on serum lipids on man. The American Journal of Clinical Nutrition 20, 198–208.

Honore, E.K., Williams, J.K., Anthony, M.S., Clarkson, T.B., 1997. Soy isoflavones enhance coronary vascular reactivity in atherosclerotic female macaques. Fertility and Sterility 67, 148–154.

Huang, X., Chen, S., Xu, L., et al., 2005. Genistein inhibits p38 map kinase activation, matrix metalloproteinase type 2, and cell invasion in human prostate epithelial cells. Cancer Research 65, 3470–3478.

Hutchins, A.M., Slavin, J.L., Lampe, J.W., 1995. Urinary isoflavonoid phytoestrogen and lignan excretion after consumption of fermented and unfermented soy products. Journal of the American Dietetic Association 95, 545–551.

Hwang, J., Sevanian, A., Hodis, H.N., Ursini, F., 2000. Synergistic inhibition of LDL oxidation by phytoestrogens and ascorbic acid. Free Radical Biology & Medicine 29, 79–89.

Kalhan, R., Smith, L.J., Nlend, M.C., Nair, A., Hixon, J.L., Sporn, P.H., 2008. A mechanism of benefit of soy genistein in asthma: inhibition of eosinophil p38-dependent leukotriene synthesis. Clinical and Experimental Allergy 38, 103–112.

Lee, C.S., Kwon, S.J., Na, S.Y., Lim, S.P., Lee, J.H., 2004. Genistein supplementation inhibits atherosclerosis with stabilization of the lesions in hypercholesterolemic rabbits. Journal of Korean Medical Science 19, 656–661.

Leri, A., Franco, S., Zacheo, A., et al., 2003. Ablation of telomerase and telomere loss leads to cardiac dilatation and heart failure associated with p53 upregulation. The EMBO Journal 22, 131–139.

Li, F., Wang, X., Capasso, J.M., Gerdes, A.M., 1996. Rapid transition of cardiac myocytes from hyperplasia to hypertrophy during postnatal development. Journal of Molecular and Cellular Cardiology 28, 1737–1746.

McVeigh, B.L., Dillingham, B.L., Lampe, J.W., Duncan, A.M., 2006. Effect of soy protein varying in isoflavone content on serum lipids in healthy young men. The American Journal of Clinical Nutrition 83, 244–251.

Mink, P.J., Scrafford, C.G., Barraj, L.M., et al., 2007. Flavonoid intake and cardiovascular disease mortality: a prospective study in postmenopausal women. The American Journal of Clinical Nutrition 85, 895–909.

Pasumarthi, K.B., Field, L.J., 2002. Cardiomyocyte cell cycle regulation. Circulation Research 90, 1044–1054.

Poolman, R.A., Brooks, G., 1998. Expressions and activities of cell cycle regulatory molecules during the transition from myocyte hyperplasia to hypertrophy. Journal of Molecular and Cellular Cardiology 30, 2121–2135.

Potter, S.M., 1995. Overview of proposed mechanisms for the hypocholesterolemic effect of soy. Journal of Nutrition 125, 606S–611S.

Rankin, S.M., Parthasarathy, S., Steinberg, D., 1991. Evidence for a dominant role of lipoxygenase(s) in the oxidation of LDL by mouse peritoneal macrophages. Journal of Lipid Research 32, 449–456.

Rivas, M., Garay, R.P., Escanero, J.F., Cia Jr., P., Cia, P., Alda, J.O., 2002. Soy milk lowers blood pressure in men and women with mild to moderate essential hypertension. Journal of Nutrition 132, 1900–1902.

Rosamond, W., Flegal, K., Furie, K., et al., 2008. Heart disease and stroke statistics – 2008 update: a report from the American Heart Association Statistics Committee and Stroke Statistics Subcommittee. Circulation 117, e25–e146.

Ross, R., 1999. Atherosclerosis – an inflammatory disease. The New England Journal of Medicine 340, 115–126.

Ross, R., Glomset, J.A., 1976a. The pathogenesis of atherosclerosis (first of two parts). The New England Journal of Medicine 295, 369–377.

Ross, R., Glomset, J.A., 1976b. The pathogenesis of atherosclerosis (second of two parts). The New England Journal of Medicine 295, 420–425.

Sacks, F.M., Lichtenstein, A., van Horn, L., Harris, W., Kris-Etherton, P., Winston, M., 2006. Soy protein, isoflavones, and cardiovascular health: an American Heart Association Science Advisory for professionals from the Nutrition Committee. Circulation 113, 1034–1044.

Schaar, J.A., Muller, J.E., Falk, E., et al., 2004. Terminology for high-risk and vulnerable coronary artery plaques. Report of a meeting on the vulnerable plaque, June 17 and 18, 2003, Santorini, Greece. European Heart Journal 25, 1077–1082.

Setchell, K.D., Brown, N.M., Desai, P., et al., 2001. Bioavailability of pure isoflavones in healthy humans and analysis of commercial soy isoflavone supplements. Journal of Nutrition 131, 1362S–1375S.

Si, H., Liu, D., 2008. Genistein, a soy phytoestrogen, upregulates the expression of human endothelial nitric oxide synthase and lowers blood pressure in spontaneously hypertensive rats. Journal of Nutrition 138, 297–304.

Steinberg, F.M., 2007. Soybeans or soymilk: does it make a difference for cardiovascular protection? Does it even matter? The American Journal of Clinical Nutrition 85, 927–928.

Steinbrecher, U.P., Witztum, J.L., Parthasarathy, S., Steinberg, D., 1987. Decrease in reactive amino groups during oxidation or endothelial cell modification of LDL. Correlation with changes in receptor-mediated catabolism. Arteriosclerosis 7, 135–143.

Thorp, A.A., Howe, P.R., Mori, T.A., et al., 2008. Soy food consumption does not lower LDL cholesterol in either equol or nonequol producers. The American Journal of Clinical Nutrition 88, 298–304.

Welty, F.K., Lee, K.S., Lew, N.S., Zhou, J.R., 2007. Effect of soy nuts on blood pressure and lipid levels in hypertensive, prehypertensive, and normotensive postmenopausal women. Archives of Internal Medicine 167, 1060–1067.

Wenzel, U., Fuchs, D., Daniel, H., 2008. Protective effects of soy-isoflavones in cardiovascular disease. Identification of molecular targets. Hämostaseologie 28, 85–88.

Willich, S.N., Maclure, M., Mittleman, M., Arntz, H.R., Muller, J.E., 1993. Sudden cardiac death. Support for a role of triggering in causation. Circulation 87, 1442–1450.

Wiseman, H., O'Reilly, J.D., Adlercreutz, H., et al., 2000. Isoflavone phytoestrogens consumed in soy decrease F(2)-isoprostane concentrations and increase resistance of low-density lipoprotein to oxidation in humans. The American Journal of Clinical Nutrition 72, 395–400.

Wu, J.M., Wang, Z.R., Hsieh, T.C., Bruder, J.L., Zou, J.G., Huang, Y.Z., 2001. Mechanism of cardio-protection by resveratrol, a phenolic antioxidant present in red wine (Review). International Journal of Molecular Medicine 8, 3–17.

Xiao, C.W., 2008. Health effects of soy protein and isoflavones in humans. Journal of Nutrition 138, 1244S–1249S.

Yang, G., Shu, X.O., Jin, F., et al., 2005. Longitudinal study of soy food intake and blood pressure among middle-aged and elderly Chinese women. The American Journal of Clinical Nutrition 81, 1012–1017.

Zhang, X., Shu, X.O., Gao, Y.T., et al., 2003. Soy food consumption is associated with lower risk of coronary heart disease in Chinese women. Journal of Nutrition 133, 2874–2878.

CHAPTER 36

Fish Oil Fatty Acids and Vascular Reactivity

K.G. Jackson*, A.M. Minihane[†]
*University of Reading, Reading, UK
[†]University of East Anglia, Norwich, UK

ABBREVIATIONS

CAVI Cardio-ankle vascular index
CVD Cardiovascular disease
DHA Docosahexaenoic acid
DVP Digital volume pulse
EPA Eicosapentaenoic acid
eNOS Endothelial nitric oxide synthase
ET Endothelin
FBF Forearm blood flow
FMD Flow-mediated dilatation
HUVEC Human umbilical vein endothelial cells
IMT Intima–media thickness
LC Long chain
LDI Laser Doppler iontophoresis
NADPH Nicotinamide adenine dinucleotide phosphate
NO Nitric oxide
PC Phosphatidylcholine
PG Prostaglandin
PUFA Polyunsaturated fatty acid
PWA Pulse wave analysis
PWV Pulse wave velocity
SFA Saturated fatty acids
TBX Thromboxane

1. INTRODUCTION

The endothelium is a single layer of cells lining the blood vessel wall, which plays a critical role in the maintenance of vascular tone and homeostasis. This active tissue releases a number of vasoactive substances, the most important being nitric oxide (NO), a potent vasodilator that causes smooth muscle relaxation and arterial dilation (Sader and Celermajer, 2002). Endothelial dysfunction, characterized by an increase in vascular tone and a reduction in vascular reactivity, is strongly associated with cardiovascular disease

Bioactive Food as Dietary Interventions for Cardiovascular Disease
http://dx.doi.org/10.1016/B978-0-12-396485-4.00033-5

© 2013 Elsevier Inc.
All rights reserved.

(CVD) risk and has emerged as a critical early modifiable event in the development of atherosclerosis (Schächinger et al., 2000). Numerous studies have highlighted the prognostic value of *in vivo* measures of vascular reactivity of both the coronary and peripheral arteries, in predicting future coronary events (Landmesser et al., 2004; Schächinger et al., 2000).

Evidence is now emerging that mechanisms involved in the control of vascular tone are influenced by dietary factors, with dietary fat composition considered to be an important modulator. The cardioprotective actions of the fish oil long chain (LC) *n*–3 polyunsaturated fatty acids (PUFAs), eicosapentaenoic acid (EPA), and docosahexaenoic acid (DHA) are now well accepted and have been attributed to a number of physiological mechanisms including their antiarrhythmic, antithrombotic, and anti–inflammatory actions, along with positive effects on the blood lipid profile and atherosclerotic plaque stability (Saravanan et al., 2010). In addition, as will be reviewed, accumulating evidence indicates positive benefits of diets rich in EPA and DHA on endothelial function and vascular reactivity, when assessed after an overnight fast (Mori et al., 2000; Nestel et al., 2002). However, individuals spend the vast majority of the day in the postprandial state and the acute impact of EPA and DHA on postprandial vascular reactivity will also be considered.

1.1 Scope of This Chapter

Data from observational, chronic supplementation, and acute postprandial test meal studies are presented together with animal and *in vitro* data to provide an insight into potential mechanisms underlying the physiological effects observed in humans. Rather than being exhaustive, the authors aim to summarize recent human studies and provide an update to the extensive review by Hall (2009), which included data published up to February 2008.

1.2 Methods Commonly Used to Assess Vascular Structure and Function in Human Studies

Structural changes in the arterial wall with aging and during the development of atherosclerotic plaques can lead to stiffening of the arteries and an increase in vascular tone. Measurement of the carotid arterial intima–media thickness (IMT) using ultrasound has been employed in a number of population-based observational (cross-sectional) studies. An increase in carotid arterial thickness (IMT and plaques) has been associated with advanced CVD (Lorenz et al., 2007).

There is currently no "gold standard" technique for measuring vascular function. Flow-mediated dilatation (FMD), involving the tracking of brachial artery dilatation by ultrasound, has been used extensively as a surrogate marker of coronary vascular function (Deanfield et al., 2005). FMD is mainly an endothelium-dependent process, predominately NO mediated, which is reflective of the ability of the artery to dilate when exposed to shear stress (Corretti et al., 2002). Forearm blood flow (FBF) measured using strain gauge plethysmography and laser Doppler iontophoresis (LDI) are other techniques to assess vascular tone in the systemic circulation and peripheral microcirculation, respectively. Both of these techniques examine the reactivity of the blood vessels in response to endothelial-dependent and –independent vasoactive substances, which are often infused into the blood vessel during the measurement of FBF and delivered through the skin to the underlying blood vessels during the LDI measurement. Arterial stiffness is commonly measured as an estimate of blood vessel elasticity and has been associated with CVD incidence (Nichols, 2005). Non-invasive methods for the assessment of arterial stiffness include pulse wave analysis (PWA), pulse wave velocity (PWV, the speed of travel of the pulse wave after the heart contracts), and digital volume pulse (DVP). Parameters calculated using these techniques, including the augmentation index (AI) measured during PWV, and the stiffness and resistance indices (SI and RI) determined using DVP, provide surrogate markers of arterial stiffness in the large and small vessels, respectively.

2. OBSERVATIONAL STUDIES EXAMINING THE RELATIONSHIP BETWEEN HABITUAL LC *n*-3 PUFA INTAKE WITH CAROTID IMT AND VASCULAR REACTIVITY

The ultrasound assessment of carotid IMT, an indicator of the presence of atherosclerotic plaques, has been performed in three studies and related to the intake of fish (assessed using a food frequency questionnaire (FFQ)) and the fatty acid composition of serum lipids and phosphatidylcholine (an indicator of short- and long-term fat intake, respectively) (Table 36.1). Although dietary intakes of LC *n*-3 PUFA in the moderate-to-high range (quartile range 0.9–3.5 g per day) did not appear to be associated with the presence of reduced atherosclerotic plaque, the daily intake of fish oil fatty acids was negatively associated with IMT in Alaskan Eskimos (Ebbesson et al., 2008). An association with higher phospholipid proportions of DHA (median value 4.8% of serum lipids), but not EPA, was also shown to be inversely associated with the mean IMT in Spanish adults with primary dyslipidemia (monogenic or polygenic disorders that lead to elevated lipid levels) (Sala-Vila et al., 2010). In a population-based cross-sectional study, the relationships between the proportion of LC *n*-3 PUFA in serum lipids and atherosclerosis in Japanese (defined as born and living in Japan), white men, and Japanese men born and living in the United States were examined. An inverse relationship between marine-derived *n*-3 PUFA and IMT was observed in the Japanese men only (Table 36.1). In addition, the Japanese men were shown to have the highest intakes of LC *n*-3 PUFA and lowest incidence of atherosclerosis relative to the Japanese and white men living in the United States (Sekikawa et al., 2008). The difference in incidence of atherosclerosis between the Japanese men living in Japan and the United States suggests that diet, as opposed to genetic factors, may be responsible for these associations.

Table 36.1 Observational Studies Investigating the Relationship between Intakes of Fish Oil Fatty Acids with Carotid Intima–Media Thickness (IMT) and Vascular Reactivity

References	Subjects	Assessment of Dietary intake	Assessment of Vascular function	Association	Outcome
Carotid IMT					
Ebbesson et al. (2008)	Alaskan Eskimos (GOCADAN study) 686 M/F 35–97 years	FFQ	Ultrasound	Yes	Higher quartiles of omega-3 fatty acid intake (quartile range 2.2–6.1 g per day) associated with lower average IMT
Sekikawa et al. (2008)	United States 281 M Japanese, 306 M White US, 281 M Japanese-American 40–49 years	Serum fatty acids	Ultrasound	Yes	Japanese men had a significant inverse association of marine-derived fatty acids with IMT
Sala-Vila et al. (2010)	Spain 261 M and 190 F with primary dyslipidemia Mean age 45 years	Serum PC	Ultrasound	Yes	DHA had a significant inverse relationship with mean common carotid artery IMT
Vascular reactivity					
Anderson et al. (2010)	United States 1500 M and 1377 F (Multi-ethnic Study of Atherosclerosis; MESA) study 45–84 years	FFQ	FMD of the brachial artery	No	No significant association between nonfried fish intake and FMD
		Plasma PC			Some associations observed when the data were split by gender
Petersen et al. (2010)	Denmark 40 Adults	FFQ Plasma PC	FMD of the brachial artery	No	No significant association among fish intake, phospholipid EPA, and DHA with FMD

DHA, docosahexaenoic acid; EPA, eicosapentaenoic acid; FFQ, food frequency questionnaire; FMD, flow-mediated dilatation; IMT, intima–media thickness; PC, phosphatidylcholine.

The relationship between fish consumption and plasma measures of LC *n*-3 PUFA with FMD has been investigated by Andersen et al. (2010) and Petersen et al. (2010) (Table 36.1). Both studies found no correlations among fish intake, plasma phospholipid levels of LC *n*-3 PUFA, EPA, or DHA with FMD in adults based in the United States (Anderson et al., 2010) or Denmark (Petersen et al., 2010). Stratification of the US adults according to gender revealed an association between the highest quartile of nonfried fish consumption (>2 potions per week) and a 0.10-mm lower brachial artery diameter in men and a 0.27% smaller FMD in women, compared with the lowest quartile of nonfried fish consumption (Anderson et al., 2010). These findings suggest that diet may have differential effects on cardiovascular outcomes in women, compared with men.

3. CHRONIC STUDIES EXAMINING THE IMPACT OF LC *n*-3 PUFA SUPPLEMENTATION ON VASCULAR FUNCTION

3.1 Combined Impact of EPA and DHA

In Hall's review (2009), data from a total of 12 chronic interventions with vascular reactivity as a study outcome (as assessed by FMD, plethysmography, LDI, or measures of arterial stiffness) were presented. In these trials, where doses of LC *n*-3 PUFA in the range of 0.5–6 g were provided for intervention periods of 2 weeks to 12 months, positive impacts on vascular reactivity and stiffness were almost exclusively reported. The more recent studies have provided less consistent findings (Table 36.2). Of the six studies that have measured fasting macrovascular function following supplementation with EPA and DHA (1.7–3.4 g per day for 6–12 weeks) (de Berrazueta et al., 2009; Rizza et al., 2009; Schiano et al., 2008; Skulas-Ray et al., 2011; Stirban et al., 2010; Wong et al., 2010), three have found a positive effect (de Berrazueta et al., 2009; Rizza et al., 2009; Schiano et al., 2008), with three reporting no change in the fasting vascular response (Skulas-Ray et al., 2011; Stirban et al., 2010; Wong et al., 2010). Schiano et al. (2008) and Rizza et al. (2009) observed a large, clinically significant, 49% and 48% increase in FMD, in patients with peripheral arterial disease and in young adults with at least one parent with type 2 diabetes, respectively, following supplementation with 1.7 g of EPA and DHA per day for 12 weeks. Using plethysmography as the assessment method, a positive impact on vascular reactivity following consumption of approximately 1.5 g of EPA and DHA per day as fish rather than capsules was also reported in elderly individuals (de Berrazueta et al., 2009). In contrast, no significant impact on vascular reactivity was observed following consumption of 1.7–3.4 g EPA and DHA per day, in type 2 diabetics or a moderately hypertriacylglycerolemic group (Skulas-Ray et al., 2011; Stirban et al., 2010; Wong et al., 2010). Both recent trials that have examined

Table 36.2 Randomized Controlled Chronic Intervention Examining the Impact of Fish Oil Fatty Acids on Fasting Vascular Function

References	Study group	Study design and duration	Intervention dose and length of washout	Measure of compliance	Vascular measurement	Impact on vascular function
Schiano et al. (2008)	PAD, $n=32$ men and postmenopausal women, mean age 66 years	Single-blind parallel, 12 weeks	2 g n-3 PUFA per day providing 1.7 g EPA+DHA (G1, $n=16$) No intervention (G2, $n=16$)	Capsule count >94%	FMD	G1: ↑ (49%) in FMD (%), $p=0.02$ G2: ↓ (4%) in FMD (%), $p=0.41$
de Berrazueta et al. (2009)	Elderly men and women, age range 62–97 years	Non-blinded parallel, 12 weeks	Four to five portions of fish per week providing 2.5 g EPA+DHA per day (G1, $n=46$) No intervention (G2, $n=23$)	60% consumption ≡ 1.5 g EPA+DHA actual intake	Reactive hyperemia by plethysmography	No impact on basal or maximum FBF
Rizza et al. (2009)	Young adults, with at least one parent with T2DM, $n=50$, mean age 30 years	Double-blind parallel, 12 weeks	2 g n-3 PUFA per day providing ≥1.7 g EPA+DHA (G1, $n=26$)	Capsule count = 94%	FMD	G1: ↑ (20%) in EDV, $p<0.001$ G2: ↓ (3%) in EDV, $p=0.62$ G1: ↑ (48%) in FMD (%), $p≤0.01$

	Subjects	Design	Intervention	Compliance	Measurement	Results
			2 g olive oil per day (G2, $n=24$)			G2: ↓ (3%) in FMD (%), $p=0.43$
Satoh et al. (2009)	Dyslipidemic adults, $n=92$, mean age 52 years	Single-blind parallel, 12 weeks	Diet[a] + 1.8 g EPA (G1, $n=46$) Diet[a] (G2, $n=46$)	Not stated	PWV and CAVI	*PWV* G1: ↓ (6%), $p<0.01$ G2: ↑ (1%), NS *CAVI* G1: ↓ (4%), $p<0.01$ G2: ↑ (1%), NS
Hallund et al. (2010)	Healthy men, $n=68$, mean age 53 years	Parallel, 8 weeks	150 g marine trout[b] per day, 3.4 g LC n-3 PUFA per day (2.9 g EPA + DHA per day) (G1, $n=23$) 150 g veg. trout[b] per day, 0.8 g LC n-3 PUFA per day (G2, $n=23$) 150 g chicken (G3, $n=22$)	Study diary >99%	PWV and AIx	*PWV* G1, ↑1%; G2, ↓1%; G3, ↑2%; NS *AIx* G1, ↓3%; G2, - 0%; G3, ↓ 9%; NS

Continued

Table 36.2 Randomized Controlled Controlled Chronic Intervention Examining the Impact of Fish Oil Fatty Acids on Fasting Vascular Function—cont'd

References	Study group	Study design and duration	Intervention dose and length of washout	Measure of compliance	Vascular measurement	Impact on vascular function
Stirban et al. (2010)	T2DM, not stated whether men or women, $n=34$, mean age 57 years	Double-blind cross over, 6 weeks with 6 weeks washout	2 g FO per day (1.7 g EPA+DHA) (T1) 2 g OO per day (T2)	Not stated	Fasting+non fasting (2, 4, 6 h) FMD and RH (microcirculation)	*Fasting* FMD and RH, NS; *Non-fasting* FMD (%) AUC: −8.24 T1 vs. −2.31 T2, $p<0.05$ LD (U.h) AUC: −705 T1 vs. 5013 T2, $p<0.05$
Wong et al. (2010)	T2DM, men and women, $n=97$, mean age 60 years	Double-blind parallel, 12 weeks	4 g FO per day (2.68 g EPA+DHA) (G1, $n=49$) 4 g OO per day (G2, $n=48$)	Not stated	FMD	G1 vs. G2: ↑ 71% vs. ↑ 53%, NS
Skulas-Ray et al. (2011)	Moderate hypertriglyceridemic, men and postmenopausal women, $n=26$	Double-blind cross over, 8 weeks with 6 weeks washout	4 g FO per day (3.4 g EPA+DHA) (T1)	Capsule count >95%	FMD, RH (microcirculation), AIx	*FMD (%)* T1, 4.14 vs. T2, 4.03 vs. T3, 5.00, $p=0.11$

| 1 g FO + 3 g CO per day (0.85 g EPA + DHA) (T2) | Red blood cell fatty acid composition | *RH* T1, 1.86 vs. T2, 1.82 vs. T3, 1.84, $p = 0.86$ |
| 4 g CO per day (T3) | | *AIx* T1, −9.25 vs. T2, −9.52 vs. T3, −9.33, $p = 0.97$ |

PAD, peripheral artery disease; FO, fish oil; EPA, eicosapentaenoic acid; DHA, docosahexaenoic acid; FMD, flow-mediated dilation; EDV, endothelial-dependent vasodilation; PWV, pulse wave velocity; CAVI, cardio–ankle vascular index; AIx, augmentation index; RH, reactive hyperemia of the microcirculation as assessed by Doppler; LC *n*-3 PUFA, long chain *n*-3 polyunsaturated fatty acids; FO, fish oil; OO, olive oil; CO, corn oil.
[a] Japanese Atherosclerosis Society Guidelines for Diagnosis and Treatment of Atherosclerotic Cardiovascular Disease.
[b] Farmed marine trout were raised on fish oil-enriched diet, while veg. trout were raised on vegetable oil-enriched diet.

the impact of chronic EPA and DHA supplementation on fasting microvascular function report no significant effect (Skulas-Ray et al., 2011; Stirban et al., 2010; Table 36.2).

In addition to vascular reactivity, two recent studies have examined the impact of chronic EPA and DHA intake on arterial stiffness (Hallund et al., 2010; Satoh et al., 2009). In dyslipidemic men supplemented for 12 weeks, a positive impact of EPA supplementation (1.8 g per day) was reported for PWV and cardio-ankle vascular index (CAVI) (Satoh et al., 2009). The CAVI is a newly developed method to assess arterial stiffness, which has been proposed to be less dependent on blood pressure relative to the traditional PWV assessment method. In a well-controlled feeding trial where participants had all their fish-containing test meals prepared for them, no difference in arterial stiffness was evident between the groups consuming 150 g farmed trout-fed marine oil (2.9 g LC n-3 PUFA per day) compared with those consuming 150 g farmed trout-fed vegetable extract (0.8 g LC n-3 PUFA per day) (Hallund et al., 2010; Table 36.2).

Therefore, although the earlier studies provided reasonably consistent evidence for a positive benefit of EPA and DHA intakes above 1.5 g per day on vascular function, the more recent studies are less consistent (Table 36.2). Further, sufficiently powered carefully controlled chronic studies are needed to provide clarification. Current dietary guidelines generally suggest a daily intake of above 500 mg per day of EPA and DHA, with doses of 1 g per day often recommended for those with diagnosed CVD (Kris-Etherton et al., 2002). Consumption of two to three portions of oily fish such as salmon, trout, and mackerel per week would typically provide a daily intake of 0.5–1 g of EPA and DHA. The impact of these levels of intake on vascular function is relatively unknown and worthy of investigation.

The trial conducted by Stirban et al. (2010), although of a different design to the other studies presented in Table 36.2, is highly physiologically relevant. In addition to fasting micro- and macrovascular function, which were unaffected by the intervention, they examined the impact of chronic EPA and DHA supplementation on postprandial vascular reactivity. At the end of the 6-week intervention (1.7 g EPA and DHA per day), participants were provided with a high-fat test meal and vascular reactivity assessed 2, 4, and 6 h later. Individuals who consumed the EPA- and DHA-containing supplement had a significantly improved postprandial vascular response relative to those on the olive oil supplement for 6 weeks.

3.2 Comparison of EPA versus DHA

To date, only a very limited number of studies have examined the individual impact of EPA versus DHA on vascular health. In 2002, Nestel et al. (2002) reported comparable 36% and 27% increases in systemic arterial compliance following supplementation with 3 g of EPA or DHA per day for 7 weeks (Nestel et al., 2002). In contrast, Mori et al. (2000) reported a positive impact of DHA supplementation (4 g per day for 6 weeks) on forearm microvascular function relative to the placebo, with no significant impact of an equivalent intake of EPA. As reviewed by Hall (2009), a number of studies, which have supplemented with EPA only (no DHA intervention arm), have reported positive benefits on vascular function. Therefore, overall, the relative impact of these two LC *n*-3 PUFA on micro- and macrovascular function is relatively unknown.

4. ACUTE STUDIES EXAMINING THE EFFECTS OF LC *n*-3 PUFA ON POSTPRANDIAL VASCULAR REACTIVITY

A number of studies conducted in healthy individuals have shown impairment in vascular reactivity 2–8 h after ingestion of moderate- to high-fat (36–80 g fat) meals. There has been considerable interest on the impact of meal fatty acid composition on postprandial vascular reactivity since transient changes in vascular function, repeated on a daily basis, undoubtedly has implications for long-term vascular health and overall CVD risk.

Before 2008, only two studies had examined the effects of LC *n*-3 PUFA on postprandial vascular reactivity, but findings were inconsistent (Jackson et al., 2008). Over the past 3 years, a growing number of studies have determined the impact of either fish oil alone or the addition of fish oil fatty acids to a high-fat test meal on vascular reactivity (Armah et al., 2008; Fahs et al., 2010; Tousoulis et al., 2010) and arterial stiffness (Chong et al., 2010; Hall et al., 2008) in healthy individuals (Table 36.3). The amount of fish oil incorporated into the test meals has varied, with one study giving 50 ml of cod-liver oil containing <10 mg of LC *n*-3 PUFA (Tousoulis et al., 2010), another study a dose equivalent to that recommended by the American Heart Association (Kris-Etherton et al., 2002) for the treatment of CVD (approximately 0.9 g; Fahs et al., 2010), whereas three studies provided between 4.7 and 5.0 g of LC *n*-3 PUFA (Armah et al., 2008; Chong et al., 2010; Hall et al., 2008), comparable to consuming two to three portions of oily fish. Of these five studies, the majority have used highly enriched fish oils containing a greater proportion of EPA.

An attenuation of the increase in postprandial arterial stiffness observed after a control high-fat meal was reported by both Hall et al. (2008) and Chong et al. (2010), following the addition of 8.3 g of an EPA-rich oil (5 g EPA) to a monounsaturated fatty acid–rich meal (high-oleic sunflower oil) (Hall et al., 2008) or 6.8 g of a DHA-rich oil (2.7 g DHA and 2.0 g EPA) to a saturated fatty acid (SFA)-rich meal (fatty acid profile similar to a typical UK diet) (Chong et al., 2010). This effect was evident whether the meal contained 51.3 or 30 g fat, with the improvement in postprandial arterial stiffness observed at 6 h after meal ingestion by Hall et al. (2008) and over the duration of the 4 h postprandial investigation by Chong et al. (2010). However, measures of arterial stiffness (PWA and PWV) were unchanged up to 4 h after consuming a high-fat meal (54 g fat) rich in SFA with three fish oil capsules (540 mg EPA and 360 mg DHA) in healthy young adults (Fahs et al., 2010; Table 36.3).

Table 36.3 Recent Studies Examining the Effects of Fish Oil Fatty Acids on Postprandial Vascular Reactivity

Reference	Study group	Study design and duration	Test meal	Vascular measurement	Significant results compared with baseline
Armah et al. (2008)	24 M, 18–70 years	Cross over, 4 h	Mixed meal (800 kcal) containing: 40 g palm olein/soybean oil or 31 g palm olein/soybean oil and 9 g fish oil (3.6 g DHA and 1.8 g EPA)	LDI in response to ACh and SNP at 0 and 4 h	Increase in vasodilatory response to SNP (47%) after fish oil-rich meal
Jackson et al. (2009)	Subdivision of the male group above 12 M (21–49 years), 12 M (55–71 years)	Single meal, 4 h	Mixed meal (800 kcal) containing 31 g palm olein and 9 g fish oil (3.6 g DHA and 1.8 g EPA)		Increase in vasodilatory response to ACh (35%) and SNP (75%) after fish oil-rich meal in men <50 years only
Hall et al. (2008)	17 M, 18–35 years	Cross over, 6 h	Mixed meal containing: 51.3 g high-oleic sunflower oil or 43 g high-oleic sunflower oil and 8.3 g EPA-rich oil (5 g EPA). A second high-fat meal (43.7 g fat) was given at 4 h	DVP at 0, 3, and 6 h	Reduction in SI greater at 6 h after the EPA-rich (9%) versus control (5%) meal
Chong et al. (2010)	25 (12 M/13 F), 19–68 years	Cross over, 4 h	Low-fat breakfast (400 kcal, 2.1 g fat) followed 5 h later by a mixed meal containing: 30 g palm olein/soybean oil, 23.2 g palm olein/soybean oil, and 6.8 g fish oil (2.0 g EPA and 2.7 g DHA)	PWA and DVP at 0, 0.5, 1, 1.5, 2, 3, and 4 h	Fish oil-enriched meal had an attenuating effect on AI and SI versus control meal
Fahs et al. (2010)	20 (10 M/10 F), 18–31 years	Cross over, 4 h	Low-fat breakfast (<10 g fat) followed 4 h later by a high-fat meal (1042 kcal; 54 g fat) with either three capsules of fish oil (540 mg EPA and 360 mg DHA) or lactose	Carotid artery stiffness, FMD of the brachial artery, FBF, PWA, PWV, 0 and 4 h	The high-fat meal with fish oil attenuated the reduction in FMD observed with the control meal

| Tousoulis et al. (2010) | 37 (26 M/11 F), age 27 years | Parallel, 3 h | 50 ml of oil (830 kcal) or water (control). The oils included: extra-virgin olive oil, maize oil, soy oil, cod-liver oil (4.1 mg EPA and 3.7 mg DHA) | FBF at 0, 1, 2, and 3 h | Relative to control, increase in reactive hyperemia with cod-liver oil (29%) and soy oil (95%), whereas decrease with maize oil (20%) at 1 h postconsumption |

AI, augmentation index; DHA, docosahexaenoic acid; DVP, digital volume pulse; EPA, eicosapentaenoic acid; FBF, forearm blood flow; FMD, flow-mediated dilatation; LDI, laser Doppler iontophoresis; PWA, pulse wave analysis; PWV, pulse wave velocity; SI, stiffness index.

Relative to their effects on arterial stiffness, the impact of fish oils on postprandial vascular reactivity are less well defined and this may be reflected in the types of vascular function measures employed in the different study designs (Table 36.3). Compared with water, 50 ml of cod-liver oil (4.1 mg EPA and 3.7 mg DHA) showed a transient improvement in FBF at 1 h postprandially, with a return to baseline levels at 2 and 3 h respectively (Tousoulis et al., 2010). Although an effect on FBF was not observed by Fahs et al. (2010), ingestion of a high-fat meal rich in SFA with three fish oil capsules was shown to attenuate the reduction in FMD observed with the high-fat meal only. Using LDI, Armah et al. (2008) reported the inclusion of 5.4 g of a DHA-rich fish oil to high-fat meal with a fatty acid profile representative of a typical UK diet to improve the vasodilatory response to sodium nitroprusside, a measure of smooth muscle reactivity (endothelium-independent vasodilation) in a group of healthy men. Interestingly, subdivision of this male group into those aged <50 and ≥ 50 years revealed the men <50 years to show greater vasodilation of the microcirculation in response to both acetylcholine (endothelium-dependent) and sodium nitroprusside (endothelium-independent) 4 h after the fish oil-enriched meal compared with baseline, with little benefit observed in the men ≥ 50 years (Jackson et al., 2009). The lack of responsiveness in the older men has been proposed to be associated with structural changes in the vascular wall with aging, which could impact on the rate of diffusion of NO to the smooth muscle layer. As far as the authors are aware, the comparative effects of EPA versus DHA on postprandial vascular reactivity have not yet been determined.

5. POTENTIAL MECHANISMS

Vascular tone and function are regulated by the production of a range of endothelial cell-derived vasoconstrictors and vasodilators (Figure 36.1). Under the action of endothelial nitric oxide synthase (eNOS), NO is produced from L-arginine and NO diffuses to the underlying vascular smooth muscle cell layer where it stimulates the cAMP-protein kinase G signaling pathway resulting in vasorelaxation. The bioavailability of NO is influenced by the oxidative status in the vascular wall. Interaction of NO with molecules, for example, superoxide (O_2^-) produced by enzymes such as nicotinamide adenine dinucleotide phosphate (NADPH) oxidase, results in the formation of peroxynitrite ($ONOO^-$), which reduces available NO concentrations and produces highly reactive nitrogen-containing compounds with opposing effects to NO (Figure 36.1).

Endothelium-derived hyperpolarizing factors describe a group of compounds (which include NO), which through hyperpolarization, also result in relaxation of the vascular smooth muscle cell layer. Endothelin (ET)-1 produced from prepro ET-1, through its interaction with specific ET receptor on endothelial cells and vascular smooth muscle cells, and through its influence on the NO signaling pathway, ultimately results in vasocontraction. Vascular tone is also regulated by a range of eicosanoid derivatives of

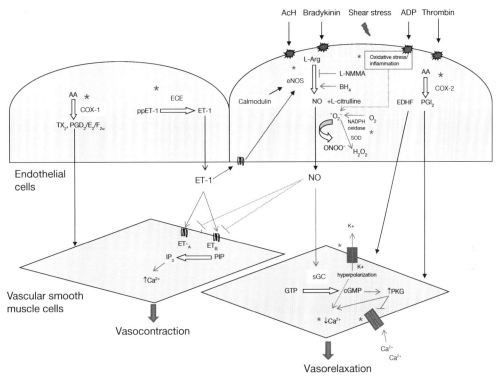

Figure 36.1 The regulation of vascular tone and potential targets of long chain (LC) *n*-3 polyunsaturated fatty acids (PUFA) in the regulatory pathways (as indicated by *). *Abbreviations*: AcH, acetylcholine; ADP, adenosine diphosphate; AA, arachidonic acid; BH_4, tetrahydrobiopterin; cGMP, cyclic guanosine monophosphate; COX, cyclooxygenase; EDHF, endothelium-derived hyperpolarizing factor; eNOS, endothelial nitric oxide synthase; ECE, endothelin converting enzyme; ET_A and ET_B, endothelin receptors; ET-1, endothelin-1; GTP, guanosine triphosphate; H_2O_2, hydrogen peroxide, a proposed EDHF; IP_3, inositol 1,4,5, triphosphate; L-Arg, L-arginine; L-NNMA, L-*NG*-Monomethylarginine; NADPH, nicotinamide adenine dinucleotide phosphate; NO, nitric oxide; O_2^-, superoxide; $ONOO^-$, peroxynitrite; ppET-1, prepro-endothelin-1; PG, prostaglandin; PGI_2, prostacyclin; PIP, phosphatidylinositol 4,5, bisphosphate; PKG, protein kinase G; sGC, soluble guanylyl cyclase; SOD, superoxide dismutase; TBX, thromboxane.

arachidonic acid (prostaglandins (PG), prostacyclin (PGI_2), and thromboxane (TBX)) produced under the action of cyclooxygenases (COX) 1 and 2 (Figure 36.1).

The available literature indicates that LC *n*-3 PUFA possesses numerous interrelated properties, which can positively influence vascular health, the most well described of which is their impact on eNOS action. Furthermore, data are suggestive than an impact of EPA and DHA on eicosanoid speciation, oxidative status, nuclear receptor activity, and cytokine production, ion channel function, and ET-1 production may in part modulate the response (Abeywardena and Head, 2001), a selection of which are described in greater detail below.

5.1 eNOS Action

The incorporation of LC *n*-3 PUFA into endothelial cell membranes, including the caveolae (where eNOS is anchored in its inactive form by caveolin-1), has been shown to displace caveolin-1 and increase cellular eNOS activity (Li et al., 2007). In a human and animal study, increased nitrite and nitrate (biomarkers of NO) in urine and plasma, respectively, have been observed following LC *n*-3 PUFA supplementation (Armah et al., 2008; Nishimura et al., 2000). In the above-mentioned acute study by Armah et al. (2008), a 32% increase in postprandial plasma nitrite (4 h) was evident following a consumption of the fish oil-enriched meal compared with an 8% decrease following the placebo meal. Furthermore, an impact of EPA and DHA on eNOS gene expression in human umbilical vein endothelial cells (HUVEC) has been reported (Stebbins et al., 2008). The ability of L-*N*-monomethylarginine (a specific eNOS inhibitor) to attenuate the impact of LC *n*-3 PUFA on vasorelaxation lends further support to the role of eNOS in mediating the positive impact of these fatty acids on vascular tone (Singh et al., 2010).

5.2 Eicosanoid Speciation

In addition to arachidonic acid, eicosanoids can be derived from EPA, with EPA-derived alternative being less potent than their arachidonic acid equivalents. In isolated mesenteric arteries (membrane surrounding the small intestine) from a type 2 diabetic rat model, prior supplementation of the animals with EPA for 4 weeks, resulted in improvements in vascular tone, normalized NO metabolism and decreased production of the deleterious TBX, PGE_2, $PGF_{2\alpha}$, and 6-keto-$PGF_{1\alpha}$ (Matsumoto et al., 2009). The ability of EPA to lower TXB_2 production has been confirmed in other studies (Yin et al., 1990).

5.3 Oxidative Status

Although the LC *n*-3 PUFAs were originally thought to be prooxidative because of their high degree of unsaturation, it is now evident that they are in fact likely to improve oxidative status. In the *APOE* knockout mouse model of atherosclerosis, diets enriched in fish oil resulted in lower superoxide production and p22^{phox} (NADPH oxidase sub unit) expression in the aortic root (Casós et al., 2010). Increased superoxide dismutase activity and lower NOX4 (NADPH oxidase subunit), hydrogen peroxide, and 8-isoprostanes (lipid peroxidation product), following LC *n*-3 PUFA administration, have also been reported in a variety of animal and cell models. The exposure of HUVEC cells to triacylglycerol-rich lipoproteins isolated from humans who had been fed a fish oil-enriched test meal resulted in a significant reduction in NOX4 mRNA expression relative to the placebo meal (Armah et al., 2008).

5.4 Ion Channel Function

The efflux of potassium ions from vascular smooth muscle cells and the simultaneous inhibition of calcium release from intracellular stores and influx from the extracellular fluid are associated with vasorelaxation. Ion channel function in cellular membranes is dependent on the fatty acid composition of the membrane phospholipids, and increased LC *n*-3 PUFA content is generally association with improved function and cation conductance resulting in lower free intracellular calcium and associated vasorelaxation (Hirafuji et al., 1998; Singh et al., 2010).

Recent *in vitro* studies have indicated that cytochrome P450 present in endothelial cells can metabolize LC *n*-3 PUFA, such as DHA, to fatty acid epoxides (Arnold et al., 2010; Wang et al., 2011), which have been proposed to promote vasodilation through activation of calcium–activated potassium channels present in vascular smooth muscle cells (Wang et al., 2011). Although the actions of these LC *n*-3 PUFA-derived fatty acid epoxides are still being elucidated, it has been proposed that these metabolites may be released in response to shear stress, as has been observed with cytochrome P450 metabolites of arachidonic acid (Huang et al., 1997).

6. CONCLUSIONS

With increasing recognition of the pivotal role of vascular dysfunction in the progression of atherosclerosis, the vasculature has emerged as an important target for dietary therapies. Data published to date provide reasonable evidence that both acute and chronic intakes of LC *n*-3 PUFA have a beneficial impact on vascular tone (Tables 36.2 and 36.3). However, the intakes of EPA and DHA in these studies are much higher than the current dietary guidelines of a minimum of 500 mg per day for healthy individuals and 1 g per day for those diagnosed with CVD. Therefore, there is a need for studies that examine the dose–response relationship between LC *n*-3 PUFA and vascular function to determine whether there is a threshold effect above which beneficial effects are observed. In addition, there is a lack of information regarding the relative potencies of the individual LC *n*-3 PUFA, EPA, and DHA, on vascular tone of the macro- and microvasculature. Determination of the individual impact of EPA and DHA on health outcomes is timely, given the recent development in plant production technologies, which in the near future will, through manipulation of plant gene expression, allow the 'tailoring' of LC *n*-3 PUFA composition of the extracted plant oils.

A number of mechanisms to explain the beneficial effects of fish oil fatty acids on endothelial function have been derived from chronic supplementation studies in both humans and animals. These include effects on eNOS action, inflammation, the oxidative status of the vascular wall, and functionality of the vascular smooth muscle layer. Therefore, it appears that LC *n*-3 PUFA possessess numerous interrelated properties, which may have synergistic effects on vascular function. Although the mechanisms of how LC *n*-3 PUFA ingestion alters postprandial vascular reactivity are relatively unknown, some studies have hypothesized that, acutely, fish oil fatty acids may lead to improvements in vascular reactivity by increasing the bioavailability of NO and reducing the oxidative status of the vascular wall. Recent *in vitro* studies have proposed that metabolites of EPA and DHA may have direct effects on the vascular smooth muscle layer during the postprandial phase. Further studies are warranted to determine the underlying mechanisms of how acute and chronic LC *n*-3 PUFAs influence vascular reactivity, with a focus on both endothelial-dependent and -independent pathways.

REFERENCES

Abeywardena, M.Y., Head, R.J., 2001. Long chain *n*-3 polyunsaturated fatty acids and blood vessel function. Cardiovascular Research 52, 361–371.

Anderson, J.S., Nettleton, J.A., Herrington, D.M., et al., 2010. Relation of omega-3 fatty acid and dietary fish intake with brachial artery flow-mediated dilatation in the Multi-Ethnic Study of Atherosclerosis. American Journal of Clinical Nutrition 92, 1204–1213.

Armah, C.K., Jackson, K.G., Doman, I., et al., 2008. Fish oil fatty acids improve postprandial vascular reactivity in healthy men. Clinical Science 114, 679–686.

Arnold, C., Markovic, M., Blossey, K., et al., 2010. Arachidonic acid-metabolising cytochrome P450 enzymes are targets of omega-3 fatty acids. Journal of Biological Chemistry 285, 32720–32733.

Casós, K., Zaragoza, M.C., Zarkovic, N., et al., 2010. A fish oil-rich diet reduces vascular oxidative stress in apoE(−/−) mice. Free Radical Research 44, 821–829.

Chong, M.F., Lockyer, S., Saunders, C.J., Lovegrove, J.A., 2010. Long chain *n*-3 PUFA-rich meal reduced postprandial measures of arterial stiffness. Clinical Nutrition 29, 678–681.

Corretti, M.C., Anderson, T.J., Benjamin, E.J., et al., 2002. Guidelines for the ultrasound assessment of endothelial-dependent flow-mediated vasodilation of the brachial artery: a report of the International Brachial Artery Reactivity Task Force. Journal of the American College of Cardiology 39, 257–265.

de Berrazueta, J.R., de Berrazueta, J.M.G., Senaris, J.A.A., et al., 2009. A diet enriched with mackerel (*Scomber scombrus*)-derived products improves the endothelial function in a senior population (Prevencion de las Enfermedades Cardiovasculares: Estudio Santona – PECES Project). European Journal of Clinical Investigation 39, 165–173.

Deanfield, J., Donald, A., Ferri, C., et al., 2005. Endothelial function and dysfunction. Part I: methodological issues for assessment in the different vascular beds: a statement by the Working Group on Endothelin and Endothelial Factors of the European Society of Hypertension. Journal of Hypertension 23, 7–17.

Ebbesson, S.O., Roman, M.J., Devereux, R.B., et al., 2008. Consumption of omega-3 fatty acids is not associated with a reduction in carotid atherosclerosis: the Genetics of Coronary Artery Disease in Alaska Natives Study. Atherosclerosis 199, 346–353.

Fahs, C.A., Yan, H.M., Ranadive, S., et al., 2010. The effect of acute fish-oil supplementation on endothelial function and arterial stiffness following a high-fat meal. Applied Physiology, Nutrition, and Metabolism 35, 294–302.

Hall, W.L., 2009. Dietary saturated and unsaturated fatty acids as determinants of blood pressure and vascular function. Nutrition Research Reviews 22, 18–38.

Hall, W.L., Sanders, K.A., Sanders, T.A.B., Chowienczyk, P.J., 2008. A high-fat meal enriched with eicosapentaenoic acid reduces postprandial arterial stiffness measured by digital volume pulse analysis in healthy men. Journal of Nutrition 138, 287–291.

Hallund, J., Overgaard Madsen, B., Bugel, S.H., et al., 2010. The effect of farmed trout on cardiovascular risk markers in healthy men. British Journal of Nutrition 104, 1528–1536.

Hirafuji, M., Ebihara, T., Kawahara, F., Nezu, A., 1998. Effect of docosahexaenoic acid on intracellular calcium dynamics in vascular smooth muscle cells from normotensive and genetically hypertensive rats. Research Communications in Molecular Pathology and Pharmacology 102, 29–42.

Huang, Y.J., Fang, V.S., Juan, C.C., et al., 1997. Amelioration of insulin resistance and hypertension in a fructose-fed rat model with fish oil supplementation. Metabolism, Clinical and Experimental 46, 1252–1258.

Jackson, K.G., Armah, C.K., Minihane, A.M., 2007. Meal fatty acids and postprandial vascular reactivity. Biochemical Society Transactions 35, 451–453.

Jackson, K.G., Armah, C.K., Doman, I., et al., 2009. The impact of age on the postprandial vascular response to a fish oil-enriched meal. British Journal of Nutrition 102, 1414–1419.

Kris-Etherton, P.M., Harris, W.L., Appel, L.J., for the Nutrition Committee, 2002. Fish consumption, fish oil, omega-3 fatty acids and cardiovascular disease. Circulation 106, 2747–2757.

Landmesser, U., Hornig, B., Dexler, H., 2004. Endothelial function – a critical determinant in atherosclerosis? Circulation 109, 27–33.

Li, Q.R., Zhang, Q., Wang, M., et al., 2007. Docosahexaenoic acid affects endothelial nitric oxide synthase in caveolae. Archives of Biochemistry and Biophysics 466, 250–259.

Lorenz, M.W., Markus, H.S., Bots, M.L., Rosvall, M., Sitzer, M., 2007. Prediction of clinical cardiovascular events with carotid intima-media thickness: a systematic review and meta-analysis. Circulation 115, 459–467.

Matsumoto, T., Nakayama, N., Ishida, K., Kobayashi, T., Kamata, K., 2009. Eicosapentaenoic acid improves imbalance between vasodilator and vasoconstrictor actions of endothelium-derived factors in mesenteric arteries from rats at chronic stage of type 2 diabetes. Journal of Pharmacology and Experimental Therapeutics 329, 324–334.

Mori, T.A., Watts, G.F., Burke, V., et al., 2000. Differential effects of eicosapentaenoic acid and docosahexaenoic acid on vascular reactivity of the forearm microcirculation in hyperlipidaemic, overweight men. Circulation 102, 1264–1269.

Nestel, P., Shige, H., Pomeroy, S., et al., 2002. The n-3 fatty acids eicosapentaenoic acid and docosahexaenoic acid increase systemic arterial compliance in humans. American Journal of Clinical Nutrition 76, 326–330.

Nichols, W.W., 2005. Clinical measurement of arterial stiffness obtained from noninvasive pressure waveforms. American Journal of Hypertension 18, 3S–10S.

Nishimura, M., Nanbu, A., Komori, T., et al., 2000. Eicosapentaenoic acid stimulates nitric oxide production and decreases cardiac noradrenaline in diabetic rats. Clinical and Experimental Pharmacology and Physiology 27, 618–624.

Petersen, M.M., Eschen, R.B., Aardestrup, I., Obel, T., Schmidt, E.B., 2010. Flow-mediated vasodilation and dietary intake of n-3 polyunsaturated fatty acids in healthy subjects. Cellular and Molecular Biology 56, 38–44.

Rizza, S., Tesauro, M., Cardillo, C., et al., 2009. Fish oil supplementation improves endothelial function in normoglycemic offspring of patients with type 2 diabetes. Atherosclerosis 206, 569–574.

Sader, M.A., Celermajer, D.S., 2002. Endothelial function, vascular reactivity and gender differences in the cardiovascular system. Cardiovascular Research 53, 597–604.

Sala-Vila, A., Cofan, M., Perez-Heras, A., et al., 2010. Fatty acids in serum phospholipids and carotid intima-media thickness in Spanish subjects with primary dyslipidaemia. American Journal of Clinical Nutrition 92, 186–193.

Saravanan, P., Davidson, N.C., Schmidt, E.B., Calder, P.C., 2010. Cardiovascular effects of marine omega-3 fatty acids. Lancet 376, 540–550.

Satoh, N., Shimatsu, A., Kotani, K., et al., 2009. Highly purified eicosapentaenoic acid reduces cardio-ankle vascular index in association with decreased serum amyloid A-LDL in metabolic syndrome. Hypertension Research 32, 1004–1008.

Schächinger, V., Britten, M.B., Zeiher, A.M., 2000. Prognostic impact of coronary vasodilator dysfunction on adverse long-term outcome of coronary heart disease. Circulation 101, 1899–1906.

Schiano, V., Laurenzano, E., Brevetti, G., et al., 2008. Omega-3 polyunsaturated fatty acids in peripheral arterial disease: effect on lipid pattern, disease severity, inflammation profile, and endothelial function. Clinical Nutrition 27, 241–247.

Sekikawa, A., Curb, J.D., Ueshima, H., et al., 2008. Marine-derived n-3 fatty acids and atherosclerosis in Japanese, Japanese-American, and white men: a cross-sectional study. Journal of the American College of Cardiology 52, 417–424.

Singh, T.U., Kathirvel, K., Choudhury, S., Garg, S.K., Mishra, S.K., 2010. Eicosapentaenoic acid-induced endothelium-dependent and -independent relaxation of sheep pulmonary artery. European Journal of Pharmacology 636, 108–113.

Skulas-Ray, A.C., Kris-Etherton, P.M., Harris, W.S., et al., 2011. Dose–response effects of omega-3 fatty acids on triglycerides, inflammation, and endothelial function in healthy persons with moderate hyper-triglyceridemia. American Journal of Clinical Nutrition 93, 243–252.

Stebbins, C.L., Stice, J.P., Hart, C.M., Mbai, F.N., Knowlton, A.A., 2008. Effects of dietary docosahexaenoic acid (DHA) on eNOS in human coronary artery endothelial cells. Journal of Cardiovascular Pharmacology and Therapeutics 13, 261–268.

Stirban, A., Nandrean, S., Gotting, C., et al., 2010. Effects of n-3 fatty acids on macro- and microvascular function in subjects with type 2 diabetes mellitus. American Journal of Clinical Nutrition 91, 808–813.

Tousoulis, D., Papageorgiou, N., Antoniades, C., et al., 2010. Acute effects of different types of oil consumption on endothelial function, oxidative stress status and vascular inflammation in healthy volunteers. British Journal of Nutrition 103, 43–49.

Wang, R.X., Chai, Q., Lu, T., Lee, H.C., 2011. Activation of vascular BK channels by docosahexaenoic acid is dependent on cytochrome P450 epoxygenase activity. Cardiovascular Research 90 (2), 344–352.

Wong, C.Y., Yiu, K.H., Li, S.W., et al., 2010. Fish–oil supplement has neutral effects on vascular and metabolic function but improves renal function in patients with type 2 diabetes mellitus. Diabetic Medicine 27, 54–60.

Yin, K., Chu, Z.M., Beilin, L.J., 1990. Effect of fish oil feeding on blood pressure and vascular reactivity in spontaneously hypertensive rats. Clinical and Experimental Pharmacology and Physiology 17, 235–239.

RELEVANT WEBSITE

http://www.americanheart.org – American Heart Association.

CHAPTER 37

Counteracting the Inflammatory Response in the Atherosclerosis Bioactive Products

F.J.O. Rios, N.O.S. Cãmara
Universidade de São Paulo, São Paulo, Brazil

1. INTRODUCTION

Atherosclerosis is a progressive cardiovascular disease (CVD), characterized by the inflammatory mechanisms and accumulation of lipids and fibrous components in the vascular wall. For many years, complications with atherosclerosis and other CVDs have been considered a public health problem related mainly to the Western societies. In fact, it is the leading cause of morbidity and mortality in these countries. However, due to changes in the pattern of social life and food habits, an increase in deaths related to CVDs in several countries in development process has been seen.

Several studies have tried to find significant risk factors associated with the atherosclerosis development. Current diagnostics observe obesity, hypertension, diabetes, and high concentration of blood cholesterol. Though, the latest data indicate that individuals without these risk factors may also develop a severe CVD, thus hindering early diagnosis and leading to myocardial infarction and hemodynamic shock.

Atherosclerosis is a very complex disease, influenced both by genetic and environmental factors. It is progressive and silent, whose lesions begin during the first decades of life. The first steps are characterized by the formation of fatty streak lesions in endothelial cells. These small lesions consist mainly of lipid-engulfed macrophages, so-called foam cells. In advanced stages of the disease, the lesion progresses to a fibrous plaque containing smooth muscle cells, calcification, deposition of extracellular lipid, and the presence of a dense and necrotic lipid core, which results in the onset of symptoms (Hansson and Libby, 2006).

2. INFLAMMATORY MECHANISMS IN ATHEROSCLEROSIS

Atherosclerosis disease affects mainly the medium- and large-sized blood vessels and rarely, affects small vessels. The research on CVD has grown considerably in the last few years and it has been assumed that the concentration in serum lipids and the oxidative

Bioactive Food as Dietary Interventions for Cardiovascular Disease
http://dx.doi.org/10.1016/B978-0-12-396485-4.00034-7

© 2013 Elsevier Inc.
All rights reserved.

modification of lipoproteins are the main responsible factors for the atherosclerosis development. Inflammatory cells from the immune system constitute the main component of the atherosclerotic plaque during the advanced stages. High risk for the atherosclerotic plaque rupture and subsequent thrombus formation in places with high number of activated inflammatory cells have been observed. Subpopulations of circulating inflammatory T lymphocytes are elevated in patients with acute coronary syndromes. Systemic inflammatory diseases are associated with the development of atherosclerosis, for example, systemic lupus erythematosus, and rheumatoid arthritis. These also support the influence of the inflammation on the atherosclerosis development (Hansson and Libby, 2006; Lusis, 2000).

The atherosclerotic process begins when the endothelium of the vessel wall suffers an injury, which induces an inflammatory response (Ross and Glomset, 1976). Thus, changes in vascular permeability lead to the migration of monocytes, T lymphocytes, and B lymphocytes to subendothelial space. The thickening of the arterial wall is caused by deposition of macromolecules, for example, lipids, cholesterol crystals, and calcium salts in the plaque. The inflammatory mechanisms in the endothelium lead to platelet aggregation and thrombus formation. Smooth muscle cells proliferate and produce extracellular matrix during advanced stages of the atherosclerosis. Proliferation is also observed in macrophages, caused by growth factors: granulocyte–macrophage-stimulating factor and macrophage colony-stimulating factors produced in the atherosclerotic plaque. The advanced stage of atherosclerotic lesions constitutes two structurally distinct components: lipid core and fibrous cape. The lipid core is rich in extracellular lipids, cholesterol esters, and crystals. The fibrous cap comprises about 70% of the total plaque size and is basically formed by inflammatory cells, smooth muscle cells, and extracellular matrix.

3. LOW-DENSITY LIPOPROTEIN

The low-density lipoprotein (LDL) particle is the most abundant lipoprotein in the human plasma and consists mainly of lipids, fat-soluble vitamins, and only one particle of apolipoprotein B-100 (apoB-100). It is responsible for the cholesterol transportation and essential for the synthesis of membrane, steroid hormones, and bile salts. It is a spherical particle with a diameter between 180 and 280 Å and density from 1.019 to 1.063 g ml^{-1}. The whole particle contains approximately 2700 molecules of fatty acids, predominantly polyunsaturated linoleic acid and arachidonic acid. With approximately six to eight molecules per LDL particle, α-tocopherol is the most abundant antioxidant. Other antioxidants are also present, such as γ-tocopherol, ubiquinol-10, α-carotene, β-carotene, lycopene, and cryptoxanthin (Hevonoja et al., 2000).

Under normal conditions, the LDL particle interacts with receptors located on the cell membrane, so-called B/E-type receptors, which recognize a specific amino acid sequence in the apoB-100 molecule. These receptors regulate the cholesterol cell uptake. Thus, when the intracellular levels of cholesterols reach optimal concentrations, the B/E-type receptors will be inhibited by feedback negative control. The extensive oxidation process affects internal lipids and protein of the LDL particle, increases the levels of toxic by-products such as malondialdehyde (MDA) and 4-hydroxy-2-nonenal (HNE). The concentration of these compounds in the plasma can also be used as markers for oxidation process. The oxidative process of the LDL particle is achieved in three main phases: an initial phase called *lag* phase, characterized by the consumption of endogenous antioxidants (e.g., α-tocopherol and β-carotene); a second phase called propagation, characterized by a linear formation of products derived from lipid peroxidation (e.g., conjugated dienes, lipid hydroperoxide, and oxysteroids), and a third phase called termination, which is characterized by constant levels of conjugated dienes (Zarev et al., 2003). Products from the lipid peroxidation also react with apoB-100 inducing its modification by glycation and/or oxidation of amino acids. The minimal modified LDL (mmLDL), where only the lipid portion is oxidized is still able to be recognized by LDL receptors (B/E-type receptors). However, the oxidized LDL (oxLDL), whose lipids and protein are extensively oxidized, is recognized mainly by a group of receptors called scavenger receptors, expressed by macrophages, endothelial cells, and smooth muscle cells (Glass and Witztum, 2001).

It is still not fully understood how, where, or when the initial point of the oxidative process of the LDL occurs *in vivo*. Some oxidant agents may be derived from cells, while others can be derived from exogenous sources such as food, pollution, or smoking. The oxidative process involves mainly reactive oxygen species (ROS) produced by endothelial cells and macrophages. Some enzymes in the arterial intimae may also contribute to the modification process, such as myeloperoxidase (MPO) and 15-lipoxygenase. It is noteworthy that the main oxidant targets usually are polyunsaturated acids of the LDL particle (Gaut and Heinecke, 2001; Figure 37.1).

Besides the crucial role in foam cell formation, the oxidative process of LDL particle brings about the formation of different compounds that can interact with several receptors and induces different effects. It has been described that these compounds can cause activation and proliferation of smooth muscle cells, expression of adhesion molecules in endothelial cells, and recruitment of monocytes and T lymphocytes into the subendothelial space, thereby initiating an immune response that will be responsible for the advancement of atherosclerotic lesions.

The modification of the LDL particle can also be mediated by several proteolytic and lipolytic enzymes present in the arterial intimae. Different proteases have been studied in this process, including plasmin, kallikrein, thrombin, trypsin, α-chymotrypsin, and pronase, which may induce anything from a small fragmentation to an extensive degradation of apoB-100, resulting in aggregation and fusion of LDL particles. Thus, the modification of the apoB-100 influences the binding with proteoglycans in the subendothelial space, thereby promoting the retention of LDL to the arterial intimae, and contributes to the beginning of the atherosclerosis lesions (Tabas et al., 2007).

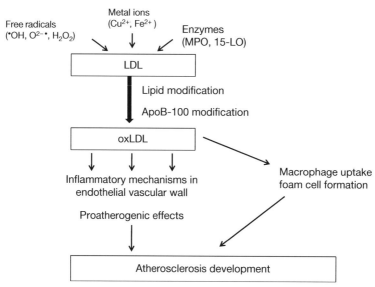

Figure 37.1 Oxidation of the low-density lipoprotein (LDL) particle leads to atherosclerosis development.

4. OXIDATIVE STRESS AND VASCULAR FUNCTION

Several risk situations have been described for the CVD development. Taking into account the tissue and cell groups involved in the beginning of atherosclerosis, the endothelium can be considered the primary target of the risk factors, which initiates the vascular inflammation . The ROS play an important and physiological role in heart function and maintenance of the vascular integrity. From the total amount of oxygen consumed by the organism, approximately 1–3% is converted in ROS. The ROS are produced mainly by the nicotinamide adenine dinucleotide phosphate–oxidase (NADPH oxidase) complex and comprises superoxide radical anion (O_2^-), hydrogen peroxide (H_2O_2), and hydroxyl radical ($^{\bullet}OH$). Another important source of ROS production includes the cytochrome p450 enzymes, flavoprotein oxidases, and peroxisomal enzymes that are involved in the metabolism of fatty acids. The ROS production is highly controlled by endogenous antioxidant mechanisms, that is, manganese and copper/zinc superoxide dismutase (MnSOD, Cu/ZnSOD), catalase, and glutathione peroxidase. However, high concentrations of ROS can exert harmful effects, contributing to vascular dysfunction associated with CVD. Together with nitric oxide (NO), the ROS may initiate the cell-signaling cascades, contributing to the inflammatory process. The NADPH oxidase complex is present in monocytes, macrophages, and cells from the vascular wall such as endothelial cells, vascular smooth muscle cells, and fibroblasts. The NADPH oxidase is formed by two subunits present in the cell membrane (p22phox and gp91phox, also called Nox2 and Nox1), the cytoplasmic subunits (p47phox, p67phox), and a G protein called rac 1. The NADPH oxidase in different cells releases superoxide anions in different locations. Leukocytes release superoxide anions in the extracellular environment, whereas the vascular cells do so intracellularly (Briones and Touyz, 2010; Cohen and Tong, 2010; Gaut and Heinecke, 2001).

The superoxide anion is the main ROS produced from the oxygen reduction. The H_2O_2 is produced from $O_2^{-\bullet}$ (superoxide radical anion), spontaneously or by reactions with superoxide dismutase (MnSOD, Cu/ZnSOD). Superoxide radical anion also reacts with NO and produces peroxynitrite (OONO$^-$), according to the reaction $O_2^{-\bullet}+NO \rightarrow ONOO^-$.

Peroxynitrite has high reactivity against lipids and proteins, initiating the oxidation of LDL, and contributes to the inflammatory mechanisms in the arterial wall. NO is a potent oxidant agent produced by endothelial cells and macrophages into the vascular intimae. The NO is able to exert anti- or proatherogenic effects, which will be dependent on where it was produced. NO produced by the enzyme endothelial NO synthase (eNOS) in the endothelial cells has vasorelaxant properties, and its deficiency is associated with hypertension and proatherogenic events. However, the NO produced during an inflammatory reaction by the inducible NO synthase (iNOS) in macrophages not only has a high microbicidal capacity but also carries out several oxidant functions and might contribute to the LDL oxidation (Luoma et al., 1998). The inhibition of iNOS decreases the inflammatory response and has anti-atherogenic effects (Detmers et al., 2000).

Besides free radicals, another large number of oxidant-generating systems have been investigated and may either directly or indirectly induce the oxidation of the LDL particle (e.g., enzymes such as 15-lipoxygenase and MPO). Indeed, it was demonstrated that the increased expression of 15-lipoxygenase in the vascular wall is associated with atherosclerosis development (Wittwer and Hersberger, 2007).

Lipoxygenases are intracellular enzymes that can catalyze the peroxidation of polyunsaturated fatty acids. *In vivo* studies and experimental results showed that the 15-lipoxygenase is increased in atherosclerotic lesions. It was observed that this enzyme may contribute to lipoprotein oxidation, producing the 13-S-hydroxyoctadecadienoic acid (13-S-HODE), present in early and advanced atherosclerotic lesions, thus suggesting that lipoxygenase may be important not only during the initial steps, but also in disease progression.

MPO is secreted by phagocytes during the inflammatory process, against invading microorganisms. It has been implicated in the atherogenic process mainly because of its high ability to produce oxidants agents, such as hypochlorous acid (HOCl) (Nicholls and Hazen, 2009). The HOCl is highly oxidative to proteins, nucleotides, and carotenoids, and it is produced according to the reaction $H_2O_2 + Cl^- + H^+ \rightarrow HOCl + H_2O$.

Some studies showed the expression of catalytically active MPO in human atherosclerotic plaques, especially in regions with high numbers of macrophages. In addition, 3-chlorotyrosine, an end-product of MPO-mediated oxidation, was observed in human atherosclerotic lesions. This suggests that MPO participates in the modification of the LDL particle, contributing to the atherogenic process.

Despite several studies about the oxidative agents and their oxidation targets, hitherto, no one knows which are the most important oxidative mechanisms or oxidative products in the atherosclerosis development. It is noteworthy that oxidative reactions are inevitable and directly associated to various physiological reactions. So, at what time are these products no longer physiological, but start to be deleterious? The oxidative agents are constantly produced. However, they are kept in balance or are inactivated by antioxidant systems in the body. In fact, the body is provided with several antioxidant defenses that are capable of inhibiting oxidation in different steps of the process: (a) Superoxide dismutase can remove transition metals and inactivate the lipid peroxidation by the superoxide anion, thereby inhibiting the peroxynitrite formation; (b) catalase reduces the hydrogen peroxide; and (c) the glutathione peroxidase system is capable of decreasing the formation lipid hydroperoxides. All these systems described are highly efficient. However, when these antioxidant defenses are in lower concentration, oxidant agents begin to exert harmful effects (Niki, 2004).

5. ANTIOXIDANTS – PROTECTIVE ROLE IN CVD

As described for the oxidant agents, the antioxidants also are a diverse group, which may act differently according to their chemical structure or site of action. Antioxidants may inactivate the oxidant agents and participate in the injured tissue recovering. The antioxidant defense system includes both endogenous and exogenous compounds. The last ones are mainly acquired from the diet, such as ascorbic acid (vitamin C), α-tocopherol (vitamin E), and β-carotene (pro-vitamin A) (Niki, 2004; Riccioni et al., 2007).

Vitamin A: Fat-soluble vitamin with three isoforms called retinoids: retinol, retinal, and retinoic acid. β-Carotene is the most important retinoid, with the highest antioxidant capacity in the group. Its antioxidant effects are associated with the blockade of free radical-mediated reactions, especially the ones where singlet oxygen is involved. It inhibits DNA damage and lipid peroxidation, inhibiting the oxidation of LDL particle. Food sources: Yellow-orange fruits, vegetables (carrots), and leafy vegetables.

Vitamin C: Water-soluble vitamin with two biologically active forms: ascorbic acid and dehydroascorbic acid. The biologic effects of the vitamin C are related to its reducing properties. Thus, the ascorbic acid is oxidized to dehydroascorbate. In this process, ascorbic acid is a hydrogen donor, which acts as a reducing agent and inactivates free radicals, preventing the oxidation process. Food sources: Fruits (citrus) and vegetables (green and red peppers, tomatoes, green and leafy).

Vitamin E: Fat-soluble vitamin, which comprises tocopherol, and tocotrienol groups that can exist as α (alpha), β (beta), γ (gamma), and δ (delta) isomers. α-Tocopherol is the most important isoform and therefore the most studied one. It has a hydroxyl group in its chemical structure and because of that the antioxidant effects are related to its ability to donate hydrogen. Studies have found that vitamin E prevents the oxidation of polyunsaturated fatty acids and the formation of conjugated dienes, which are present in the oxidation of the LDL particle. Food sources: Vegetable oil (soybean, corn, olive), grains, nuts and seeds, green and leafy vegetables.

Among the antioxidants present in the LDL particle, α–tocopherol and β–carotene are the most abundant ones, contributing to the integrity of the chemical structure. This explains why several research groups have high interest in these antioxidants. The deficiency in α–tocopherol contributes to the atherosclerotic lesion formation. Thus, it is plausible to believe that the enrichment of the LDL particle with these antioxidants might increase the resistance to oxidative reactions. However, a large number of randomized studies have shown that supplemental enrichment of the diet with α–tocopherol did not show improvement in atherosclerotic disease treatment (Rock et al., 2001).

Several studies have reported prevention in CVD associated with consumption of antioxidant-rich foods, such as fruits, vegetables, walnuts, red palm oil, and flavonoids. It is easily observed that diets rich in fruits and vegetables containing high levels of vitamin C, vitamin E, and β–carotene are associated with reduced risk for CVD. However, the main question still remains to be answered: If the consumption of antioxidant-rich food prevents CVDs, why does daily supplemental intake of the antioxidants has failed to show protective characteristics of these compounds? One possible answer to this tricky question is that fruits and vegetables have different amounts of different compounds and also several other antioxidants found naturally (e.g., flavonoids), which are not present in chemically synthesized supplements.

Regarding the benefits of antioxidants, the discrepancy observed between the results might be explained by the methodology applied during the study: observational studies or randomized trials using dietary supplements. For most part of health professionals, the methodology designed for the study would not interfere in the main result. However, it can be seen below that it makes all the difference.

5.1 Randomized Studies

Most studies and randomized clinical trials have failed to prove the benefits of antioxidant supplement therapy in the treatment of CVD. However, to analyze the data obtained in different studies is a very difficult work. Different studies use different doses of supplements and vitamins. Another difference observed is the population studied.

To complicate the understanding about antioxidant therapies, some side effects regarding the use of antioxidant supplements also have been observed. One study performed in 2001, using statin therapy in combination with several antioxidants (vitamin E, β–carotene, vitamin C, and selenium), reported an increase in cardiovascular events compared with the group treated only with statin (Brown et al., 2001). This indicates that antioxidant supplements, somehow, interfered with the effectiveness of statins. Similarly, one study of 34 486 postmenopausal women showed that the use of supplements containing vitamin E and vitamin C, associated with hormone replacement therapy, unexpectedly resulted in increased mortality associated with CVDs in postmenopausal women (Kushi et al., 1996).

In summary, from the studies mentioned above and several others with similar results, the use of antioxidant dietary supplements to prevent CVD should not be recommended until their effect is proven in well-designed clinical trials (randomized, placebo-controlled) that directly test their impact on CVDs end points.

5.2 Observational Studies

Although several studies have shown conflicting results regarding the antioxidant therapy, the American Heart Association still defends that some micronutrients may have benefits against risks for CVD (vitamin E, vitamin C, and β-carotene). The recommendation is based on several epidemiological and population studies.

A large number of results that indicate an importance in the consumption of diet rich in antioxidants to prevent CVDs come from observational studies, including case–control and cohort studies. In most part of these studies, a reduced risk for CVDs associated with the intake of antioxidants in the diet, especially vitamin E, β-carotene, or vitamin C, compared with the group where these oxidants were not part of the diet, has been observed. In addition, clinical reports of individual cases have shown significant reduction in death risks related to cardiovascular events in patients with antioxidant-rich diets (Esposito et al., 2006).

Even though antioxidant supplements did not prove beneficial in preventing heart problems, foods that are sources of antioxidants are still recommended. There are benefits in getting vitamins of the food that might not occur in supplement form. For example, foods rich in antioxidants may have nutrients such as flavonoids and lycopenes, which are not included in vitamin supplements. In addition, several studies have observed the dietary intake of antioxidant nutrients in combating atherosclerosis (wine, olive oil, etc.). Dietary factors based on cereals, dark green vegetables, citrus fruits, crude palm oil, soybean oil, cod-liver oil, whole grain, and walnuts can significantly reduce the concentration of oxidants in the blood and the risk for CVD. Phenolic compounds, like flavonoids present in fruits and vegetables, can also improve endothelial function and inhibit platelet aggregation in humans, thus preventing the thrombus formation (Seifried et al., 2007).

A healthy diet is based mainly on food quality rather than quantity ingested. The fatty acid concentration versus total fat in the diet can be crucial to cholesterol levels in serum. Fatty acids can be divided into four categories: Saturated, monounsaturated, polyunsaturated, and trans-fatty acids. Within these categories, the saturated fatty acids and trans-fatty acids are associated with increased risk for CVD. However, monounsaturated fatty acids (MUFA, ω–9) and polyunsaturated fatty acids (PUFA, ω–3, ω–6) are associated with a reduced risk for CVD, as discussed below.

Monounsaturated fatty acids: The consumption of food rich in this fatty acid is able to decrease risk factors for CVD (lipoprotein levels, blood pressure, glucose, and antithrombotic properties), contribute to a better functioning of the endothelium, interfere with the proliferation of smooth muscle cells, and also has some antioxidant properties. These effects were first observed in Mediterranean-type diet, which has olive oil as the main source of fat in the diet.

Polyunsaturated fatty acids: Alpha linolenic acid (ALA, ω–3) and linoleic acid (LA, ω–6). They can be converted to long-chain fatty acids, such as arachidonic acid, eicosapentaenoic acid (EPA)/docosahexaenoic acid (DHA). Seafood and fatty fish, vegetable oils, cereals, and walnuts are the main sources of ω–3 and ω–6. The intake of foods containing ω–3 has been associated with a decreased risk for the primary and secondary CVD, preventing arrhythmias, lowering heart rate and blood pressure, decreasing platelet aggregation, improving vascular reactivity, and lowering plasma triglyceride levels. EPA and DHA can also decrease the production of hepatic triglycerides and increase the clearance of plasma triglycerides (Badimon et al., 2010).

6. CONCLUDING REMARKS

Despite the knowledge of the role of oxidants in the CVD development, little is known about the oxidative mechanisms that are actually involved in the initial steps in disease progression. It is plausible to admit that the lack of knowledge can be the reason for the difference between the results found in several studies. As the crucial mechanisms are not known, it is difficult to find targets that ensure the use of specific antioxidant supplements. In addition, more homogeneous studies are needed in order to obtain a correct efficiency of antioxidant supplements, such as characteristics of the study population, dose and correct isomer of the molecule used, as well as adequate time for supplementation and duration of the study. It is important to recognize that atherosclerosis may proceed by different mechanisms, and it is probably difficult for any antioxidant to be effective for all mechanisms. However, the collective results suggest that antioxidant-rich fruits, vegetables, nuts, and whole grain have biological activities mainly because their action does not depend on a single compound, but a combination of vitamins, fatty acids, flavonoids, and other antioxidants that might act synergically and counteract the atherosclerosis and other CVDs.

REFERENCES

Badimon, L., Vilahur, G., Padro, T., 2010. Nutraceuticals and atherosclerosis: human trials. Cardiovascular Therapeutics 28 (4), 202–215.

Briones, A.M., Touyz, R.M., 2010. Oxidative stress and hypertension: current concepts. Current Hypertension Reports 12 (2), 135–142.

Brown, B.G., Zhao, X.Q., Chait, A., et al., 2001. Simvastatin and niacin, antioxidant vitamins, or the combination for the prevention of coronary disease. The New England Journal of Medicine 345 (22), 1583–1592.

Cohen, R.A., Tong, X., 2010. Vascular oxidative stress: the common link in hypertensive and diabetic vascular disease. Journal of Cardiovascular Pharmacology 55 (4), 308–316.

Detmers, P.A., Hernandez, M., Mudgett, J., et al., 2000. Deficiency in inducible nitric oxide synthase results in reduced atherosclerosis in apolipoprotein E-deficient mice. Journal of Immunology 165 (6), 3430–3435.

Esposito, K., Ciotola, M., Giugliano, D., 2006. Mediterranean diet, endothelial function and vascular inflammatory markers. Public Health Nutrition 9 (8A), 1073–1076.

Gaut, J.P., Heinecke, J.W., 2001. Mechanisms for oxidizing low-density lipoprotein. insights from patterns of oxidation products in the artery wall and from mouse models of atherosclerosis. Trends in Cardiovascular Medicine 11 (3–4), 103–112.

Glass, C.K., Witztum, J.L., 2001. Atherosclerosis. the road ahead. Cell 104 (4), 503–516.

Hansson, G.K., Libby, P., 2006. The immune response in atherosclerosis: a double-edged sword. Nature Reviews Immunology 6 (7), 508–519.

Hevonoja, T., Pentikainen, M.O., Hyvonen, M.T., Kovanen, P.T., Ala-Korpela, M., 2000. Structure of low density lipoprotein (LDL) particles: basis for understanding molecular changes in modified LDL. Biochimica et Biophysica Acta 1488 (3), 189–210.

Kushi, L.H., Folsom, A.R., Prineas, R.J., Mink, P.J., Wu, Y., Bostick, R.M., 1996. Dietary antioxidant vitamins and death from coronary heart disease in postmenopausal women. The New England Journal of Medicine 334 (18), 1156–1162.

Luoma, J.S., Stralin, P., Marklund, S.L., Hiltunen, T.P., Sarkioja, T., Yla-Herttuala, S., 1998. Expression of extracellular SOD and iNOS in macrophages and smooth muscle cells in human and rabbit atherosclerotic lesions: colocalization with epitopes characteristic of oxidized LDL and peroxynitrite-modified proteins. Arteriosclerosis, Thrombosis, and Vascular Biology 18 (2), 157–167.

Lusis, A.J., 2000. Atherosclerosis. Nature 407 (6801), 233–241.

Nicholls, S.J., Hazen, S.L., 2009. Myeloperoxidase, modified lipoproteins, and atherogenesis. Journal of Lipid Research 50 (Suppl.), S346–S351.

Niki, E., 2004. Antioxidants and atherosclerosis. Biochemical Society Transactions 32 (Pt 1), 156–159.

Riccioni, G., Bucciarelli, T., Mancini, B., et al., 2007. Antioxidant vitamin supplementation in cardiovascular diseases. Annals of Clinical and Laboratory Science 37 (1), 89–95.

Rock, E., Winklhofer-Roob, B.M., Ribalta, J., et al., 2001. Vitamin A, vitamin E and carotenoid status and metabolism during ageing: functional and nutritional consequences (VITAGE PROJECT). Nutrition, Metabolism, and Cardiovascular Diseases 11 (Suppl. 4), 70–73.

Ross, R., Glomset, J.A., 1976. The pathogenesis of atherosclerosis. The New England Journal of Medicine 295, 369–377.

Seifried, H.E., Anderson, D.E., Fisher, E.I., Milner, J.A., 2007. A review of the interaction among dietary antioxidants and reactive oxygen species. The Journal of Nutritional Biochemistry 18 (9), 567–579.

Tabas, I., Williams, K.J., Boren, J., 2007. Subendothelial lipoprotein retention as the initiating process in atherosclerosis: update and therapeutic implications. Circulation 116 (16), 1832–1844.

Wittwer, J., Hersberger, M., 2007. The two faces of the 15-lipoxygenase in atherosclerosis. Prostaglandins, Leukotrienes, and Essential Fatty Acids 77 (2), 67–77.

Zarev, S., Bonnefont-Rousselot, D., Jedidi, I., et al., 2003. Extent of copper LDL oxidation depends on oxidation time and copper/LDL ratio: chemical characterization. Archives of Biochemistry and Biophysics 420 (1), 68–78.

CHAPTER 38

Cardioprotective Efficacy of Alternative and Complementary Therapeutics

R. Arora[*,†], B. Goswami[†], A.R. Shivashankara[‡], D.M. Periera[‡], M.S. Baliga[‡]

[*]Staff Officer to Chief Controller Research and Development (Life Sciences and International Cooperation), New Delhi, India
[†]Institute of Nuclear Medicine and Allied Sciences, Delhi, India
[‡]Father Muller Medical College, Kankanady, Mangalore, India

1. INTRODUCTION

Despite significant progress in medical research, cardiovascular diseases (CVDs; comprising ischemic heart disease (IHD), stroke, and congestive heart failure) continue to be the largest contributors to morbidity and mortality in both developed and developing countries (Dabhadkar et al., 2011). Of all the CVDs, the focus for both clinicians and researchers is primarily IHD, stroke, and congestive heart failure, which contribute most to the burden. In the context of these observations, most people living in developing countries rely on plant-based traditional medicines, which are not part of conventional modern medicine and are now termed complementary and alternative medicine.

India is a biodiversity hot spot and reports indicate that nearly 45 000 plant species indigenous to the region are useful as medicinal agents in the various traditional and folk systems of medicine. Scientific studies carried out over the past three decades have validated many of the ethnomedicinal claims of plants used in the Indian traditional systems of medicine, Ayurveda, Siddha, and Unani. The cardioprotective effects the plants provide may be due to their ability to increase the blood supply to heart muscle, their antihypertensive and anticoagulant properties, their potential to steady the heartbeat and improve the tone of the vessels, their antilipidemic properties, and their antioxidant effects. Preclinical studies carried out in the recent past have confirmed that the Ayurvedic medicinal plants *Acorus calamus*, *Aegle marmelos*, *Allium cepa*, *Allium sativum*, *Centella asiatica*, *Commiphora wightii*, *Emblica officinalis*, *Ocimum sanctum*, *Picrorhiza kurroa*, *Terminalia arjuna*, *Terminalia chebula*, *Tinospora cordifolia*, *Withania somnifera*, and *Zingiber officinale* possess cardioprotective effects (Figure 38.1; Dwivedi and Chaturvedi, 2000). These plants also possess diverse pharmacological properties, which are addressed in Table 38.1. This chapter collates the scientific observations supporting their ethnomedicinal validation.

© 2013 Elsevier Inc.
All rights reserved.

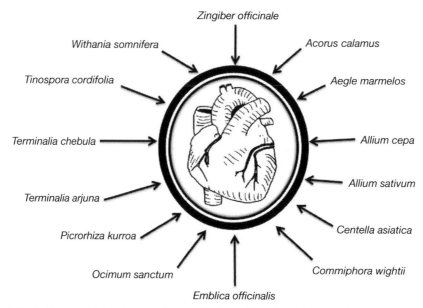

Figure 38.1 Indian medicinal plants with scientifically validated cardioprotective properties.

2. *ACORUS CALAMUS*

A. calamus commonly known as vacha in Hindi and belonging to the family Acoraceae is an important psychotropic drug. With regard to the cardioprotective effects of *A. calamus*, studies have shown that extracts of this plant sensitize the cells to insulin and prevent weight gain (Wu et al., 2009), block platelet aggregation, exhibit antioxidant properties, and ameliorate hyperlipidemia (D'Souza et al., 2007). *A. calamus* has been shown to contain certain phytochemicals that inhibit the key enzyme of cholesterol biosynthesis, HMG CoA reductase (D'Souza et al., 2007).

3. *AEGLE MARMELOS*

Commonly known as bael, *A. marmelos* is a tree originally indigenous to India but is today found growing in Pakistan, Sri Lanka, and other Southeast Asian countries. With regard to the cardioprotective effects of bael, studies have shown that bael has antidiabetic, anti-hyperlipidemic, antioxidant, and direct cardiocytoprotective actions. Preclinical studies have observed that treatment with bael seed, fruit, and leaf extracts caused a reduction in blood glucose, improved glucose tolerance and glycemic control, corrected dyslipidemia, and improved the antioxidant status (Kamalakkannan and Prince, 2003) in diabetic animals. Bael enhanced the levels of superoxide dismutase (SOD), catalase (CAT), and glutathione peroxidase (GPx) and lowered the glutathione content in the heart in

Table 38.1 The Main Phytochemicals and Medicinal Uses of the Important Cardioprotective Indian Medicinal Plants

Scientific name and family	Colloquial name	English name	Phytochemicals present	Medicinal uses
Acorus calamus Acoraceae	Vacha	Sweet flag	Dehydrodiisoeugenol, linalool, apigenin 4′,7-dimethyl ether, 2,2,5,5-tetramethyl-3-hexanol, bornyl acetate, galgravin, retusin, isoeugenol methylether, dehydroabietic acid, acetophenone, elemicin, camphor, butyl butanoate, borneol, 2-allyl-5-ethoxy-4-methoxyphenol, linolenic acid, isoelemicin, geranylacetate, furyl ethyl ketone, epieudesmin, asarone, acetic acid, á-ursolic acid, (9e,12e,15e)-9,12,15-octadecatrien-1-ol, sakuranin, nonanoic acid, (-)-spathulenol, (-)-4-terpineol, and lysidine	Bronchodialator; improves cognition and helps in wound healing
Allium cepa Alliaceae	Pyaz	Bulb onion	Allicin, allin, alliospiroside, allyl-propyl-disulfate, α-amyrin, α-linolic acid, capaene, ferulic acid, kaempferol, mevalonic acid, zymostenol, quercetin, α-sitosterol and 4-methyl-zymostenol, ianshic acid, N-trans-feruloyl tyramine, β-sitosterol-3 β-glucopyranoside-6′-palmitate, sitosterol, daucosterol, tryptophane, adenine riboside, 5-hydroxy-3-methyl-4-propylsulfanyl-5H-furan-2-one, 5-(hydroxymethyl) furfural, acetovanillone, methyl 4-hydroxyl cinnamate, and ferulic acid methyl ester	Anti-inflammatory, anticancer, antioxidant; prevents osteoporosis

Continued

Table 38.1 The Main Phytochemicals and Medicinal Uses of the Important Cardioprotective Indian Medicinal Plants—cont'd

Scientific name and family	Colloquial name	English name	Phytochemicals present	Medicinal uses
Allium sativum Alliaceae	Lashun	Garlic	Allicin, ajoene, allylpropl, diallyl, trisulfide, sallylcysteine, vinyldithiines and S-allylmercaptocystein, allium fructan, allisatin, hexand, β-carotene, allium lectin, ascorbic acid, allin, and kaempferol	Antibacterial, antiviral, antifungal, antiparasitic, anticancer, antioxidant and anti-inflammatory; increases osteoporosis
Commiphora wightii Burseraceae	Guggul		Myrrhanol A, myrrhanone A, myrrhanol B, myrrhanones B, A acetate, 20(S),21-epoxy-3-oxocholest-4-ene, 8 β-hydroxy-3,20-dioxopregn-4,6-diene, 5-(13′ Z-nonadecenyl)resorcinol, Z-guggulsterones, and E-guggusterones	Anti-inflammatory and antiproliferative
Withania somnifera Solanaceae	Ashwagandha	Winter cherry	Alkaloids, steroidal lactones, anhydrine, withanine, somniferine, somnine, somniferinine, withananine, pseudo-withanine, tropine, pseudo-tropine, cuscohygrine, anferine, anhydrine, sitoindoside VII, sitoindoside VIII, and withanolides	Anticarcinogenic, antioxidant, diuretic, anti-inflammatory, anti-stress, immunomodulator, hemopoietic, and is indicated in neurodegenerative diseases
Tinospora cordifolia Menispermaceae	Guduchi		Giloin, gilenin, gilosterol, columbin, chasmanthin, palmarin, sesquiterpenes, diterpenes, norditerpene furan glycosides cordiofolisides A, B, and C, tinocordifolin, tinocordifolioside, palmatosides C and F, amritosides, cordioside, tinosponone, tinocordioside, tinosporaside, tinocordiside, syringin, cordiol, cordioside, cordifoliosides A and B, berberinelignan, octacosanol,	Immunostimulatory, anti-inflammatory, immunoprophylactic, and hepatoprotective

		nonacosan-15-one, heptacosanol, β-sitosterol, tinosporidine, cordifol, cordifolone, magnoflorine, tembetarine, syringine, syringine apiosylglycoside, isocolumbin, palmatine, tetrahydropalmatine, magnoflorine, and jatrorrhizine	
Picrorhiza kurroa Scrophulariaceae	Kutki	Picroliv, kutkin, apocynin, drosin, picrosides I, II, III, D-mannitol, vanillic acid, and cucurbitacin glycosides	Antioxidant, anti-apoptotic, hepatoprotective, antiasthmatic, and choleretic
Centella asiatica Mackinlayaceae	Brahmi	Madecasoside, asiaticoside, madecasic acid, asiatic acid, asiaticoside G, asiaticoside F, quadranoside IV, 2α,3β,6β-trihydroxyolean-12-en-28-oic acid, kaempferol, quercetin, astragalin and isoquercetin, indocentellosides, brahmoside, brahminoside, asiaticoside, thankuniside, triterpene acids (indocentoic, brahmic, thankunic and isothankunic), isobrahmic acid, betulic acid, bicoside A & B, centellose, stigmasterol, terpene acetate, camphor, and cineole	Anticonvulsant, adaptogen, antibacterial, antiviral, anti-inflammatory, antiulcerogenic, anxiolytic, a cerebral tonic, a circulatory stimulant, a diuretic, nervine, and vulnerary; promotes the proliferation of granulation and increases tensile strength of wounds
Emblica officinalis Punicaceae	Amla Indian gooseberry	Alkaloids, tannins, flavonoids, kaempferol, phyllembic acid, emblicol, ellagic acid, ascorbic acid, and gallic acid	Antipyretic, analgesic, antitussive, antiatherogenic, adaptogenic, cardioprotective, gastroprotective, antianemic, antihypercholesterolemic, antidiarrheal, antiatherosclerotic, hepatoprotective, nephroprotective, and neuroprotective; helps in wound healing

Continued

Table 38.1 The Main Phytochemicals and Medicinal Uses of the Important Cardioprotective Indian Medicinal Plants—cont'd

Scientific name and family	Colloquial name	English name	Phytochemicals present	Medicinal uses
Zingiber officinale Zingiberaceae	Ginger	Adhrak	β-sesquiphelladrene, bisabolene, β-phelladrene, cineol, citral, farnesene, curcumin, sesquiterpenoids, 6-gingerol, 6-shogaol, borneol, caffeic-acid, camphor, capsaicin, chlorogenic-acid, eugenol, ferulic-acid, gingerol, myrcene, p-cymene, quercetin, shogaol, farnesol, ferulic-acid, kaempferol, limonene, and linalool	Antibacterial, antiasthmatic, neuroprotective, analgesic, sedative, and antipyretic
Ocimum sanctum Lamiaceae	Tulsi	Holy basil	Ursolic acid, eugenol, β-elemene, β-caryophyllene, germacrene D, methyl chavicol, linalool, bicyclogermacrene, α-terpineol, 1,8-cineole, camphor, limonene, camphene, and (E)-β-ocimene	Anticancer, antidiabetic, antifungal, antimicrobial, antiemetic, hepato-protective, cardioprotective, antispasmodic, analgesic, adaptogenic, and diaphoretic
Terminalia chebula Combretaceae	Haritaki	Black Myrobalan	Gallic acid, ethyl gallate, ellagic acid, chebulinic acid, 2,4-chebulyl-b-D-glucopyranose, luteolin, and tannic acid	Antiulcerogenic, anticancer, and antimicrobial
Aegle marmelos Rutaceae	Bael	Stone apple	Skimmianine, aegelin, lupeol, cineole, citral, citronellal, cuminaldehyde (4-isopropylbenzal-dehyde), eugenol, marmesinin, marmelosin, luvangetin, aurapten, psoralen, marmelide, fagarine, marmin, and tannin	Astringent, antidiarrheal, antidysenteric, demulcent, antipyretic, and anti-inflammatory
Terminalia arjuna Combretaceae	Arjuna	Arjuna	Flavonoids, oligomeric proanthocyanidins, saponin glycosides, tannins, calcium, magnesium, triterpenoid glycosides, arjunoside III, arjunoside IV, arjunglucoside I, arjunetin, leucocyanidin, ellagic acid, and gallic acid	Decreases the level of thyroid hormones; antiasthmatic and diuretic; decreases the level of thyroid hormones

experimental diabetes (Kamalakkannan and Prince, 2003). Bael has also been found to be useful in diabetes associated with IHD (Dwivedi and Aggarwal, 2009).

4. *ALLIUM CEPA*

A. cepa is commonly known as the bulb onion and is an important culinary and medicinal plant in various traditional systems of medicine to treat respiratory diseases, anemia, skin disorders, cholera, bleeding piles, common cold, and heart diseases. Preclinical and clinical studies have shown that *A. cepa* reduced blood glucose levels, improved glucose tolerance (Campos et al., 2003; Taj Eldin et al., 2010), and increased insulin secretion in diabetic rats fed a high-fat diet (Islam et al., 2008). Onion is also reported to exert an antihyperlipidemic effect by decreasing the total serum lipid, triglyceride, and atherogenic index and increasing the high-density lipoprotein (HDL)-cholesterol/total cholesterol ratio in diabetic rats (Bang et al., 2009). It is also observed to reduce systolic blood pressure in both L-NAME induced-hypertensive and spontaneously hypertensive rats (Kawamoto et al., 2004). The methanolic extract of onion was also demonstrated to exert a cytoprotective effect on heart cells and to decrease reactive oxygen species (ROS), mitochondrial membrane depolarization, cytochrome C release, and caspase-3 activation during hypoxia in heart cells *in vitro*, and it significantly reduced the infarct size, the apoptotic cell death of the heart and the plasma malondialdehyde (MDA) level *in vivo* in rats (Park et al., 2009).

5. *ALLIUM SATIVUM*

A. sativum, commonly known as garlic, is a plant belonging to the family Alliaceae and has both culinary and medicinal use. Studies have shown that garlic possesses antidiabetic, hypolipidemic, antihypertensive, antioxidant, anti-inflammatory, and antiplatelet actions. *In vitro* studies have shown that garlic extracts and some phytochemicals scavenge free radicals (Banerjee and Maulik, 2002). Garlic also possesses antidiabetic properties and is effective in reducing the blood glucose levels in diabetic rats, rabbits, and mice (Banerjee and Maulik, 2002). Feeding garlic to cholesterol-fed, hyperlipidemic, or diabetic animals is shown to improve the plasma antioxidant activity and to decrease lipid peroxidation (LPO) and LDL oxidation (Gorinstein et al., 2007).

Several studies have shown that garlic reduces the plasma levels of total cholesterol, triglycerides, and LDL cholesterol, and increases the levels of HDL-cholesterol in plasma (Banerjee and Maulik, 2002; Gorinstein et al., 2007). Mechanistic studies have shown that garlic reduces cholesterol biosynthesis, inhibits lipogenic enzymes, and controls cholesterol esterification in cells (Banerjee and Maulik, 2002). Garlic is shown to inhibit platelet aggregation and to possess fibrinolytic activity. Multiple studies with both raw and aged garlic have shown them to be effective at restoring the endothelial function of arteries and to possess hypotensive and vasodilatory effects (Banerjee and Maulik, 2002; Gorinstein et al., 2007). Clinical studies have also shown that garlic reduces both systolic and diastolic blood pressure in hypertensive subjects (Banerjee and Maulik, 2002; Gorinstein et al., 2007), thereby validating the experimental and ethnomedicinal observations.

6. *CENTELLA ASIATICA*

C. asiatica commonly known as brahmi is a small herbaceous annual plant of the family Mackinlayaceae. It is a mild adaptogen, is mildly antibacterial, antiviral, anti-inflammatory, antiulcerogenic, and anxiolytic, a cerebral tonic, a circulatory stimulant, and a diuretic, nervine, and vulnerary. Studies have shown that brahmi possesses antioxidant action (Gnanapragasam et al., 2007), improves microcirculation in patients suffering from venous hypertension (De Sanctis et al., 2001), and stabilizes hypoechoic, low-density arteriolar plaques (Cesarone et al., 2001). Brahmi reversed the toxic manifestations of adriamycin-induced cardiomyopathy in rats, restored the cardiac tissue levels of cardiac marker enzymes (lactate dehydrogenase (LDH), aspartate aminotransferase (AST), and creatine kinase (CK)), enzymes of the citric acid cycle and electron transport chain, and the antioxidant enzymes, and the cellular architecture of cardiac tissue (Gnanapragasam et al., 2007).

7. *COMMIPHORA WIGHTII*

C. wightii, commonly known as guggal, the guggul or mukul myrrh tree, is a flowering plant of the family Burseraceae (Deng, 2007; Sharma et al., 2009). Guggul possesses potent antihyperlipidemic effects, and guggulsterone, its principal phytochemical, is reported to be an antagonist of the farnesoid X receptor (FXR) and to upregulate the bile salt export pump, thereby contributing to a cholesterol-lowering effect (Deng, 2007). Randomized, double-blind clinical studies with hypercholesterolemic patients have shown that administering guggul reduced the total cholesterol, triglycerides, and LDL, and also decreased the plasma lipid peroxides (Singh et al., 1993). Guggulsterone ameliorated the prodiabetic changes such as increased serum glucose, cholesterol, and triglyceride levels and concomitantly increased the insulin resistance and enhanced the expression and activity of peroxisome proliferator-activated receptor gamma (PPARγ) in high fat-induced diabetic rats (Sharma et al., 2009). The hydroalcoholic extract of guggul is also shown to improve cardiac function and prevent myocardial ischemic impairment (Ojha et al., 2008).

8. *EMBLICA OFFICINALIS*

E. officinalis, which is commonly known as the Indian gooseberry or amla, belongs to the family Phyllanthaceae (Shri and Arora, 2010). Amla has antioxidant, anti-inflammatory, antihyperglycemic, and antihyperlipidemic effects (Shri and Arora, 2010). Preclinical studies have observed that amla ameliorated hyperlipidemia (Antony et al., 2006; Nampoothiri et al., 2011), reduced the activity of HMG CoA reductase (rate limiting enzyme of cholesterol biosynthesis) in heart and liver tissues, inhibited LDL oxidation (Nampoothiri et al., 2011), and reversed the progression of atheromatous plaques (Antony et al., 2006). The antiatherogenic properties of amla have been attributed to corilagin and its analog 1,6-di-O-galloyl-β-D-glucose. They are proposed to inhibit the progression of atherosclerosis by alleviating oxidation injury or by inhibiting ox-LDL-induced vascular smooth muscle cell (VSMC) proliferation (Duan et al., 2005).

9. *OCIMUM SANCTUM*

O. Sanctum, commonly known as tulsi in various Indian languages and as Holy Basil in English is an aromatic plant of the family Lamiaceae. Tulsi provides cardioprotection because of its antidiabetic, antihyperlipidemic, antioxidant, and hypoglycemic effects in both normal and diabetic animals (Rai et al., 1997). Feeding tulsi to both normal and diabetic rats is shown to reduce the total cholesterol, LDL cholesterol, triglycerides, and total lipids in plasma and liver (Rai et al., 1997). Tulsi oil contains high levels of linoleic acid and linolenic acid, the polyunsaturated fatty acids that are known to reduce serum cholesterol and offer cardioprotection (Suanarunsawat et al., 2010). Tulsi decreases blood glucose and restores the blood antioxidant enzymes, zinc, and selenium in diabetic rats (Chandra et al., 2008). Tulsi is also reported to cause significant reduction in plasma glucose, HbA1c, lipid profile, and LPO and to increase GPx, SOD, CAT, and glutathione S-transferase (GST) in rats (Eshrat and Mukhopadhyay, 2006).

10. *PICRORHIZA KURROA*

P. kurroa, commonly known as kutki and belonging to the family Scrophulariaceae, is a herb native to the Himalayan regions of India, Pakistan, and Nepal. It is a very effective hepatoprotective plant and also possesses antihyperlipidemic and antioxidant actions. The aqueous extract of kutki is also effective in decreasing fasting blood glucose and hyperlipidemia, increasing glucose tolerance and liver glycogen content, and preventing body weight loss in type 1 diabetic rats (Husain et al., 2009). Oral administration of kutki also prevented isoproterenol-induced myocardial infarction and maintained the normal status of rats (Senthil Kumar et al., 2001). Picroliv, the ethanolic extract of the roots, is reported to prevent hydrazine-induced increase in serum levels of triglycerides, cholesterol, free fatty acids and total lipids in rats (Vivekanandan et al., 2007).

11. *TERMINALIA ARJUNA*

T. arjuna, commonly known as Arjuna in Hindi, is arguably the most important cardioprotective medicinal plant in the Indian traditional system of medicine, Ayurveda.

Scientific studies have shown that the aqueous extract prepared from the bark is useful in treating angina, high blood pressure, hypertension, and atherogenesis. It is also effective in ameliorating the pain of angina pectoris, cardiac failure, hypercholesterolemia, coronary artery diseases and in strengthening the heart muscles. The cardioprotective effects of Arjuna are attributed to its antioxidant, antihyperlipidemic, and antiatherogenic potentials (Dwivedi, 2007; Dwivedi and Chaturvedi, 2000).

The bark powder is shown to impart beneficial effect in patients with stable angina by marginally decreasing anginal frequency, blood pressure, body mass index, blood sugar, cholesterol and increasing HDL-cholesterol. The bark extract and the phytochemical balcein significantly scavenged superoxide radicals and inhibited LPO in cardiac tissue homogenates. The bark extract is also reported to inhibit the oxidative degradation of lipids in human low-density lipoprotein and rat liver microsomes and to scavenge the superoxide and hydroxyl radicals *in vitro* (Dwivedi, 2007; Dwivedi and Chaturvedi, 2000).

Preclinical studies have shown that Arjuna was effective in enhancing glucose utilization, reducing blood glucose, and improving glucose tolerance and glycemic control in the diabetic animals. The bark extract corrected dyslipidemia in animal models of study and reduced the serum levels of total cholesterol, triglycerides, very-low-density lipoprotein, and LDL cholesterol, increased HDL-cholesterol level, fecal bile acid excretion and plasma lecithin–cholesterol acyltransferase activity, and reduced the atherosclerotic lesions in the aorta. Similar observations were observed in clinical studies with diabetic and hypercholesterolemic patients (Dwivedi, 2007; Dwivedi and Chaturvedi, 2000).

Arjuna is also reported to mitigate isoprenaline-induced myocardial fibrosis, oxidative stress, and cardiac hypertrophy in rats. Additionally, the phytochemical arjunolic acid was also effective in preventing isoproterenol-induced myocardial necrosis in rats and in restoring the levels of various antioxidant molecules. In patients with stable angina, Arjuna reduced the anginal episodes, improved the performance of patients in the treadmill test, and improved the left ventricular ejection fraction; it also lowered systolic blood pressure and the body mass index (Dwivedi, 2007; Dwivedi and Chaturvedi, 2000).

12. *TERMINALIA CHEBULA*

T. chebula, commonly known as haritaki in Hindi, belongs to the family Combretaceae. The seed of the fruit is regarded as the 'universal panacea' of Ayurvedic medicine as it has a lot of medicinal value. The peel of the dry nut is used in various ailments. Administration of haritaki produces a dose-dependent reduction in blood glucose levels, reduces cholesterol levels, and prevents atherosclerosis (Thakur et al., 1988). It also increases the amount of insulin released from the pancreatic islets (Rao and Nammi, 2006). Haritaki ameliorated isoproterenol-induced myocardial injury; it reversed histological abnormalities, mitigated oxidative stress, and prevented the release of cardiac marker enzymes to serum (Suchalatha and Shyamala Devi, 2004).

13. *TINOSPORA CORDIFOLIA*

T. cordifolia, commonly known as guduchi, is a herbaceous vine of the family Menispermaceae. It is an important medicinal plant in Ayurveda for treating various ailments. The alcoholic extract of the guduchi root is shown to reduce blood and urine glucose and increase serum insulin levels in type 1 diabetic rats (Stanely et al., 2003). Guduchi increases antioxidants in the heart, reduces lipid peroxidation, and prevents LDL oxidation; it possesses antiyperlipidemic effects, and prevents atherogenesis and oxidative damage to the heart (Rao et al., 2005; Umamaheswari and Mainzen Prince, 2007). Treatment with *T. cordifolia* also resulted in a dose-dependent reduction in myocardial infarct size (Rao et al., 2005).

14. *WITHANIA SOMNIFERA*

W. somnifera, also known as ashwagandha in Hindi, and as Indian ginseng and winter cherry in English, is a plant of the Solanaceae family. In the Ayurvedic system of medicine, ashwagandha is considered beneficial in treating many diseases, including cardiac ailments. Ashwagandha also has hypoglycemic effect, improves insulin sensitivity and glycemic control, and stimulates hepatic glucose metabolizing enzymes (Anwer et al., 2008; Ojha and Arya, 2009). It has significant antihyperlipidemic and antiatherogenic potential (Hemalatha et al., 2004; Ojha and Arya, 2009). It has been shown to reduce serum cholesterol, triglycerides, and the atherogenic index, and to increase HDL in post myocardial infarction patients (Dwivedi et al., 2000). The phenolic compounds present in ashwagandha have antioxidant properties, which decrease lipid peroxidation, and improve the antioxidant status in the myocardial tissue (Hemalatha et al., 2004; Mohanty et al., 2008). *In vitro* studies have shown that treatment with ania extract restores the myocardial oxidant–antioxidant balance, exerts anti-apoptotic effects, and reduces myocardial damage (Mohanty et al., 2008).

15. *ZINGIBER OFFICINALE*

Ginger, the rhizome of the plant *Z. Officinale*, has both culinary and medicinal uses in the various traditional and folk systems of medicine. Ginger provides cardioprotective effects mainly through prevention of atherogenesis. It decreases serum levels of total cholesterol, LDL cholesterol, and triglycerides, and increases serum HDL level; thus, ginger corrects dyslipidemia and prevents the accumulation of 'bad' cholesterol and formation of small dense LDL in blood vessel lining. Mechanistic studies have shown that ginger induces bile acid synthesis, represses cholesterol synthesis, inhibits LDL oxidation and aggregation, and promotes the uptake and catabolism of the bad cholesterol LDL (Fuhrman et al., 2000; Nammi et al, 2010). Ginger possesses antihyperlipidemic, antioxidant, anti-inflammatory, and antiplatelet properties, as well as antihyperglycemic and insulino-tropic effects, to increase insulin sensitivity and to prevent the formation of advanced gly-cation end products. Ginger possesses antioxidant property; ginger extracts resulted in reduced capacity of macrophages to oxidize LDL and reduced uptake of oxidized LDL as a result of the strict modification of plasma lipoprotein receptors (Fuhrman et al., 2000). Ginger also possesses antiplatelet and fibrinolytic effects and reduces athero-sclerotic lesions (Verma et al., 2004).

16. CONCLUSIONS

Preclinical studies with experimental animals suggest that certain Ayurvedic medicinal plants are effective as cardioprotective agents. Scientific studies indicate that the herbs exercise their pharmacological effects by stimulating the function of specific organs pos-sibly by altering hormones, affecting immunity and the neurotransmitters, and increasing antioxidant activities. The mechanism of action of herbal drugs is always polyvalent, and the final effect is either additive or synergistic and mostly devoid of adverse effects. Certain phytochemicals present in the plants stimulate the desired effect, while others may enhance the potency of these active compounds. Of the medicinal plants investi-gated, *T. arjuna*, garlic, onion, and guggul have been shown to possess potent effects, which validates their extensive use in both Ayurvedic and other Indian folk systems of medicine. However, with other plants, further explorations are necessary to elucidate their pharmacological activities and clinical utility.

ACKNOWLEDGMENTS

The authors RA and BG are grateful to Director, INMAS, Delhi for support. Funding and support received from the Defense Research and Development Organization (DRDO), Government of India is acknowl-edged. The authors DMP, ARS, and MSB are grateful to Rev. Fr. Patrick Rodrigus (Director), Rev. Fr. Denis D'Sa (Administrator) and Dr. Jaya Prakash Alva, (Dean) of Father Muller Medical College for providing the necessary facilities and support. The authors declare no conflict of interest.

REFERENCES

Antony, B., Merina, B., Sheeba, V., Mukkadan, J., 2006. Effect of standardized Amla extract on atheroscle-rosis and dyslipidemia. Indian Journal of Pharmaceutical Sciences 68, 437–441.
Anwer, T., Sharma, M., Pillai, K.K., Iqbal, M., 2008. Effect of *Withania somnifera* on insulin sensitivity in non-insulin-dependent diabetes mellitus rats. Basic and Clinical Pharmacology and Toxicology 102 (6), 498–503.
Banerjee, S.K., Maulik, S.K., 2002. Effect of garlic on cardiovascular disorders: a review. Nutrition Journal 1, 4.
Bang, M.A., Kim, H.A., Cho, Y.J., 2009. Alterations in the blood glucose, serum lipids and renal oxidative stress in diabetic rats by supplementation of onion (*Allium cepa*. Linn). Nutrition Research and Practice 3 (3), 242–246 Fall.

Campos, K.E., Diniz, Y.S., Cataneo, A.C., Faine, L.A., Alves, M.J., Novelli, E.L., 2003. Hypoglyc-aemic and antioxidant effects of onion, *Allium cepa*: dietary onion addition, antioxidant activity and hypoglycaemic effects on diabetic rats. International Journal of Food Science and Nutrition 54 (3), 241–246.

Cesarone, M.R., Belcaro, G., Nicolaides, A.N., et al., 2001. Increase in echogenicity of echolucent carotid plaques after treatment with total triterpenic fraction of *Centella asiatica*: a prospective, placebo-controlled, randomized trial. Angiology 52 (Supplement 2), S19–S25.

Chandra, A., Mahdi, A.A., Singh, R.K., Mahdi, F., Chander, R., 2008. Effect of Indian herbal hypoglyce-mic agents on antioxidant capacity and trace elements content in diabetic rats. Journal of Medicinal Food 11 (3), 506–512.

Dabhadkar, K.C., Kulshreshtha, A., Ali, M.K., Narayan, K.M., 2011. Prospects for a cardiovascular disease prevention polypill. Annual Review of Public Health 32, 23–38.

De Sanctis, M.T., Belcaro, G., Incandela, L., et al., 2001. Treatment of edema and increased capillary fil-tration in venous hypertension with total triterpenic fraction of *Centella asiatica*: a clinical, prospective, placebo-controlled, randomized, dose-ranging trial. Angiology 52 (Supplement 2), S55–S59.

Deng, R., 2007. Therapeutic effects of guggul and its constituent guggulsterone: cardiovascular benefits. Cardiovascular Drug Review 25 (4), 375–390.

D'Souza, T., Mengi, S.A., Hassarajani, S., Chattopadhayay, S., 2007. Efficacy study of the bioactive fraction (F-3) of *Acorus calamus* in hyperlipidemia. Indian Journal of Pharmaceutical Sciences 39, 196–200.

Duan, W., Yu, Y., Zhang, L., 2005. Antiatherogenic effects of phyllanthus emblica associated with corilagin and its analogue. Yakugaku Zasshil 125 (7), 587–591.

Dwivedi, S., 2007. *Terminalia arjuna* Wight & Arn. – a useful drug for cardiovascular disorders. Journal of Ethnopharmacology 114 (2), 114–129.

Dwivedi, S., Aggarwal, A., 2009. Indigenous drugs in ischemic heart disease in patients with diabetes. Journal of Alternative and Complementary Medicine 15 (11), 1215–1221.

Dwivedi, S., Chaturvedi, A., 2000. Cardiology in ancient India. Journal of Indian College of Cardiology 1, 8–15.

Dwivedi, S., Chaturvedi, D., Sharma, K.K., 2000. Modification of coronary risk factors by medicinal plants. Journal of Medicinal and Aromatic Plant Sciences 22, 616–620.

Eshrat, H.M., Mukhopadhyay, A.K., 2006. Effect of *Ocimum sanctum* (tulsi) and vitamin E on biochemical parameters and retinopathy in streptozotocin induced diabetic rats. Indian Journal of Clinical Biochemistry 21 (2), 181–188.

Fuhrman, B., Rosenblat, M., Hayek, T., Coleman, R., Aviram, M., 2000. Ginger extract consumption reduces plasma cholesterol, inhibits LDL oxidation and attenuates development of atherosclerosis in atherosclerotic, apolipoprotein E-deficient mice. Journal of Nutrition 130 (5), 1124–1131.

Gnanapragasam, A., Yogeeta, S., Subhashini, R., Ebenezar, K.K., Sathish, V., Devaki, T., 2007. Adriamycin induced myocardial failure in rats: protective role of *Centella asiatica*. Molecular and Cellular Biochem-istry 294, 55–63.

Gorinstein, S., Zenon, J., Namiesnik, J., Leontowicz, H., Leontowicz, M., Trakhtenberg, S., 2007. The atherosclerotic heart disease and protecting properties of garlic: contemporary data. Molecular Nutrition and Food Research 51, 1365–1381.

Hemalatha, S., Wahi, A.K., Singh, P.N., Chansouria, J.P., 2004. Hypoglycemic activity of Withania coa-gulans Dunal in streptozotocin induced diabetic rats. Journal of Ethnopharmacology 93 (2–3), 261–264.

Husain, G.M., Singh, P.N., Kumar, V., 2009. Antidiabetic activity of standardized extract of *Picrorhiza kurroa* in rat model of NIDDM. Drug Discoveries and Therapeutics 3, 88–92.

Islam, M.S., Choi, H., Loots du, T., 2008. Effects of dietary onion (*Allium cepa* L.) in a high-fat diet streptozotocin-induced diabetes rodent model. Annals of Nutrition and Metabolism 53 (1), 6–12.

Kamalakkannan, N., Prince, S.M., 2003. Effect of *Aegle marmelos* Correa. (Bael) fruit extract on tissue an-tioxidants in streptozotocin diabetic rats. Indian Journal of Experimental Biology 41 (11), 1285–1288.

Kawamoto, E., Sakai, Y., Okamura, Y., Yamamoto, Y., 2004. Effects of boiling on the antihypertensive and antioxidant activities of onion. Journal of Nutrition Sciences and Vitaminology (Tokyo) 50 (3), 171–176.

Mohanty, I.R., Arya, D.S., Gupta, S.K., 2008. *Withania somnifera* provides cardioprotection and attenuates ischemia–reperfusion induced apoptosis. Clinical Nutrition 27 (4), 635–642.

Nammi, S., Kim, M.S., Gavande, N.S., Li, G.Q., Roufogalis, B.D., 2010. Regulation of low density lipoprotein receptor and 3-hydroxy-3-methyl glutaryl coenzyme A reductase expression by *Zingiber officinale* in the liver of high fat diet fed rats. Basic and Clinical Pharmacology and Toxicology 106 (5), 389–395.

Nampoothiri, S.V., Prathapan, A., Cherian, O.L., Raghu, K.G., Venugopalan, V.V., Sundaresan, A., 2011. In vitro antioxidant and inhibitory potential of Terminalia bellerica and *Emblica officinalis* fruits against LDL oxidation and key enzymes linked to type 2 diabetes. Food and Chemical Toxicology 49 (1), 125–131.

Ojha, S.K., Arya, D.S., 2009. *Withania somnifera* Dunal (Ashwagandha): a promising remedy for cardiovascular diseases. World Journal of Medical Sciences 4 (2), 156–158.

Ojha, S.K., Nandave, M., Arora, S., et al., 2008. Effect of Commiphora mukul extract on cardiac dysfunction and ventricular function in isoproterenol-induced myocardial infarction. Indian Journal of Experimental Biology 46 (9), 646–652.

Park, S., Kim, M.Y., Lee, D.H., et al., 2009. Methanolic extract of onion (*Allium cepa*) attenuates ischemia/hypoxia-induced apoptosis in cardiomyocytes via antioxidant effect. European Journal of Nutrition 48, 235–242.

Rai, V., Iyer, U., Mani, U.V., 1997. Effect of Tulasi (*Ocimum sanctum*) leaf powder supplementation on blood sugar levels, serum lipids, and tissue lipids in diabetic rats. Plant Foods for Human Nutrition 50 (1), 9–16.

Rao, P.R., Kumar, V.K., Viswanath, R.K., Subbaraju, G.V., 2005. Cardioprotective activity of alcoholic extract of *Tinospora cordifolia* in ischemia-reperfusion induced myocardial infarction in rats. Biological and Pharmaceutical Bulletin 28, 2319–2322.

Rao, N.K., Nammi, S., 2006. Antidiabetic and renoprotective effects of the chloroform extract of *Terminalia chebula* Retz. seeds in streptozotocin-induced diabetic rats. BMC Complementary and Alternative Medicine 6, 17.

Senthil Kumar, S.H., Anandan, R., Devaki, T., Santhosh, K.M., 2001. Cardioprotective effects of Picrorrhiza kurroa against isoproterenol-induced myocardial stress in rats. Fitoterapia 72 (4), 402–405.

Sharma, B., Salunke, R., Srivastava, S., Majumder, C., Roy, P., 2009. Effects of guggulsterone isolated from Commiphora mukul in high fat diet induced diabetic rats. Food and Chemical Toxicology 47, 2631.

Shri, R., Arora, D., 2010. Effect of *Emblica officinalis* diet in streptozotocin diabetic mice. In: Gupta, V.K., Singh, G.D., Singh, S., Kaul, A. (Eds.), Medicinal Plants: Phytochemistry, Pharmacology and Therapeutics 1, 413–420.

Singh, R.B., Niaz, M.A., Ghosh, S., 1993. Hypolipidemic and antioxidant affects of Commiphora mukul as an adjunct to dietary therapy in patients with hypercholesterolemia. Cardiovascular Drugs and Therapy 8, 659–664.

Stanely, M., Prince, P., Menon, V.P., 2003. Hypoglycaemic and hypolipidaemic action of alcohol extract of *Tinospora cordifolia* roots in chemical induced diabetes in rats. Phytotherapy Research 17, 410–413.

Suanarunsawat, T., Boonnak, T., Na Ayutthaya, W.D., Thirawarapan, S., 2010. Anti-hyperlipidemic and cardioprotective effects of *Ocimum sanctum* L. fixed oil in rats fed a high fat diet. Journal of Basic and Clinical Physiology and Pharmacology 21, 387–400.

Suchalatha, S., Shyamala Devi, C.S., 2004. Protective effect of *Terminalia chebula* against experimental myocardial injury induced by isoproterenol. Indian Journal of Experimental Biology 42, 174–178.

Taj Eldin, I.M., Ahmed, E.M., Elwahab, H.M.A., 2010. Preliminary study of the clinical hypoglycemic effects of *Allium cepa* (Red Onion) in type 1 and type 2 diabetic patients. Journal of Environmental and Health Insights 4, 71–77.

Thakur, C.P., Thakur, B., Singh, S., Sinha, P.K., Sinha, S.K., 1988. The Ayurvedic medicines Haritaki, Amala and Bahira reduce cholesterol-induced atherosclerosis in rabbits. International Journal of Cardiology 21, 167–175.

Umamaheswari, S., Mainzen Prince, P.S., 2007. Antihyperglycemic effect of 'Ilogen-Excel', an ayurvedic herbal formulation in streptozotocin-induced diabetes mellitus. Acta Poloniae Pharmaceutica 64, 53–61.

Verma, S.K., Singh, M., Jain, P., Bordia, A., 2004. Protective effect of ginger, *Zingiber officinale*·Rosc on experimental atherosclerosis in rabbits. Indian Journal of Experimental Biology 42, 736–738.

Vivekanandan, P., Gobianand, K., Priya, S., Vijayalakshmi, P., Karthikeyan, S., 2007. Protective effect of picroliv against hydrazine-induced hyperlipidemia and hepatic steatosis in rats. Drug and Chemical Toxicology 30 (3), 241–252.

Wu, H.S., Zhu, D.F., Zhou, C.X., et al., 2009. Insulin sensitizing activity of ethyl acetate fraction of *Acorus calamus* L. in vitro and in vivo. Journal of Ethnopharmacology 123, 288–292.

CHAPTER 39

Effect of *Terminalia arjuna* on Cardiac Hypertrophy

S. Kumar*, S.K. Maulik†
*University of Pittsburgh, Pittsburgh, PA, USA
†All India Institute of Medical Sciences, New Delhi, Delhi, India

ABBREVIATIONS

MHC Myosin heavy chain
SOD Superoxide dismutase

1. *TERMINALIA ARJUNA*: A CARDIOPROTECTIVE PLANT

Terminalia arjuna (Roxb.), commonly known as *Arjun* in India, is an evergreen tree. It belongs to the family Combretaceae and is a large tree attaining a height of 20–30 m. In ancient Indian literature, *Ayurveda* (traditional medical practice of India), *T. arjuna* has been mentioned for cardiac disease; it has also been mentioned by *Charaka* in his treatise *Charak Samhita* and practiced by the descendent *Ayurvedic* practitioners like *Chakradatta* and *Bhava-Mishra* (Kirtikar et al., 1935).

The stem bark of the plant, which is generally used for medicinal purposes, is described in *Ayurvedic* terms as being acrid, sweet, cooling, styptic, tonic, antidysenteric, and febrifuge in nature. It has been proposed to be used as powder, decoction, hydroalcoholic extract, bark powder with *Ghrita* (fat), or bark powder boiled in milk (*kshirpaak*), according to the pathophysiological condition. Different formulations having *T. arjuna* bark have been reviewed earlier (Kumar and Prabhakar, 1987). Formulations with special mention for cardiac ailments are summarized in Table 39.1.

With the evolution of modern science, phytochemical investigations were carried out for different chemical compounds present in stem bark, root bark, leaves, and fruits (Anjaneyulu and Ramaprasad, 1982; Kandil and Nassar, 1998; Singh et al., 1995). Stem bark of *T. arjuna* contains oleane-type triterpenes like arjunic acid, arjunolic acid, arjungenin, arjunetin, tannins, glycosides, and very large amounts of flavonoids (quercetin, kaempferol, luteolin, and pellargonidin), ellagic acids, phytosterols, and minerals such as calcium, magnesium, zinc, and copper (Ali et al., 2003; Cheng et al., 2002; Dwivedi and Udupa, 1989; King et al., 1954; Row et al., 1970; Singh et al., 2002). The estimated total flavonoid content is 5.7 ± 0.5 g/100 g tree bark (Nair and Gupta, 1996).

Bioactive Food as Dietary Interventions for Cardiovascular Disease
http://dx.doi.org/10.1016/B978-0-12-396485-4.00036-0

© 2013 Elsevier Inc.
All rights reserved.

Table 39.1 Formulations with Special Mention for Cardiac Ailments

Name of formulations	Indications
Arjunatvagadi kasayam	Heart disease due to *pitta*
Arjunatvak churnam	Heart disease, chronic fever, *raktapitta*
Godhumakakubha churnam	Severe heart disease
Godhumakakubhatvak churnam	Heart disease
Kakubhadi churnam	All types of heart disease
Nagabaladi churnam	Heart disease, rheumatism, rejuvenation
Nagarjunabhram	Heart disease, colic, piles, tuberculosis
Cintamanirasam	Heart disease, prameha, cough
Hrdayarnavarasam	Heart disease
Sankaravadi	Heart disease, chronic fever, uterine bleeding
Trinetrarasam	Heart disease due to *tridosa*
Visvesaram	Heart disease

In recent years, *T. arjuna* has been screened for its various pharmacological properties, in particular cardioprotective, and has been found to be effective in both experimental and clinical studies (Dwivedi, 2007; Maulik and Katiyar, 2010). In preclinical studies, the bark extract of *T. arjuna* produced a fall in blood pressure (Singh et al., 1982). In studies by Gauthaman et al. (2001, 2005), the bark powder of *T. arjuna* augmented the endogenous antioxidants in the heart. Moreover, in clinical studies, it has been shown to have antioxidant properties comparable to that of vitamin E, and there is also encouraging evidence of its beneficial effects in patients of refractory heart failure as well as coronary artery disease (Bharani et al., 1995; Dwivedi and Jauhari, 1997; Gupta et al., 2001). However, there have been only three reports mentioning the effect of *T. arjuna* on heart weight (a measure of cardiac hypertrophy), and, out of three studies, only one provides details about its effect on cardiac hypertrophy. Here, the general findings regarding the use of *T. arjuna* in cardiovascular disorder with are summarized special reference to its effect on cardiac hypertrophy.

The first study on the effect of *T. arjuna* on the heart weight, a small clinical trial (number of patients = 10) conducted in patients with coronary artery disease having myocardial infarction and angina, was reported by Dwivedi and Jauhari (1997). Patients were prescribed bark powder of *T. arjuna* along with the standard treatment protocol of nitrates, aspirin, and/or calcium channel blocker. A significant reduction in the left ventricular mass was noted along with an increase in ejection fraction in patients receiving *T. arjuna*. In another more recent study by Parveen et al. (2011), administration of hydroalcoholic extract of *T. arjuna* prevented the increase in heart weight due to isoproterenol-induced cardiac failure. However, none of these studies specifically targeted cardiac hypertrophy, which is a direct risk factor toward myocardial dysfunction.

The study by Kumar et al. (2009) is the only one investigating the effect of *T. arjuna* on cardiac hypertrophy. A standardized aqueous extract of the bark powder of

T. arjuna was evaluated against the isoproterenol-induced cardiac hypertrophy in rats. Apart from assessing the key hypertrophic markers, changes in heart weight/body weight and cardiomyocyte diameter, the study also focused on other characteristic pathologies associated with isoproterenol-induced cardiac hypertrophy such as myocardial fibrosis, decrease in myocardial endogenous antioxidant, and switching of alpha to beta myosin heavy chain (MHC).

2. *TERMINALIA ARJUNA* AND CARDIAC HYPERTROPHY

In a study by Kumar et al. (2009), *T. arjuna* prevented myocardial fibrosis, decrease in myocardial endogenous antioxidant, and switch of alpha to beta MHC. However, contrary to other reports (Dwivedi and Jauhari, 1997; Parveen et al., 2011), it did not prevent the increase in hypertrophic markers (fractional wall thickening, heart weight/body weight, left ventricular mass, cardiomyocyte diameter).

2.1 Effect of *Terminalia arjuna* on Oxidative Stress and Cardiac Hypertrophy

In ancient literature, *T. arjuna* has been reported to have a therapeutic effect in cardiac disorders, and its cardioprotective effect has also been observed in modern investigational studies (Maulik and Katiyar, 2010). The phytochemical analysis of the bark extract showed the presence of different polyphenols, tannins, along with triterpenoids, which are known to have antioxidant property. Arjunolic acid, which is one of the chemical entities in the bark extract, has been reported to protect the heart against isoproterenol-induced necrosis (Sumitra et al., 2001). The free radical scavenging property of *T. arjuna* has also been observed in *in vitro* studies, which reflects its direct antioxidant property (Munasinghe et al., 2001; Pawar and Bhutani, 2005). In later studies with *T. arjuna*, it has been found to protect heart against ischemic–reperfusion injury (Gauthaman et al., 2001). Administration of *T. arjuna* also leads to induction of heat shock protein 72 (HSP 72), which is recognized as a cardioprotective heat shock stress protein (Gauthaman et al., 2005; Guisasola et al., 2006). In recent reports, *T. arjuna* prevented the carbon tetrachloride-induced increase in cardiac oxidative stress markers (Manna et al., 2007) as well as protected the heart against doxorubicin-induced cardiomyopathy (Singh et al., 2008).

In line with earlier studies, administration of *T. arjuna* prevented the decrease in myocardial endogenous antioxidants (glutathione, superoxide dismutase (SOD), and catalase) associated with cardiac hypertrophy (Kumar et al., 2009). A recent study by Parveen et al. (2011) reported the protective effect of *T. arjuna* against the decrease in myocardial antioxidants and was associated with improvement in myocardial performance. To defend the increased oxidative stress, antioxidant enzymes, SOD, and catalase work in coherence (Mao et al., 1993). Dismutation of superoxide radicals by SOD generates hydrogen peroxide, which is detoxified by catalase and glutathione peroxidase into water. Hence, the correct proportion of the two enzymes is very important for their antioxidant effect. Iso-proterenol administration induced disproportionate decrease in SOD and catalase, which was corrected by administration of *T. arjuna*. Administration of *T. arjuna* prevented the depletion of myocardial levels of SOD and catalase without disturbing the relative proportion of these two enzymes. These findings support the previous reports that *T. arjuna* augments myocardial endogenous antioxidant level as well as prevents oxidative stress. However, in the same study, *T. arjuna* failed to prevent the development of cardiac hypertrophy following chronic isoproterenol administration.

The discrepancy among the existing reports on the effect of *T. arjuna* on cardiac weight or mass may be due to many of the following reasons. The foremost reason to be considered is the standardization of the plant material and the dose and dosage forms used. In a study by Dwivedi and Jauhari (1997), the crude bark powder was used, while in a study by Kumar et al. (2009) and Parveen et al. (2011), the aqueous and hydroalcoholic extracts were used, respectively. Hence, the variation in response could be due to the possible different chemical profiles of the drugs used, which has been recently highlighted by Oberoi et al. (2011). The comparative evaluation of aqueous and organic extracts of the bark in rat ventricular myocytes showed positive inotropic effect of aqueous extract of *T. arjuna* bark; however, the organic extract had a detrimental effect on myocardial function. The finding supports the beneficial effects observed in earlier studies in a situation of heart failure where improving myocardial performance may help in improving the pathological state. In a study by Kumar et al. (2009), isoproterenol was used to induce cardiac hypertrophy, which is itself cardiotonic. Oberoi et al. (2011) used the aqueous extract of *T. arjuna* in a study, which also showed the cardiotonic effect. Hence, it appears rational that *T. arjuna* did not offer any protection against isoproterenol-induced cardiac hypertrophy.

Another possible explanation for the failure of *T. arjuna* to prevent the increase in hypertrophic markers even after preventing the oxidative stress may be due to the activation of different pathways in isoproterenol-induced hypertrophy. Along with increased oxidative stress, stimulation of beta-adrenoceptor by isoproterenol leads to the activation of nuclear factor of activated T-cells signaling via glycogen synthase kinase 3-beta ultimately causing increased protein synthesis. Hence, it can be suggested that *T. arjuna* could have prevented the oxidative stress mediated via beta-adrenoceptor activation due to its antioxidant properties sparing the other pathways mediating the induction of cardiac hypertrophy. Earlier experimental studies have also reported the differences regarding the efficacy of antioxidants in cardiac hypertrophy. Drugs with antioxidant properties, for example, statin and tempol, have been shown to prevent hypertrophy, that is, reduction in heart weight/body weight, as well as oxidative stress in pressure overload hypertrophy (Chess et al., 2008; Takemoto et al., 2001). However, in isoproterenol-induced cardiac hypertrophy, tempol (a cell membrane-permeable free radical scavenger) failed to prevent the increase in heart weight/body weight even if it prevented the activation of mitogen-activated protein kinases (Zhang et al., 2005). It supports the later hypothesis that the prevention of oxidative stress by *T. arjuna* was not sufficient enough to block the isoproterenol-induced hypertrophic signaling.

The present findings together with the earlier reports suggest that isoproterenol-induced cardiac hypertrophy may be mediated via different pathways and, hence even after prevention of oxidative stress and necrosis by *T. arjuna*, the increased heart weight/body weight and cardiomyocyte diameter did not change.

2.2 *Terminalia arjuna* and Myocardial Fibrosis and Myocardial Alpha/Beta-MHC

Increased myocardial fibrosis is considered a hallmark of pathological cardiac hypertrophy and has been associated with cardiac functional abnormality as well as making the heart more arrhythmogenic (Noorman et al., 2008). The antifibrotic effect of *T. arjuna* in cardiac hypertrophy reported by Kumar et al. (2009) is a significant finding. Coadministration of *T. arjuna* prevented the increase in myocardial fibrosis (L-hydroxyproline content), which was also evident in the histopathological evaluation as reduced replacement fibrosis.

Reduction of myocardial fibrosis has been achieved by administration of other plant products as well (Seymour et al., 2008). In separate studies, plants having terpenes or flavonoids have been reported to reduce the fibrosis in liver diseases (Lee et al., 2008; Liu et al., 2005). *T. arjuna* bark also contains triterpenoids and flavonoids in plenty and hence it can be suggested that these might have contributed to *T. arjuna*-mediated decrease in myocardial collagen content (fibrosis).

Another important finding was the effect of *T. arjuna* on the proportion of MHC isoforms in the heart. The two isoforms of cardiac MHC, alpha and beta, differ significantly with respect to their adenosine triphosphate (ATP)-hydrolyzing capacity, in spite of having more than 93% homology. The expression of alpha/beta-MHC isoforms changes with induction of cardiac hypertrophy and also with aging (Reiser et al., 2001). Increased expression of beta-MHC has been reported to be associated with pathological hypertrophy (Frey and Olson, 2003). Isoproterenol-induced cardiac hypertrophy has also been reported to be associated with increased expression of beta-MHC (Saadane et al., 1999). *T. arjuna* prevented the increase in myocardial beta-MHC mRNA as well as facilitated the reduction in beta-MHC mRNA in isoproterenol-induced cardiac hypertrophy (Kumar, 2009).

Recently, a correlation between fibrosis and modulation of beta-MHC expression has been reported. A detailed *in vitro* study showed the colocalization of the collagen deposition and expression of beta-MHC in cardiomyocytes (Pandya et al., 2006). In the present study, increased fibrosis was observed in parallel with increased expression of beta-MHC mRNA, which is in tune with the previous report where beta-MHC has been reported to be associated with increased fibrosis. Hence, it appears plausible to hypothesize that the antifibrotic effect and the effect on beta-MHC mRNA of *T. arjuna* might have some correlation.

3. CONCLUSION AND FUTURE PERSPECTIVE

Although the available literature is not sufficient to provide a concluding remark on the effect of *T. arjuna* on cardiac hypertrophy, these findings do highlight its protective effect against pathological changes associated with cardiac hypertrophy. Moreover, these preliminary reports do suggest some rational for further evaluation of *T. arjuna* for its therapeutic potential in cardiac hypertrophy as many of the questions are still to be answered. Similar to other herbal/natural products, the question of dose and dosage form is also associated with *T. arjuna* and has been more clearly raised in a study by Oberoi et al. (2011). It also supports the traditional way of prescribing the same herb/drug in the different dosage forms for different disease conditions, which needs to be addressed in modern scientific ways. Another important aspect to study will be to unravel the effect of *T. arjuna* on other potential molecular target(s) involved in cardiac hypertrophy. As it appears from the discussion, it is still required to be evaluated by using different *in vitro* and *in vivo* models of cardiac hypertrophy to conclude on its effect on cardiac hypertrophy.

REFERENCES

Ali, A., Abdullah, S.T., Hamid, H., Ali, M., Alam, M.S., 2003. Two new pentacyclic triterpenoid glycosides from the bark of *Terminalia arjuna*. Indian Journal of Chemistry 42B, 2905–2908.

Anjaneyulu, A.S.R., Ramaprasad, A.V., 1982. Chemical examination of roots of *Terminalia arjuna* (Roxb.) Wight & Arnot. Part-I: characterization of two new triterpenoid glycosides. Indian Journal of Chemistry 21B, 530–533.

Bharani, A., Ganguly, A., Bhargava, K.D., 1995. Salutary effect of *Terminalia arjuna* in patients with severe refractory heart failure. International Journal of Cardiology 49, 191–199.

Cheng, H.Y., Lin, C.C., Lin, T.C., 2002. Antiherpes simplex virus type-2 activity of casuarinin from the bark of *Terminalia arjuna* Linn. Antiviral Research 55, 447–455.

Chess, D.J., Xu, W., Khairallah, R., et al., 2008. The antioxidant tempol attenuates pressure overload-induced cardiac hypertrophy and contractile dysfunction in mice fed a high-fructose diet. American Journal of Physiology – Heart and Circulatory Physiology 295, H2223–H2230.

Dwivedi, S., 2007. *Terminalia arjuna* Wight & Arn. – a useful drug for cardiovascular disorders. Journal of Ethnopharmacology 114, 114–129.

Dwivedi, S., Jauhari, R., 1997. Beneficial effects of *Terminalia arjuna* in coronary artery disease. Indian Heart Journal 49, 507–510.

Dwivedi, S., Udupa, N., 1989. *Terminalia arjuna*: pharmacology, phytochemistry, pharmacology and clinical use. A review. Fitoterapia 60, 413–420.

Frey, N., Olson, E.N., 2003. Cardiac hypertrophy: the good, the bad and the ugly. Annual Review of Physiology 65, 45–79.

Gauthaman, K., Banerjee, S.K., Dinda, A.K., Ghosh, C.C., Maulik, S.K., 2005. *Terminalia arjuna* (Roxb.) protects rabbit heart against ischaemic-reperfusion injury: role of antioxidant enzyme and heat shock protein. Journal of Ethnopharmacology 96, 403–409.

Gauthaman, K., Maulik, M., Kumari, R., et al., 2001. Effect of chronic treatment with bark of *Terminalia arjuna*: a study on the isolated ischemic-reperfused rat heart. Journal of Ethnopharmacology 75, 197–201.

Guisasola, M.C., Descomdel, M., Gonzalez, F.S., et al., 2006. Heat shock proteins, end effectors of myocardium ischemic preconditioning? Cell Stress and Chaperones 11, 250–258.

Gupta, R., Singhal, S., Goyle, A., Sharma, V.N., 2001. Antioxidant and hypocholesterolaemic effects of *Terminalia arjuna* tree-bark powder: a randomised placebo-controlled trial. Journal of the Association of Physicians of India 49, 231–235.

J Munasinghe, T.C., Seneviratne, C.K., Thabrew, M.I., Abeysekera, A.M., 2001. Antiradical and antilipo-peroxidative effects of some plant extracts used by Sri Lankan traditional medical practitioners for cardioprotection. Phytotherapy Research 15, 519–523.

Kandil, F.E., Nassar, M.I., 1998. A tannin anticancer promoter from *Terminalia arjuna*. Phytochemistry 47, 1567–1568.

King, F.E., King, T.J., Ross, J.M., 1954. The extractives from hardwoods. Part XVIII. The constitution of arjunolic acid, a triterpene from *Terminalia arjuna*. Journal of the Chemical Society 3995–4003.

Kirtikar, K.R., Basu, B.D., Combretaceae, N.O., 1935. Terminalia arjuna. In: Kirtikar, K.R., Basu, B.D. (Eds.), second ed. Indian Medicinal Plants, vol. II. LM Basu, Allahabad, pp. 1023–1028.

Kumar, S., 2009. Effect of *Terminalia arjuna* on cardiac hypertrophy in rats. Unpublished Thesis (Ph.D.) All India Institute of Medical Sciences, New Delhi, India.

Kumar, S., Enjamoori, R., Jaiswal, A., et al., 2009. Catecholamine-induced myocardial fibrosis and oxidative stress is attenuated by *Terminalia arjuna* (Roxb.). Journal of Pharmacy and Pharmacology 61, 1529–1536.

Kumar, D.S., Prabhakar, Y.S., 1987. On the ethnomedical significance of the arjuna tree, *Terminalia arjuna* (Roxb.) Wight & Arnot. Journal of Ethnopharmacology 20, 173–190.

Lee, M.K., Yang, H., Yoon, J.S., et al., 2008. Antifibrotic activity of diterpenes from Biota orientalis leaves on hepatic stellate cells. Archives of Pharmacal Research 31, 866–871.

Liu, C.Y., Gu, Z.L., Zhou, W.X., Guo, C.Y., 2005. Effect of Astragalus complanatus flavonoid on anti-liver fibrosis in rats. World Journal of Gastroenterology 11, 5782–5786.

Manna, P., Sinha, M., Sil, P.C., 2007. Phytomedicinal activity of *Terminalia arjuna* against carbon tetrachloride induced cardiac oxidative stress. Pathophysiology 14, 71–78.

Mao, G.D., Thomas, P.D., Lopaschuk, G.D., Poznansky, M.J., 1993. Superoxide dismutase (SOD)-catalase conjugates. Role of hydrogen peroxide and the Fenton reaction in SOD toxicity. Journal of Biological Chemistry 268, 416–420.

Maulik, S.K., Katiyar, C.K., 2010. *Terminalia arjuna* in cardiovascular diseases: making the transition from traditional to modern medicine in India. Current Pharmaceutical Biotechnology 11, 855–860.

Nair, S., Gupta, R., 1996. Dietary antioxidant flavonoids and coronary heart disease. Journal of the Association of Physicians of India 44, 699–702.

Noorman, M., van Rijen, H.V., van Veen, T.A., de Bakker, J.M., Stein, M., 2008. Differences in distribution of fibrosis in the ventricles underlie dominant arrhythmia vulnerability of the right ventricle in senescent mice. Netherlands Heart Journal 16, 356–358.

Oberoi, L., Akiyama, T., Lee, K.H., Liu, S.J., 2011. The aqueous extract, not organic extracts, of *Terminalia arjuna* bark exerts cardiotonic effect on adult ventricular myocytes. Phytomedicine 18, 259–265.

Pandya, K., Kim, H.S., Smithies, O., 2006. Fibrosis, not cell size, delineates beta-myosin heavy chain reexpression during cardiac hypertrophy and normal aging in vivo. Proceedings of the National Academic of Science of the United States of America 103 (45), 16864–16869.

Parveen, A., Babbar, R., Agarwal, S., Kotwani, A., Fahim, M., 2011. Mechanistic clues in the cardioprotective effect of *Terminalia arjuna* bark extract in isoproterenol-induced chronic heart failure in rats. Cardiovascular Toxicology 11, 48–57.

Pawar, R.S., Bhutani, K.K., 2005. Effect of oleanane triterpenoids from *Terminalia arjuna* – a cardioprotective drug on the process of respiratory oxyburst. Phytomedicine 12, 391–393.

Reiser, P.J., Portman, M.A., Ning, X.H., Schomisch Moravec, C., 2001. Human cardiac myosin heavy chain isoforms in fetal and failing adult atria and ventricles. American Journal of Physiology – Heart and Circulatory Physiology 280, H1814–H1820.

Row, L.R., Murty, P.S., Rao, G.S.R.S., Rao, C.S.P., Rao, K.V.J., 1970. Chemical examination of Terminalia species: Part XIII-Isolation and structure determination of Arjunetin, from *Terminalia arjuna*. Indian Journal of Chemistry 8, 772–775.

Saadane, N., Alpert, L., Chalifour, L.E., 1999. Expression of immediate early genes, GATA-4, and Nkx-2.5 in adrenergic-induced cardiac hypertrophy and during regression in adult mice. British Journal of Pharmacology 127, 1165–1176.

Seymour, E.M., Singer, A.A., Bennink, M.R., et al., 2008. Chronic intake of a phytochemical-enriched diet reduces cardiac fibrosis and diastolic dysfunction caused by prolonged salt-sensitive hypertension. Journals of Gerontology. Series A, Biological Sciences and Medical Sciences 63, 1034–1042.

Singh, N., Kapur, K.K., Singh, S.P., et al., 1982. Mechanism of cardiovascular action of *Terminalia arjuna*. Planta Medica 45, 102–104.

Singh, G., Singh, A.T., Abraham, A., et al., 2008. Protective effects of *Terminalia arjuna* against doxorubicin-induced cardiotoxicity. Journal of Ethnopharmacology 117, 123–129.

Singh, B., Singh, V.P., Pandey, V.B., Rucker, G., 1995. A new triterpene glycoside from *Terminalia arjuna*. Planta Medica 61, 576–577.

Singh, D.V., Verma, R.K., Singh, S.C., Gupta, M.M., 2002. RP-LC determination of oleane derivatives in *Terminalia arjuna*. Journal of Pharmaceutical and Biomedical Analysis 28, 447–452.

Sumitra, M., Maniknandan, P., Kumar, D.A., et al., 2001. Experimental myocardial necrosis in rats: role of arjunolic acid on platelet aggregation, coagulation and antioxidant status. Molecular and Cellular Biochemistry 224, 135–142.

Takemoto, M., Node, K., Nakagami, H., et al., 2001. Statins as antioxidant therapy for preventing cardiac myocyte hypertrophy. Journal of Clinical Investigation 108, 1429–1437.

Zhang, G.X., Kimura, S., Nishiyama, A., et al., 2005. Cardiac oxidative stress in acute and chronic isoproterenol-infused rats. Cardiovascular Research 65, 230–238.

CHAPTER 40

Plant Sterols and Artery Disease

H. Gylling, T.A. Miettinen[†]
University of Helsinki, Helsinki, Finland

ABBREVIATIONS

ACAT- 2 Acyl-CoA cholesterol acyltransferase-2
CAD Coronary artery disease
HDL High-density lipoprotein
hsCRP Highly sensitive C-reactive protein
IDL Intermediate density lipoprotein
LDL Low-density lipoprotein
NPC1L1 Niemann–Pick C1-like 1 protein
TICE Transintestinal cholesterol efflux
VLDL Very low-density lipoprotein

1. WHAT ARE PLANT STEROLS?

Plant sterols and plant stanols (collectively called phytosterols in the following) are normal components of plants. They are present in all vegetable foods, especially in vegetable oils, seeds, nuts, and cereals. Corn oil is rich in plant sterols amounting up to 900 mg/100 g of oil; rapeseed oil, up to 700 mg/100 g; soybean oil and sunflower oil, about 300 mg/100 g; but olive oil, <200 mg/100 g. Sesame seeds are rich in plant sterols containing about 700 mg/100 g of plant sterols/seeds; peanuts, about 200 mg/100 g; rye, 100 mg/100 g; and wheat, 70 mg/100 g. The amount of plant sterols in vegetables, fruits, and berries is lower varying from 40 mg/100 g in cauliflower to that of 20 mg/100 g in oranges and 10 mg/100 g in carrots. The mean intake of phytosterols in normal Western diet is about 300 mg day^{-1} for men and 240–290 mg day^{-1} for women (Klingberg et al., 2008a; Valsta et al., 2004). There are also small amounts of stanols in plants so that their amount in diet is about 13–20 mg day^{-1} (Klingberg et al., 2008a; Valsta et al., 2004). The most abundant plant sterols in human diet are sitosterol and campesterol. Sitosterol contributes to 60–66% of total phytosterol intake; campesterol, 22%; stigmasterol, 3–8% (Klingberg et al., 2008a; Valsta et al., 2004); and avenasterol, 3%. The intake of plant stanols represents about 4–8% of the total phytosterol intake (Valsta et al., 2004). Women have higher phytosterol intake density than men, 35–36 mg/100 kJ versus 32 mg/1000 kJ (Klingberg

[†]Deceased.

Bioactive Food as Dietary Interventions for Cardiovascular Disease
http://dx.doi.org/10.1016/B978-0-12-396485-4.00038-4

© 2013 Elsevier Inc.
All rights reserved.

et al., 2008a; Valsta et al., 2004). The intake is also related to the educational level of the person so that subjects with the lowest educational level also have the lowest intake of phytosterols (Valsta et al., 2004).

The main food sources of phytosterols are vegetable oils, vegetable-fat spreads and margarines, cereals and cereal products (bread), and vegetables, and these sources contribute to 50–80% of the total phytosterol intake (Klingberg et al., 2008a; Valsta et al., 2004). The role of fruits as the phytosterol source is small, about 12%.

Phytosterols are steroid alcohols. The chemical structure of plant sterols is closely related to cholesterol, and the differences are located in the side chain. However, these minor structural alterations between plant sterols and cholesterol make the plant sterols metabolically and functionally completely different substances from cholesterol, and even different plant sterols have their own metabolic characteristics. Plant stanols differ from plant sterols by the saturated $\Delta 5$ double bond in the steroid ring B, which again changes their functional characteristics from the respective plant sterols and from cholesterol.

The most important differences between phytosterols and cholesterol are (1) phytosterols are not synthesized in the human body, (2) phytosterols have their intestinal absorption much lower than that of cholesterol, and (3) large doses of phytosterols in diet diminish the absorption of cholesterol. Since phytosterols are completely derived from diet and because of their low absorption percentage, normally their serum concentrations are very low. In general population, serum plant sterol levels vary from 100 to 800 $\mu g\,dl^{-1}$ (2–21 $\mu mol\,l^{-1}$) and those of plant stanols from 2 to 10 $\mu g\,dl^{-1}$ (0.05–0.3 $\mu mol\,l^{-1}$) (Miettinen, unpublished observations 2011). The recommended serum cholesterol level, 190 $mg\,dl^{-1}$ (5.0 $mmol\,l^{-1}$), is much higher when compared with the serum phytosterol levels.

The mankind has been consuming plant sterols throughout its existence. In an analysis of fecal steroids in 1000–2000-year-old human coprolites found in dry caves of Nevada, the plant sterol to cholesterol content was comparable to that of people today (Lin and Connor, 2001). However, in a Greenland Eskimo mummy from AD 1475, the amount of fecal plant sterols was only 0.4% of that of the Americans at present, suggesting that the dietary intake of plant sterols varied a lot between ancient populations (Lin and Connor, 2001).

The naturally occurring intake of dietary phytosterols has only a small effect of about 3% on serum total and low-density lipoprotein (LDL) cholesterol levels (Klingberg et al., 2008b). However, already in the 1950s, the hypolipidemic effect of large doses of phytosterols has interested scientists as a dietary, nonpharmacological means to lower serum cholesterol by interfering with cholesterol absorption. The first food product enriched with phytosterols was plant stanol ester margarine (Benecol®), and it was launched to market in 1995. It was demonstrated that consuming 1.8–2.6 g of plant stanols everyday as esters lowered LDL cholesterol about 10% in a 1-year study (Miettinen et al., 1995). Since then, a large amount of different phytosterol products in different food matrixes have entered the market. There is a large body of information regarding the hypocholesterolemic efficacy and safety of these 'functional foods,' the daily consumption of which has been included in several international recommendations as an additive dietary means to lower serum total and LDL cholesterol level. In recent meta-analyses, the efficacy of plant sterol and plant stanol products has turned out similar with daily doses of 2 g of plant sterols or plant stanols (Demonty et al., 2009; Musa-Veloso et al., 2011), but with larger doses, plant stanol ester products are more effective than those of plant sterols (Musa-Veloso et al., 2011). In these meta-analyses, the 2.0–2.5 g daily dose of plant sterols or plant stanols lowers LDL cholesterol by 9% (Demonty et al., 2009; Musa-Veloso et al., 2011), whereas the maximal LDL cholesterol lowering with plant stanol esters was 18% (Musa-Veloso et al., 2011). While reducing total and LDL cholesterol levels, consumption of foods enriched with plant sterols and plant stanols increases their serum levels. During customary plant-sterol-enriched margarine consumption, the serum plant sterol concentrations increase from 19 to 30 μmol l^{-1} (730–1158 μg dl^{-1}) with no change in serum plant stanol values (Fransen et al., 2007). When plant-stanol-enriched margarine is customarily used, the serum plant stanol concentrations increase from 0.2 to 0.7 μmol l^{-1} (from 8 to 27 μg dl^{-1}), but serum plant sterols decrease by 16–23% (Fransen et al., 2007).

The role of phytosterols in human artery disease was emerging from the clinical findings in phytosterolemia, a human disease with extremely high serum (0.3–1 mmol l^{-1}) and tissue phytosterol levels, usually only moderately elevated serum total and LDL cholesterol levels, and very aggressive atherosclerosis (Bhattacharyya and Connor, 1974). In addition, in animal experiments, ingestion of large daily doses of plant sterols increased serum plant sterol levels several-fold together with increasing atherosclerosis in these animals in spite of normal serum cholesterol level (Weingärtner et al., 2008). In clinical studies, the consumption of plant sterols 2 g daily increase serum plant sterols levels 1.7–2.0-fold, but in general, they still are lower than observed in phytosterolemia. In the following, first the metabolism of plant sterols and plant stanols in man is presented, after which the chapter deals with their roles in atherosclerosis and artery disease concentrating in human clinical studies.

2. METABOLISM OF PHYTOSTEROLS IN HUMANS

2.1 Intestinal Absorption of Unsaturated Plant Sterols

Normal human diet contains free and esterified plant sterols. After entering the upper part of the small intestine, pancreatic cholesterol hydrolase splits the esters into free sterols, but apparently plant sterol glycosides remain mainly intact. Free plant sterols, initially of dietary origin, form the bulk of intestinal plant sterols, but they are mixed with biliary plant sterols and those originated from transintestinal cholesterol efflux (TICE). Biliary daily secretion of sitosterol plus campesterol is around 10 mg day^{-1} (Miettinen and Gylling, 2000), the contribution of that of TICE may be only about 500 μg, assuming that direct intestinal cholesterol secretion is 300 mg day^{-1} (van der Velde et al., 2010) and its phytosterol contents according to plant sterols transported by serum cholesterol is only 1.8 µg mg^{-1} of cholesterol (Vanhanen and Miettinen, 1992). During the intestinal motility, the plant sterols are mixed with intestinal cholesterol to oil phase and micellar phase. The absorbable amount of micellar plant sterols are actively transported by a membrane protein, the Niemann-Pick C1-like 1 protein (NPC1L1), through the enterocyte membrane inside the cell, where the sterols are esterified with acyl-CoA cholesterol acyltransferase-2 (ACAT-2) to sterol esters and incorporated with triglycerides and apolipoprotein B-48 to chylomicrons to be released to lymph. However, the brush border membranes of the enterocytes contain other transporters, such as ABCG5 and ABCG8, that pump free sterols from enterocytes back into the intestinal lumen. Thus, the two transporter systems regulate the level of sterols in the enterocyte indicating, for example, that if the efflux activity is impaired, the plant sterols accumulate in the enterocyte and increase their serum concentration resulting finally in phytosterolemia. Some of the sterols can be effluxed via the ABCA1 transporter to apolipoprotein A-I for formation of nascent high-density lipoprotein (HDL) of intestinal origin.

2.2 Metabolism of Plant Sterols

Chylomicrons are normally losing their triglycerides in circulation and are converted to very low-density class lipoproteins (VLDL) being finally eliminated by the liver. It has been shown, however, that chylomicrons contribute directly to the development of arterial atheromatosis showing a way to plant sterol accumulation in arterial wall. The bulk of dietary plant sterols can enter into the hepatic sterol pool being then partly released during the synthesis of VLDL and released to circulation. Even though about 60% of plant sterols are transported by LDL, the plant sterol ratio to cholesterol is usually lowest in VLDL and highest in chylomicrons, intermediate density lipoproteins (IDL), and HDL. It appears that intestinal plant sterols appear to circulation in chylomicrons and nascent HDL, the major proportion being transferred further through VLDL metabolism to IDL, LDL, and HDL, of which they are randomly equilibrated with tissue sterols, for example, vessel wall sterols. Since the ratio of serum plant sterols to cholesterol are related to those in arterial tissues (Helske et al., 2008; Miettinen et al., 2005; Weingärtner et al., 2008), high dietary intake and high absorption efficiency of plant sterols effectively increase their serum contents, which then equilibrate with arterial wall sterols. In fact, the proportions of serum campesterol and sitosterol to cholesterol were similar to respective ratios of endarterectomized carotid artery (Miettinen et al., 2005, 2011).

The LDL catabolism by its hepatic uptake apparently removes its plant sterols to the liver. The high plant sterol contents of HDL might also mean that in reversed sterol transport, HDL brings also plant sterols back to the liver or to the TICE. Acute administration of statins reduces markedly serum plant sterols mainly because of lowering of the transport effect of LDL complex. It is probable that several hundred micrograms of plant sterols are rapidly transferred from serum, red cells, and endothelial vascular cells to the liver, some being probably secreted into the bile, during the few hours after acute LDL cholesterol lowering by hydroxyl-methyl-glutaryl CoA reductase inhibition. As shown above (Miettinen and Gylling, 2000), about 10 mg of plant sterols are normally secreted in bile and probably an additional small amount in the TICE. Plant sterol secretion in small amount of skin sterols may be very low. Since intestinal plant sterol absorption is very low, at most 5% of dietary intake, and since plant sterols are not synthesized in human tissues, their major route of elimination is biliary secretion and ultimate excretion in stools. The biliary secretion rate of plant sterols similarly to cholesterol is regulated by the transporter proteins under the expression of ABCG5 and ABCG8 genes. In enterocytes, these transporters decrease high-sterol contents, and in hepatocytes, they stimulate sterol secretion to the biliary tract.

2.3 Metabolism of Plant Stanols

As shown above, the amounts of dietary plant stanols are very small, and they appear to mix completely with other intestinal sterols being incorporated to micellar and oil phases. They effectively inhibit cholesterol and plant sterol absorption. As compared to plant sterols (<5% absorbed), they are almost unabsorbable, <0.3% being absorbed, and only trace amounts are seen in serum even after plant-stanol-enriched food consumption with no harmful accumulation to tissues (Miettinen et al., 2011). In serum, plant stanols are transported mainly by the LDL lipoprotein density, but as for plant sterols, the ratios to cholesterol are highest in chylomicrons and HDL. Mutations of genes regulating the ABCG5 and ABCG8 transport proteins increase markedly also serum plant stanols in phytosterolemic patients, even though less than that of plant sterols. Plant stanols are secreted in bile, the daily amount for sitostanol being <2 μmol.

Intestinal bacteria hydrolyze the remaining plant sterol or plant stanol esters to the respective free ones and convert most of the plant sterols to coprostanols (5-beta) and also to coprostanones (3-keto, 5-beta), while plant stanols are usually resistant to bacterial action. Fecal plant sterols are quantitatively equal with dietary plant sterols because sterol structure is not opened during intestinal passage. Thus, their measurement can be used for quantitation of dietary plant sterol intake. Intestinal bacteria can saturate the delta-5 double bond also to the 5-alfa form in some conditions.

3. PLANT STEROLS AND ARTERY DISEASE IN HUMANS

3.1 Effects on Risk Factors

There is a unanimous agreement based on a large body of randomized, controlled clinical trials that dietary phytosterols 2–3 g day^{-1} decrease serum total and LDL cholesterol levels by about 8–10% (Demonty et al., 2009; Musa-Veloso et al., 2011). Most of the documentation is based on studies with the esterified products of plant stanols or plant sterols. The efficacy has been documented in different study populations and patient cohorts, including normolipidemia, primary hypercholesterolemia, familial hypercholesterolemia, type 1 and type 2 diabetes, metabolic syndrome, and coronary artery disease, and the studies have included different age groups, even children. Phytosterols are effective in both men and women, and when added to statin treatment, they have an additive cholesterol lowering efficacy of about 10% (Gylling and Miettinen, 2010). The LDL particle size does not diminish during phytosterol consumption. It has been calculated that the 10% LDL cholesterol reduction with long-term phytosterol consumption about 2 g day^{-1} is expected to reduce coronary events by 20% (Gylling and Miettinen, 2010) suggesting that at least 2 g of phytosterols per day is an excellent dietary means to interfere with arterial disease. The amount of phytosterols in regular diet is not large enough to reduce significantly LDL cholesterol level even though cholesterol metabolism is interfered (Linn et al., 2010).

Regarding other risk factors of artery disease, there are recent data demonstrating that plant stanol esters reduced high-sensitive C-reactive protein (hsCRP) values by 17% in a population of noncoronary subjects with mean baseline values about 2 mg l^{-1}, but in several other studies with hsCRP of similar or lower mean value, no effect has been observed (Gylling and Miettinen, 2010). In some populations, phytosterol consumption has reduced serum triglyceride levels. Phytosterol consumption has no effect on HDL cholesterol level.

Accordingly, daily consumption of 2–3 g of phytosterols decreases the most important risk factor of artery disease, the LDL cholesterol level, to such an extent that it can be assumed to lower the atherosclerosis burden. In addition, there are some indications that they also reduce inflammation and serum triglyceride levels. However, it remains to be shown whether the doubled serum and tissue plant sterol levels during chronic plant sterol consumption have any effect on arterial wall. On the contrary, plant stanol consumption decreases plant sterol levels is serum and in tissues, and the levels of plant stanols, even though increased during plant stanol consumption, remain very low in serum and were not increased in arterial wall (Miettinen et al., 2011).

3.2 Effects on Arterial Wall

The effects of phytosterols on arterial wall has been studied in seven studies (Gylling and Miettinen, 2010) using the surrogate risk markers of cardiovascular health (intima–media thickness, flow-mediated dilatation, and arterial stiffness). The studies have evaluated noncoronary subjects in short- and long-term studies with controversial results.

In children with familial hypercholesterolemia, in short-term studies and in a 1-year study in hypercholesterolemic adults, and in type 1 diabetes phytosterols had no effect on vascular properties despite cholesterol lowering (Gylling and Miettinen, 2010). On the other hand, customary plant stanol ester consumption at least for 2 years was associated with beneficial changes in carotid artery compliance. In addition, plant stanol esters improved carotid artery compliance and flow-mediated dilatation in subjects with initially reduced respective values. Accordingly, it seems evident that sufficiently long treatment is needed for beneficial effects in the vascular wall, but it seems also evident that plant stanol ester consumption is not harmful to vascular health.

3.3 Effects on Artery Disease

The knowledge of the relationship between phytosterols and artery disease in humans is limited to association studies in different population cohorts. There are only a few intervention studies, but the outcomes have focused on changes in endothelial function (Gylling and Miettinen, 2010) or in arterial wall sterols (Miettinen et al., 2011) instead of the coronary events. Accordingly, we have no information whether there is a causality between serum and whole-body plant sterol contents and atherosclerosis.

In a recent genome-wide study, it was demonstrated that common variants in the sterol transporter ABCG8 gene and in the blood group ABO locus are strongly associated with serum plant sterol levels and coronary artery disease (CAD) (Teupser et al., 2010). Genetic variants in ABCG8 and ABO related to increased serum plant sterol levels displayed significant associations with increased CAD risk, while other alleles at ABCG8 and ABO are associated with reduced serum plant sterol levels and reduced CAD risk.

There are ten cross-sectional (Fassbender et al., 2008; Glueck et al., 1991; Gylling et al., 2010; Matthan et al., 2009; Silbernagel et al., 2009; Sudhop et al., 2002; Sutherland et al., 1998; Weingärtner et al., 2008; Wilund et al., 2004; Windler et al., 2009) and three follow-up (Assman et al., 2006; Escurriol et al., 2010; Pinedo et al., 2007) cohort studies, in which the association between serum plant sterol levels and the presence or the risk or the severity of CAD or coronary calcification has been evaluated. The cross-sectional cohort studies include population cohorts, case–controls, or subjects referred to hospital for coronary angiography. The three follow-up studies included population cohorts, one including only men.

In seven of all studies, lipid-lowering medication and/or plant sterol/stanol consumption were exclusion criteria, but in the rest of studies, these aspects were not taken into consideration. The age of the study subjects varied from 30 to 89 years. One study included only subjects of old age (65–89-year old), and the study population contained not only home dwelling but also institutionalized subjects (Fassbender et al., 2008). The mean age in the different cohorts varied from ~55 years to ~65 years when Fassbender et al. (2008) was excluded. Two studies (Gylling et al., 2010; Windler et al., 2009) included only women, and one (Assman et al., 2006) only men. The presence of diabetes was significantly higher in cases versus controls in four studies, but the presence of diabetes was not reported in five studies. Background diet was not evaluated in nine studies.

In eight studies (Assman et al., 2006; Glueck et al., 1991; Gylling et al., 2010; Matthan et al., 2009; Silbernagel et al., 2009; Sudhop et al., 2002; Sutherland et al., 1998; Weingärtner et al., 2008), high serum plant sterol levels or high cholesterol absorption assessed with serum noncholesterol sterols were associated with high risk of CAD, with more frequent presence of CAD, or with more versus less severe coronary disease. In five studies (Escurriol et al., 2010; Fassbender et al., 2008; Pinedo et al., 2007; Wilund et al., 2004; Windler et al., 2009), no association or an inverse association between serum plant sterol levels and the presence of CAD, with coronary calcinosis, or with the risk of CAD was demonstrated.

In addition, there are three studies evaluating the relationship of serum plant sterol levels with all-cause or cardiovascular mortality (Silbernagel et al., 2010; Strandberg et al., 2010; Tilvis et al., 2011). In the study by Strandberg et al., a high-risk male cohort of the age 57–64 years ($n = 232$) had been followed for 22 years, and it turned out that higher serum plant sterol levels in middle age predicted lower long-term mortality risk (Strandberg et al., 2010). Similar results were obtained in a study with subjects over 75-year old at the baseline ($n = 623$) and followed for 17 years (Tilvis et al., 2011). In this study, low serum cholesterol, low serum lathosterol (cholesterol synthesis marker), and low serum sitosterol level were all associated with impaired survival. Completely different results were obtained with the LURIC population of German coronary subjects with a mean age of 62.8 years at baseline and followed for 7.3 years (Silbernagel et al., 2010). In this study, high-cholesterol absorption assessed with serum noncholesterol sterols predicted increased all-cause and cardiovascular mortality. Similar results were obtained with statin-treated Finnish 4S population (Gylling and Miettinen, 2010).

Accordingly, regarding the present knowledge, the situation is confusing between plant sterols and artery disease, and it is impossible to conclude whether plant sterols have a role in human atherosclerosis. In addition, there are several problems related to some of these studies. Lipid-lowering medication or consumption of plant sterol/plant stanol products were not taken into consideration in 6 of 13 studies. Statins, in addition to interfering with cholesterol metabolism, elevate serum plant sterol levels. On the other side, consumption of plant sterols increases their serum levels, but consumption of plant stanol products decreases serum and tissue plant sterol levels (Gylling and Miettinen, 2010). Furthermore, in some case–control studies, the presence of obesity or type 1 or type 2 diabetes were not controlled, and the possible presence of diabetes was ignored in several studies. Obesity, insulin resistance, fatty liver, and type 2 diabetes interfere with cholesterol and plant sterol metabolism, so that the serum levels of plant sterols are lower compared with healthy controls. On the contrary, serum plant sterol levels are higher in type 1 diabetes than in controls. These aspects, if not taken into consideration, would lead to misinterpretation of the results. In only 4 of 13 studies, the background diet was controlled. Except the dietary amount of plant sterols, there are also other components in the diet; for example, the amount and type of fat and cholesterol affect the absorption and serum levels of plant sterols. When dietary components are studied, background diet need to be evaluated and even controlled in long-term studies. In old age, institutionalization (and poor health) decreases not only serum cholesterol but also the serum plant sterol levels (Tilvis et al., 2011). Epidemiologic studies can never reveal causality. And finally, the assessment of serum plant sterols in different laboratories was not validated, and the measured levels varied a lot between studies. Accordingly, it is difficult to compare the results between studies, and a high level in one study was a median or even a low level in another study.

4. CONCLUSIONS

In humans, serum plant sterols vary from low to high values depending on heredity, diet, medication, metabolic circumstances, and concomitant diseases, which all interfere with sterol metabolism. Plant sterols are taken into tissues, including arterial wall and plaques in relation to their serum concentrations. However, at the moment, it is not clear whether they have an active atherogenetic role beyond cholesterol in the endothelial cell or in the plaque. The concern of atherogenesis does not deal with plant stanols, because their serum levels remain very low, about 1:10 000 of that of cholesterol, they reduce plant sterols, and they are not taken up into arterial wall.

REFERENCES

Assman, G., Cullen, P., Erbey, J., et al., 2006. Plasma sitosterol elevations are associated with an increased incidence of coronary events in men: results of a nested case-control analysis of the Prospective Cardiovascular Münster (PROCAM) Study. Nutrition, Metabolism, and Cardiovascular Diseases 16, 13–21.

Bhattacharyya, A.K., Connor, W.E., 1974. Beta-sitosterolemia and xanthomatosis. A newly described lipid storage disease in two sisters. Journal of Clinical Investigation 53, 1033–1043.

Demonty, I., Ras, R.T., van der Knaap, H.C.M., et al., 2009. Continuous dose–response relationship of the LDL-cholesterol–lowering effect of phytosterol intake. Journal of Nutrition 139, 271–284.

Escurriol, V., Cofán, M., Moreno-Iribas, C., et al., 2010. Phytosterol plasma concentrations and coronary heart disease in the prospective Spanish EPIC cohort. Journal of Lipid Research 51, 618–624.

Fassbender, K., Lütjohann, D., Dik, M.G., et al., 2008. Moderately elevated plant sterol levels are associated with reduced cardiovascular risk – The LASA Study. Atherosclerosis 196, 283–288.

Fransen, H.P., de Jong, N., Wolfs, M., et al., 2007. Customary use of plant sterol and plant stanol enriched margarine is associated with changes in serum plant sterol and stanol concentrations in humans. Journal of Nutrition 137, 1301–1306.

Glueck, C.J., Speirs, J., Tracy, T., et al., 1991. Relationship of serum plant sterols (phytosterols) and cholesterol in 595 hypercholesterolemic subjects, and familial aggregation of phytosterols, cholesterol, and premature coronary heart disease in hyperphytosterolemic probands and their first-degree relatives. Metabolism 40, 842–848.

Gylling, H., Miettinen, T.A., 2010a. The effects of plant stanol ester in different subject groups. European Cardiology 6, 18–21.

Gylling, H., Hallikainen, M., Rajaratnam, R.A., et al., 2010b. The metabolism of plant sterols is disturbed in postmenopausal women with coronary artery disease. Metabolism 58, 401–407.

Helske, S., Miettinen, T.A., Gylling, H., et al., 2008. Accumulation of cholesterol precursors and plant sterols in human stenotic aortic valves. Journal of Lipid Research 49, 1511–1518.

Klingberg, S., Andersson, H., Mulligan, A., et al., 2008a. Food sources of plant sterols in the EPIC Norfolk population. European Journal of Clinical Nutrition 62, 695–703.

Klingberg, S., Ellegård, L., Johansson, I., et al., 2008b. Inverse relation between dietary intake of naturally occurring plant sterols and serum cholesterol in northern Sweden. American Journal of Clinical Nutrition 87, 993–1001.

Lin, D.S., Connor, W.E., 2001. Fecal steroids of the coprolite of a Greenland Eskimo mummy, AD 1475: a clue to dietary sterol intake. American Journal of Clinical Nutrition 74, 44–49.

Linn, X., Racette, S.B., Lefevre, M., et al., 2010. The effects of phytosterols present in natural food matrices on cholesterol metabolism and LDL-cholesterol: a controlled feeding trial. European Journal of Clinical Nutrition 64, 1481–1487.

Matthan, N.R., Pencina, M., LaRocque, J.M., et al., 2009. Alterations in cholesterol absorption/synthesis markers characterize Framingham Offspring Study participants with CHD. Journal of Lipid Research 50, 1927–1935.

Miettinen, T.A., Gylling, H., 2000. Cholesterol absorption efficiency and sterol metabolism in obesity. Atherosclerosis 153, 241–248.

Miettinen, T.A., Nissinen, M., Lepäntalo, M., et al., 2011. Non-cholesterol sterols in serum and endarterectomized carotid arteries after a short-term plant stanol and sterol ester challenge. Nutrition, Metabolism, and Cardiovascular Diseases 21, 182–188.

Miettinen, T.A., Puska, P., Gylling, H., Vanhanen, H., Vartiainen, E., 1995. Reduction of serum cholesterol with sitostanol-ester margarine in a mildly hypercholesterolemic population. The New England Journal of Medicine 333, 1308–1312.

Miettinen, T.A., Railo, M., Lepäntalo, M., Gylling, H., 2005. Plant sterols in serum and in atherosclerotic plaques of patients undergoing carotid endarterectomy. Journal of the American College of Cardiology 45, 1792–1801.

Musa-Veloso, K., Poon, T.H., Elliot, J.A., Chung, C., 2011. A comparison of the LDL-cholesterol lowering efficacy of plant stanols and plant sterols over a continuous dose range: results of a meta-analysis of randomized, placebo-controlled trials. Prostaglandins, Leukotrienes and Essential Fatty Acids 85, 9–28.

Pinedo, S., Vissers, M.N., von Bergmann, K., et al., 2007. Plasma levels of plant sterols and the risk of coronary artery disease: the prospective EPIC-Norfolk Population Study. Journal of Lipid Research 48, 139–144.

Silbernagel, G., Fauler, G., Hoffmann, M.M., et al., 2010. The associations of cholesterol metabolism and plasma plant sterols with all-cause and cardiovascular mortality. Journal of Lipid Research 51, 2384–2393.

Silbernagel, G., Fauler, G., Renner, W., et al., 2009. The relationships of cholesterol metabolism and plasma plant sterols with the severity of coronary artery disease. Journal of Lipid Research 50, 334–341.

Strandberg, T.E., Gylling, H., Tilvis, R.S., Miettinen, T.A., 2010. Serum plant and other noncholesterol sterols, cholesterol metabolism and 22-year mortality among middle-aged men. Atherosclerosis 210, 282–287.

Sudhop, T., Gottwald, B.M., von Bergmann, K., 2002. Serum plant sterols as a potential risk factor for coronary heart disease. Metabolism 51, 1519–1521.

Sutherland, W.H.F., Williams, M.J.A., Nye, E.R., et al., 1998. Associations of plasma noncholesterol sterol levels with severity of coronary artery disease. Nutrition, Metabolism, and Cardiovascular Diseases 8, 386–391.

Teupser, D., Baber, R., Ceglarek, U., et al., 2010. Genetic regulation of serum phytosterol levels and risk of coronary artery disease. Circulation. Cardiovascular Genetics 3, 331–339.

Tilvis, R.S., Valvanne, J.N., Strandberg, T.E., Miettinen, T.A., 2011. Prognostic significance of serum cholesterol, lathosterol, and sitosterol in old age; a 17-year population study. Annals of Medicine 43, 292–301.

Valsta, L.M., Lemström, A., Ovaskainen, M.L., et al., 2004. Estimation of plant sterol and cholesterol intake in Finland: quality of new values and their effect on intake. British Journal of Nutrition 92, 671–678.

van der Velde, A.E., Brufau, G., Groen, A.K., 2010. Transintestinal cholesterol efflux. Current Opinion in Lipidology 21, 167–171.

Vanhanen, H., Miettinen, T.A., 1992. Effects of unsaturated and saturated dietary plant sterols on their serum contents. Clinica Chimica Acta 205, 97–107.

Weingärtner, O., Lütjohann, D., Shengbo, J., et al., 2008. Vascular effects of diet supplementation with plant sterols. Journal of the American College of Cardiology 51, 1553–1561.

Wilund, K.R., Tu, L., Xu, F., et al., 2004. No association between plasma levels of plant sterols and atherosclerosis in mice and man. Arteriosclerosis, Thrombosis, and Vascular Biology 24, 2326–2332.

Windler, E., Zyriax, B.C., Kuipers, F., Linseisen, J., Boeing, H., 2009. Association of plasma phytosterol concentrations with incident coronary heart disease. Data from the CORA study, a case-control study of coronary artery disease in women. Atherosclerosis 203, 284–290.

CHAPTER 41

Antiatherogenic Effects of Ginger (*Zingiber officinale* Roscoe): Scientific Observations and Ethnomedicinal Validation

A.N. Prabhu*, A.R. Shivashankara*, R. Haniadka*, P.L. Palatty*, D. Prabhu[†], M.S. Baliga*

*Father Muller Medical College, Mangalore, Karnataka, India
[†]Manipal University, Manipal, Karnataka, India

ABBREVIATIONS

ABTS 2,2′-Azino-bis(3-ethylbenzthiazoline-6-sulphonic acid)
ACE Angiotensin-converting enzyme
ADP Adenosine diphosphate
CAD Coronary artery disease
COX-1 Cyclooxygenase-1
COX-2 Cyclooxygenase-2
HDL High-density lipoprotein
IL-1β Interleukin-1beta
IL-6 Interleukin-6
LDL Low-density lipoprotein
5-LOX 5-Lipooxygenase
PGE2 Prostaglandin E2
TNF-α Tumor necrosis factor alpha
TXA2 Thromboxane A2
VLDL Very low-density lipoprotein

1. INTRODUCTION

Chronic noncommunicable diseases are assuming increasing importance among the adult population in both developed and developing countries. Currently, cardiovascular diseases (CVDs) account for about 16.7 million deaths worldwide and are responsible for about 25% of disability-adjusted life years lost due to noncommunicable diseases in the southeast Asian region countries (Libby, 2008). Of these, atherosclerosis remains the major cause of death and premature disability. Current predictions are that by the year 2020, CVDs, and notably atherosclerosis, will probably become the leading cause of global disease burden and its prevention will be very important (Libby, 2008).

Bioactive Food as Dietary Interventions for Cardiovascular Disease
http://dx.doi.org/10.1016/B978-0-12-396485-4.00267-X

© 2013 Elsevier Inc.
All rights reserved.

Atherosclerosis, characterized by intimal lesions (called *Atheromas*) protruding into and obstructing the vascular lumen, is a prolonged process and occurs over a period of many years. Symptomatic atherosclerosis most often involves the arteries supplying blood to the heart, brain, kidneys, and lower extremities, resulting in myocardial infarction, stroke, aortic aneurysms, and peripheral vascular diseases as its major consequences (Libby, 2008).

2. ETIOPATHOGENESIS OF ATHEROSCLEROSIS

Atherosclerosis is a multifocal progressive chronic inflammatory response of arterial wall initiated by injury to endothelium and sustained by interaction between modified lipoproteins, macrophages, lymphocytes, and cellular constituents of the arterial wall. It is characterized by focal lipid-rich deposits of atheroma that remain clinically silent until they became large enough to impair arterial perfusion or certain lesions result in thrombotic occlusions of affected vessels. It is now well established that hypercholesterolemia, high levels of low-density lipoprotein (LDL), low levels of high-density lipoprotein (HDL), hypertension, diabetes mellitus, familial history of coronary artery disease (CAD), smoking, obesity, and sedentary lifestyle with decreased physical activity are the major risk factors contributing to atherosclerosis (Libby, 2008).

Atherosclerosis is a prolonged process and, although beginning in early life, the clinical manifestations appear only in the fifth or sixth decade. Early atherosclerotic lesions scientifically termed as fatty streaks occur at sites of altered arterial shear stress (such as bifurcations), and are associated with abnormal endothelial function. The fatty streaks develop when inflammatory cells, predominantly monocytes, bind to endothelial cells, migrate into the intima, and take up oxidized LDL from the plasma to become lipid-laden foam cells or macrophages (Libby, 2008).

Extracellular lipid pools appear in the intimal space when these foam cells die and release the contents. Moreover, in response to cytokines and growth factors produced by activated macrophages, smooth muscle cells from media of the arterial wall migrate into the intima, and change from contractile to repair phenotype in an attempt to stabilize the atherosclerotic lesion. If they are successful, the lipid core will be covered by smooth muscle cells and matrix, producing a stable atherosclerotic plaque or atheroma. This remains asymptomatic until it becomes large enough to obstruct the arterial blood flow. In advanced atheroma, macrophages mediate inflammation and smooth muscles promote repair; if inflammation predominates, plaque becomes unstable and may be complicated by ulceration and superadded thrombosis (Libby, 2008).

The treatment of dyslipidemia in modern medicine is multifarious and depending on the need and clinical condition may involve more than one type of drug. Niacin (nicotinic acid), bile acid-sequestering resins (cholestyramine, colestipol, and colesevelam), statins (lovastatin, simvastatin, atorvastatin, pravastatin, rosuvastatin, etc.), fibric acid derivatives (gemfibrozil, fenofibrate, and bezafibrate), and ezetimibe are some of the most commonly used drugs in the treatment of dyslipidemia. Unfortunately, regular use of these drugs is associated with untoward side effects (Libby, 2008), thereby necessitating the search for novel nontoxic agents.

3. PLANTS IN THE PREVENTION OF ATHEROSCLEROSIS

Various studies have suggested that dietary agents like *Allium sativum* and *Zingiber officinale*, and medicinal plants like *Eugenia Jambolana*, *Aegle marmelos*, *Syzygium cuminii*, and *Asparagus racemosus* possess hypolipidemic, anti-inflammatory, and antioxidant properties that contribute to the prevention of atherogenesis. *Z. officinale* (ginger; Figure 41.1) is a popular culinary ingredient and also occupies an important place in Ayurvedic, Chinese, Greek, and Arabic systems of medicine, where it is used for treating rheumatism, gout,

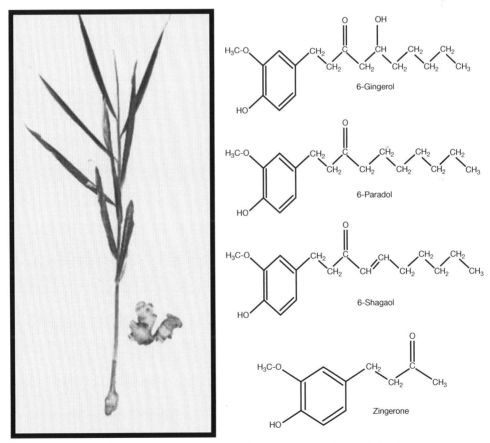

Figure 41.1 Ginger plant and structures of some important phytochemicals in ginger rhizome.

and asthma and to stimulant gastrointestinal tract (GIT; Ali et al., 2008; Schulick, 1994). Scientific studies by various investigators have shown that ginger possesses cardioprotective effects and delays/prevents atherosclerosis. This chapter addresses the various observations and mechanisms contributing to the prevention of atherosclerosis by ginger.

4. PROTECTIVE EFFECTS OF GINGER AGAINST ATHEROSCLEROSIS

4.1 Ginger Possesses Antihyperglycemic and Antidiabetic Effects

Reports indicate that most patients with diabetes mellitus die of atherosclerosis and its associated complications. The abnormal lipoprotein profile associated with insulin resistance, known as diabetic dyslipidemia, accounts for cardiovascular risk in type 2 diabetes (Figures 41.2 and 41.3). Furthermore, in diabetic patients, the LDL particles tend to be smaller and denser, and therefore more atherogenic. Hypertension also frequently accompanies central obesity, insulin resistance, and dyslipidemia, and the cluster of risk factors is termed metabolic syndrome (Libby, 2008).

Preclinical studies have shown that ginger possesses antidiabetic effects in both type I and II preclinical models of study. Administering ginger either as juice or aqueous or ethanolic extract is shown to produce antihyperglycemic and insulinotropic effects (Akhani et al., 2004; Al-Amin et al., 2006; Bhandari et al., 2005; Islam and Choi, 2008; Kadnur and Goyal, 2005; Ojewole, 2006). Additionally, studies have also shown that [6]-gingerol, the active principle of ginger, is also shown to decrease the fasting blood glucose and improve the glucose tolerance in genetically programmed type II diabetic mice (db/db mice; Singh et al., 2009).

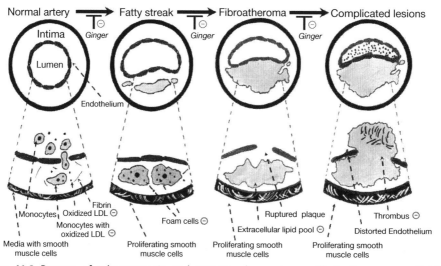

Figure 41.2 Process of atherogenesis and targets where ginger affects the process (inhibits/retards = $\ominus$).

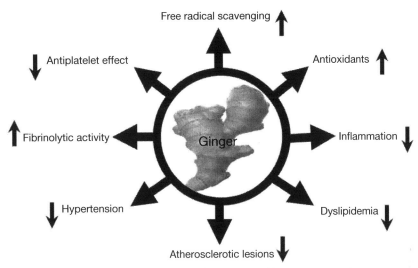

Figure 41.3 Targets of ginger in preventing atherogenesis (down arrows = decrease; up arrows = increase).

Ginger has been shown to reduce diabetic hyperlipidemia, one of the key risk factors of atherosclerosis, stimulate synthesis of insulin (insulinotropic effects), increase antioxidants, inhibit the carbohydrate-digesting enzymes, and prevent formation of sorbitol and advanced glycation end products (Alizadeh-Navaei et al., 2008; Bhandari et al., 1998; El Rokh et al., 2010; Fuhrman et al., 2000; Madkor et al., 2010; Thomson et al., 2002). Gingerol, the phytochemical present in ginger, is also reported to interact with adipocytes and pancreatic cells, to activate peroxisome proliferator-activated receptor γ and NF-E2-related factor 2 signaling pathways leading to downregulation of adipokines, tumor necrosis factor (TNF)-α, leptin, resistin, and monocytes chemotatic protein-1 (Aggarwal, 2010). Together, all these properties may have contributed to the prevention of atherosclerosis and macrovascular damage.

4.2 Ginger Ameliorates Dyslipidemia

Dyslipidemia, characterized by elevated serum levels of total cholesterol, triglycerides, and LDL, and decreased serum level of HDL, is an independent but major risk factor for atherosclerosis. Dyslipidemia leads to the formation of small dense LDL particles and LDL oxidation, which in turn are responsible for the fatty streak and atherosclerotic plaque (Libby, 2008).

Preclinical studies have shown that ginger reduces the serum levels of cholesterol, LDL, and triglycerides, and concomitantly increases the levels of HDL (Alizadeh-Navaei et al., 2008; Bhandari et al., 1998; El Rokh et al., 2010; Fuhrman et al., 2000; Madkor et al., 2010; Thomson et al., 2002). Feeding raw ginger (500 mg kg^{-1}, i.p., 7 weeks) to diabetic rats is also reported to decrease the serum cholesterol and triacylglycerol level (Al-Amin et al., 2006). Additionally, supplementing ginger in a cholesterol-enriched diet is also shown to decrease the expression of retinoid-binding protein and fatty acid-binding protein genes in the liver and adipose tissue of rats (Matsuda et al., 2009).

Oral feeding of the ethanolic extract of ginger (200 mg kg^{-1} for 20 days) to streptozotocin-induced diabetic rats decreased the levels of serum total cholesterol, triglycerides, and concomitantly increased the levels of HDL cholesterol (Thomson et al., 2002). The administration of methanolic and ethanolic extracts of ginger to fructose-induced type II diabetic rats is also shown to decrease the serum levels of cholesterol, triglycerides, LDL, and very low-density lipoprotein (VLDL; Kadnur and Goyal, 2005). Administering the aqueous extract of ginger (200 mg kg^{-1} body weight) for a month to rats on high-fat diet was also effective in reducing serum cholesterol, atherogenic index, and enhancing the levels of serum HDL (Unnikrishnan et al., 2009).

Clinical trials have also shown that ginger was effective in reducing hyperlipidemia in nondiabetic individuals. In a double-blind clinical trial, Alizadeh-Navaei et al. (2008) have observed that when compared to placebo treatment, administration of fine powder of ginger (3 g day^{-1} in three divided doses for 45 consecutive days) caused a significant decrease in the levels of triglyceride and cholesterol, and also decreased the levels of LDL and concomitantly increased the levels of HDL (Alizadeh-Navaei et al., 2008).

Mechanistic studies indicate that ginger attains its hypolipidemic effect by inducing the synthesis of bile acid, repressing cholesterol synthesis, promoting the uptake and catabolism of LDL, and inhibiting LDL oxidation and aggregation (Bhandari et al., 2005; Fuhrman et al., 2000; Kadnur and Goyal, 2005; Nammi et al., 2009, 2010; Srinivasan and Sambaiah, 1991). Studies with apolipoprotein E-deficient mice have shown that administering ginger extract (250 mg day^{-1} for 10 weeks) reduces the atherosclerotic lesions in aorta; reduces the plasma levels of triglycerides, cholesterol, and LDL; and inhibits the cholesterol biosynthesis rate in peritoneal macrophages (Fuhrman et al., 2000).

Administering ethanolic extract of ginger (400 mg kg^{-1} for 6 weeks) to rats fed on high-fat diet upregulated LDL receptor messenger ribonucleic acid and downregulated 3-hydroxy-3-methylglutaryl-coenzyme A reductase protein expression in liver (Nammi et al., 2010). Ginger is also shown to stimulate the conversion of cholesterol to bile acids by increasing the activity of hepatic cholesterol 7-alpha hydroxylase (Srinivasan and Sambaiah, 1991). The ginger phytochemical (E)-8β, 17-epoxylabd-12ene-15,16-dial is also reported to inhibit the cholesterol biosynthesis in the liver of hypercholesterolemic mice (Tanabe et al., 1993).

4.3 Ginger Possesses Antioxidant Property

Oxidative stress resulting from an imbalance due to increased free radical generation and decreased antioxidants is implicated in the pathogenesis of many diseases including atherosclerosis. Reactive oxygen species generated mainly due to hyperlipidemia and hyperglycemia cause oxidation of LDL, which is the key trigger in the uptake of LDL by macrophages and smooth muscle cells and formation of foam cells (Libby, 2008).

The free radical scavenging and antioxidant potential of ginger has been validated by both *in vitro* (Ali et al., 2008; Chrubasik et al., 2005; El-Ghorab et al., 2010; Stoilova et al., 2007), and *in vivo* systems of study (Afshari et al., 2007; Shanmugam et al., 2011). Cell-free assays have shown that ginger and its phytochemicals, gingerol, paradol, zingerone, and shogol (Figure 41.1), possess free radical scavenging properties in various assays like 1,1-diphenyl-2-picrylhydrazyl (DPPH), 2,2′-azino-bis(3-ethylbenzthiazoline-6-sulphonic acid) – ABTS, hydroxyl, superoxide, nitric oxide, peroxyl radicals *in vitro* (Ali et al., 2008; Chrubasik et al., 2005).

Studies have also shown that administering ginger to diabetic rats increased the levels of the antioxidant glutathione and the enzymes superoxide dismutase (SOD), catalase, glutathione peroxidase, and glutathione reductase, and concomitantly reduced the levels of malondialdehyde in blood (Madkor et al., 2010), liver (Shanmugam et al., 2011; Thomson et al., 2002), brain (Shanmugam et al., 2010), pancreas (Thomson et al., 2002), and renal (Afshari et al., 2007) tissues. These findings conclusively show that ginger exerts a protective effect in diabetes by decreasing oxidative stress and promoting the levels of antioxidants in tissues.

Seminal studies by Fuhrman et al. (2000) have also shown that the extract of ginger decreased macrophage oxidative responses in both animal and *in vitro* assay systems. Ginger extract reduced the capacity of macrophages to oxidize LDL and decreased the uptake of oxidized LDL due to steric modification of plasma lipoprotein receptors. This concomitantly reduced the development of atherosclerotic lesions in apolipoprotein E-deficient mice and imparted its beneficial effects (Fuhrman et al., 2000).

4.4 Ginger Has Antiplatelet Effect and Increases Fibrinolytic Activity

Platelet aggregation and thrombosis are the key phenomena in atherosclerosis and CVD. Platelets stick to the damaged vessel wall to form a plaque, and then stick to each other (aggregate) and release adenosine diphosphate (ADP) and thromboxane A2 (TXA2), which promote further aggregation. Platelet plug thus formed causes partial or complete obstruction at the site of the lesion and distal embolization, resulting in ischemia/infarction of the affected organ. Antiplatelet drugs used in clinical practice act by inhibiting the key process of platelet aggregation (Frederick, 2004).

Studies have shown that ginger reduces platelet aggregation and has an antithrombotic effect. Gingerol, the major phytochemical of ginger, is reported to inhibit the synthesis of TXA2 and prostaglandin D2 from arachidonic acid, and also to inhibit platelet aggregation (Guh et al., 1995). Oral administration of aqueous extract of ginger in high doses (500 mg kg^{-1}) is shown to decrease the levels of serum prostaglandin E2 (PGE2) and

TXA2 (Thomson et al., 2002). Clinical studies have also shown antiplatelet activity of ginger in both healthy individuals and in patients with CAD (Verma et al., 1993; Bordia et al., 1997). A single dose of powdered ginger produced a significant reduction in the platelet aggregation induced by ADP and epinephrine in CAD patients (Bordia et al., 1997).

With respect to the fibrinolytic actions of ginger, studies have shown that administering air-dried ginger powder (0.1 g kg^{-1} body weight orally for 75 days) to rabbits fed on high-cholesterol diet caused distinct enhancement in fibrinolytic activity (Verma et al., 2004). In a randomized, placebo-controlled trial with healthy adult males, addition of ginger to a fatty meal (5 g orally) prevented fat-induced decrease in fibrinolytic activity and enhanced fibrinolysis (Verma and Bordia, 2001).

4.5 Ginger Reduces Atherosclerotic Lesions

Atherosclerosis may manifest as CAD, cerebrovascular disease, or peripheral vascular disease. These entities often coexist and the pathogenesis of disease is similar. Conventionally atherogenisis can be prevented or retarded through lifestyle modification and by regular consumption of medications. In early stages, practice of regular exercise/physical activity, abstinence from smoking and alcohol consumption, and dietary modification is suggested. Secondary prevention intended to prevent recurrence of atherosclerosis-related complications like myocardial infarction is based on risk factor modification such as control of hypertension and diabetes, weight reduction, and, most importantly, lowering total and LDL cholesterol levels while increasing HDL. In this direction, the use of medications, especially hypolipidemic drugs like statin and antihypertensive drugs like angiotensin-converting enzyme (ACE) inhibitors, is recommended (Libby, 2008). Ginger, apart from hypolipidemic and antihypertensive effects, has direct effect on atherosclerotic lesions and preclinical studies have shown that, when compared to cholesterol-alone-fed rabbits, coadministering ginger reduced the degree of atherosclerotic lesions in the aorta (Bhandari et al., 1998). Similar observations were seen when dry ginger powder (0.1 g kg^{-1} body weight for 75 days) was also fed to rabbits on high-cholesterol diet (Verma et al., 2004), and in mice on high-cholesterol diet (Al-Tahtawy et al., 2011; Fuhrman et al., 2000).

4.6 Ginger Has Anti-Inflammatory Effect

Recent reports indicate that the inflammatory process aggravates and speeds up the process of atherosclerosis and that anti-inflammatory drugs reduce/delay the process. Mechanistic studies have shown that ginger suppresses prostaglandin synthesis by inhibiting cyclooxygenase-1 (COX-1), COX-2, and leukotriene biosynthesis by inhibiting 5-lipooxygenase (5-LOX; Grzanna et al., 2005; Srivastava, 1984, 1986). Additionally, the ginger constituents [8]-paradol and [8]-shogaol are also reported to possess strong inhibitory effects on COX-2 enzyme activity *in vitro* (Tjendraputra et al., 2001). The COX-1 inhibitory activity of [8]-paradol was more potent than the gingerol analogs (Tjendraputra et al., 2001). The diarylheptanoid with catechol group was the most active compound against 5-LOX (Kiuchi et al., 1992).

Aqueous extract of ginger (500 mg kg^{-1}) when administered to rats through either oral or intraperitoneal routes decreased the levels of PGE2 in blood and hyperalgesia that cause vasodilatation and inflammation (Thomson et al., 2002). The phytochemical [6]-gingerol is also shown to modulate the levels of COX and other inflammatory mediators (Bhattarai et al., 2001; Ojewole, 2006; Priya Rani et al., 2011). Molecular studies have shown that ginger and its phytochemicals decrease the levels of proinflammatory cytokines (TNF-α, interleukin-1beta (IL-1β), IL-6, and interferon γ) and reduce the elevated expression of nuclear factor kappaB (Aggarwal and Shishodia, 2004). Two major phytochemicals [6]-gingerol and [6]-shaogaol were shown to inhibit TNF-α expression (Isa et al., 2008).

4.7 Ginger Has Antihypertensive Effect

Hypertension (blood pressure) is a major risk factor for atherosclerosis and is regulated by the autonomic nervous system and renin–angiotensin system. ACE is the key enzyme in the formation of angiotensin-II which has vasoconstrictory effect and helps in sodium retention. ACE inhibitors are used in the treatment of hypertension. Preclinical studies with anesthetized rats have shown that the crude extract of ginger induces a dose-dependent (0.3–3 mg kg^{-1}) decrease in the arterial pressure, inhibits ACE, and concomitantly reduces the blood pressure (Ghayur and Gilani, 2005). *In vitro* studies in the guinea pig paired atria have shown that ginger extract exhibited cardio-depressant effect on the rate and force of contraction. Additionally, in the rabbit thoracic aortic preparations, ginger is shown to relax phenylephrine-induced and potassium-induced contraction and the vasodilatory effect was comparable to the effect of verapamil, a standard calcium channel-blocking drug (Ghayur and Gilani, 2005). Together, all these observations indicate the usefulness of ginger in reducing hypertension.

5. CONCLUSION

Ginger rhizomes have a long history for their health benefits and use as traditional medicine, and recently published reports clearly indicate that consumption of ginger extracts attenuates atherogenesis. Ginger possesses strong hypolipidemic activity and mediates these effects by reducing plasma total cholesterol, LDL cholesterol, triglycerides, and phospholipid levels, promotes bile acid synthesis, represses cholesterol synthesis, and promotes catabolism of LDL cholesterol. Ginger is also shown to possess antidiabetic activity and to ameliorate diabetic dyslipidemia. Ginger is a scavenger of free radicals, possesses antiinflammatory and antiplatelet effects, promotes fibrinolysis, decreases lipid peroxidation, and increases the levels of antioxidants, all of which contribute to its anti-atherosclerotic action. The information available from the limited pilot clinical studies although encouraging strongly suggest the need for larger clinical trials (Alizadeh-Navaei et al., 2008; Bordia et al., 1997; Verma and Bordia, 2001; Verma et al., 2004).

ACKNOWLEDGMENT

The authors are grateful to Rev. Fr. Patrick Rodrigus (Director), Rev. Fr. Denis D'Sa (Administrator), and Dr. Jayaprakash Alva (Dean) of Father Muller Medical College for providing the necessary facilities and support.

REFERENCES

Afshari, A.T., Shirpoor, A., Farshid, A., et al., 2007. The effect of ginger on diabetic nephropathy, plasma antioxidant capacity and lipid peroxidation in rats. Food Chemistry 101, 148–153.

Aggarwal, B.B., 2010. Targeting inflammation induced obesity and metabolic diseases by curcumin and other nutraceuticals. Annual Review of Nutrition 30, 173–199.

Aggarwal, B.B., Shishodia, S., 2004. Suppression of the nuclear factor-kappaB activation pathway by spice-derived phytochemicals: reasoning for seasoning. Annals of the New York Academy of Sciences 1030, 434–441.

Akhani, S.P., Vishwakarma, S.L., Goyal, R.K., 2004. Antidiabetic activity of Zingiber officinale in streptozotocin induced type 1 diabetic rats. Journal of Pharmacy and Pharmacology 56, 101–105.

Al-Amin, Z.M., Thomson, M., Al-Quttan, K.K., Peltonen-Shalaby, R., Ali, M., 2006. Anti diabetic and hypolipidaemic properties of ginger in streptozotocin-induced diabetic rats. Bristish Journal Nutrition 96, 660–666.

Ali, B.H., Blunden, G., Tanira, M.O., Nemmar, A., 2008. Some phytochemical, pharmacological and toxicological properties of ginger (Zingiber officinale Roscoe): a review of recent research. Food and Chemical Toxicology 46, 409–420.

Alizadeh-Navaei, R., Roozbeh, F., Sarvi, M., Pouramir, M., Jalali, F., Moghadamnia, A.A., 2008. Investigation of the effect of ginger on the lipid levels A double blind controlled clinical trial. Saudi Medical Journal 29, 1280–1284.

Al-Tahtawy, R.H.M., El-Bastawesy, A.M., Monem, M.G.A., et al., 2011. Antioxidant activity of volatile oils of Zingiber officinale (Ginger). Spatula DD 1, 1–8.

Bhandari, U., Kanojia, R., Pillai, K.K., 2005. Effect of ethanolic extract of Zingiber officinale on dyslipidaemia in diabetic rats. Journal of Ethnopharmacology 97, 227–230.

Bhandari, U., Sharma, J.N., Zafar, R., 1998. The protective action of ethanolic ginger (Zingiber officinale) extract in cholesterol fed rabbits. Journal of Ethnopharmacology 61, 167–171.

Bhattarai, S., Tran, V.H., Duke, C.C., 2001. The stability of gingerol and shogaol in aqueous solutions. Journal of Pharmaceutical Science 90, 1658–1664.

Bordia, A., Verma, S.K., Srivastava, K.C., 1997. Effect of ginger (Zingiber officinale Rosc.) and fenugreek (Trigonella foenumgraeum L.) on blood lipids, blood sugar and platelet aggregation in patients with coronary artery disease. Prostglandins Leukot Essent fatty Acids 56, 379–384.

Chrubasik, S., Pittler, M.H., Roufogalis, B.D., 2005. Zingiberis rhizoma: a comprehensive review on the ginger effect and efficacy profiles. Phytomedicine 12, 684–701.

El Rokh, el-SM, Yassin, N.A., El-Shenawy, S.M., Ibrahim, B.M., 2010. Antihypercholesterolaemic effect of ginger rhizome (Zingiber officinale) in rats. Inflammopharmacology 18, 309–315.

El-Ghorab, A.H., Nauman, M., Anjum, F.M., Hussain, S., Nadeem, M., 2010. A comparative study on chemical composition and antioxidant activity of ginger (Zingiber officinale) and cumin (Cuminum cyminum). Journal of Agricultural and Food Chemistry 58, 8231–8237.

Frederick, J.S., 2004. Blood vessels. In: Kumar, V., Abbas, A.K., Fausto, N. (Eds.), Robbins and Cotran Pathologic Basis of Disease, seventh ed. 511–554.

Fuhrman, B., Rosenblat, M., Hayek, T., Coleman, R., Aviram, M., 2000. Ginger extract consumption reduces plasma cholesterol, inhibits LDL oxidation and attenuates development of atherosclerosis in atherosclerotic, apolipoprotien E-deficient mice. Journal of Nutrition 130, 1124–1131.

Ghayur, M.N., Gilani, A.H., 2005. Ginger lowers blood pressure through blockade of voltage dependent calcium channels. Cardiovascular Pharmacology 45, 74–80.

Grzanna, R., Lindmark, L., Frondoza, C.G., 2005. Ginger – an herbal medicinal product with broad anti-inflammatory actions. Journal of Medicinal Food 8, 125–132.

Guh, J.H., Ko, F.N., Jonq, T.T., Tenq, C.M., 1995. Antiplatelet effect of gingerol isolated from *Zingiber officinale*. Journal of Pharmacy and Pharmacology 47, 329.

Isa, Y., Miyakawa, Y., Yanagisawa, M., Goto, T., Kang, M.S., Kawada, T., 2008. 6-Shogaol and 6-gingerol, the pungent of ginger, inhibit TNF-alpha mediated downregulation of adiponectin expression via different mechanisms in 3T3–L1 adipocytes. Biochemical and Biophysical Research Communication 373, 429–434.

Islam, M.S., Choi, H., 2008. Comparative effects of dietary ginger (*Zingiber officinale*) and garlic (*Allium sativum*) investigated in a type II diabetes model of rats. Journal of Medicinal Food 11, 152–159.

Kadnur, S.V., Goyal, R.K., 2005. Beneficial effects of *Zingiber officinale* Roseoe on fructose induced hyperlipidaemia and hyperinsulinemia in rats. Indian Journal of Experimental Biology 43, 161–164.

Kiuchi, F., Iwakami, S., Shibuya, M., Hanaoka, F., Sankawa, U., 1992. Inhibition of prostaglandin and leukotriene biosynthesis by gingerols and diarylheptanoids. Chemical and Pharmaceutical Bulletin 40, 387–391.

Libby, P., 2008. The pathogenesis, prevention and treatment of atherosclerosis. In: Fauci, A.S., Braunwald, E., Kasper, D.L. et al., (Eds.), Harrison's Principles of Internal Medicine, seventeenth ed. 1501–1508.

Madkor, H.R., Mansour, S.W., Ramadan, G., 2010. Modulatory effects of garlic, ginger, turmeric and their mixture on hyperglycemia, dyslipidaemia and oxidative stress in streptozotocin-nicotinamide diabetic rats. British Journal of Nutrition 10, 1–8.

Matsuda, A., Wang, Z., Takahashi, S., Tokuda, T., Miura, N., Hasegawa, J., 2009. Upregulation of mRNA of retinoid binding protein and fatty acid binding protein by cholesterol enriched-diet and effect of ginger on lipid metabolism. Life Sciences 84, 903–907.

Nammi, S., Kim, M.S., Gavande, N.S., Li, G.Q., Roufogalis, B.D., 2010. Regulation of low density lipoprotein receptor and 3-hydroxy-3-methyl glutaryl coenzyme A reductase expression by *Zingiber officinale* in the liver of high fat diet fed rats. Basic and Clinical Pharmacology and Toxicology 106, 389–395.

Nammi, S., Sreemantula, S., Roufogalis, B.D., 2009. Protective effects of ethanolic extract of *Zingiber officinale* rhizome on the development of metabolic syndrome in high fat diet-fed rats. Basic and Clinical Pharmacology and Toxicology 104, 366–373.

Ojewole, J.A., 2006. Analgesic, anti-inflammatory and hypoglycaemic effects of ethanol extract of *Zingiber officinale* (Roscoe) rhizomes in mice and rats. Phytotherapy Research 20, 764–772.

Priya Rani, M., Padmakumar, K.P., Sankarikutty, B., Lijo Cherian, O., Nisha, V.M., Raghu, K.G., 2011. Inhibitory potential of ginger extracts against enzymes linked to type 2 diabetes, inflammation and induced oxidative stress. International Journal of Food Sciences and Nutrition 62, 106–110.

Schulick, P., 1994. Ginger-Common Spic and Wonder Drug. Herbal Free Press Ltd, Brattleboro, VT p 111.

Shanmugam, K.R., Ramakrishna, C.H., Mallikarjuna, K., Reddy, K.S., 2010. Protective effect of ginger against alcohol-induced renal damage and antioxidant enzymes in male albino rats. Indian Journal of Experimental Biology 48, 143–149.

Shanmugam, K.R., Mallikarjuna, K., Kesireddy, N., Sathyavelu Reddy, K., 2011. Neuroprotective effect of ginger on anti-oxidant enzymes in streptozotocin-induced diabetic rats. Food and Chemical Toxicology 49, 893–897.

Singh, A.B., Akanksha, Singh, N., Maurya, R., Srivatsava, A.K., 2009. Anti-hyperglycaemic, lipid lowering and anti-oxidant properties of [6]-gingerol in db/db mice. International Journal of Medical Sciences 1, 536–544.

Srinivasan, K., Sambaiah, K., 1991. The effect of spices on cholesterol 7 alpha hydroxylase activity on serum and hepatic cholesterol levels in the rat. International Journal for Vitamin and Nutrition Research 61, 364–369.

Srivastava, K.C., 1984. Aqueous extracts of onion, garlic and ginger inhibit platelet aggregation and alter arachidonic acid metabolism. Biomedica Biochimica Acta 43, S335–S346.

Srivastava, K.C., 1986. Isolation and effects of some ginger components on platelet aggregation and eicosanoid biosynthesis. Prostaglandins, Leukotrienes, and Medicine 25, 187.

Stoilova, I., Krastanv, A., Stoyanova, A., Denev, P., Gargova, S., 2007. Antioxidant activity of ginger extract (*Zingiber officinale*). Food Chemistry 102, 764–770.

Tanabe, M., Chen, Y.D., Saito, K., Kano, Y., 1993. Cholesterol biosynthesis inhibitory component from *Zingiber officinale* Roscoe. Chemical and Pharmaceutical Bulletin 41, 710–713.

Thomson, M., Al-Qattan, K.K., Al-Sawan, S.M., Alnaqeeb, M.A., Khan, I., Ali, M., 2002. The use of ginger (*Zingiber officinale* Rose.) as a potential anti inflammatory and antithrombotic agent. Prostaglandins Leukot Essential Fatty Acids 67, 475–478.

Tjendraputra, E., Tran, V.H., Liu-Brennan, D., Roufogalis, B.D., Duke, C.C., 2001. Effect of ginger constituents and synthetic analogues on cyclooxygenase-2 enzyme in intact cells. Bioorganic Chemistry 29, 156–163.

Unnikrishnan, G., Indu, K.M., Ozarkar, K., 2009. Hypercholesterolemic effect of *Zingiber officinale* (Rosc) in high fat diet fed rats. Journal of Herbal Medicine Toxicology 3, 19–22.

Verma, S.K., Bordia, A., 2001. Ginger, fat and fibrinolysis. Indian Journal of Medical Sciences 55, 83–86.

Verma, S.K., Singh, M., Jain, P., Bordia, A., 2004. Protective effect of ginger *Zingiber officinale* Rosc on experimental atherosclerosis in rabbits. Indian Journal of Experimental Biology 42, 736–738.

Verma, S.K., Singh, J., Khemasra, R., Bordia, A., 1993. Effect of ginger on platelet aggregation on man. Indian Journal of Medical Research 98, 240.

Note: Page numbers followed by *b* indicate boxes, *f* indicate figures and *t* indicate tables.

G

Printed and bound by CPI Group (UK) Ltd, Croydon, CR0 4YY

15/05/2025

01872389-0002